"The framework presented about neurorelationships is highly relevant to all disciplines focused on early development. This integration of theories about brain function within context, and particularly within relationships, is vitally important for understanding development, behavior, assessment, and intervention for all professionals in early learning, early intervention, parenting, and mental health. Numerous tables and guidelines summarize clinical applications. No one reading this will ever think or act without the perspective of brain, behavior, context, and relationships as the integrating framework for assessment and treatment of developmental concerns."
—**Kathryn E. Barnard, RN, PhD**, Professor Emeritus, School of Nursing, University of Washington

"This book is beautifully written and applies a nonlinear dynamic systems approach to neurobiology, weaving together neurobiological concepts and contextual development into a coherent and integrated framework. It provides the theoretical foundation for professionals to shift from singular diagnostic categorizations in infant-parent work to a dimensional approach, where multiple dynamics that underlie all diagnostic categories can be considered simultaneously by professionals. The most significant contribution of this truly stunning book is the interdisciplinary nature of the tone, discussion, and clinical applications, paired with a new perspective and new language. This book provides the complexity and cohesiveness that can advance all professionals endeavoring to shift from multidisciplinary to interdisciplinary theory and practice."
—**Kristie Brandt, RN, CNM, MSN, DNP**, Parent-Infant & Child Institute, Napa, CA, Director of the Infant-Parent Mental Health Post-Graduate Certificate Program, in collaboration with Dr. Ed Tronick, at the University of Massachusetts, Boston

"This is a timely book that offers us all a chance to do better work for children and families."
—**T. Berry Brazelton, MD**, Professor Emeritus of Pediatrics, Harvard Medical School and Founder, Brazelton Touchpoints Center

"This book is visionary! The authors have brought a depth of understanding to child mental health that is informed by their creativity, brilliance, and unwillingness to be confined to the views of any one discipline. Their work elaborates a new analytic model capable of integrating data critical to diagnosis and treatment as never before. The book offers exciting opportunities for meaningful collaboration in this complex field."
—**Sara Latz, JD, MD**, Clinical Faculty, David Geffen School of Medicine, Psychiatry and Biobehavioral Sciences, Child/Adolescent Division, The Semel Institute of Neuroscience and Human Behavior, University of California, Los Angeles

"Given the increasing interest in accountability in health care, one often hears of the need for 'evidence-based practice.' This is certainly a message imparted by the authors in their excellent review of the literature supporting their framework. However, what is truly impressive is their 'practice-based evidence,' with which they convincingly demonstrate the value of the clinical process in driving scientists' search for new knowledge. This is clearly a win-win situation for clinical practice and basic research.

The authors are highly articulate in melding the clinician's 'art' with neuro 'science' in a way that will help to more clearly understand early developmental processes."
—**Patrice L. (Tamar) Weiss, PhD**, Faculty of Social Welfare & Health Sciences, University of Haifa, Israel

"The authors have spanned the chasms between neurodevelopment, relational contexts, and clinical practice to describe a new and visionary model of comprehensive interventions for challenged infants and young children and their parents. This unique and brilliantly conceived book provides a groundbreaking and in-depth framework for the integration of neuroscience research, early childhood mental health, and early intervention services. The clarity, yet complexity, of this described model, along with its clinical application, combine to make this work revolutionary for the study of interdisciplinary, team-based care. This book will inspire all to adopt the neurorelational framework as a guide for individualized and comprehensive brain and relationally-based interventions."
—**David W. Willis, MD, FAAP**, Behavioral-Developmental Pediatrics, Northwest Early Childhood Institute, Portland, OR

Infant/Child Mental Health,

Early Intervention, and

Relationship-Based Therapies

The Norton Series on Interpersonal Neurobiology
Allan N. Schore, PhD, Series Editor
Daniel J. Siegel, MD., Founding Editor

The field of mental health is in a tremendously exciting period of growth and conceptual reorganization. Independent findings from a variety of scientific endeavors are converging in an interdisciplinary view of the mind and mental well-being. An interpersonal neurobiology of human development enables us to understand that the structure and function of the mind and brain are shaped by experiences, especially those involving emotional relationships.

The Norton Series on Interpersonal Neurobiology will provide cutting-edge, multidisciplinary views that further our understanding of the complex neurobiology of the human mind. By drawing on a wide range of traditionally independent fields of research—such as neurobiology, genetics, memory, attachment, complex systems, anthropology, and evolutionary psychology—these texts will offer mental health professionals a review and synthesis of scientific findings often inaccessible to clinicians. These books aim to advance our understanding of human experience by finding the unity of knowledge, or consilience, that emerges with the translation of findings from numerous domains of study into a common language and conceptual framework. The series will integrate the best of modern science with the healing art of psychotherapy.

A Norton Professional Book

Infant/Child Mental Health, Early Intervention, and Relationship-Based Therapies

A Neurorelational Framework for Interdisciplinary Practice

Connie Lillas

Janiece Turnbull

W. W. Norton & Co., Inc.

New York • London

For information about permission to reproduce selections from this book,
write to Permissions, W. W. Norton & Company, Inc.,
500 Fifth Avenue, New York, NY 10110

For information about special discounts for bulk purchases,
please contact W. W. Norton Special Sales at
specialsales@wwnorton.com or 800-233-4830

Manufacturing by Courier Westford
Production manager: Leeann Graham

Library of Congress Cataloging-in-Publication Data

Lillas, Connie.
    Infant/child mental health, early intervention, and relationship-based
therapies : a neurorelational framework for interdisciplinary practice /
Connie Lillas, Janiece Turnbull.—1st ed.
        p. ; cm.—(The Norton series on interpersonal neurobiology)
    Includes bibliographical references and index.
    ISBN 978-0-393-70425-9 (hardcover)
    1. Infant psychiatry.   2. Child psychiatry.   I. Turnbull, Janiece.   II.
Title.   III. Series.
    [DNLM: 1. Infant.   2. Mental Disorders—therapy.   3. Child.   4. Early
Intervention (Education)   5. Interdisciplinary Communication.   6.
Interpersonal Relations. WS 350.2 L729i 2009]
    RJ502.5.L55 2009
    618.92'89—dc22   2008042468

ISBN 13: 978-0-393-70425-9

W. W. Norton & Company, Inc., 500 Fifth Avenue, New York, N.Y. 10110
www.wwnorton.com
W. W. Norton & Company Ltd., Castle House, 75/76 Wells St., London W1T 3QT
3 4 5 6 7 8 9 0

To my beloved Trevor, Alexander, and Nicholas, whose support, love, patience, and endurance made this book possible for me. I will always be grateful for your steady holding through this process.

In memory of Emily Fenichel, who was a bright beam of support and encouragement at a pivotal point in my career.

—C.L.

In memory of my dearly missed father, Duane Turnbull, who died on December 6, 2007. He was generous with everything he had to give, especially laughter and love.

Dedicated to my family, who are a joy to know and love and whose affections mean the world to me.

—J.T.

Contents

Part III: Bringing It All Together

Acknowledgments

CONNIE LILLAS

Several aspects of my work contributed to and made possible the creation of this book. I am very grateful to those who attended my infant mental health study groups during the 1990s, as they were a salient part of my efforts to consolidate theory, clinical practice, and personal experience. The information taught during this time subsequently became foundational material for the curriculum that was used during the multidisciplinary training programs I had the privilege of directing. Actually, the impetus for the 2-year training program emerged from a group member, Carol Blake, who caught the vision for what bringing disciplines together could do. Training across systems of care by inviting teams from agencies to apply, rather than single professionals, was a concept initiated by Janis Minton. Without the funding, primarily driven by Richard Atlas, the experience of training across disciplines and systems of care would not have been possible.

In addition to the 2-year training program, a 1-year training program was conceived and implemented to bridge the gap between L.A. County's Department of Mental Health and Child Protective Services by offering combined training to their practitioners. Bill Arroyo, Carol Blake, Sam Chen, Marilyn Garrison, John Hatakeyama, Phil Moser, Jeanne Smart, Zohreh Zarnegar, and others were instrumental in forging the groundwork to make this training possible. Adopted children and children in foster care are often our most vulnerable kids. A large portion of the inspiration for writing this book comes from my experiences with these infants and young children.

I am grateful to all the agencies that supported these extensive trainings. The many graduates from the training programs are a continual source of inspiration to me as they work for change and implement programs of their own that have far-reaching effects upon Los Angeles County's child services profile. Indeed, their efforts now extend worldwide.

One of the wonderful outgrowths of the 2-year training program was the emergence of a core interdisciplinary faculty during the actual training program itself. When the grant projects were no longer funded, the Interdisciplinary Training Institute (ITI) was formed as a way to keep an integrated training approach moving forward in smaller venues, whether by training an entire agency's staff over a period of months, conducting an in-service training to a specialized discipline, or informing parents and professionals in short-term, 1-, 2-, and 3-day intensives. I am especially grateful to a core group of professionals across disciplines who participated in a variety of ITI projects through the years: Valerie Copelan, LCSW; Kate Crowley, OT; Marilee Hartling, MFT, RN; Patricia Lakatos, PhD; Margaret Moritmore, PT; Richard Perkins, SLP; and Janiece Turnbull, PhD. In working together, they are a wonderful example of interdisciplinary practice in action. A special thanks goes to Jeanne and Robert Segal; through the Segal Foundation, they have been key supporters of bringing interdisciplinary concepts to the local parenting communities in Los Angeles.

One person who stands out as a source of encouragement during the early formation of these training programs is Emily Fenichel. I recall that she was the fastest person I had ever known to return an e-mail. Years before I met her in person, she was responsive, quick-witted, and enthusiastic. I was struck by one conversation we had in which she commented that an essential challenge perpetually before us is answering the question, "What is the meaning of the behavior(s) we see?" This question became an inspiration for me and an organizing principle for this book.

A warm and heartfelt thanks to Serena Wieder, who, as a busy professional, was willing to bridge the East Coast–West Coast time frame, providing reflective and creative facilitation and mentorship during late-night hours. Her observations of videotapes of my work were pivotal as I shifted from working primarily with adults to working with young and very young children.

Dan Siegel's invitation to be a part of the series on interpersonal neurobiology came at a transitional time in my life when my answer could only be a "yes." We are grateful for his generous and gracious donation of time as we met in his office for lunch meetings. Dan was the catalyst who suggested that Janiece and I integrate our distinctive models in writing the manuscript as an integrated whole. Special thanks to Cori Linder for her editorial help in the early years of this project.

Becoming a part of the ZERO TO THREE family as a Leadership Fellow, I was honored to have had the privilege of being mentored by Kathryn Barnard. One of the difficulties in writing this book was finding a way to organize large amounts of complex material into a comprehensible format. Kathryn consistently followed the evolution of this project and was very helpful in providing feedback throughout. Sheri L. Hill was also central in helping us find a basic structure for our brain system chapters.

Janiece Turnbull, my coauthor, has been invaluable to the creation of this book. Without her expertise, this book would lack the solid foundation in neuroscience theory that is so critical for our interdisciplinary endeavors to move forward. Janiece is gifted with a pristine mind that can hold an enormous number of complex concepts while bringing precision and clarity to the degrees of distinctions that lie among them. Our collaboration has involved the richest combination of learning through relationship that one could have. She not only brought neuroscience and neuropsychological assessment skills to this endeavor, she also made an enormous contribution with her writing skills. Again, her conceptual precision and her insistence on achieving the highest possible quality brought a rigorousness to the project that is cherished. This rigor was not without a humorous side, however. Many a time she would shift from the intensity of working through a conceptual glitch to refreshing us with a funny story. The combination of a gifted mind, a kind heart, and playful spontaneity is rare. She is a treasure.

It is likely no coincidence that a framework that can be used for interdisciplinary teamwork would need a team of folks to organize and edit it. Our conference calls with our two editors were always stimulating and would eventually resolve a complex problem that was facing us. Margaret Ryan, our West Coast editor, kept pulling us toward an articulation of complex information that transcended the jargon it was so easy to fall into. She and I spent many a late night on the phone outlining, editing, and reediting chapters. I will always remember her spontaneous laughter as a wonderful sound that still brings a smile to my face. Mary Gawlik, our East Coast editor, kept our feet to the ground with organizational and structural issues. She steadied the ship, both finding problems we hadn't noticed, while also helping us solve them.

Deborah Malmud of W. W. Norton provided guiding feedback to help us pull together the structure of the book and extended much patience to us in the long, arduous process of bringing it to fruition.

The families who have come to me over the years are a precious gift. I cannot thank them enough for allowing me to share in their journey and to learn with them through the gains and mistakes we have made along the way.

My family and friends have participated in, and withstood, the pains-taking efforts this project required. Without their support through all the ups and downs, this book would have never come to pass. Thank you for your enduring love and enormous patience and perseverance.

JANIECE TURNBULL

I owe a great deal to clients, colleagues, friends, and especially family, all of whom have inspired, enlightened, and supported me in writing this book.

First and foremost, I want to acknowledge the heroic spirit of parents who have children with developmental problems. You sometimes hear derogatory comments about parents who "just want to fix things with a pill" or "don't know how to discipline their kids" or "are overpro-tective," but I must say that I rarely meet these parents. The parents that I know are doing the absolute best they can to respond to difficult and often overwhelming circumstances. If it appears that they don't know how to discipline, it is often because the child far exceeds the boundaries of typical parenting skills and requires a level of skill that none of us pos-sesses naturally. If they appear to be doting, it is because they sense and empathize with the child's vulnerabilities, which may be hard to see for those who are not as connected to the child. And as for medication, I have yet to meet a single parent who was eager to medicate his or her child. In my opinion, the parents who move in that direction show tremendous courage. They are willing to make a tough decision in favor of the child's needs despite their own dreams for what would be, and despite knowing that others may not understand or support them. It is exactly this type of self-sacrificing devotion that I feel deserves to be recognized and respected, and this book represents my attempts to do so.

I am grateful to the many mentors and supervisors who helped to shape my thinking and also inspired me with their dedication and passion. There were many but I can name only a few: my graduate school mentor, Dr. Warren Brown, who managed to be an exacting neuroscientist, an in-novative philosopher of mind, and a fun human being all rolled into one; and my residency mentor, Dr. Paul Satz, who never ceased to amaze me with his mind and his open heart. Dr. Satz approached every client with the same interest and intellectual energy, and he was never one to allow numbers on a page to define the person. He sat with every data sheet and cycled through it until a living, breathing person emerged and all the pieces fit together into a meaningful whole. Dr. Satz was the quintessential professional father, seeing each resident as capable of great things and full

of promise and providing direction in that spirit. I am also grateful to my friend and former supervisor, Dr. Lorie Humphrey, for her many contributions to my professional development. One that stands out in the context of this book was her persistence in translating assessment into treatment. In her mind, our work was not done until the "what to do about it" question was fully answered in a meaningful way for the individual child and family.

During the slow evolution of this book, I have accumulated many debts to colleagues, friends, and family. Professional colleagues and friends, too many to mention, were willing to give time and mental effort to think through ideas, share insights, give feedback on portions of text, or just be a sounding board for ideas. Our two editors, Margaret Ryan and Mary Gawlik, were especially pivotal to the sometimes arduous process of wrestling with cohesion of concepts. They offered a degree of intellectual energy and passion that I am quite certain went well beyond the call of duty.

A very special thanks to my family and friends, who gave endless support and were so gracious and understanding when my time so often went to the book instead of them. I know you are all happy that "the damn book" is now done! In addition to being tolerant and considerate, my adorable husband, Skip Rizzo, always accorded epic-proportion importance to this work. When I would run out of steam, he would emerge with an impassioned sermon that made me feel like I was curing cancer. Thanks to the affections of all of you, my life resonates with meaning. And I must also acknowledge my kitties, who were major players in keeping me fueled. They kept me company, curled up by my side, occasionally nudged me for petting, and were sometimes quite inconsiderate and impatient, forcing my hand by simply lying down across my keyboard.

This book is all about parents, and mine, Kathy and Duane, deserve special attention. They brought so much more to parenting than the handbook of personal experience. Determined to forge a better path, they worked to break free from patterns that they knew well but did not want for their own children. They were courageous and giving and taught their children to get past barriers, take risks, and laugh. My mother gave me the freedom to pursue my own interests and at the same time provided both practical and emotional support. My father was interested in everything I did and always wanted to hear all the details. Once he was far enough along with Alzheimer's disease, I found myself recounting the same details over and over, but I never minded. He was eager to read this book and told me many times that he might not be around long enough to read it, and sadly he was right. Interestingly, given our central theme of relationships in this book, it was my dad who understood from the start (long before I did!) that my relationship with Connie would be at the heart of this effort. He couldn't have been more right.

Which brings me to my heartfelt thanks to my friend and coauthor, Connie Lillas. We worked hard to fashion a cohesive integration from start to finish instead of each serving up alternating slices of our own professional pie. This was not easy, and we agreed fairly early on to relinquish any notion that we could shape the content without emotion. In this effort, Connie lived by the principles of this book, whereby maintaining a sense of safety in the relationship, an attitude of openness to learning, and a balance between flexibility and stability were paramount. In my mind, the authenticity of the collaborative journey that went on behind the scenes lends a sincerity and credibility to this work that goes far beyond its instructional elements.

It is my hope that this book will make a difference.

Preface

CONNIE'S STORY

Every book has its own back story. Taking on a project with the size and scope of creating an interdisciplinary framework with neuroscience underpinnings demands enormous passion. My energy for collaborating in the creation of this book has grown from several key experiences in my life in which I witnessed some type of fragmentation in health care, whether as a clinical practitioner delivering care or as a recipient of early intervention services.

During my first career, from 1976 to 1986, I worked as a high-risk maternal–child nurse. In the early years of this professional life, I was fortunate to work at a university hospital setting that was implementing Drs. Kathryn Barnard's and T. Berry Brazelton's work. I attended in-service trainings that brought new understandings from infant research regarding infant physiology and maternal–child bonding into labor and delivery room practices and newborn and postpartum settings. It was during one of those in-services that I saw the film *The Amazing Newborn*, which connected the range of infant states of arousal with behavior and the attainment of a particular infant state of arousal with the ability to build healthy relationships. This film opened up a whole new world of awareness for me. During this time, expert thinking was evolving from a view of infants as neurologically inept to a realization that even newborns were active participants in learning about their world.

During this time I had the privilege of following patients from their prenatal days to their labor and delivery to their postnatal period, participating in some of the most intimate experiences my patients could have.

I realized that this type of ongoing connection felt very important, not only to me, but to them as well. As a professional, I wanted to find a way to have even more continuity with families in supporting them through the intensely emotional sequelae that their birthing experiences were stimulating. With this hope in mind, I decided to pursue a mental health degree in marriage, family, and child therapy.

As I shifted from a medical setting to a mental health setting, I found myself working with adults who, as infants and young children, had experienced physiological compromises such as prematurity, exposure to toxins in utero, and regulatory disorders, in conjunction with varying degrees of trauma in their early relationships. I had shifted from a population of newborns and their moment-to-moment formation of early relationships to an adult population whose problems I was convinced had salient, early physiological and relational components that needed to be addressed as part of the therapeutic process. Although my family systems training emphasized the value of viewing illness in terms of a relational context—an invaluable perspective—there was no physiological component to my mental health training, and early development was not necessarily emphasized. Thus, during this professional transition, I experienced the consequences of the divide that still existed between the mind and the body in the clinical world, as well as a clinical disconnect between early developmental processes and later outcomes.

What I observed was that many of my adult clients with early physiological and relational difficulties were continuing to struggle, unable to cultivate anything more than sparse relationships, and some were unable to sustain a connection to anyone. The degree of despair and angst voiced by these patients prompted me to investigate more deeply the psychological origins of the self. I wanted to learn more about early development, so that perhaps I could find a way to make links among physiology, early childhood relational patterns, and later outcomes. I began psychoanalytic training and was enthralled to find practitioners who were dedicated to making connections among early development, relational processes, and adult functions. I was fortunate to participate in a program that promoted a wide variety of psychoanalytic approaches. I slowly realized, however, that although psychoanalysis was unified in its commitment to an emphasis on early childhood development and a belief in unconscious processes, each psychoanalytic theory offered a different view of what constituted a healthy mother–infant or mother–father–infant unit, what constituted developmental breakdowns, and hence, how to repair these problems in the early years as well as in the adult arena. Some of these theories naturally leaned toward what the infant brought to the family relationships and others leaned toward what the parents brought to the baby.

The history of psychoanalytic institutes has been characterized by periods of creativity, but also by acrimony and divisiveness over theoretical and clinical disagreements. These divisions exemplify how help-oriented professionals can become extremely fragmented in their views of what constitutes the problem and the solution. As the nature-vs.-nurture pendulum had swung from one side to the other in theory development, the physiology of the body was yet to be found in my psychoanalytic search.

While the family systems movement gathered momentum during the 1980s, the field of infant mental health was being birthed, a field in which early relationships were deemed as critical to the literal life and death of a child's physical body and emotional self. Infant mental health theories now began to emerge from these aforementioned psychoanalytic theory bases. Many of the pioneers in infant mental health were psychoanalysts or influenced by psychoanalytic concepts. Due to these strong ties to psychoanalysis, the relationship-based approaches that emerged in infant mental health often followed similar emphases. Some focused on quietly allowing the internal psychological world of the child or parent to unfold as a curative strategy. Some stressed the interpersonal engagement in the here-and-now within the parent–child relationship. Yet others leaned toward actively fostering self-reflection in the parent to better understand how the past affects the present assumptions and projections onto the child.

Within this body of infant mental health literature I was thrilled to discover the infant states of arousal (physiology) that had been so foundational in my day-to-day nursing practice. Delving into this infant mental health literature, I had the experience of coming home. I was excited to begin a synthesis from my nursing, family systems, and psychoanalytic careers that would be broad enough to hold the tension between what the child contributed, what the parents brought, and the co-created capacities that emerged for building a healthy relationship.

While completing my psychoanalytic training in the early 1990s, I began to work on creating a model that would contain the important interconnections among physiology, interpersonal relationships, and the private, internal psychological world. An early interventionist caught sight of this perspective and soon I found myself presenting a framework that came to be known as the *diamond model*. Without completely realizing the implications, I was being introduced to the realm of practitioners known as early interventionists, who most often work with developmental delays and disabilities in infants and young children. While these practitioners may focus on learning and cognitive delays, they are often more naturally connected to bodily functions because of their work with physical and genetic disabilities. During this time, infant mental health principles

were beginning to be introduced into early intervention settings, and these professionals welcomed a model that brought the mind, the body, and the relational world into a coherent perspective. In a timely yet challenging twist of fate, just as I was beginning to teach my model in early intervention centers, I found myself beginning a parallel personal journey into the need for early intervention. I began to relive my professional life from the side of being a high-risk pregnant patient, and then consumer of services for my premature child. Now I was a parent with a child who needed help from both the early intervention and mental health domains. I knew that my child had what is now classified as a regulatory disorder in the *Diagnostic Classification of Mental Health and Developmental Disorders of Infancy and Early Childhood, Revised* (DC:0–3R, 2005), but diagnosing my child and knowing what to do with my child as a parent were two vastly different matters (in the same way assessment and intervention can be). This intensely personal situation dramatically shifted my experience. Now, instead of viewing the existing fragmentations from a professional perspective on the side of providing services to others, I was living the fragmentations on the receiving end, from what felt like being in the trenches. The impact of this systemwide fragmentation became a visceral entity in my daily life as I searched for help. My passion to unite the fragments that composed our disconnected service delivery system into a working whole, once a flame, now burst into a bonfire.

Each professional whom I had encountered along the way was lovely and helpful. Yet I realized two important matters. First, I noticed that in early intervention settings, parents dropped off their infants and children for therapy and came back to pick them up at the end of the appointment, regardless of the service specialty. I was saddened to realize that early intervention professionals were not being trained to work within the context of the parent–child relationship. Second, I realized that what I most needed—a cohesive team of professionals that used a common language or framework from which to understand the multiple services that my child and our family required during the first 5 years of his life—was nowhere to be found in my community. If it was this hard for me to understand my child's behaviors—a professional who had spent some 20 years studying child development and working with at-risk populations—I knew it must be incredibly difficult for those who had little or no training in these matters.

This daunting but transforming experience inspired me to expand my clinical practice to work with at-risk children, from birth to age 5 years, and their parents. It also inspired wonderful visions that turned into concrete opportunities. By the early 2000s, I was able to direct some grant-funded training programs. The largest of these included bringing together

19 different agencies representing 14 different disciplines in Los Angeles County. That training program was designed to foster a shift from multidisciplinary functioning to interdisciplinary practice and to create a web of professional relationships and services in the county that was held together by a common language and vision of the big picture. We were fortunate to have many presenters who were luminaries in their field, including Allan Schore and Dan Siegel. At the end of 2 years, 59 professionals graduated from the training program. The momentum for collaboration continued when the Department of Mental Health and the Department of Child and Protective Services selected employees to attend a 1-year course with a special emphasis on foster care children (self-selected practitioners from a regional center also joined); this program graduated 47 professionals.

Next, the privilege of becoming a ZERO TO THREE Leadership Fellow proved pivotal in shifting me from a large county perspective to a national one. From this vantage point, I could see with even greater precision the gap between professionals identified with infant mental health (with a focus on the socioemotional and relational aspects of development) and early interventionists (with a focus on developmental milestones and cognitive delays). Although I had a model of physiological, interpersonal, and internal processes that applied to both groups of practitioners, it seemed imperative to ground these concepts in neurodevelopment. I realized at that point that I needed to collaborate with someone trained specifically in the neuroscience field.

Janiece Turnbull, a pediatric neuropsychologist, was a part of the emergent core faculty that had formed from my earlier 2-year training program, and I was captivated by her lectures on the brain, which highlighted the global, interconnected processes on which brain functioning rests. I intuitively believed that neuroscience theories, which conceptualize the brain as large-scale networks, could provide a unifying foundation on which to create a solid theoretical framework that could undergird the existing model I had developed, and likewise, could be used to link all the fragmented parts of the systems of care. Janiece and I began a long, arduous, and rewarding journey together, from which the neurorelational framework emerged. Interdisciplinary collaboration requires a tremendous amount of dedication. The fruitful outcome, which involved much bumping into each other along the way resolving, disorganizing, and reorganizing many issues and concepts together—is far beyond what either of us could have achieved individually. We hope this book contributes to the interdisciplinary movement by linking current efforts with neuroscience theories, enriching the foundation on which we can continue to learn, practice, and advocate for the use of interdisciplinary approaches collectively in our efforts to support young children and their families.

JANIECE'S REFLECTIONS

I was recently telling a psychiatrist friend of mine that my husband is developing a virtual reality application for diagnostic interviewing. In this VR environment, a student can learn diagnostic criteria and practice interviewing skills by talking with a virtual patient, a patient who has been programmed to fit the *DSM-IV* criteria. She laughed and said, "Now if we could just get *real* patients to be like that!" Her response sums up one of my primary reasons for wanting to write this book. Diagnosis, regardless of the nomenclature used, is certainly a reasonable place to start with assessment or treatment—but it is just a start. People are simply too complex to be neatly packaged into a predefined construct. Some certainly fit these constructs better than others, and some respond more readily and robustly to treatments, as well. But there will always be those who are not so easy to define and not so responsive to treatment, those who not only challenge our usual ways of thinking but also encourage our professional growth.

In my experience, it is somewhere in this territory that communication across disciplinary boundaries begins to break down. Once professionals step away from the language of nomenclature and begin to speak in terms of "a little bit of this and a little bit of that" or begin to ponder *why* questions, the language can be more confounding than clarifying. We have different areas of focus and expertise, our terms may have nuanced or vastly different meanings, and we are trained to think through issues in different ways with fundamentally different starting points. This means that with our most challenging cases, when professionals most need to join forces to enhance assessment and intervention, we actually have the most hurdles to overcome in terms of effective communication. We do the best that we can and we make it work using various strategies, but the situation is certainly not optimal, and it is rarely acknowledged or discussed openly. The barriers to communication across disciplinary boundaries become hard to tolerate once one has a taste for how rich the assessment and intervention process can be with true collaboration.

Since my introduction to neuropsychology, the desire to understand the brain had some fundamental connection to the promise of a unifying theory. Just as physicists and cosmologists seek that one unifying theory that will provide understanding of the world around us and its origins, the brain seemed to hold the promise of unlocking both fundamental principles and ever-expanding insights with respect to human development and potential. Now, 20 years later, I am convinced that a shared knowledge of brain functioning and brain development across disciplines has the potential to lay out a common pathway for true interdisciplinary

collaboration. I am further convinced that this pathway will *not* be paved with the shared knowledge of hundreds or thousands of discrete associations between brain areas and body/behavior functions but rather with the broad and unifying principles that are informed by these discrete associations. In other words, it is a shared knowledge of the brain as a *whole* that will allow us to traverse disciplinary boundaries with comfort and ease, not islands of brain–behavior associations.

My other primary reason for wanting to write this book stems from my belief that all disciplines should have some grounding in neuroscience. Despite one's area of expertise with children, be it teaching in a classroom, assessing a learning problem, or treating a mood disorder with medication, professional efforts cannot and should not be separated from a developing brain. At a practical level, this vision would require that training across disciplines include learning about the brain as a whole, as well as learning about the brain parts that are specific to that discipline. On a deeper level, what I am actually advocating is a shift toward placing how we think within a neuroscience context. A brain-based perspective encourages a new way of doing clinical work, a way that I believe respects human differences, values the complexity of behavior, and holds an unwavering belief in change and enhancing outcomes. It compels a fundamental transition from answering *what* questions to contemplating *why* questions as a routine application of emerging neuroscience insights, which in and of itself is a major thrust toward progress.

We already know a lot about what comprises a disability or a disruption to development, how one type of disruption is different from another, and often even what is likely to be an effective treatment. However, we know much less about *why* we see the symptoms that we do, and neuroscience sheds light on the best places to look for answers. A child on the autistic spectrum may not make eye contact, may be hypersensitive to sound, or may lack language altogether, but *why*? What are the brain mechanisms involved in these symptoms? Is there a single intrinsic mechanism or several? How do features of the extrinsic environment influence the trajectory of intrinsic mechanisms? Currently, the answers to such questions about autism and other disorders that disrupt development are being pursued vigorously in research labs around the globe and, no matter the disciplines represented, there is a common goal: to discover, describe, further elucidate or expand upon, either directly or indirectly, the brain mechanisms involved.

With every child, we are presented with a novel combination of features, and we set about judging the coherence of those features in order to make decisions about treatment. In this context, rapid decisions are not a good thing. When we are too eager to arrive at a conclusion, we run the

risk of overrelying on cook book answers and, in the process, we may side-step the potential for improving the intervention plans for the individual child and family. Principles of brain development remind us that no child will fit perfectly into predetermined models; there are simply far too many intrinsic and extrinsic factors at play during the prolonged course of brain development for such simple models or decision trees to be possible. Thus, an important component of our work involves challenging our assumptions and slowing down the decision-making process in order to adequately consider the alternatives.

In this context, a professional's innovation and creativity become a standard component of making sound clinical decisions. Grounded in an understanding of brain mechanisms, we have the freedom to speculate about *why* a particular behavior is present or absent and how that situation emerged with greater confidence and stability than we are allowed by using our discipline's constructs and clinical experience alone. Such an approach with each individual may present a challenge, but it is also a source of professional vitality and inspiration.

In summary, there are two related ideas that fueled the passion for this effort. The first is the idea that neuroscience has the potential to reshape how the various disciplines that work with children function in relation to one another. The second is the idea that science, and neuroscience in particular, is likely to completely reshape the future tools and treatments of early intervention. The reason for this *neuroscience* focus is straightforward: neural plasticity. Neural plasticity is the promise that we can make a difference, we just have to figure out how. Thus, the more we understand about what is going on in the brain (for both typical and atypical brains), the more we can develop rational hypotheses about what to do to improve interventions and, ultimately, enhance quality of life. As long as we use the brain (and, hopefully, theory) as our guide, our "misses" can contribute to further understanding of the brain and continue to shape further insights and progress. For over a decade, we have seen ample evidence of this type of neuroscience influence across developmental disorders.

The neurorelational framework is our attempt to meet the parallel goals of using neuroscience to develop a common language for collaboration and using neuroscience to enhance our clinical work. Because these are lofty goals, we view the framework as a work in progress. The framework may be overdone and begging for simplicity at some points and underdone and lacking enough complexity at others. In addition, when seen through others' eyes, the framework is likely to reveal biases in particular directions, despite our efforts to the contrary by inviting regular feedback from other disciplines. As we are not specialists in all of the

areas discussed, there are certain to be a few errors or inconsistencies. Our wish is that our readers will provide feedback, collaborate in this effort, and contribute to ongoing efforts to adapt and reshape the neurorelational framework to become an increasingly relevant, useful, and cohesive resource for all disciplines.

WHO MIGHT BENEFIT FROM THIS BOOK?

Professionals from many diverse fields—child and adult mental health practitioners, infant mental health specialists, early interventionists (occupational, physical, speech and language therapists), educational therapists, teachers, pediatric medical practitioners, and teachers of master's- and doctoral-level programs in any of these fields—might find material of value to them in this book. In general, this book will appeal to the following types of readers:

- Professionals who are looking for ways to integrate an understanding of the body, the mind, and relationships.
- Professionals who value the brain as a template for providing a common language and framework for child development for all pediatric disciplines to use.
- Professionals who value the context of relationships as a primary focus for assessment as well as a primary healing medium.
- Professionals who value the need to understand early developmental processes, recognizing a link between early development and adult development and relationships.
- Researchers who are looking for clinical resources to help them enhance the clinical relevance of their work (bench to bedside).
- Professionals involved in interdisciplinary study and/or practice.
- Students and professionals interested in interdisciplinary approaches to clinical work.

OVERVIEW OF THE BOOK

Because the neurorelational framework is a whole-to-part-to-whole type of framework, the book's sections are structured to complement this same process. Part I, The Big Picture, presents the global picture of the neurorelational framework. In Chapter 1, we explore the problems of fragmentation, isolation, hierarchy, and specialization in how professionals view, understand, and treat concerns in infant, child, and family development.

In attempting to resolve this basic fragmentation, the neurorelational framework draws on several salient clinical approaches. Chapter 2 examines the neuroscientific underpinnings of the neurorelational framework and introduces the four major brain systems (which serve as a touchpoint for the more detailed material in Chapters 4–11). Chapter 3 focuses on the use of the socioemotional milestones, paired with the four brain systems, as one way to assess and work with dyads.

Part II, The Brain Systems, provides an in-depth exploration of each brain system in the neurorelational framework. Chapters 4–11 take the reader into the complex workings of each of the four brain systems: the regulation system, the sensory system, the relevance system, and the executive system. Each brain system is divided into two chapters. The first addresses the key structures, function, and behaviors of the brain system. The second addresses assessment and intervention priorities and strategies. Clinical applications of each brain system are demonstrated through the use of composite case studies. Each pair of chapters on a brain system shares such a case study.

Part III, Bringing It All Together, provides a synthesis of the material presented and a vision for future directions. Chapter 12 holds the parts of each brain system in relation to the whole, reaching insights about the complex functioning of the child, the parent, and the dyad. This synthesis then guides a discussion of future directions for professional development across academic, research, and clinical settings.

Infant/Child Mental Health,

Early Intervention, and

Relationship-Based Therapies

1

The Big Picture

1

In Search of New Approaches
to Complex Problems

Perhaps the biggest problem facing parents of young children with physical, learning, or mental health problems is not the various conditions affecting those children, but the service delivery of the treatments they encounter. Children are routinely denied the help they need due to policy and funding regulations, or limitations imposed by assessment and diagnostic practices. Most of us have had the experience of realizing that a child who is just starting treatment with us has needs that went unnoticed, were noticed but not understood, or maybe were understood but not well enough for the benefits of intervention to be sustained. The story unfolds in a multitude of variations, but the ending is typically the same: the child's issues worsen. The typical predicament in which parents find themselves was expressed by one exasperated father, who said, "Sorry if I'm skeptical, it's just that I'm starting to see the pattern here. In the beginning, everyone says they know what to do, and we feel hopeful, but in the end, things get worse, I get angry, and my wife gets a whole new wave of guilt."

If we did a postmortem examination on such a case, each of us in the helping profession would come up with a different answer, likely led by very discipline-specific ideas. As such, each comment would generate a diverse set of genuinely passionate responses. If we could all speak our minds at once, the resulting cacophony would provide a vivid metaphor for why these problems persist. To extend the metaphor, perhaps we should not shield our ears from the dissonance but rather learn to listen for patterns that would allow us to see what was actually wrong, begin to work together, and move from dissonance into a full-fledged song.

The neurorelational framework described in this book emerged as our response to this need for a cross-disciplinary approach that could

serve as the catalyst for a systems-wide integration of treatment services. The most important and fundamental aspects of the framework are in its title—"neuro" and "relational" are an integrated whole. The brain is embedded within and modified by relational experiences, and the nature of relationships cannot escape the opportunities afforded or the limits imposed by the brains involved in the relationship. We use the brain as our guide because it is the perfect model of a complex and dynamic system that is able to "hold" child development, adult functioning, primary relationships, the concerns of all disciplines, and the process of change in real time. We draw on neuroscience as a starting point for the analysis of behavior because the language of the brain allows for a more neutral description of behaviors and competencies, accessible across disciplines.

DEFINING THE PROBLEMS

We begin with defining the problems that countless parents and professionals have experienced.[1] Simply stated, when there is progress there will be problems. Our view is that despite advances in knowledge and tools for assessment and intervention across the pediatric disciplines, significant problems with cross-disciplinary communication and collaboration remain, and perhaps in some respects have even worsened. We have structured these problems according to four overarching (and sometimes overlapping) terms: fragmentation, isolation, hierarchy, and specialization.

With the explosion of pediatric disciplines to treat "new" disorders over the past century, these four challenges to collaboration influenced our professional advancements (and not always negatively). A unifying characteristic of these four challenges has to do with our inability to integrate "part-to-whole" and "whole-to-part" approaches. By omitting other possible views, training within specific disciplines often encourages students to look at their domain as defining the individual child's, the parents', or the parent–child's (dyad's) needs. This tendency within training approaches prepares us for our part but does not allow for an understanding of our contribution within the whole. Imagine that a group of people were told to build the different parts of a house in different places, without communicating with each other. Someone is told to build a roof, another to build staircases, and others each build individual rooms, an entranceway, and a fireplace. When they finally come together with their various parts to put the house together, you can imagine the mess; the stairs would lead to nowhere, the fireplace wouldn't fit the chimney, the roof might not cover all the rooms, and the entryway might open into a wall. This kind of disparity—the inability to build a staircase that fits within

the overall dimensions of the house (part-to-whole), or the inability to see a house as a sum of its integral parts (whole-to-part)—can be a source of many problems that emerge during treatment.

A major contributor to this problem is the idea that individual disciplines tend to emphasize their focus as primary. A real-world example lies within the fragmented service delivery system for pre-birth to 5-year-olds. One large segment of professionals in that system identifies with the umbrella term *infant mental health* (IMH), whereas the other identifies with *early intervention* (EI). Professionals who identify with IMH are primarily concerned with the social and emotional aspects of the development of infants and young children and the well-being of the parent–child relationship (Sameroff, 2004; ZERO TO THREE, 2008). This parent–child relationship is referred to as a dyad. IMH professionals strongly identify with the goal of developing the *emotional mind* of the child through relationships. These professionals are typically specialists recognized as having attended additional training in infant mental health. Depending on the site, this training may or may not be open to all disciplines. Often, those who attend are mental health practitioners (e.g., social workers, marriage/family/child therapists, psychologists).

Professionals who identify with EI are concerned with the broad range of a child's health and well-being—usually with a focus on physical and developmental delays, disabilities, or both—that are expressed through lags in the attainment of age-appropriate sensory, motor, communication, and cognitive milestones in the context of family functioning (Meisels & Shonkoff, 2000). Early intervention professionals focus primarily on the body and how it interfaces with the *learning mind*. Professionals who identify with EI typically include nurses, pediatricians, teachers (including preschool and special education teachers), physical therapists, occupational therapists, speech and language pathologists, and those working in Early Head Start and Head Start programs. The term *early intervention* is a source of some linguistic confusion because it represents both an identified group of professionals, as defined here (in a professional sector), as well as an action—to intervene early—as it is understood in the public sector.

The gap between research and practice also contributes to the parts-to-whole problem. Often, research evidence is held up as representing the "whole" in and of itself, and thereby driving decisions about clinical and educational interventions. However, all too often, researchers and practitioners alike frequently fail to consider the research findings in terms of the other "parts"—that is, other evidence that emerges from family, professional wisdom, and consumer values (Buysse & Wesley, 2006)—to realize a more integrated whole. Buysse and Wesley define evidence-based practice for the early childhood field as "a decision-making process that integrates

the best available research evidence with family and professional wisdom and values" (2006, p. 12). An important and often delicate balance must be maintained between evidence-based research, professional wisdom, and a family's values. Any one of these can become skewed (i.e., not keeping up with research-based literature and treatments, disregarding peer-reviewed clinical expertise, or not being culturally sensitive).

Individual practitioners, in their part-oriented roles, generally are not exposed to the whole—a result of the disciplinary isolation that is accepted as status quo. This deficit, common within professional training/education programs, inhibits individual professionals from realizing their need to span boundaries through collaboration. The neurorelational framework provides a part-to-whole and a whole-to-part theory base for all disciplines working across all diagnostic categories. This framework has a dual purpose: to address the need for individual practitioners to incorporate the whole picture in relation to their part in assessment and intervention with each individual child, parent, and dyad, as well as the need to provide a global framework for team collaboration. We believe that as individual practitioners grasp the whole picture, they will be inspired to build tighter links with other disciplines to achieve the best outcome in the context of the whole.

As we elaborate on the problems of fragmentation, isolation, hierarchy, and specialization—all of which have accompanied advancements in development and mental health—we highlight not only the difficulties that result from holding only a part of the picture but also the problems that arise from lack of interdisciplinary collaboration and therefore preclude any success over the part-to-whole problem. Each of these problems has a particular underlying theme:

- *Fragmentation*: Rapid growth across pediatric disciplines continually expands the number of players and possibilities; there is little connection among the parts; there is no overall structure or cohesion.
- *Isolation*: Professional training and personal philosophy tend to set us on separate paths; no matter how sharp the professional lens, we cannot "see" the whole landscape from our path; on a personal note, we like to travel with those who are like-minded.
- *Hierarchy*: Culture assigns degrees of value to professions and approaches, setting up a pecking order of dominance in groups where multiple disciplines are represented; in hierarchical situations, some voices are amplified while others are silenced.
- *Specialization*: As we learn within a particular domain, we integrate and speak the language of that knowledge base; as we grow, the "new" language becomes more elaborated and integrated with the structure of our thinking; the more we learn, the more complex, rich, and nuanced the meanings behind our terms become.

Problem 1: Fragmentation

Over the past 50 years, there has been an explosion of professional disciplines and services that are dedicated to promoting well-being for children and families. However, disciplines that evolve this rapidly lack a grand design. There is no plan in place to connect the various branches in a way that would reduce repetition and promote efficiency within and across disciplinary boundaries. Only after sufficient expansion and progress have occurred is there even the possibility of reflecting on where duplications and inefficiencies may exist.

Although rapid and spontaneous expansion creates the potential for flexibility and creativity among participants to develop solutions, often the effects of such expansion are problematic for both individual practitioners and team collaboration. Without a working knowledge of the other branches, each individual professional starts from scratch with each case, performing the prescribed assessment approach, informed by philosophical and theoretical influences that tend toward a preference for seeing a particular (and often singular) causal domain. Such a myopic view tends to promote repetitive, inefficient, and fragmented assessment and treatment. Often families end up enlisting the help of a variety of practitioners in serial fashion, presenting their child's same problems yet hearing interpretations through a different professional lens—inadvertently culminating in a confusing, distressing, and disheartening scenario.

The fragmentation between IMH and EI has led to significant problems in assessment and treatment. A given professional's training and context of practice will often determine what issues are recognized as problems. For example, a child's lack of eye contact may be of primary concern to a psychologist during an observation but is completely unnoticed by the pediatrician during a regular checkup. When there is agreement among the different professionals that the same problem exists, the cause of the problem may be conceptualized very differently, and even unpredictably by those distinct disciplines. For example, a child "acting out" in the classroom may be perceived as having an attention problem by the teacher, but as suffering from a lack of adequate parental structure and discipline by the pediatrician. The subject and details of interest, the content of what is deemed relevant, the methods of assessment, and the prescription for a solution can all be expected to differ relative to the professional domain. Personal preferences toward one's own theoretical and clinical training tend to form the lens through which any given symptom is approached. Although this narrow focus is a boon to the expansion of knowledge, it is a bane of the parent seeking help.

A second effect of rapid disciplinary expansion is that it inhibits the potential for team collaboration. The lack of a holistic infrastructure that

bridges pediatric specialties prevents adequate communication and collaboration across disciplinary boundaries and thus limits each professional's capacity to consider factors that lie outside his or her sphere of knowledge. For example, the child specialist, working only within his or her professional boundary, has limited ability to recognize and understand how other disciplines may offer benefits to a child's optimal development. This limitation promotes a kind of inertia toward oversimplification. Currently, most disciplines have evolved to the point where serving children requires specialized or additional training, especially in medical and mental health arenas (e.g., pediatric occupational therapists, pediatricians, developmental psychologists, pediatric neuropsychologists, child psychiatrists, marriage, family, and child therapists). In addition, specialization into particular issues has led to further professional branching (e.g., special education teachers, developmental pediatricians, foster care/adoption social workers, psychologists specializing in trauma or autism).

Although disciplinary boundaries support the need for expertise, they have not facilitated the flow of disciplinary collaboration. Categorical diagnostics provide a glaring example of such a barrier. Diagnoses are useful and necessary but present a type of logistical catch-22: the expertise is intended to enhance treatment, but the discipline-specific and categorically specific details actually preclude the type of global view necessary for this population. Across a broad spectrum of potential categorizations, from trauma to autism or relationship disorders, an exclusive focus provides an unintentional way of eclipsing the more global aspects of behavior that can occur within and across all diagnostic categories.

Problem 2: Isolation

Across professional domains, there remains a very strong tendency to treat one's area of specialty as an isolated entity, somehow cut off from the whole. The effects of isolation can undermine the individual practitioner's capacity to integrate multiple causal factors contributing to the presenting problem behavior(s). A social worker may address a child's aggressive behaviors without ever considering the possibility of a learning disorder; a speech and language pathologist may treat an articulation disorder without considering the possibility of an emotional problem; a dentist may treat temporomandibular joint syndrome without considering the possibility of stress. In other words, assessment and treatment of a child often take place in an isolated manner, which means that many important contributions to the problem (possibly even the primary contributions) are left unaddressed. There may be little consideration of the

child's developmental history, the family context, relationship issues, social and community factors related to poverty or violence, and so on. Yet children's presenting problems usually do not have a single cause. Without including the whole picture, an individual practitioner's assessment is likely to be inadequate, and treatment gains are less likely to be sustained. The same tendency can occur with professional relationships that form into isolated, like-minded groups, discussing cases or referring only among others in the same group.

How one frames a solution very much depends on how one defines the problem. Disciplinary collaboration can be compromised when various disciplines view a particular aspect of the child as holding the etiology for any given problem. Some disciplines are weighted toward biology and bodily mechanisms, some are weighted toward the mind and mental functions, and others are weighted toward the environment and relational dynamics. Such preferences strongly influence the course of assessment and treatment, both with each particular child and family as well as with the nature of the professional alliances that are formed over time. In other words, professionals tend to function in isolation; when they do collaborate, it tends to be with like-minded professionals. Once the stated intervention goals are obtained, it may be the "end of story." If the goals are not met, there are limited alternatives.

Problem 3: Hierarchy

Across professional domains, our culture and educational training influence how we define status, and status may drive decision making about a child's assessment and treatment. When presented with conflicting views from a teacher and a pediatrician, a parent will tend to go with the individual perspective and advice of the pediatrician. This cultural hierarchy tends to win out even in the face of commonsense arguments to the contrary (e.g., "I know that my child's teacher should know more about learning problems, but the pediatrician said she's fine"). Although wanting to believe the doctor, parents are left in a quandary about whom to believe and how to assess their child and family situation.

Within the context of disciplinary collaboration, issues of hierarchy can impact the course of assessment and intervention. Those with higher status tend to be dominant in terms of planning and goals, and those with lesser status may "go along" to avoid interpersonal conflicts or career consequences. Thus, despite clear arenas of knowledge specialty within particular disciplines (e.g., speech and language pathologists should know the most about speech and language development and problems), the

"disciplinary pecking order" (Klein, 2005, p. 32) can present a major obstacle to effective assessment and intervention.

A hierarchy of personal and cultural values may also have strong influence. Some hold information that is derived from measurable data as being more accurate and reliable; others hold speculative hypotheses emerging from theory as being more beneficial and progressive. How a particular hierarchy influences the course of assessment and intervention is very much dependent on the particular family and professional culture. Although some parents would run from the professional who speculates beyond the data, others would embrace him or her.

Problem 4: Specialization

As professional specializations have emerged, novel terms and descriptions of new (or old) phenomena and theories have been established. Within disciplines, individual professionals tend to communicate with one another using discipline-specific jargon, and they know what the other means. The further one travels beyond the professional boundary, however, it is less likely that the other understands the meaning of terms. When professionals are weighted toward similar domains, they may incorrectly assume that the terms used are mutually understood. For example, one mental health professional may only use the term *depression* when referring to a clinical condition with a set of specific symptoms and parameters for intensity and duration, whereas another mental health professional may use the term more loosely as an emotional state of persistent sadness. When professionals are weighted toward different domains, they may not be aware that their use of a term is defined in a way that is distinctive to their profession and does not hold the same meaning for others. When the same term is defined in different ways, misunderstanding or confusion is sure to follow. For example, the term *representation* in neuroscience refers to the translation of firing patterns of neurons into information for the organism; in developmental circles, the term *representation* refers to a symbolic recreation of experience; and in infant mental health circles, the parent's internal *representation* of what the infant represents to him or her (based on past and present relationships) is critical in determining whether the infant is imbued with positive or negative attributions (Fraiberg, 1980; Lieberman, Silverman, & Pawl, 2000; Weatherston, 2005). Communication among discipline-specific professionals and communication from one professional discipline to another often becomes quickly complicated by language, where mistaken assumptions about the meanings of terms run rampant.

Another difficulty related to professional language is the use of short-hand terminology within disciplines. A single word or phrase encompasses a rich and complex meaning, whereby a quick translation tends to compromise nuance and clarity. In other words, there are times when extensive background knowledge is necessary to adequately understand and apply a term or a concept; it may not be possible to unpack the meaning of a term or phrase in one sitting and do it justice. At this point, the direct participation of a professional from that domain becomes necessary, at least to whatever extent the concept is involved in a particular child's problem. This particular professional should have a more central role so that the depth of his or her understanding can influence the assessment and treatment process. Clearly, this type of involvement across disciplines, wherein roles may shift relative to area of specialization, is not possible without collaboration.

A more complicated problem arises when different disciplines apply different terminology in diagnosis. Further, the different terminology (or diagnosis) often denotes different assumptions or implications as to underlying causal factors. Each discipline is necessarily weighted toward a specific domain in its focus (e.g., psychiatry toward mental health, physical therapy toward motor enhancement) and there is, of course, overlap where different disciplines focus within the same general domain (e.g., occupational therapy with auditory hypo/hypersensitivities and language therapy with auditory processing). Similar to the problem just noted with shorthand terminology, it creates confusion and frustration for professionals when diagnostic labels are assigned or causal attributions are made that may have little or no meaning outside of the particular discipline. The situation is far worse for the parent who receives different diagnoses from different disciplines but is given no help in reconciling the meaning of these differences.

For example, consider a child who presents with inattention and hyperactivity. The neuropsychologist concludes that this indicates an attention-deficit/hyperactivity disorder (ADHD) and suggests that the child's hyperactivity and inattention reflect differences in the brain related to dopamine pathways and the areas involved in attention, motor, and executive functioning. With the same child, the occupational therapist concludes a sensory processing disorder and suggests that the child's hyperactivity is due to under-responsiveness of the vestibular system and the inattention to difficulties with discriminating sensory stimuli. The psychologist recommends medication and psychotherapy, the occupational therapist recommends occupational therapy. Add a speech-language pathologist or audiologist to the picture and we may have a third diagnosis of a central auditory processing disorder. So where does this leave the

parent? At this juncture, the typical response of a professional is to take sides—support one conclusion and dismiss the others, and cite the research or arguments to support it. But, again, where does this leave the parent? The professional may have only succeeded in changing the problem domain from one of trying to understand the child's disorder to one of choosing whom to trust.

Recent studies have begun to examine the issue of differentiating between disorders from different nomenclatures, for example, using vignettes to determine how occupational therapists and psychologists differentiate sensory overresponsivity from anxiety disorder (Ben-Sasson, Cermak, Orsmond, Carter, & Fogg, 2007). Whereas this work is important in further defining and clarifying diagnostic issues, it does not resolve the larger problem that our different labels denote different etiologies and different treatments. What we lack is an efficient way to return to the same playing field to discuss areas of overlap and difference, and from there determine the optimal treatment priorities and sequence.

A BRIEF HISTORY OF ASSESSMENT AND INTERVENTION APPROACHES

A primary value that underlies the development of the neurorelational framework is the importance of understanding behavior within a global context. With this overarching goal in mind, it is fitting to place the neurorelational framework within a historical perspective. The current state of affairs has deep historical roots that we review here in broad strokes.

Professional and popular interest in child development is a relatively recent phenomenon, going back a little more than a century. A review of the history reveals a few general themes: (1) an ebb and flow in viewing either nature or nurture as dominant in influencing development; (2) a progression of emphasis on physical issues, moving to cognitive issues, and then to emotional issues in understanding children's needs; (3) increasing awareness that early intervention can change outcomes; and (4) an ebb and flow in the commitment of the political community in addressing the needs of children.

Charles Darwin is often credited as one of the first to focus on development with the publication of his diary logging his own child's development (Darwin, 1877). Not until the late 1800s, however, were any formal studies of child development undertaken. Using questionnaires with children, Stanley Hall and his students examined topics such as anger, fears, mathematics, and dreams, and concluded that the normal growth of the

mind occurs as a series of evolutionary stages (Watson, 1978). During the early 1900s, Gesell was the first to directly catalog and study infant development (Gesell, 1929). The data he produced influenced the construction of assessment instruments that were based on a linear model of development. It was thought that long-term outcomes could be predicted by the rate at which developmental milestones where achieved in early childhood.

During this period, due in part to the influence of Galton (1892) and his views on hereditary genius, the view of biological determinism (nature) held sway. By reading federal publications, parents learned that too much play or stimulation early in their child's development would disrupt nature's unfolding. In terms of children with special needs, Caldwell (1973) dubbed the first half of the 20th century the "forget and hide" period, when children with significant physical or mental problems were typically institutionalized or kept out of public view. It was believed that no change and very little quality of life were possible.

This extreme view of nature's importance was countered by behaviorism, as championed by Watson (1928), who posited that developmental outcomes in children were largely controlled by environmental forces (nurture). Although behaviorism is criticized for its mechanistic approach, the research generated during this time made it exceedingly difficult to discount the impact of experience and thus helped pave the way for early intervention. During this same period, Sigmund Freud drew attention to the importance of childhood experiences for adult emotional health (Jolibert, 1993).

Around the time of World War II, professional views of children with disabilities began to change, largely stimulated by the results of massive testing of military personnel. The testing revealed a striking prevalence of young persons with physical, mental, or behavioral disabilities. At the same time, large numbers of veterans were returning from war with physical impairments. These events raised awareness and stimulated changes in public attitudes about disabilities. During the 1950s and 1960s, children with disabilities were tested and identified in greater numbers, but they continued to be isolated if their problems were severe and were mainstreamed without help if they were not. Many of these children eventually dropped out of school. This period was dubbed "screen and segregate" (Caldwell, 1973).

Largely due to the influence of Piaget (1960), the 1960s was also a time of focus on cognitive development. Piaget's view supported a nature perspective, with a linearly unfolding cognitive blueprint, as well as a nurture perspective, and a focus on movement and interaction with the environment. The emotional world of the child was considered to develop on a separate track from cognitive development.

The next phase (1970s) brought the importance of early intervention to the forefront. Children's needs could be identified and thereby something more could be done in response. In some circles, this news was not new. Spitz coined the term *hospitalism* in the 1940s to describe the destructive impact that sustained isolation (absence of a loving and consistent caregiver) and understimulation had on children in institutions (Spitz, 1945). Parallel to this development, a series of studies that began with institutionalized children with mental retardation suggested that the sequelae of early deprivation were modifiable (Skeels & Dye, 1939). Bowlby (1969, 1973, 1978) examined the mental health consequences of early deprivation and highlighted the importance of the mother–child relationship for healthy development. His work led to the now well-known construct of attachment and later studies of social-emotional adaptation. In education, this period was dubbed "identify and help," initiated by special education legislation (Meisels & Shonkoff, 2000).

The 1970s was also a time of great political and public enthusiasm and support. For this reason, there was a surge in activity across several levels (public awareness campaigns, community initiatives, academic research, education reforms, and interdisciplinary programs in clinical settings), and priority was placed on efforts to identify and screen children for special needs during early years to provide intervention services. As some outcome analysis (Meisels & Shonkoff, 2000) began to indicate equivocal or meager results, however, the wave of enthusiastic support waned. It appeared that how programs were organized and then later evaluated was a much more complex issue than expected. This analysis initiated interest and spurred research into more comprehensive programs and more complex methods of analysis.

While emotional disorders and the importance of emotional health were increasingly coming into public awareness in the 1970s and 1980s, an emotional focus was (and continues to be) slowly and clumsily integrated into children's services. The area of family relationships and emotional health was included in many early intervention program goals and special education initiatives, but actual means for identifying and treating emotional issues were rare. The primary focus of most programs continued to be cognitive and academic.

The decade of the 1990s presented a massive surge in brain research and dissemination of knowledge about the brain. For a time, these events created a resurgence of public and political enthusiasm for early intervention, but the efforts wavered with political priorities and failed to give way to a strong commitment of funding support (Meisels & Shonkoff, 2000).

Brain research escorted in a way to integrate the nature and nurture sides of child development. We have a better understanding of the genetic mechanisms that drive and influence brain development as well as how

critically important interaction with sensory information from the environment is for the brain to develop normally. Brain research has also presented us with ways to understand our emotional world without having to be severed from our thinking world. More recently, brain research has provided fascinating accounts of functioning that integrate the body-mind-environment sphere into a seamless whole.

TODAY'S MOVEMENT FROM SINGULAR TO MULTIPLE CAUSES

In the context of the vast specialization within multiple disciplines, there are clusters of different communities that have vested interests in specialized areas. Some professional communities within a discipline focus on academic research, others on public policy, and others on clinical practice (Shonkoff, 2000). Each community inside each discipline also has its own language and its own goals that attempt to address systems failures. Thus, each particular discipline has its own research division that often does not speak to the clinical practitioners and others working to promote public policy for the discipline's professional advancement and who may not understand the complexities of either research or practice. Parents are affected by each of these communities and conversely influence public policy, research, and clinical practice by applying public pressure.

If it wasn't enough to contend with the various layers of communication breakdown between research, public policy, and clinical approaches, we have an added limitation: the developmental theories that both clinicians and researchers use hold "a number of damaging dualities that have plagued the study of development" (Keating & Miller, 2000, p. 390). Common dualities that most of us have "inherited" by virtue of our training include (1) assumptions that causal factors for poor outcomes oscillate between nature (innate factors) versus nurture (environment); (2) an emphasis on developmental constraints (diagnosis) versus opportunities (strengths); (3) the struggle over the importance of cooperative (peer interactions) versus competitive (individualistic) efforts involved in learning; and (4) whether development unfolds in a linear fashion with continuity and stability or nonlinearly though change and instabilities (Keating, 1999). These dualities tend to generate research on development that looks for singular (rather than multiple) causes. Although current thinking contends that the nature–nurture debate no longer exists, the fact remains that many clinical theories and research designs are weighted toward unidirectional causalities, for example, those dealing with temperament versus attachment (Karen, 1994) and person versus situation influence (Funder, in press).

Dynamic systems theory has affected a broad range of fields from biology to the social sciences. A vital aspect of dynamic systems models, especially in their application to development, is their goal to achieve "a coherent integration across numerous levels, subsystems, or components" (Keating & Miller, 2000, p. 378; see also Bertalanffy, 1968; Howe & Lewis, 2005). Its emphasis on understanding complex systems and moving away from dualistic paradigms has provided timely theoretical support for comprehensive models that are "more accurately rooted in the complexities of mutually causal dynamic systems" (Keating & Miller, 2000, p. 390).

In the following sections, we share descriptions of some of the ways that public policy, academic scientific research, and theoretical and clinical approaches are recognizing and using the idea that outcomes result from multiple causes, not singular ones (Sameroff & Fiese, 2000a). This idea is at the core of the movement to embrace complexity. In our view, the neurorelational framework builds on this emerging zeitgeist, which accepts the reality of complexity in all arenas.

Public Policy

Part C of the Individuals with Disabilities Education Act (IDEA), passed in 1990 and reauthorized in 1997, stipulates that children from birth to age 3 years who have disabilities should be referred to the Individualized Education Programs (IEPs). This regulation, in large part, is how the term *early intervention* became primarily associated with physical disabilities as well as disciplines working with disabilities, even though all professionals providing services to children from birth to age 3 years are providing early intervention per se. The early intervention programs inadvertently contributed to the creation of a split between physical disabilities and emotional disabilities—the mental health diagnostic categories that focus on children's socioemotional health and the mental health of the caregiver.

An opportunity for integration arose, however, when the Child Abuse Prevention and Treatment Act (CAPTA; Pub. L. No. 93-247), originally enacted in 1974, was amended and reauthorized as the Keeping Children and Families Safe Act of 2003 (Pub. L. No. 108-36), mandating that all children from birth to 3 years are required to be referred for a thorough evaluation when there is substantiated abuse, neglect, or illegal substance use in the home. A public policy that directly links developmental disabilities with prenatal risk factors and emotional and physical abuse and neglect provides another chance for building bridges between disciplines to address the interface between emotional health, physical health, and family relationships.

Academic Research

Academic research often leads the way toward new trends. In May 2002, Elias A. Zerhouni, director of the National Institutes of Health (NIH), convened a series of meetings to chart a roadmap for medical research in the 21st century.[2] These meetings included input from more than 300 nationally recognized leaders in academia, industry, government, and the public. The purpose was to identify major opportunities for and gaps in biomedical research that NIH must address as a whole to optimize its entire research portfolio. Research areas of the future were identified as (1) high-risk research, (2) interdisciplinary research, and (3) public–private partnerships. The "Overview of the NIH Roadmap" (NIH, 2008) includes the following explanation for this vision:

> The scale and complexity of today's biomedical research problems increasingly demands that scientists move beyond the confines of their own discipline and explore new organizational models for team science. . . . NIH wants to stimulate new ways of combining skills and disciplines in both the physical and biological sciences . . . will encourage investigators to take on creative, unexplored avenues of research that carry a relatively high potential for failure, but also possess a greater chance for truly groundbreaking discoveries. In addition, novel partnerships, such as those between the public and private sectors, will be encouraged to accelerate the movement of scientific discoveries from the bench to the bedside.

Interdisciplinary research can been defined as the *integration* of several disciplines to create a *unified outcome* that is sustained and substantial enough to enable a new hybrid discipline to develop over time. Integration of multiple disciplines requires collaboration in designing new types of (experimental) approaches and analyses that combine methods and concepts from each participating discipline.[3] As part of this interdisciplinary vision, the NIH Exploratory Centers for Interdisciplinary Research offers funding for interdisciplinary approaches. The success of an interdisciplinary approach is defined as "combining aspects of individual disciplines to provide a new approach to solving a problem that is likely to yield insights that could not have been achieved by an isolated laboratory or using a multi-disciplinary approach" (U.S. Department of Health and Human Services, 2003).

Complementing this shift in conceptual framework was a large investment of funds. In March 2003, the National Academies and the W. M. Keck Foundation announced a 15-year $40 million grant (from the Keck Foundation) to underwrite the National Academies Keck Futures Initiative, a program designed to realize the untapped potential of interdisciplinary research.

The intent is "to stimulate new modes of inquiry and break down the conceptual and institutional barriers to interdisciplinary research that could yield significant benefits to science and society" (W. M. Keck Foundation, 2003). Stated outcome goals are to provide recommendations to academic institutions and public and private sponsors of research as to how to better kindle and support interdisciplinary research.

This trend toward interdisciplinarity has tremendous potential to change the landscape of how research and theory building are conducted in the 21st century. This movement toward collaboration in research should be mirrored in practice. The surge of interest within major funding sources clarifies and supports the notion that complex problems require complex approaches. This understanding of complexity must extend to a parallel movement within clinical professions to merge and integrate the contributions from multiple disciplines. A clinical framework that extends its boundaries broadly enough to allow the infusion of current research findings from across disciplines can provide a common global template with a common language to support the integration of specialized knowledge domains across early intervention and infant mental health. That, indeed, is the goal of our neurorelational framework.

Current Clinical Approaches That Are Salient to the Neurorelational Framework

As mentioned, the neurorelational framework is grounded in a dynamic systems approach and equally inspired by the schools of thought described in the following sections. These theories reflect complex and integrated approaches to the assessment and treatment of at-risk clinical populations.

Sameroff's Transactional Model

As research on a national level shifts away from isolated endeavors, a parallel process has occurred in the clinical arena, supported by clinical research investigating causal factors that lead to poor child outcomes. For example, in contrast to isolating variables to find the one "main problem," Sameroff and Fiese, researchers and developmental psychologists at the University of Michigan, bring a complex view to research and clinical practice that they call the *transactional model*. The model provides a paradigm for child development across research, academic, and clinical communities (Sameroff & Fiese, 2000a, 2000b). Sameroff's longitudinal research dismantles any remaining notion of one single individual or environmental factor that has major consequences for developmental outcomes.

His perspective is that *no one factor* is causal. Rather, it is the *accumulation of a variety* of risk factors, independent of their specific qualities, that determines influence (Sameroff & Fiese, 2000a, 2000b). Sameroff's transactional model is now being used in research endeavors that influence public health and public policy (Halfon & Hochstein, 2002). His research supports the need for clinical conceptual frameworks that can incorporate multiple variables for all team members to use as a shared theory base, so no single discipline holds the only lens through which to evaluate and understand a child's distress signals. A premise of multiple causalities sets the stage for more complex clinical models.

Sameroff identifies three assumptions that are required for successful implementation of interventions that support child development (Sameroff & Fiese, 2000b, p. 135):

1. Child development has multiple contributors at multiple levels.
2. At each level, multiple processes are represented in family thought and cultural symbols.
3. Intervention processes "must be targeted at a particular problem for a particular child in a particular family in a particular culture."

A child's presenting behavioral and developmental problems are more likely than not to be a result of multiple variables. Assessing across multiple functional domains most often requires a team effort, rather than the isolated endeavors of a solo practitioner. Sameroff's transactional model reflects the assumptions of the neurorelational framework, which holds that multiple interconnected systems contribute to the complexities inherent in a child's and family's behaviors. The neurorelational framework considers multiple domains in the context of multiple diagnostic categories, rather than narrowing the focus to a singular causal domain.

Within the transactional model lies a complex process approach to child development in which "the child is seen as a product of the continuous dynamic interactions of the child and the experience provided by his or her family and social context" (Sameroff, 2004, p. 7). This transactional process is depicted in Figure 1.1.

This visual description shows the impact that parent and child have on each other in real time. The series of transactions show how development is rarely the sole consequence of immediate causes or previous events, but rather the cumulative effects that converge as a result of what a child brings, what a parent brings, and the co-created dynamics between the two.

Despite the mutual influence that parent and child exert on each other, a natural asymmetry exists in the ration of child's degree of need to parent's degree of need. Obviously a child needs considerably more

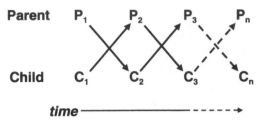

Figure 1.1. Transactional process with reciprocal effects between the child and the parent across time. (From "Ports of Entry and the Dynamics of Mother-Infant Interventions," by A. J. Sameroff, 2004, in *Treating Parent-Infant Relationship Problems,* p. 8, by A. J. Sameroff, S. C. McDonough, & K. L. Rosenblum [Eds.], New York: Guilford Press. Copyright 2004 by The Guilford Press. Reprinted with permission.)

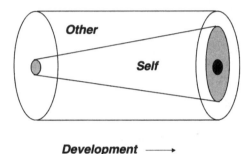

Figure 1.2. Changing balance between other-regulation and self-regulation as a child develops into an adult. (From "Ports of Entry and the Dynamics of Mother-Infant Inter-ventions," by A. J. Sameroff, 2004, in *Treating Parent-Infant Relationship* Problems, p. 12, by A. J. Sameroff, S. C. McDonough, & K. L. Rosenblum [Eds.], New York: Guilford Press. Copyright 2004 by The Guilford Press. Reprinted with permission.)

assistance from a parent for healthy development to progress. Self and other regulation are important vehicles through which development oc-curs. The developmental changes in child's and parent's need for each other are depicted in Figure 1.2 (Sameroff, 2004). As development pro-gresses, a balanced dynamic of self and other regulation occurs through maturation, although these dynamics are subject to shifts at various points along the life cycle (e.g., adolescence, medical illness, aging).

Tronick's Mutual Regulation Model and Dyadic Expansion of States of Consciousness

As an extensive infant–parent researcher, Tronick developed key concepts, two of which include his mutual regulation model and the dyadically expanded states of consciousness model, in which self and interactive

regulation functions optimally within open systems. Tronick builds on a dynamic system's principle in which any open biological system functions in a paradoxical way to "incorporate and integrate increasing amounts of meaningful information into more coherent states" (Tronick, 2007, p. 406). As more information is integrated into our biological systems, we gain more complexity; as there is an increase in coherence, we gain more organization. As we shall see, the successful maturation of states of arousal (also referred to as states of consciousness which include the work of Als, 1984, 2002; Als & Gibes, 1986; Barnard, 1999; Brazelton, 1973, 1984, 1992; Prechtl, 1977) can also be understood as the growth of energy and information that maintains, increases, and expands the complexity and coherence of the organization and structure of these states of consciousness. Tronick proposes three ways of expanding coherence and complexity: "(1) interacting and communicating with people, (2) acting on things, and as Modell (1993) would argue, (3) engaging our private selves" (Tronick, 2007, p. 3). The interaction of these three factors is pivotal to the continued growth and development of a healthy, open self-organizing system.

Als's Synactive Theory of Development

Heidelese Als (1982) developed a systems oriented, relationship-based, integrative theory—the synactive theory of development—that identifies the overlapping systemic forces that provide the basis for how to understand the behavior we see in vulnerable infants. Individualized, highly attuned bedside care is provided by a variety of trained hospital staff for both individual professionals and teams, including physicians and nurses; physical, respiratory, and occupational therapists; social workers, and so on (Als et al., 1994). Parents are viewed as members of the health care team and as the infant's most important nurturers and comforters. Als's Neonatal Individualized Developmental Care Assessment Protocol (NIDCAP) (Als, 1984, 2002; Als & Gibes, 1986) is an integrated approach to tracking an infant's physiological, motor, attentional, and state-regulation capacities. Daily care, interventions, and interactions are based on following the infant's states—that is, his or her need for rest or recovery following a stressful event—before attempting interactions or further invasive procedures. Environmental demands from lights and sounds are carefully monitored, as are individualized needs for motor and physical support, and aids for self-regulation and containment are provided. Als's integrative theory base is one of the few that has gone through various forms of evidence-based outcome research. Although the need for research outcomes is ongoing, "evaluations have found that NIDCAP babies had less need for certain medical treatments, better behavioral outcomes at key stages,

earlier initiation of oral feeding, better average daily weight gains, shorter hospital stays, more activity in the brain's frontal lobe, and a lower incidence of developmental delays than babies in a comparison group" (Pathways, 2008; see also Als et al., 2003; Als et al., 2004). NIDCAP has also been shown (Als et al., 2004) to enhance brain structure and function with significance in MRI results (see www.nidcap.org).

Greenspan and Wieder's Developmental, Individual, Relationship Model (DIR/Floortime)

Continuing the focus on individualized, developmental approaches that support interpersonal interactions, Greenspan and Wieder's (1998) developmental, individual, relationship (DIR) model brings a clinical interdisciplinary perspective to older newborns and young children in IMH and EI settings, holding multiple factors across multiple developmental domains in tension with each other while promoting team cross-fertilization. This clinical model provides a complex organization for individual practitioners as well as for those who work on teams. The DIR model assesses each infant or child across sensory (sight, hearing, etc.), motor (movement and balance), affective (emotional), speech and language, and cognitive systems (Wieder & Greenspan, 2005). Assessments are used to prioritize the functional aspects of a child's behavior, the parent's interpersonal style, and the functional interactions between the two; treatment focuses on changing the interactions in the present through guidance, coaching, and modeling. Relational-interpersonal development is assessed across functional emotional milestones that serve as the basis for Axis V of the diagnostic classification system DC:0–3R (ZERO TO THREE, 1994, 2005) (more fully described in Chapter 3). A functional approach does not rely solely on the set parameters provided by test measurements but allows the practitioner to take into account evidence from multiple sources and views observable behaviors as integrated from multiple domains. This theoretical approach is another advanced and complex clinical model that bridges IMH (socioemotional) and EI (sensory, motor, speech/language, and cognitive domains), thereby creating one large playing field.

The DIR/Floortime™ clinical perspective has a strong play-based component, and the emotional relationship between the child and the parent(s), exhibited through naturalistic interactions, is at the core of assessment, diagnosis, and intervention. Parents are always included in the process and are given as much information as they can assimilate to function as the healing agents with their children. Whereas the origins of DIR/ Floortime emerged from working with low-income families, due to its inherent holistic approach it has attracted families who have children with

developmental delays and learning disabilities. In fact, the DIR approach is applicable to all healthy and at-risk children.

Bagnato's Convergent Model of Assessment

From a psychoeducational perspective, Bagnato, Neisworth, and Munson (1997) applied the interdisciplinary concept to assessment tools and instruments used in early intervention educational settings (such as preschools). Their convergent model brings together parents, discipline-specific professionals working in early intervention, and teachers to collaborate in the collection of information in authentic, natural ways. Input about the children is gathered in multiple settings, on various occasions, from many sources, using a variety of assessment instruments. Because there is no singular causation, there can be no single assessment tool. Because there are multiple variables, infants and young children should be observed in multiple settings.

Bagnato and associates critiqued and evaluated standardized measurement tools used in infant mental health and early intervention circles according to multiple factors (e.g., sensitivity, authenticity, equity, and congruence). Assessment that occurs across a variety of settings, using multiple tools that are oriented to real-life events, is a necessary aspect of team and individual practice. No single discipline is viewed as possessing the proper assessment instruments that can determine the sole cause of a child and family's concerns.

Guralnick's Team Frameworks and Guidelines

Guralnick's (2000) work leads the way in promoting interdisciplinary teamwork by providing guidelines for setting up a functional team for complex assessment processes within academic and university settings. Parents who have children with developmental delays and disabilities come from local, rural, and outlying areas for a comprehensive assessment process that usually is completed in 1 or 2 days. These interdisciplinary teams service children and families that otherwise would not have access to proper assessment, ultimately developing plans and recommendations, including locating community resources to meet the identified needs of the child and family. Specifically, the teams (1) ensure that team members from each discipline are able to gather information and understand thoroughly, in relation to their domains of expertise, child and family functioning; (2) identify areas where additional information is needed; (3) help establish a diagnosis or provide the probable source or sources of the child's difficulties and communicate that information clearly to

parents; (4) recommend and suggest interventions; and (5) create a foundation for a framework that can guide more detailed, intervention-oriented assessments.

LIVING THE EFFECTS OF OUR SHORTCOMINGS

The following scenario may be familiar to many health professionals and is an attempt to illustrate the practical application of the aforementioned observations and approaches.

At his yearly checkup, 5-year-old Joseph is given a clean bill of health. He is within normal height and weight limits for a boy his age and appears healthy and happy. He is potty-trained and has long ago met the accepted age-related milestones for walking and talking. By all appearances, the pediatrician reports that Joseph is more than ready to enter kindergarten. Joseph's mother, Rachel, responds to this news with apprehension but can't articulate why. As the appointment continues, a few unusual behaviors come to light. First, Joseph shows no pain when he receives his shots; his eyes glaze over during the procedure and he fails to make eye contact with Rachel. She remembered that he does this whenever he receives a shot. As soon as the shot is over, he bolts off Rachel's lap, ignoring her shrill yell, and trips on the way out the door. This fall fails to deter him because he is so focused on getting to the front desk and rigidly adhering to his routine of picking out a sticker. Rachel is aware of his many other routines that require similar strict adherence. After gathering her two other children, she wearily chases after Joseph, struggling to get him under control.

  Rachel is reluctant to share her worry about her son's concerning behavior and unconventional delays. She finally mentions to the pediatrician that Joseph doesn't pay attention to her, is clumsy, and has few friends. But these concerns are only the tip of the iceberg for her. What she does not (or cannot) share is that she feels frustrated and exhausted. Her day is so consumed with Joseph that by the time her husband returns home from work she is despondent, irritable, and quiet, which is creating a strain on her marriage. She mentions none of this. She answers the pediatrician's questions and listens intently to his advice, agreeing to be more consistent in her discipline and to provide increased social opportunities. In the end, the pediatrician provides reassurance: "Don't worry, Joseph is a healthy, lively boy. . . . Let's see if these things have improved by the time of his next visit." Rachel feels a surge of cheerfulness but it is short-lived. Leaving the office, unsettling feelings creep in. Rachel thinks about all the things she *didn't* say and realizes that she cannot cling to his optimism when she didn't give the whole picture. She wonders once again if her son really is healthy, if he really is ready for school. A few months later, when Joseph falls

behind in school and has two aggressive incidents with his peers, she realizes that her concerns were valid.

In an assessment process, practitioners in each discipline would look at Joseph and Rachel and highlight different aspects of the scene. One mental health specialist would emphasize Joseph's poor eye contact and lack of reciprocal communication and consider an autistic spectrum disorder. Another would note these things as well as Joseph's glazed eyes and failure to seek comfort from his mother and interpret these as signs of an attachment disorder. Another may acknowledge these possibilities but feel that Joseph's chaotic actions and aggression suggest an acute or cumulative traumatic history. Thus, even under the same general domain of mental health, we see that very different meanings can emerge from the same clinical phenomenon.

A specialist concerned with processing abilities (e.g., a psychologist, occupational therapist, speech-language pathologist, or educational therapist) might suspect a visual processing problem because Joseph does not "see" where he is going and does not "read" faces or other social cues. This does not mean that Joseph does not have adequate sight; it means that how he processes visual information is problematic. Another professional suspects an auditory or language processing problem because Joseph does not seem to "hear" his mother talking to him and may not follow her directives because he cannot filter her words from background noise or perhaps understand her language. Another professional suspects difficulties with sensory discrimination or modulation because Joseph shows poor postural control and doesn't seem to perceive his body position in space accurately. The teacher wonders why no one is talking about ADHD.

With so many different views, what is the best way to proceed with assessment? All of these disciplines are typically spread out in various settings, such as community agencies, private treatment facilities, schools, and private practice, so most often there is no forum where so many different voices can come together and plan out an assessment strategy. Currently, the assessment path is largely determined by the child's age (i.e., 0–3, 3–5, and 6 and above are served by different approaches and state agencies), the setting where the problem behaviors occur (e.g., mostly at school, mostly at home, mostly in groups), and how the concerns are raised (e.g., by the parents, a caring friend, a frustrated teacher, the pediatrician). For the family, if choices were available, they would be very confusing. Should they obtain a neuropsychological assessment, a psychoeducational evaluation, an occupational therapy evaluation, or a parent–child socioemotional (dyadic) assessment first? Further, will the assessment obtained tell us if Joseph's lack

26 Infant/Child Mental Health

of eye contact is due to a problem in the relationship with his mother, a genetic predisposition such as Asperger syndrome, a visual processing problem, or all of these? If there are problems in both mental health and processing domains, which intervention should go first if there are limited resources and time constraints?

These and additional professional voices expand into a very long list of possible treatments. A specialist focused on the relational dynamics would be alarmed and want to work with Rachel and Joseph as a pair. A behaviorist would immediately see Rachel's lack of consistency in her approach, her lack of setting consequences to inappropriate behavior, and her lack of rewards for his appropriate behavior as a core structural problem. A family systems therapist might see Joseph's problems as indeterminable due the disruptive effect of chronic stress caused by the problems in the marriage, and insist on marital therapy. Joseph's behavior may be viewed as resulting from an overinvolved mother and an underinvolved father, leaving no strong male role model or marital dyad to parent this child. Another mental health professional would pick up on the mother's agitated depression and suggest individual therapy for her to process her emotional distress and her possible projection of disappointments with her husband and past relationships onto her son. Someone else from within mental health might disagree, stating that the only viable treatment for depression is medication.

If by now you are beginning to feel overwhelmed and agitated at all the possibilities, one can only imagine how unsettling the confusion must be for parents when the well-being of their child is at stake. In sum, these are the potential diagnostic categories and intervention strategies that have been noted:

- a possible trauma response for Joseph (as indicated by his lack of connection to his mother), with individual or dyadic treatment recommended;
- regulatory and sensorimotor processing problems for Joseph, with occupational therapy recommended;
- a mood component of either anxiety or depression for Joseph or Rachel, with individual therapies or medications recommended;
- an attachment disorder, with individual therapies recommended for both Joseph and Rachel as a way to explore their internal worlds, which they project onto each other;
- an attentional disorder for Joseph, with medication and behavioral therapy recommended if his parents are willing to use medication, and neurofeedback (Monastra, 2005; Strehl et al., 2006) or sensory-integration treatment (Mangeot et al., 2001; Miller & Fuller, 2007;

Miller, Schoen, James, & Schaaf, 2007) if they prefer to use alternatives or in conjunction with medical measures;
- an autistic spectrum disorder or Asperger syndrome for Joseph,
  with a recommendation for a full team of professionals working
  10–20 hours a week across a variety of therapies;
- a lack of proper parental consequences and reinforcements requiring in-home behavioral therapy;
- a painful relational history for Rachel with probable trauma, with
  individual therapy recommended;
- a relational problem in the parent–child dyad, with dyadic therapy
  recommended;
- a marital problem for the couple, with couple therapy recommended.

Most practitioners are under pressure to identify the most "accurate" diagnostic code for financial purposes, often after the first visit. However, it
is very likely that more than one diagnostic category is correct—in which
case, how would an individual or team practitioner organize interventions? Where does one begin when more than one problematic condition
is going on at the same time? As Rachel frantically goes from one professional to the next, searching for answers, she is left with more questions as
each specialist offers his or her version of what is "wrong" and recommends his or her brand of intervention as a top priority. Even if Rachel
were capable financially of affording all of the treatments (a capability
that is unlikely for most clients), there would not be enough time for her
and Joseph to attend them.

BRAIN FUNCTIONING AS A TEMPLATE FOR THE NEURORELATIONAL FRAMEWORK

The overarching goal of this book is to present a conceptual framework for
individual practitioners and interdisciplinary collaboration that addresses
the four common problems (i.e., fragmentation, isolation, hierarchy, and
specialization). To be adequate for this purpose, the neurorelational framework must (1) be broad enough to contain the theories and approaches
represented across all pediatric disciplines, (2) provide a core knowledge
base and set of referents that bear relevance across all disciplines, and (3)
provide professionals with a part-to-whole view of the clinical picture to
help them see distinctions and areas of overlap with other disciplines. The
brain is the ideal model for the neurorelational framework presented in this
book for many reasons.

First, the principles of brain development and functioning provide a template for considering the multiple determinants of behavior. A brain map is all encompassing because it represents the culmination of all individual experience with the self, others, and the world and as such provides a global map for all possible contributions to a problem. It does not exclude the contributions from any single system. It contains the history of the individual and the mechanisms that drive behavior (e.g., from hunger to status to revenge), relationships, and the prevailing context within one's environment. The neurorelational framework holds the complexity of multiple underlying sources of causality through its global and systemic view of brain functioning.

Second, knowledge of brain development and functioning provides relevant and useful information for any pediatric professional, regardless of discipline. Every discipline has an affiliation toward certain functional domains of the brain. As such, practitioners from each discipline should be familiar with not only the neural underpinnings of their domain but also the relationship of that domain to others. The brain as template for clinical intervention both preserves and opens disciplinary boundaries. The neurorelational framework, as described in the following chapters, provides an integrated infrastructure for all individual practitioners and team disciplines to share. Specialization is preserved, and boundary crossing can occur within an organized and thoughtful approach that parallels brain development and brain functioning. Consider the scenario presented above where the same child obtained three different diagnoses from three different professionals: attention-deficit/hyperactivity disorder (neuropsychologist), sensory processing disorder (occupational therapist), and central auditory processing disorder (speech-language pathologist). Rather than tossing the conundrum into the lap of the parent, it makes much more sense, both logically and ethically, for the three professionals to work through the possibilities for etiology, anticipate the implications of each for treatment or nontreatment, and decide on the treatment approach that is most likely to be effective. Without some type of shared framework, there is a good chance that such a conversation would not be productive or would not even take place.

Third, the neurorelational framework provides a process for both individual and team practitioners that reduces the hierarchical turf battles by leveling the playing field. Who goes first, second, and third is determined by developmental and clinical considerations rather than preconceived cultural hierarchy. In addition, the neurorelational structure allows for flexibility and creativity in problem solving, clarification of thinking, and the weighting and prioritizing of contributions across systems. When evidence-based research is not yet available, sound neurodevelopmental

theory and guiding principles can be used to guide decisions. At the same time, clinical practices that do not make sense or are dangerous, from a brain development and brain functional point of view, can be challenged as necessary.

Principles of brain functioning provide a foundation for the neurorelational framework presented in this book; the neurorelational framework, in turn, provides a response to the four common problems faced by individual practitioners and team collaborators noted here and summarized in Table 1.1.

Chapter 2 presents an overview of the neurorelational framework and its underpinnings. This global framework identifies four major brain

Table 1.1.   Responses to the Four Common Problems

Brain Template	Neurorelational Framework
Fragmentation	
The brain is not fragmented in its functioning; it functions as an integrated and interdependent system.	The neurorelational framework reduces fragmentation by offering an integrated approach for assessment and intervention and by bridging disciplines through a reliance on brain processes, as a way to understand the meaning of behavior, irrespective of diagnostic categorization.
Isolation	
The brain is not an unsituated, disembodied entity; its functions are reciprocally interconnected with the body and the environment.	The neurorelational framework provides a holistic container whereby multiple causes and multiple treatment options across a wide range of disciplines can be considered at the same time. Bodily processes, emotional processes, and mental and educational processes are always held in dynamic interchange and in the context of the child's most important relationships, environmental challenges, and opportunities.
Hierarchy	
The brain does not "play favorites"; the dominance of activity in any area is relative solely to the task at hand (i.e., no ego issues clutter the task-allocation process).	The neurorelational framework does not favor any one brain system or discipline over another. All disciplines are guided by the clinical need and the associated brain system(s). Ego issues are more easily revealed for what they really are and less likely to elicit collusion or opposition when team members hold true to the value-neutral approach.

(Continued)

Table 1.1. Continued

Brain Template	Neurorelational Framework
Specialization	
The brain does not have a unitary central processor; different regions of the brain take on specialized functional roles within the context of distributed large-scale networks (Mesulam, 1998).	The neurorelational framework provides a common language and approach for use by both individual practitioners and team collaborators, in which the part-to-whole perspective is always held in mind.

systems that are viewed as being in continual interaction with the "other" and with the environment; these represent the neuro components of *neuro*relational framework. In addition, we describe how the neuroscience theories of sensory–motor plasticity, embodied cognition, connectionism, and allodynamic regulation allow us to avoid the common pitfalls of fragmentation, isolation, hierarchy, and specialization discussed here.

NOTES

1. Throughout this book, the term *parent* refers neither to biological nor gender-related meanings but signifies the caregiver who is emotionally capable of meeting the demands of parenting that require providing protection, nurturance, and training to one's child (Ruddick, 1994). Whenever possible, it is crucial to include the parent not only on the team but also in the intervention setting.

2. The results of these meetings produced a roadmap that can be found at http://nihroadmap.nih.gov/overview.asp.

3. It is important to note that the term *interdisciplinary* does not mean the same thing as *multidisciplinary*. Multidisciplinary efforts involve sharing information and working toward goals, but they do not involve *integrating* one (or more) discipline's approach with another.

2

An Overview of the Neurorelational Framework

The neurorelational framework pulls from global theories of brain development and functioning with four primary goals in mind. The first is to consolidate large amounts of neurodevelopmental information into four brain systems and a relational context that gives footing to all disciplines (i.e., any discipline should be able to "find itself" within a brain system context). Through consolidation of information that embraces all disciplines, our second purpose and ultimate hope is to provide a common language and approach that supports interdisciplinary collaboration. Having such a common language is a critical component in moving toward collaboration, because it provides clarity and promotes communication within and across disciplinary boundaries. In this sense, the neurorelational framework is a conceptual support structure for holding multiple domain-specific disciplines side by side as they merge their efforts in a single case. Much like a freeway system, practitioners may enter and exit the conceptual flow of assessment and intervention as needed, but when they are on the freeway, they can move forward together in the same direction and with the same purpose. The consolidation of neurodevelopmental information and provision of a common language supports our third goal of assisting practitioners across disciplines to be aware of and to hold the *whole* child or adult, including the ongoing issues and needs that are outside one's purview. Our perceptions and conclusions represent parts that may expand or shift in meaning when viewed against the whole, and the whole often involves the perceptions and conclusions of others. Each practitioner has the freedom to begin with the primary responsibilities of his or her discipline, but eventually the domain-specific information will be situated within the larger context of functioning across

all brain systems. Finally, our fourth goal is to use these four brain systems to promote insight into the fundamental mechanisms that underlie behavior, regardless of diagnostic category, which can then stimulate a number of solid strategies for intervention that prioritize the needs of a particular child.

The neurorelational framework is organized according to four global systems—regulation, sensory, relevance, and executive—each representing a collection of related brain functions. The four systems are viewed as being in dynamic, interdependent, and reciprocal relationship with each other, the body, and the world. Each brain develops and lives within a context that has universal and unique properties, shaping the expression of individual behavior. Relationships largely define the context of the child's world—"Human existence is social existence" (Sameroff & Emde, 1989, p. 221). The quality of nurturance and type of stimulation experienced interact with the child's brain to shape development and behavior. The dynamic and reciprocal nature of brains in relationship reminds us that the parent's brain is also not isolated but is continually affected by the child. In essence, the four systems of the brain are embedded in a context, and conversely, that context shapes and is represented within the four systems.

- The regulation system describes those brain mechanisms that are involved in bodily processes and the regulation of energy. The primary constructs presented within the regulatory system include states of arousal (such as sleep and alertness), stress responses (such as to challenge and threat) and stress recovery, and efficient and adaptive energy regulation.
- The sensory system describes how the brain translates energy in the world into our integrated experience of sights and sounds and bodily feelings. The primary constructs discussed within this system include individual differences in sensory processing, reflecting the hierarchical emergence of abilities such as language and visual recognition, as well as sensory modulation, reflecting sensitivities and preferences for certain types of sensory information.
- The relevance system describes the mechanisms involved in the determination of salience, which is what motivates and drives one behavior over another. The primary constructs discussed within this system include positive and negative emotion, emotional "blends," learning and memory, and the emergence of private and shared meanings.
- The executive system describes the components involved in real-time, real-world flexible and adaptive action—what to do, how to

do it, and when to do it. The primary constructs discussed within this system include the activation and inhibition of behavior (which include thoughts, emotions, and actions), the balance of thought and emotion, the balance of self and other, and the self in relation to achievement of goals.

In using the four brain systems, the process of assessment and intervention involves flexibly shifting from whole to parts and back again to keep pace with change and emerging insights as a case unfolds. Assessment and intervention also involves cycling back and forth between content and process. Among professionals, each of us brings domain-specific knowledge to the picture and a unique and specialized perspective (the "content"), but then we must return to the team of professionals and compare insights as we determine what to do with the collective information (the "process"). The process of assessment and intervention is also a bidirectional, hypothesis-driven approach whereby assessment *is* intervention and intervention *is* assessment. The processes of seeking and offering help, asking and answering questions, and gathering and providing data begin to prompt "aha!" moments of insight for both the parent and the professional. The seeds of change are planted at first contact. For the professional, evaluating the response to intervention in real time provides additional data that continually feed back into the assessment.

Assessment and intervention are learning processes. Assessment should not be a one-time effort that initiates a fixed treatment plan. Assessment should result in solid findings, to be sure, but it should also involve a plan for unpacking the important uncertainties that remain. Intervention is where the learning process unfolds. It is about *learning your way toward effective intervention* for the individual child, adult, and dyad. Even for treatment models that have a very prescribed, specific approach (e.g., discrete trials training, or following an established protocol), there are still a multitude of decisions to be made that require good judgment and clinical acumen, especially when the child's more global needs within his or her specific context are considered. In other words, even the most regimented approach requires good clinical acumen to accommodate for the variations in context and to keep the big picture in mind.

In our efforts to observe behavior as an expression of underlying brain mechanisms, we are attempting to link up two different levels of analysis: brain and behavior.[1] Although brain imaging gives a glimpse into possible links, we cannot impose a one-to-one correspondence between behavior X and brain area X. What we can do through our understanding

of various brain processes, however, is gain insight into potential causes for behaviors that can drive hypothesis-driven intervention. This type of neuroscience information often comes to us in little nuggets. For example, say you learn that stress disrupts cortisol levels and excess cortisol can damage brain areas that regulate circadian rhythms. With this information, you might think about the child you treat who has rage episodes, and, forming the connection from rage to stress to cortisol to sleep, you decide to take a closer look at sleep patterns. However, such nuggets of information are far too numerous for any one person to accumulate, and furthermore, not everyone will interpret the implications of the research findings in the same way. Thus, to strengthen the bridge from bench to bedside, we suggest that it is most efficient and useful to first grasp the large-scale dynamics of brain function rather than multiple, domain-specific, micro-level mechanisms. With large-scale processes as the foundation of knowledge, the more domain-specific micro-level mechanisms can then be integrated within the larger context.

NEUROSCIENCE THEORIES

The following sections provide a review of the neuroscience theories that both inspired and influenced the neurorelational framework:

- sensory–motor plasticity;
- embodied cognition;
- behavioral neuroanatomy/connectionism; and
- allodynamic regulation.

These theories are introduced here and are referenced in the brain system chapters (4–11). The first two theories reflect the conceptual fundamentals of the brain's adaptive interaction with its surroundings, highlighting the central importance of movement to the brain's development and functioning. These reflect our outside-in–inside-out influences. The latter two theoretical accounts bring us inside the skull to explore the global aspects of autonomic and central nervous system structure and function. These reflect our top-down–bottom-up influences. The first two are more concerned with *what* the brain does, the latter two with *how* the brain does it. Each theory consolidates and integrates a large amount of data from the neurosciences into a manageable conceptualization of how the brain, as a whole, does its job. Finally, each theory highlights a perspective that illustrates a core assumption of the neurorelational framework.

Sensory–Motor Plasticity

We start at the evolutionary level by asking the basic question, what is the brain for? Many species have one, so what are the brain's most fundamental purposes? A task universal to the brains of all organisms is to convert sensory information into motor behavior and motor behavior into sensory information—that is, to perform sensory–motor transformations (Tweed, 2003). Organisms that must navigate the world to reproduce and survive, be they insects (yes, insects have brains) or mammals, rely on their brains to translate energy in the world into sensory information and propel effective motor behaviors. Conversely, living things that do not need to change location to reproduce and survive do not have brains. To illustrate this point, think of plant life. Some plants move, like the walking palm, but plants do not pull up roots in search of food and a mate, so they do not need a brain. Thus, we can consider motor responses to sensory stimuli and sensory responses to motor stimuli to be among the fundamental and universal features of brains. Even visceral activity follows the same fundamental process (i.e., organs are activated or deactivated by particular stimuli). All brain activity can be traced back to this "what for" capacity at some level. To emphasize the fundamental importance of movement to brains, some theorists have asserted that the very formation and evolution of brains across species is the product of movement, that the brain evolved "from the motor periphery all the way back to the sensors" (Tweed, 2003).

In addition, the variations among brains are a reflection of the sensory and motor capacities necessary for a particular species' survival. For humans, vision is a very important sense for survival, so human brains devote a lot of space to the processing of visual stimuli and the integration of visual information with motor capacities (e.g., the frontal lobes dedicate a respectable amount of space to eye movements). For dogs, smell is a very important sense for survival, so dog brains accord much more neural real estate to associating and elaborating olfactory stimuli than do human brains. As a result, we have the capacity to see and respond to a broader range of visual stimuli in the world than dogs, but dogs can make a better living sniffing luggage at the airport than we can. In essence, when an organism must rely more heavily on a particular sense (or aspect of a sense) for reproduction and survival—for example, smelling reproductive readiness, hearing a predator, seeing the necessary colors or contours of food, or detecting shifts in the wind—then its brain devotes more neurons to processing those sensory details and representing those details with the appropriate motor programs.

Building on the concept of sensory–motor transformations, we use the term *sensory–motor plasticity* to highlight the formative and interactive

influences between human brains and the environment. Sensory–motor plasticity emphasizes that human brains support an open learning system in the service of greater flexibility for behavioral adaptation. In lower organisms, the links between sensations and actions are more rigidly coupled than in humans (e.g., a single sensory cue activates a single behavioral sequence) (Mesulam, 1998). Furthermore, any disruption to these links greatly reduces the chances for survival. For example, bodily damage that compromises an animal's movement, or an environmental event that results in loss of a food source, would likely result in death. In contrast, higher-level organisms, especially humans, have much more flexibility. The path from stimulus to response is not obligatory; rather, processing across multiple levels allows our behavior to be guided by the context (Mesulam, 1998). Thus, disruptions such as changes in the environment, damage to the body, and even damage to the brain itself need not result in death. For humans, there is a great deal of flexibility among the systems involved in sensing and moving; this flexibility allows for learning that services adaptation to both internal and external change. Importantly, human brains also support an incredible capacity for anticipation of change (Fuster, 2002; Tranel, 2002) (discussed in more detail later).

The neurorelational framework uses the idea of sensory–motor plasticity as a basis for the behaviors we see throughout each brain system, behaviors that are modifiable through sensorimotor experience. Although the various sensorimotor functions tend to get segmented according to certain disciplines (i.e., occupational science, speech and language, physical therapists), they are not similarly segmented in the brain. All are important for all professionals because these functions represent a fundamental task of the brain as well as a fundamental tool for change. Sensory–motor *plasticity* reminds us that the human brain supports an open learning system, whereby sensory–motor processes can be learned and expanded. The treatment goals of the neurorelational framework all share a focus on adaptive flexibility in the functioning of both intra- and interpersonal behaviors. This theme is developed as the framework unfolds.

Embodied Cognition

The theory of embodied cognition highlights the central role of movement and environmental interaction in both shaping the developing brain and promoting adaptive success. In this view, the brain is most adept at supporting real-time, goal-directed interactions between organisms and their environment; therefore, any understanding of the relationship of

behavior to brain activity must acknowledge this fact: Thinking beings are acting beings. The theory of embodied cognition emerged from several arenas of the cognitive sciences (i.e., developmental psychology, artificial life and robotics, linguistics, philosophy of mind) but makes two common assumptions: (1) a necessary condition for cognition is embodiment, which is broadly understood as the unique way an organism's sensorimotor capacities enable it to successfully interact with its particular environmental niche; and (2) cognitive explanations must capture the manner in which mind, body, and world mutually interact and influence one another to promote an organism's adaptive success (Cowardt, 2006). We are mainly influenced by the work of Andy Clark (1997, 2003), a cognitive scientist and philosopher currently at the University of Edinburgh, because he presents support for the theory of embodied cognition by drawing on and integrating insights across multiple scientific domains and often associates ideas with developmental issues.

For our purposes, the important aspect of embodied cognition is in coming to view the brain as an active, adaptive organ versus a passive, "rational" organ. In other words, the brain is not in a box and not all about thinking. In the real world, human brains confront challenges that unfold rapidly within the context of ongoing behavior (action and inhibition of action). We are active creatures. If we think in terms of variety of actions, we may well be the most active creatures. We are also adaptive creatures. We do not stop and think thousands of times a day as we go about our lives; rather, the greater part of brain work remains automatic, outside of our awareness, and seamlessly integrated within our ongoing movements as we adapt to contexts and goals.

Our brains are embodied and embedded, active and adaptive, and these fundamental properties have important implications for understanding how our brains work and why they sometimes don't work. Are we giving enough consideration to the fact that the vast majority of our brain functioning occurs in real time in the real world? Although focused thought is presumably uniquely human, is it really a good starting point for understanding how our brains work? Some researchers have investigated the nature of learning in the context of movement in the environment. In a series of studies conducted by Thelen and Smith (1994), the researchers examined the progression of motor competencies in children. Infants, still crawling, learned through experience how to negotiate slopes of varying degrees of tilt. However, once these infants transitioned to walking, they had to learn these same lessons again, now through experience with walking on slopes of varying degrees of tilt. The point is that these findings suggest that action in the real world played the greater role in acquiring motor skills than the "cognitive" storing of information. These children

did not appear to have stored a "slopes and degrees" file that they could access from the appropriate slot, apply to the task, and thereby avoid falling. They had to work it out in the real world relative to the new developmental context—walking. To elaborate a bit more, the brain does not appear to function like a passive, rational organ that gathers and stores information about the world into a massive database to be retrieved as needed. To be sure, a great deal of learning and information is stored and retrieved like this, but the brain is actually *most* adept at learning and adapting within a behavioral context. Much of what it does is worked out in real time and in the real world.

A second important aspect of embodied cognition theory for our purposes is its implications of a continuous and cooperative interplay between brain, body, and world. We are in constant interaction with external props (e.g., language, symbols, tools) to the point that they become seamlessly integrated into our ongoing cognitive processes. For example, consider language. Clark refers to language as "the ultimate artifact: so ubiquitous it is almost invisible, so intimate it is not clear whether it is a kind of tool or a dimension of the user" (Clark, 1997, p. 218). This point broadens the scope of how we define cognitive processes and opens up, quite literally, a world of tools for intervention. If we truly grasp the idea of an extended mind, external supports take on a whole new meaning for remediation and accommodation.

A few examples will help illustrate the extension of cognition into the world (Clark, 1997). In completing a jigsaw puzzle, we do not figure out how to solve it with pure thought and then proceed to carry out the solution already achieved in the head. Rather, we group pieces, move them around, pick them up, rotate them, try them out, and so on, as we make steady progress toward the solution. Each successive movement along the path to the goal changes the problem domain. Other examples include grouping grocery items for packing, arranging Scrabble tiles to cue words, and consolidating and writing down a child's history according to categories. The latter example reflects the use of external props to ease the demands on our "thinking" brains. We make notes in margins, keep to-do lists, and put appointments in calendars to both scaffold our thinking and "offload" demands on our thinking. Our everyday use of tools, whether tangible (e.g., pens, computers) or symbolic (e.g., signs, language), is a reflection of this interactive process, as well as a sort of communal sharing of cognitive resources. In these examples, the boundary between thought and action becomes difficult to identify; they become mingled together in a problem-solving loop (Clark, 1997). Viewed through this lens, our capacities start to appear much more distributed—not isolated in the head, but continually emerging and adapting in real time and in

interaction with the environment. Note the important parallel here to assessment and intervention. If each successive movement with static tasks, such as puzzles, creates a shift in the problem domain, then what type of shifts in the problem domain might occur with each successive change in a system as dynamic as a child's world? It illustrates the point that assessment and intervention should reflect a similar iterative and dynamic process.

Much traditional behavioral neuroscience research resulted from studies of brains engaged in relatively motionless and often purely rational tasks. For this reason, embodied cognition theory is a reminder for how we might think critically about the research when trying to understand the functioning of an individual child. If a child does not demonstrate good reasoning on a pure thought task, perhaps we should be cautious in generalizing this finding across modalities. For example, maybe a child who has difficulty coming up with an alternate strategy on a conceptual task would be able to generate multiple strategies if it were a visual-motor task.

The neurorelational framework uses the theory of embodied cognition to support our emphasis on the importance of functional assessments and intervention goals in real-world, real-time settings. Tests are definitely informative and most often crucial to a good assessment, but they cannot tell us everything there is to know about a child's abilities. In addition, relationships are the dominant influence for the developing brain, so the parent–child relationship sets the interpretive context for assessment in the neurorelational framework. To this end, the next chapter considers (1) the socioemotional milestones and (2) the heart, hand, and head relational paradigm that provides a metalevel organization for interpersonal dynamics.

Behavioral Neuroanatomy: Connectionism

Behavioral neuroanatomy is the analysis of the brain's structural and functional systems, and it provides much of our current understanding about how brain activity is linked to behavior. This section brings us into the brain but remains oriented toward understanding global principles. For this perspective, we rely on the work of M. Mesulam (1998, 2000b), a behavioral neurologist at Northwestern University who provided a rich and brilliant consolidation and conceptualization of neuroscience data in the first chapter of *Principles of Behavioral and Cognitive Neurology* (2000b). His work provides us with a deeper understanding of the complex webs of interconnectivity within the brain, on one hand, and the amazing simplicity of overall structure and function, on the other. In the process of

assessment and intervention, it is useful to have an understanding of how the brain works at this level when trying to isolate areas of compromise and think critically about the implications of that compromise.

Mesulam asserts that one of the primary tasks of the brain is to discharge the needs of the internal milieu (the body) according to the opportunities and restrictions presented by the environment (Mesulam, 1998). Within the highest levels of the brain, he details a global organization according to several "selectively distributed networks," whereby each network has a particular functional preference (e.g., for managing spatial attention, language, memory), and each network relies on "specialized nodes" that handle particular core aspects of processing (e.g., visual, auditory). These networks may be activated simultaneously by any particular event, and will eventually settle into a "state of best fit (or least conflict)" (Mesulam, 1998, p. 1038) where one or more networks take on selected and distributed roles. This organization elucidates both the specialized and distributed aspects of brain functioning in real time; it provides a framework for preserving the specialized roles of the parts, for example, as multiple instruments in a symphony, without losing the dynamics of the whole concerto that is unfolding in real time (an organization that is analogous to optimal interdisciplinary collaboration).

The data processed within these large-scale networks come from both the internal (body) and the external (world) milieu (Mesulam, 1998). To manage and integrate these data, different brain regions are affiliated with the body, the environment, and regions in between. The latter inform the brain's overall goal of coordinating biological and contextual information according to personal relevance and behavioral adaptation. The data processed within these large-scale networks are, to some extent, processed in a hierarchical sequence. To illustrate this point, Mesulam begins at the neuronal level by grouping brain regions according to histological differences. According to this organization, regions that are affiliated with the body (the inner and lower terrain of the brain) contain neurons that are more randomly distributed and have broad response properties, whereas regions affiliated with the world (at the sensory and motor periphery) contain neurons that have an intricate and complex organization and have much narrower response properties. These highly organized regions are commonly referred to as *primary areas* (however, not all primary sensory regions have this organization, which is discussed later).

The development of the neurorelational framework began here. We took this histological organization of brain regions having affiliations with internal milieu, external milieu, and personal significance and behavioral adaptation, to develop the rubric of the four functional brain systems, with each system being both specialized and distributed in their functions.

Roughly, our regulation system reflects the regions affiliated with the internal milieu, our sensory system reflects the regions affiliated with the external milieu, our relevance system reflects the regions affiliated with personal significance, and our executive system reflects the regions affiliated with behavioral adaptation.

These four brain systems can be viewed in a linear fashion, intended to reflect a very general developmental progression of increasing abilities as well as increasing specialization (see Figure 2.1). Brain development proceeds in a general hierarchical manner with many functions emerging and developing in parallel fashion. At birth, the regulation system is dominant in the sense that the bodily functions are maturing rapidly, basic regulatory systems such as sleep and hunger are both organizing and becoming more stable, and the behaviors associated with the regulation system are most prominent. Many aspects of the sensory system are online at birth and mature rapidly in the first year of life, especially the auditory and visual senses. The relevance system is functioning from birth in the form of establishing associations and implicit memories and begins to take off in a more conscious form in the toddler years (e.g., with emergence of self-awareness and explicit memories). The building blocks of the executive system are also forming early, especially those related to movement and the early representations of goal-oriented behavior. The executive abilities show rapid development in early childhood and continue to develop throughout life.

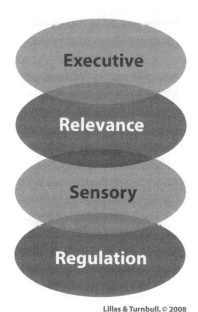

Lillas & Turnbull, © 2008

Figure 2.1.   A developmental hierarchical progression of brain systems.

With development also comes increasing specialization. Initially, pre-set biases guide behavior, and brain systems are also responsive to environmental features. With experience and time, inputs become increasingly honed to respond to the particular features that make up the world for the individual brain. For example, infants exposed exclusively to their native language lose the capacity to detect phonemes of other languages by the second year (Werker & Polka, 1993; Werker & Tees, 1984; see also Kuhl, Williams, Lacerda, & Stevens, 1992). Over time, as more is learned, each system is increasingly shaped to specialize to its unique context. The brain systems lower on the hierarchy are more stable than those higher up, and this hierarchy remains loosely intact throughout life in the sense that lower systems are more stable in their specialization than higher ones (Huttenlocher, 2002).

The four brain systems can also be viewed in a nonlinear fashion that reflects their functional integration (see Figure 2.2). Early in life, the needs of the body dominate and an infant's behavior is guided solely from the bottom up. Bottom-up processes are seen in behaviors that are not willful, not conscious, and not easily controlled. An infant cannot choose to inhibit an impulse to cry. Although very early forms of intent can be detected in the first year, a child's capacity for intentional behavior and goals becomes more apparent in the second year. As the child matures, there is increasing capacity for top-down control and more flexible bottom-up and top-down interactions (Berntson, Cacioppo, & Sarter, 2003; Berntson, Sarter, & Cacioppo, 2003a). The regulation and sensory systems

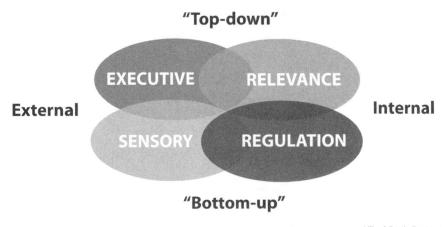

Lillas & Turnbull, © 2008

Figure 2.2. A nonlinear perspective of the four brain systems, showing two sets of potential relationships: those between top-down and bottom-up processes and those between internal and external domains.

are considered more bottom-up systems. The regulation system can trump other systems easily at any time (e.g., headache, food poisoning), and most regulatory functions are not capable of being controlled or modified by sheer will (e.g., sleep, hunger). The sensory system is more open to control in the sense that higher-level sensory processes can be influenced by decision; however, lower-level sensory inputs are less modifiable and sensory capacities may be lost if not exercised early.

Top-down is synonymous with attentional guidance (be it conscious or unconscious) and with "conscious control." The relevance system is considered top-down in the sense that personal *meanings* have a strong influence on what we attend to, which means that the information that is ultimately "delivered" to the brain for processing relies largely on what and whom we attend to in the environment (Koivisto & Revonsuo, 2007). Our brains are limited and cannot absorb everything in our surroundings; only those things that find our attention will be further elaborated and engaged. The rest goes unprocessed. The information that is engaged then influences our arousal, emotions, and thoughts and continues to shape what we attend to and react to. This point is important because it illuminates (1) the very powerful influence of past experience (e.g., a traumatized child continually tunes in to cues of potential threat), and (2) the very powerful influence of selective attention on current experience (e.g., the child's brain is continuing to elaborate and engage cues associated with threat and thus will miss the opportunity to process cues associated with safety).

The top-down influence can be positive, as well. For example, experiences of success can shift attention to seeing opportunities, and falling in love can make the world look full of promise. The trauma situation exemplifies a bidirectional process within the relevance system. A trigger for potential danger may come out of the blue, and the subsequent emotional response is both intense and unexpected. This bottom-up influence, which travels the "the quick-and-dirty subcortical pathway" (LeDoux, 2002, p. 399), is obviously crucial for survival, but can have devastating consequences when triggered in error and too often. This highlights the importance of taking a much closer look at what a child is attending to and absorbing and what can be done to shift the focus to things that are beneficial to the child's development. The executive system is more obviously about top-down control. It involves functions such as inhibiting impulses, pushing to sustain attention, setting goals, taking another's perspective, showing empathy, negotiating a conflict, and social graces.

The four brain systems can also be thought of in terms of their internal and external affiliations. The regulation and relevance systems are more internal in the sense that they are concerned with the self (e.g., bodily

drives, emotions, personal memories). The sensory and executive systems are more geared toward the external because the sensory, while also involved in processing internal sensory information, is concerned with absorbing and processing the environment and the executive is concerned with acting within and on the environment.

Whereas there are multiple regions in the brain dedicated to processing specific sensory perceptions and specific motor movements, the *flow* of information throughout the local and global connections ultimately determines behavior. In the brain, the pathways that carry this flow "are replete with lateral interactions within organizational levels, and with parallel processing routes between levels" (a heterarchical organization; Berntson, Cacioppo, & Sarter, 2003, p. 1106). There are also connections that do not respect the hierarchy and bypass intermediary levels with direct connections between lower and higher brain regions (a bypass hierarchy; Berntson et al., 2003, p. 1106; see Figure 2.3).

Although we have presented three potential patterns for the direction of influence among the brain systems (Figures 2.1, 2.2, and 2.3), these are not intended as static categorical formats. It is clinically useful to view a child's or adult's behaviors according these patterns of influence, albeit within the context that the four brain systems are always integrated in their functioning.

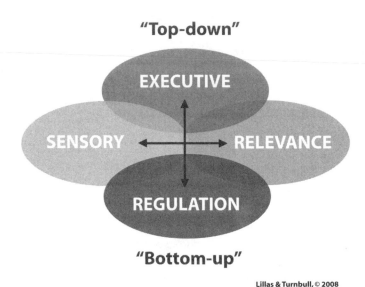

Figure 2.3. Another nonlinear perspective of the four brain systems showing the lateral (heterarchical) pathways and the bypass hierarchy that directly connects top-down and bottom-up processes.

Connectionism's overlapping large-scale networks provides conceptual support for the neurorelational framework's emphasis on functional assessment. The importance of networks leads us to ask our core assessment question: "What is the meaning of the behavior we see in terms of each brain system and in terms of the individual and the dyad?" Answering this question gives us functional types of information that can enhance the information that traditional diagnostic categories provide. The four brain systems provide a dimensional approach to assessment, diagnosis, and intervention along concurrent multiple continuums. Such a dimensional approach has the potential to capture the underlying meaning of behaviors by simultaneously considering a wide range of symptoms across multiple behavioral domains (Rosenblum, 2004). In contrast, the categorical and hierarchical method traditionally used in diagnosis assumes that (1) a failure to "meet criteria" means there is not a problem "big enough" to be treated, and (2) it is most important to find a single "primary" diagnosis that rises to the top of the categorical list. The first emphasis lacks appreciation for the functional impact of symptoms that do not "cross the threshold," and the second emphasis reinforces assumptions of singular causality, which obscures other relevant behavioral concerns (Rosenblum, 2004). Further, this approach reinforces a view of health that is reactive versus proactive. Although we value a dimensional approach to clients of all age ranges, we find its use of utmost importance in identifying how to intervene effectively and comprehensively with our youngest population, when intervening early has the potential to make a more dramatic difference.

Allodynamic Regulation

To understand allodynamic regulation, it is easiest to start with its more familiar precursor, homeostasis. The term *homeostasis* (Cannon, 1929) was coined to refer to those processes that maintain the relative constancy of the internal environment. For any particular visceral function (e.g., heart rate), disruptions from the mean position, or setpoint, are brought back toward the mean before extremes are reached. This concept was expanded to "allostasis" (Sterling & Eyer, 1988) to incorporate higher neural systems in visceral regulation. Allostasis (*allo* = variable; *stasis* = stable) reflects a more flexible and dynamic type of regulation whereby higher-level brain mechanisms support rapid and large shifts across multiple interacting physiological variables and subsequent recovery back to baseline. Allostasis also encompasses the regulatory capacity to anticipate the need

for adjustments. With anticipation, the target physiological parameters can "ready themselves" for change such that overall energy expenditure can be regulated more efficiently than it can in conditions of surprise. Surprises, or the absence of anticipation, can certainly be handled, but at a greater overall energy cost.

Berntson and Cacioppo expand the concept of allostasis into their theory of allodynamic regulation (Berntson & Cacioppo, 2000, 2007; Cacioppo & Berntson, 2007) to highlight the reciprocal interactions between the central (top-down) and autonomic (bottom-up) nervous systems that support behavioral flexibility and adaptability (Berntson et al., 2003). Allodynamic regulation explains that higher neural controls can bypass, inhibit, or modulate regulatory mechanisms, thereby altering regulatory setpoints. The concept of allodynamic regulation accords more complex connectivity and greater flexibility to the target visceral parameters. For example, higher-level control means that internal and external conditions can influence visceral regulation and vice versa (e.g., thoughts can affect physiology and vice versa).

When this flexibility is lost, however, systems become stuck in chronic or malfunctioning stress responses, leading to risk factors for allostatic load. In general, allostatic load conditions can be assumed when one of the three primary stress states of autonomic arousal—the hypoalert, hyperalert, or flooded state—dominates the landscape. (These states are described more fully in the coming chapters on the four brain systems.) In short, because of their persistence, *states* become *traits* (Perry, Pollard, Blakely, Baker, & Vigilante, 1995).

In exploring an aspect of allodynamic regulation, Berntson and colleagues (Berntson, Boysen, & Cacioppo, 1991; Berntson, Cacioppo, & Quigley, 1991; Berntson, Cacioppo, Quigley, & Fabro, 1994) proposed an alternative to the previously held all-or-nothing view in which energy either goes up or down (Koizumi & Kollai, 1992). In conducting and reviewing human and animal studies, empirical research supports their proposal of a dynamic systems alternative that translates into a variety of patterns and movements between the two main forces of autonomic energy: the sympathetic (activating) and parasympathetic (inhibiting) nervous systems. In addition to the well-known inverse action of sympathetic and parasympathetic branches (one goes up, the other goes down—called a *reciprocal* pattern), they propose two other patterns that expand into multiple modes of autonomic control: *uncoupled* patterns (one changes while the other stays the same) and *coupled* patterns (both go up or both go down). The uncoupled mode of control "may represent a *midpoint* along a continuum extending from reciprocal" to coupled control (Berntson,

Hans, & Percansky, 1991, p. 176). The autonomic modes of control allow for much more dynamic variation and gradation than the more static patterns that are typically thought to underlie arousal states and emotions. As we will explore in Chapter 4, there are multiple states of arousal as well as varying combinations that can occur with activating and inhibiting energy.

The properties of allodynamic regulation combine flexibility with stability. The neurorelational framework uses this paradox to describe a well-functioning open brain system, which we refer to as allodynamic coordination, or simply coordination. *Coordination* is a foundational concept throughout this book. It is defined as the ability to function predominantly within a state of arousal that allows for open learning and flexibility (supported with an alert processing state) while also efficiently responding to stressful situations with recovery in a timely manner according to the context. Coordination is supported by the following features: (1) adequate development of the expected capacities within each brain system, (2) conditions of real or perceived safety, and (3) the process of modulation. Modulation supports the ability to maintain an alert processing state and recover from a stress response. Each brain system contributes in specific ways to manage the overall modulated response (this concept will be elaborated within each brain system chapter).

Responses to stress can take the forms of hypoalert, hyperalert, or flooded responses during awake states. In addition, a sleep-related stress response is the inability to cycle into deep sleep. Stress responses are, in and of themselves, not unhealthy; in fact, they are an intrinsic part of typical development and are necessary for adaptive functioning. However, when the underlying activating and inhibiting processes within the stress response cycle (1) occur too frequently, (2) do not accommodate to situations that should no longer be stressful, (3) stay on too long or do not shut down after the stressor is removed, or (4) are inadequate in their stress recovery, allodynamic load creates wear and tear on internal organs (which we refer to as *load conditions*) (Berntson & Cacioppo, 2007; Cacioppo & Berntson, 2007; Kaltsas & Chrousos, 2007; McEwen, 2002). Furthermore, certain risk factors increase the likelihood that stress reactions can become load conditions. Risk factors include (1) brain capacities that are not present or poorly functioning (each of the four brain systems has designated capacities that are further elaborated in Chapters 4–11), (2) an individual's experience of real or perceived challenge that is beyond his or her reach, and (3) an individual's experience of real or perceived threat.

THE FOUR BRAIN SYSTEMS

In the neurorelational framework, each of the four brain system heuristics captures a fundamental influence underlying behavior: arousal (the regulatory system); sensory processing and modulation (sensory system); emotional reactivity, memory, and meaning making (the relevance system); and motor activity and behavioral control (the executive system). Each system is affiliated with general and specific anatomical regions in the brain as well as general and specific behavioral states. The structural interconnectivity among systems allows for infinite patterns of interaction to support and drive behavior. In other words, no single brain system could ever stake a claim for always initiating or completely governing any given behavior.

In terms of assessment, the functional behaviors across the four brain systems provide multiple contributions to understanding the behavior we are observing in the child, parent, and dyad. In terms of treatment priorities, we can look both for strengths and concerns within and across all brain systems as a way to organize the resiliencies and risk factors within each child, parent, and dyad. In addition, the four brain systems provide a way for professionals to organize the parts up against the big picture. This parts-to-whole process can serve another important purpose. Typically, professionals tend to notice the parts with which they are most familiar (usually what is closely related to their disciplinary training). The neurorelational framework is attempting to provide bridges into unfamiliar territory that may encourage professionals to notice the parts that they otherwise might have overlooked in the assessment and intervention process. Traversing unfamiliar territory can inspire professional development and can expand and enrich collegial relationships.

The Regulation System

Regulation is considered the foundation that influences all developmental domains and all learning and relationships. The regulation system ensures that the body has the energy it needs to carry out the goal of behavioral adaptation. For any organism to survive, it must acquire more energy than it expends, which means that it should be in tune with the environmental context (reacting to opportunities and risks), and its energy expenditures should be purposeful. In the service of these goals, the regulation system manages arousal levels and is primarily affiliated with the body. The information this system receives about current needs

comes from the body. For example, when the body sends a signal indicating hunger or pain, the regulation system reacts. The other systems are heavily dependent on optimal functioning of the regulation system. In fact, physical discomfort of any kind can quickly hijack attention and trump other goals. Thus, supporting optimal regulation and understanding what deviations from optimal look like are primary goals of intervention.

Brain Components of the Regulation System

The primary structures of the regulation system include the hypothalamus, autonomic substrates in the brainstem, and the neurochemical factories within the brainstem and basal forebrain. The regulation system has general and specific influences on all systems through both selective connections and widely distributed connections that bathe the brain with chemical messengers. It has primary connections with the amygdala (in the relevance system) and the prefrontal cortex (in the executive system). The top-down connectivity (i.e., the connections coming from the other systems) allows the regulation system to be influenced by context, behavioral significance, and learning. Some of these top-down connections bypass the intermediary autonomic controls and head straight for autonomic motor neurons, allowing much faster responses (Berntson & Cacioppo, 2007). The bottom-up connections allow visceral activity to prime or bias feelings, thoughts, and behaviors. For example, the area of the brainstem that receives visceral information (the nucleus tractus solidaris) connects directly to the amygdala, which links sensory information with emotions, and to the basal forebrain, which distributes chemical messages throughout the cortex (enhances cortical activity) (Iversen, Iversen, & Saper, 2000).

Five major chemical messenger systems originate in the brainstem and the base of the brain. They work together to influence cortical arousal, but some chemicals have regional preferences. Four sensory modalities feed directly into these messenger systems: touch (including pain), vestibular (balance), taste, and auditory. A quick review of these mechanisms follows (Kapp & Cain, 2001).

- Norepinephrine or noradrenergic system: Originates in brainstem, has greater affinity with the sensory system, supports sensory alertness.
- Dopamine system: Most pathways originate in brainstem, has greater affinity with the relevance and executive systems, supports prediction of reward and motor activity.

- Serotonin: Originates in brainstem, affiliated with the regulation and relevance systems, supports autonomic controls and emotion.
- Cholinergic: Originates in basal forebrain, widely distributed throughout systems, supports everything.
- Histamine: Originates in the hypothalamus, widely distributed throughout systems, supports everything.

The hypothalamus is the hub of the regulation system. Its role is to ensure optimal functioning of bodily needs in both the short and long run. The hypothalamus is tuned in to very specific body–world negotiations, such as sleep (with day–night cycles) and hunger (with increased movement of the gut and the body). The hypothalamus is the apex of the autonomic nervous system (ANS; also known as the visceral motor system) and connected to all the bodily organs (Truex & Carpenter, 1964). The ANS is divided into the sympathetic nervous system (SNS) and the parasympathetic nervous system (PNS), each connected to multiple organs. The SNS and PNS are organized differently in terms of their primary chemical messengers, influence on target organs, and connectivity to the spinal cord and brain. Autonomic adjustments are ongoing and responsive to internal cellular processes, temporal cycles, orthostatic changes, and psychological challenge and stress (Berntson & Cacioppo, 2000).

The autonomic reflex provides a description of a basic regulatory mechanism. For a given visceral parameter, a deviation from a central tendency sends a signal that activates a compensatory response. For example, an elevated blood pressure reflexively causes blood pressure to decrease; similarly, decreased blood pressure depresses the baroreflex, causing blood pressure to rise (Sleight, 1995). This process is a feedback loop. More broadly, however, autonomic control mechanisms regulate multiple interacting parameters that are influenced by internal, external, and temporal conditions. Expanding into higher-level controls, autonomic adjustments are not merely reflexive; they are also learned, as when a physiological response occurs to some conditioned external stimuli (e.g., Pavlov's dog). Appropriate, conditioned (learned) autonomic adjustments may function as an energy-conserving mechanism to minimize or preclude autonomic disturbances and adjustments (Dworkin, 2000) not unlike, for example, the idea that bracing oneself for bad news makes it easier to manage. Autonomic adjustments also result from psychological stress, even from very mild stressors (e.g., mental arithmetic slows heart rate) (Backs, 1998; Sharply, 1992).

The reciprocal (or inverse), coupled, or uncoupled patterns of SNS and PNS activity may vary according to type of challenge (orthostatic versus psychological) and learning characteristics (habituation versus sensitization). The phrase "autonomic modes of control" refers to these various response patterns of the SNS and PNS under conditions of challenge (Berntson, Cacioppo, & Quigley, 1991). Individual variations in SNS and PNS response patterns appear to have important implications for immune responses. For example, the high SNS reactivity to psychological stress is predictive of poorer immune reactions (Hawkley & Cacioppo, 2004).

Regulation is not only controlled by the central nervous system (CNS); it also involves autoregulatory processes—peripheral physiological or hormonal mechanisms that are always at work to maintain a steady internal state (e.g., kidney regulation of blood pressure) (Berntson & Cacioppo, 2000). These set the background on which CNS autonomic regulatory mechanisms must operate; however, the relationship is reciprocal because the CNS can also affect autoregulation.

Behavioral Components of the Regulation System

The regulatory system can be thought of as the oldest or most primitive of the systems because it controls arousal, the fundamental ingredient of all behavior. Whereas *arousal* is a frequently used and easily understood word, a clear and consistent definition has been elusive (Pfaff, 2006). In very general terms, we define arousal according to the degree of energy expenditure. A person in a coma is at the lowest level of energy expenditure and arousal; a person in fight–flight survival mode is at the highest level of energy expenditure and arousal. An operational definition of generalized arousal that fits nicely into our four-system framework was recently put forth by Donald Pfaff (2006), a neuroscientist at Rockefeller University in New York. Pfaff defined arousal according to the degree of sensory alertness, emotional reactivity, and motor activity. With this definition, arousal can be precisely measured according to its behavioral correlates. In essence, arousal functions as a distributed property and supports the functions of each of our brain systems (for more on this discussion see CD-ROM Section 2.1).

Applying this definition of arousal to development, we adopt the behavioral correlates of arousal used in infant research (Als, 1984, 2002; Als & Gibes, 1986; Barnard, 1999; Brazelton, 1973, 1984, 1992; Prechtl, 1977), which categorized states of arousal according to clusters of particular bodily cues and temporal patterns observable in behavior, emerging from distinct target muscles and organs in the body (see Table 2.1).

Table 2.1.   Arousal States as Indicated by Bodily Cues and Observable Behavior

Target Sites	Behavior
Eyes	Condition of eyelids, quality of eyes, pupils, eye movement
Facial muscles	Facial expressions through muscle positions
Heart	Pinkish skin and mucosa, accelerations and decelerations of pulse rate
Lungs	Breathing patterns, shallow/deep, slow/rapid
Vocal cords	Quality of tone, vocal rhythm and rate, intensity and timing
Muscle tone and movement of the body	Muscle tone (floppy, rigid, relaxed), type of movement (smooth, jerky, awkward, sluggish), quality of attention (distracted, sustained, fixated)
Gut	"Tummy" sensations from relaxed, to butterflies, to sinking; type of intestinal muscular contractions, from regular peristalsis, to more frequent (diarrhea), to slowed down (constipation)
Gestures	Type of movement of extremities

The arousal states are located along a continuum from low to high energy expression:

LOW sleep ↔ drowsy ↔ hypoalert ↔ alert ↔ hyperalert ↔ flooded HIGH

As noted, regulation is considered the foundation that influences all domains of development and all learning and relationships. Once arousal states can be identified, the task is to (1) understand what constitutes a deviation from optimal, and then (2) begin to formulate hypotheses regarding the mechanisms that might be driving the deviation. To identify a deviation, it is important to understand what "optimal regulation" looks like:

- *Cycling and frequency patterns:* Optimal regulation is the capacity to cycle between deep sleep and alert processing as the predominant states; when disrupted, the capacity to achieve a timely return to the appropriate predominant state occurs.
- *Gradual state changes:* Optimal regulation includes the capacity to smoothly transition from one state of arousal to another.
- *Sudden state changes:* When confronted with challenge and threat, optimal regulation demonstrates the capacity to have an appropriate and abrupt state change and recover back to baseline.
- *Modulation:* Optimal regulation is the capacity for a variety of subtle arousal gradations *within* states, which allows for behavioral

flexibility without abrupt state changes (sets the background for smooth transitions with state changes; this allows for a broad range of affect expression within the alert processing state).

For younger children, more assistance is required from a caretaker to sustain optimal regulation. When a baby begins to dysregulate due to hunger, the arousal state will not return to baseline until someone assists with feeding. This other-assisted regulation (Sameroff, 2004) is known as *interactive regulation* (or mutual regulation) (Beebe & Lachmann, 2002; Tronick, 2007). As an infant grows, conditions of safety allow the child to begin to establish increasing capacities for self-regulation. A 1-month-old infant has awakened hungry many times and has been sated every time, so there is no need for the large energy expenditure that comes with a flooded arousal state. The baby may even begin to tolerate hunger sensations without distress or be distracted from them by a spinning mobile.

This capacity for interactive regulation translates into a vital skill for the parent of a baby with an immature or otherwise vulnerable nervous system. Vulnerability in a child (or parent's) nervous system is defined by poor regulation of arousal states and requires more interactive regulation. In this situation, learning to decode the infant's cues and respond with the relevant supports becomes a crucial ingredient to optimizing his or her regulation. An infant's environment can also be the source of chronic dysregulation. For the abused and neglected infant, chaotic surroundings or a dysregulated parent can throw off an otherwise healthy physiology. Without intervention, development becomes layered on unhealthy regulatory patterns caught in unending cycles of compensation, meaning that the foundation for learning and relationships is now shaky.

Interactive regulation also means that the infant or child can affect the adult's regulatory capacities. Consider the teenage mother living in poverty with no solid social supports whose infant cries constantly. No matter what she does to soothe him, the crying never seems to stop. She is already depleted from the pregnancy, has chronically poor nutrition, and now rarely sleeps. This infant is exposed to a dysregulated parent and is at high risk for abandonment or abuse. As tragic as this situation is for the child, it also carries considerable psychological repercussions for the mother.

With intervention, this mother could learn how to read her baby's cues and, like a detective, figure out through trial and error how to move him or her toward more optimal regulation. Each small success along the way increases her sense of usefulness, puts a smile on her face, and gives her a surge of energy. Her sense of being a good mother boosts her toward optimal regulation. She tolerates the sleepless nights much better and brings increased warmth and problem-solving capacities to each crying

spell. Able to sustain her own regulation, she can better nurture her baby's path toward optimal regulation.

The Sensory System

Brains translate energy in the world into sensory information. The developmental integrity of the brain regions that participate in translation provide crucial contributions to behavioral competencies. The sensory regions are differentiated according to their respective "obligatory portals" for entry of sensory information into the brain (Mesulam, 1998, p. 1015). These include the visual, auditory, and somatosensory processing regions in the occipital, temporal, and parietal lobes, respectively, and the vestibular, gustatory, and olfactory processing regions in the limbic regions. The regions where sensory information from each modality first enters the brain are called *primary areas*. With the exception of the primary areas in the limbic/paralimbic regions, the primary areas protect the fidelity of incoming sensory information such that earliest stages of processing are thought to occur in a manner that is distanced from the mediating influences of emotion, memory, and goals (Mesulam, 1998, p. 1023). As the sensory modalities integrate with each other and with other brain systems, the sensory information becomes represented within personal meanings and contextual significance. Variations in physiology or environment from person to person set the stage for vast individual differences in sensory processing parameters. What is music to one is noise to another. Disruptions within sensory systems may lead to mild delays or severe deficits. In general, processing issues are more severe when the disruption has a broad impact at the initial stages of sensory processing. The outcome is related to internal, external, and temporal factors (e.g., genetics, environmental opportunities, age). As providers, we can optimize outcome by providing optimal intervention and intervening early.

Brain Components of the Sensory System

Our bodies are surrounded with various forms of energy that the brain translates into sensory information. The energy sources are thermal, mechanical, chemical, and electromagnetic, and they activate sensors called *receptor sites* in the body (e.g., skin, ears, tongue, eyes). These receptor sites are specialized to pick up specific types of energy and send the sensory message along a nerve path to areas in the brain (the primary areas) that are specialized to begin the translation process into sensory information (e.g., as temperature, sound, taste, light) (Gardner & Martin, 2000).

Most often, we are not conscious or aware of all the available sensory information, but we can quickly bring it to consciousness if we choose or
quickly be reminded of it with any disruption. For example, you are using
light to read, but, at least before I mentioned it, you were not likely aware
of or "experiencing" light. Sensory processing activities are really quite
remarkable in that way; they hang out in the wings of the conscious stage
indefinitely, yet leap into the spotlight with a simple shift of attention.

Once a sensory message reaches the brain, the translation process
proceeds in a hierarchical fashion (Amaral, 2000). For the systems located
in higher cortical areas (visual, auditory, and somatosensory), the initial
decoding of the fundamental sense properties occurs in the primary cortical regions (which contain point-to-point projections that map the sensory field), then proceeds, again in point-to-point fashion, to secondary
areas that combine the fundamental properties into relatively elementary
attributes of the sensory modality (e.g., color, motion, pitch). From here,
the information is passed on to association areas (in parietal, temporal,
and frontal areas), where sensory data combine to support perceptions
such as objects, faces, word forms, spatial locations, and sound sequences.
As sensory modalities are integrated, meaning begins to take shape. Finally, transmodal areas (i.e., where association areas combine) translate
perception into recognition, word forms into meaningful communications, scenes and events into experiences, and spatial locations into targets
for exploration (Mesulam, 1998, p. 1041).

Sensory information is not processed in a purely bottom-up hierarchical fashion; context also determines the meaning of perception. In
other words, the meaning that an object or event being perceived holds
for the individual is dependent on its contextual significance and personal
relevance. For example, a cup may represent its traditional meaning in
one context (something to drink from), but may serve an entirely different function as well (an object used upside down to trace a circle). In this
way, one's past experience with sensory information and one's contextual
goals in the moment also influence the ultimate "meaning" that is shaped
from sensory data.

Neuroscience research has traditionally focused on how the brain
processes visual and auditory stimuli, and other senses have received far
less attention. This emphasis reflects the fact that visual and auditory regions are dominant senses in the human brain as well as the easiest to
explore, both in humans and in animals (especially the visual system).
More recently, the brain regions that process bodily sensations, such as
touch and "gut feelings" (viscera), have gained more attention, largely due
to a renewed interest in emotional processes, the body as it relates to mind,
and connections among emotions and actions (Damasio, 1999; Dolan, 2007;

Freeman, 2000). Taste, smell, and balance also have their own respective ports of entry in the brain (or primary areas), but these areas do not have the same organization as the senses just described (Mesulam, 1998). Being situated within the limbic, or older regions of the brain, these senses are translated by neuronal groups that are more loosely organized, often multisensory, and more open to influence from other regions. Table 2.2 traces the sequence of sensory processing from energy in the world, to sensory organ, brain, and sensory experience.

The primary sensory areas are more fully formed at birth than are other areas. The immature cortical maps are largely genetically programmed and then increasingly tuned by experience and practice. Early in development, these tuning curves are broad; that is, the sense properties of the point-to-point projection cells are generalized across a sensory dimension. With experience, or sensory stimulation, cells begin to change their properties to match the range and complexity of the input, and the tuning curves become more specialized and organized (Huttenlocher, 2002; O'Leary, 1989; Wiesel & Hubel, 1965). In the end, the tuning process forms individually specific maps of the sensory environment. The size, specificity, and number of neurons of a map region may be preset by genetic predispositions, but the subsequent expansion or contraction of the tuning process is influenced by (and, during certain stages of development, depends on) experience and practice (de Haan & Johnson, 2003; Huttenlocher, 2002; Jones, 1990; Leonard, 2003). Thus, sensory development involves the dynamic interaction of nature and nurture. Nature endows us with preset biases that amplify the relevant sensory features (species-specific), and nurture provides the sensory stimulation that induces expansion or contraction in the sensory maps (individual-specific) (de Haan & Johnson, 2003; Leonard, 2003).

Table 2.2.   Pathways from Energy to Sensory Information

Energy	Receptor Site	Primary Area	Sensory Information
Thermal	Skin	Somatosensory	Temperature, pain
Mechanical	Ears, skin, muscle	Heschel's gyrus, somatosensory, vestibular	Sound, balance, touch, proprioception, pain
Chemical	Skin, tongue, nose	Somatosensory, gustatory, olfactory	Pain, itch, taste, smell
Electromagnetic	Eyes	Calcarine fissure	Sight, vision

Note. From "Coding of Sensory Information" by E. P. Gardner and J. H. Martin, 2000, in *Principles of Neural Science* (4th ed., p. 414) by E. R. Kandel, J. H. Schwartz, and T. M. Jessell (Eds.), New York: McGraw-Hill. Copyright 2000 by the McGraw-Hill Companies. Adapted with permission.

Brain development follows the same progressive sequence as the processing pathways already described. The sensory primary areas mature before the motor primary area, with auditory a step ahead of visual at birth (babies can hear more than they can see in the womb). The older interior areas of the brain mature before the newer exterior areas. The projections from higher cortical areas to lower brain and spinal cord areas (that link the body and viscera) mature early and continue throughout the first year. Several reflexive links between sensory stimulus and motor response, largely controlled by brainstem mechanisms, are present in early infancy. These reflexes begin to disappear as cortical development takes over the sensory processing (Johnson, 2005). The areas that mediate percepts (association areas) mature before the areas that mediate concepts (transmodal areas). The prefrontal cortex, one of the last areas to mature, includes the region that receives information from regulatory mechanisms. On both global and specific levels, the hierarchical sequence means that the quality of development early on affects later developing regions.

Behavioral Components of the Sensory System

The importance of sensations is twofold. First, sensory experiences provide the core foundation for how we perceive our bodies and the world. Just as we each have a unique fingerprint, we also have a unique makeup of sensory receptors and pathways (influenced by nature and nurture) that underlies individual differences in perception and experience. Because of these individual sensory prints, the same sensory event could yield a broad range of responses across individuals—an experience that is pleasurable to one and repulsive to another, novel to one and boring to another, safe to one and challenging or threatening to another. For example, the sensory information that accompanies the up-and-down motion of a swing may be quite pleasurable for one child but uncomfortable, or even painful, for another.

Second, a sensory processing disruption, from mild to severe, can trigger subsequent adjustments to development that may throw off the quality of the sensory information, both within and across systems. As developmental progress falls further from the mean (i.e., the age-appropriate gap widens), the areas of specific and global delay become cumulative. For example, language delays may restrict understanding of others, self-expression, and conceptual thinking (Huttenlocher, 1998; Shevell, Majnemer, Webster, Platt, & Birnbaum, 2005; Waisman Center, 2008); visual delays may complicate spatial awareness, language development (oral–motor imitation, labeling of objects and actions), and social learning ("seeing" gestural communication and emotions) (Atkinson & Braddick, 2007; Sonksen & Dale, 2002). However, because human brains have a flexible

and open organization that promotes plasticity (through compensatory mechanisms or learning), providing the appropriate environmental stimulation can go a long way toward addressing disruptions (e.g., Ludington-Hoe & Swinth, 1996; Shaywitz et al., 2004).

The progression of behavioral competencies that we observe in children is dependent on the integrity and quality of development within and across sensory systems (de Haan & Johnson, 2003; Greenough & Alcantara, 1993; Leonard, 2002; Molfese, 2000). With an understanding of sensory processing, it becomes clear that behavior is intimately related to the integration of sensory modalities and the quality of processing within the sensory system. Sensory processing begins with separate sensory modalities but the pathways are soon integrated and expressed in functional abilities. As such, it does not really make sense to examine functional abilities that are weighted toward one sensory modality (e.g., language and the auditory modality) without considering the quality of the functional abilities weighted toward other sensory modalities (e.g., visual perception and the vision modality). Furthermore, with an understanding of the hierarchical progression of sensory development, it becomes clear that the quality of current abilities is dependent on the quality of prior abilities. Thus, the current state of any sensory system can only be understood within the context of history.

The Relevance System

The relevance system determines what is salient through the three large domains of emotion, memory, and meaning-making. Our memories of events and their emotional impact form the meanings that are shaped throughout life, and conversely, we tend to remember and be more emotionally sensitive to things that are meaningful to us. The things that are deemed relevant might be species-specific, meaning important to all humans (e.g., things related to survival), or individual-specific, meaning important to "me" (e.g., things related to preferences). For example, when directing attention to the same spatial location or witnessing the same event, two people can (and often do) focus on and recall different things. Certainly, one would get two different responses from asking two different people to share the meanings associated with the same witnessed event. For humans, what is deemed relevant to the individual and what personal meanings emerge lead to tremendous variability in behaviors, as well as tremendous complexity in unraveling the contributions to any given behavior.

The relevance system is situated between the newer and older regions of the brain; it has dense reciprocal connections with both, which

link it to the state of the body and the state of the environment (Mesu-lam, 2000b). The relevance system is informed by emotions, which determine what is worth expending energy and attention on, and what to approach and what to avoid. Emotions exert this influence reflexively (e.g., fight–flight) by relying on prior experience or learning. Emotions inform memory by "tagging" what is important to remember; memory informs emotion through the capacity to recall the valence and meaning of a past experience (see LaBar & Cabeza, 2006, for review). This capacity to pull from past experience to inform current and future behaviors is valuable to efficient regulation. When something is deemed relevant, it will be both influenced by and reflected through processes of arousal and emotion, which serve to direct and sustain our attention to what is most relevant *for us*, both internally and externally. The relevance system integrates both internal bodily needs and whatever is salient in the external environment to promote purposeful behaviors. It also assists in the encoding and consolidation of experiences, from among all systems, into memories to promote adaptive behaviors. Memories allow us to learn more each day about where and how our needs are met most readily as well as how we might better avoid trouble in the future. The integration of emotions and memories shapes the ongoing and dynamic process of meaning-making. Meaning emerges through positive and negative emotions and through implicit and explicit memories. Sharing these meanings connects us to others and creates social bonds. Private meanings may not be shared or shared only in the context of intimate relationships. Public meanings are those that may be more easily observed in behavior and create social connections (e.g., hobbies, politics, traditions).

Brain Components of the Relevance System

The relevance system is associated with the limbic system—that is, with regions of cortex tucked under and between the two hemispheres. The limbic system is situated between the higher cortical areas, which are affiliated with the functions of representing and acting on the environment, and lower subcortical regions, which are affiliated with autonomic functions. The primary structures included in this region are the hippocampus, amygdala, insula, orbitofrontal cortex, and temporal pole. These structures are reciprocally linked (directly or indirectly) with major sensory hubs from the viscera (e.g., hypothalamus) and from the environment (e.g., cortical sensory association areas), including the limbic sensory regions (gustatory, olfactory, and vestibular). The limbic system has been characterized as the "visceral brain" due to its intermediary role among autonomic and mental functions (MacLean, 1955).

We call this brain system the relevance system because its primary role is to link up sensory and motor information with emotional and behavioral significance—the linking process is all about what is *relevant*. It has to do with an organism's state (its needs, drives, goals) as well as the opportunities and constraints present within the environment (Mesulam, 1998). Thus, what is relevant is always changing. If I am hungry, then I am likely either moving toward the kitchen or the phone, to order take-out. If I am sleepy, then I am likely either moving toward the bedroom or sitting here at my laptop, which makes the point that long-term goals can override an organism's drives.

Earlier we discussed the fundamental task of the brain as one of establishing the necessary sensory–motor transformations for reproduction and survival. To do this, the brain needs to emphasize species-specific features of the sensory world and associate that information with the appropriate motor programs. The honeybee brain detects detailed sensory features of a flower and then initiates the motor program that will successfully extract the nectar (Churchland, Ramachandran, & Sejnowski, 1994; Clark, 1997). In other words, that particular sensory–motor link is quite relevant to that particular species. The human infant detects the sensory features of a face, and this biased motor program promotes eye contact (Farroni, Csibra, Simion, & Johnson, 2002; Farroni, Johnson, Brockbank, & Simion, 2000; Johnson & Morton, 1991). No one teaches an infant to orient and sustain ocular motor movements on faces and eyes or to engage the appropriate motor program for crying when hungry.

How, then, does a brain "know" what is relevant? As you may have suspected, this is nature's contribution. Exactly what aspects of the sensory world are amplified has to do with preset biases toward specific sensory–motor links. At birth, a healthy organism in a sustaining environment will begin to exercise these prewired stimulus–response chains (e.g., face gazing in human babies, flower gazing in bee babies). The higher evolved the brain, the greater the capacity for stretching, branching, and adjusting these chains—which is where individual differences come into the picture (Quartz & Sejnowski, 1997). For humans, preset biases are only the beginning. From there, how the brain knows what is relevant is related to individual-specific mechanisms of stimulus–response reinforcement (i.e., sensitization, habituation, conditioning). Relevance emerges in the brain by means of nature *and* nurture from the ground up, for example:

- Individual-specific relevance based on external cues: An infant in an orphanage may initially respond according to the brain's preset biases to orient toward faces and cry when hungry (nature).

However, if the environment does not sustain those behaviors, the infant may stop fixing his or her gaze on faces and stop crying in response to discomfort (nurture).

- Individual-specific relevance based on internal cues: An infant with severe reflux may cry throughout feeding rather than relaxing; the meaning of feeding becomes associated with discomfort and fear.

The relevance system negotiates the ever-expanding web of sensory–motor links by means of emotions and memory, functions that correspond to the amygdala and hippocampus. In general, the amygdala links the appropriate emotional response to sensory information. The rhesus monkey with an ablated amygdala on one side will show the species-typical aggressive response when perceiving a human presence through the eye that is linked with the intact amygdala, but no aggressive response when perceiving a human presence through the eye that is linked with the ablated amygdala (Downer, 1962). The hippocampus is the critical structure for learning and memory. The expansion in memory capacities with development is not so much about the hippocampus per se, but the increasing maturity and integrity of the surrounding cortical structures. It does not store memories but is better thought of as a "nursery" for memories (Mesulam, 1998, p. 1042). The hippocampus promotes connectivity for relevant and repeated sensory–motor experiences. Once the connections of a path are sufficiently stable, the hippocampus has done its job and can bow out. Implicit memory is more dependent on lower brain structures (e.g., brainstem, cerebellum) and the sensory systems than later developing cortical areas (McCormick & Thompson, 1984; Petri & Mishkin, 1994). Thus, certain types of learning, such as habituation, and can be detected very early, even in the womb (Hepper, 1997a, 1997b).

Finally, none of this activity would happen without the help of the midbrain dopamine system. It is well established that dopamine is integral to the experience of reward. For example, several studies have found that animals will forgo satisfying basic drives such as eating and sex in lieu of performing an action (e.g., pressing a lever) that stimulates dopamine release in their brains (Olds & Milner, 1954; Wise & Bozarth, 1981). In the human brain, dopamine pathways project to multiple areas that mediate goals and value of reward. More recently, studies have shown that this system is also involved in reward expectation and errors in reward prediction, which has a clear role in the process of learning (see Montague & Quartz, 1999, for review). The dopamine system is fully functional early in development; however, some of the projection pathways go to regions that are the latest to mature (e.g., the prefrontal areas that continue to develop through adolescence) (Benes, 2001). Based on principles of hierarchical

development, discussed earlier, this organization suggests that not only very early learning but also ongoing learning is intricately involved in the entire developmental process.

Behavioral Components of the Relevance System

Aspects of the relevance system that are functional from birth enable infants to detect and respond to novel sensory events, become accustomed to repeated sensory events (habituation), improve detection and processing for recent sensory events (sensitization or priming), and strengthen associations for the sequence of sensory events. The latter involves the infant's capacity to anticipate—for example, predict where a visual event will occur based on prior experience (Haith, Benson, Roberts, & Pennington, 1994; Haith, Hazen, & Goodman, 1998).

In the memory literature, the terms *implicit* and *explicit* refer to differences in awareness or in the availability of stored information to consciousness. Implicit memory is expressed through autonomic changes and behavioral responses that are not conscious, such as gut feelings or motor procedures (e.g., walking or driving); explicit memory is expressed through cognitive activities whereby retrieval is a conscious process, such as facts or events. Because implicit memory relies on earlier developing brain regions, it is functional early on. During the first year of life, infants can retain learning from experiences of habituation, sensitization, and conditioning for increasing durations. Infants can repeat or try to avoid previous stimulus–response experiences, anticipate the next movement during a diaper change, and anticipate the next peek-a-boo. Because explicit memory relies on later developing regions, it is not *fully* functional until adolescence. Novelty detection (an immature type of explicit memory) is present at birth, but the types of explicit memory requiring retrieval emerge at about 1 year. With age, the infant becomes increasingly adept at acquiring new sensory information (e.g., mobility opens up new possibilities), establishing associations (e.g., now initiating multiple favored routines), and linking them to meanings (e.g., these people are called "Mommy" and "Daddy"). The graded expansion of memory abilities is related to increasing functional capacities across systems, not just to the limbic system. Notably, the executive system assists in the organization, search, and retrieval of relevant memories, as well as the anticipation of what will need to be recalled in the future.

An emotion results from a change, internal or external, that has some type of reinforcement value. Emotions can be simply classified as having a positive or negative valence, and this valence is influenced by arousal level as well as environmental context. With a sufficient degree of arousal

to support the action, animals typically approach something that is likely to safely satisfy a drive and avoid something that threatens safety. For example, when female mice were injected with a hormone to stimulate arousal, they increased their locomotion when placed in a safe environment (appropriate for courtship behaviors) but reduced their motor activity when placed in a novel or otherwise challenging or threatening environment (Morgan & Pfaff, 2001). In other words, whether the heightened arousal state resulted in sex or fear was dependent on the context (safe or threatening), which influenced what meaning was created.

Approach–avoid behaviors are also expressed when something is *anticipated* to be positive or negative, a type of meaning-making that can be encoded by means of implicit or explicit memory. For example, a child with a history of trauma may exhibit extreme fear responses to otherwise neutral sensory information that have been associated with threat. The arousal levels that underpin positive and negative emotions are also responsive to external context. For example, novelty and unpredictability in the environment heighten arousal, whereas repetition and predictability decrease arousal (Pfaff, 2006). The former situation would have a positive valence given safe circumstances (e.g., explore) but would have a negative valence given challenging or threatening circumstances (e.g., hide), and vice versa for the latter situation. The parameters of sensory information from the environment, such as sounds and movement, may also affect arousal. For a full-term healthy infant, a typical level of sensory information may sustain alertness and interest and has a positive valence, although too much or for too long would eventually push arousal too high and change the valence. For a premature or unhealthy infant, what would be typical sensory information constitutes a sensory overload (pushing arousal too high) and has a negative valence.

In keeping with the focus on global principles, this overview of emotion, memory, and meaning-making provides a solid starting point for understanding the spectrum of underlying mechanisms and influences of the relevance system, as noted in the following points. The relevance system primes:

- regulation in the form of anticipatory adjustments, autonomic patterns of activation–deactivation;
- sensory alertness via internal bodily sensations, external orienting, and attention to sensory information;
- emotional reactivity in relation to internal comfort and discomfort as well as appraisals of external safety, challenge, and threat; and
- behavioral action or inhibition via approach, avoid, and freeze reactions.

Looking at a child, adult, or dyad through the lens of the relevance system brings us back to a basic point, where emotional reactivity (or lack thereof) is viewed as a reflection of what is *relevant* for the child and the dyad. From here, we can begin to decode the child's first language, which is the nonverbal communication of arousal (states of arousal), sensory responses (type and level of reactivity and processing associated with sensory information), emotional reactivity (range and intensity of positive and negative affects), and motor activity (high–low, toward–away–against). This information can be most accurately interpreted within the context of history for both internal (physiological) and external (environment) conditions.

By understanding each individual in the dyad through the lens of the relevance system, you can begin to decode the co-created relational patterns. As noted, triggers for threat can arise from internal physiology or external context, or both. As a general rule, the more vulnerable or disrupted the physiology (of child or parent), the more the environment has to compensate; alternatively, the more constraints or disruptions in the environment, the more physiology has to compensate. With both, the risk for chronic dysregulation and disrupted sensorimotor patterns is extremely high. Intervention brings the potential to develop increasing conditions of internal and external safety for the child, the parent, and the relationship, increasing the potential for optimal regulation and sensory–motor plasticity.

The Executive System

The executive system is concerned with real-world, real-time behaviors—what to do, how to do it, and when to do it. To answer these questions, the executive system relies on the other systems to provide information about internal conditions (regulation of bodily states), information about external conditions (environmental and visceral sensory information), and personal and contextual relevance (personal associations and social meanings) and integrates this information in the service of adaptive action. In the end, the executive system is about *movement*—its initiation or inhibition—that promotes the achievement of goals. These movements include, for example, speaking, shifting the eyes, and the muscle tension that accompanies inhibition of an emotional expression. Even thinking, typically considered a purely cognitive task, is ultimately concerned with some type of action (Tweed, 2003).

The areas of the brain involved in the executive system are among the first and the last to mature fully (Henson et al., 2008; Huttenlocher, 1990; Johnson, 2005). Each system feeds major pipelines of information

into the prefrontal cortex, which is not only the last to fully mature but also the latest "addition" to the human brain. A major task of optimal prefrontal development involves its capacity to orchestrate a synchrony among the four systems, with each system honoring its affiliations and responding to its goals within the context of overall adaptation.

Brain Components of the Executive System

The functions of the executive system primarily involve top-down control of goal-oriented behavior (actions, emotions, and thoughts) in real time and are primarily associated with the frontal lobes of the brain (Mesulam, 2002). In terms of motor capacities, the frontal cortex contains the primary motor area that activates large motor movements, the association area that is involved in guiding and sequencing movements, the hand area that is involved in coordinating fine motor movements, the frontal eye fields that direct ocular movements, and Broca's area that controls oral–motor and speech movements (Miller & Cummings, 2007). These areas are reciprocally connected with all lower brain structures involved in motor activity as well as all modalities of sensory information (Mesulam, 2000b). These reciprocal loops allow for the establishment of tight sensory–motor links (e.g., ocular movements) up through sensory–motor transformations of ever-expanding complexity (e.g., carrying out a long-term action plan).

The motor areas reveal hierarchical stages of motor representation and processing (Fuster, 2002). When movement sequences are first attempted, the corresponding motor areas are active along with the cerebellum and multiple other regions. As the motor behaviors are learned, however, the multiple participating regions drop out as deeper and older motor structures (e.g., basal ganglia, striatum) take over motor control (Pascual-Leone, Grafman, & Hallet, 1995). These movements are now automatic, meaning that they can be carried out without having to think about them, as with walking. However, once we have to think about walking again, such as making our way through slippery mud, higher levels of control and other participating regions are called into play to assist with the increased effort of intentional action guidance. This capacity for storing automatic action programs is highly adaptive in that it frees up higher-level resources for other pursuits and allows for the layering of adjustments that comes with learning highly skilled behaviors.

Just in front of the motor areas is the dorsolateral cortex, a large region that is reciprocally connected with nearly all brain regions. It is densely connected with the orbitofrontal cortex and structures of the relevance system, the areas that integrate and elaborate sensory information, and the hypothalamus and chemical messengers of the regulatory system

(Kaufer, 2007). The mass integration of reciprocal connectivity from nearly all areas of the brain into the foremost regions of the frontal lobes brings personal and contextual significance together to coordinate immediate and long-term purposeful behaviors (Mesulam, 2002; Picton, Alain, & McIntosh, 2002). In a way, the prefrontal areas bring organization to the entire system. This region is associated with the highest levels of human capacities, such as social acumen, foresight, creativity, abstract thought, and complex planning and problem solving.

The developmental sequence of the executive system largely follows the hierarchical stages of processing already noted. At birth, the motor functions involving motor reflexes and elemental large motor movements are present due to maturity of the primary motor cortex (and deeper structures), including the preset biases that set the stage for a "social brain" (e.g., ocular motor toward faces). The early stages of prefrontal development allow for emergence of intentional (top-down) behaviors, such as directing attention, eliciting attention, obtaining a toy, holding a goal in mind, or lying to avoid trouble. Prefrontal regions also bring order to a rapidly increasing mass of percepts, sensory–motor links, and cause–effect associations, allowing for the emergence and expansion of meaning, planning, and problem solving throughout adolescence.

Behavioral Components of Executive System

The executive system is concerned with behaviors that are both personally and socially adaptive. As noted, it coordinates what to do, how to do it, and when to do it. The "what to do" involves engaging in behaviors or selecting goals that satisfy personal needs, sustain optimal regulation, form relevant memories, and promote social learning and adaptation. For the infant, the "what to do" involves exercising and expanding sensory–motor chains as well as learning to tolerate mild discomfort. With increasing age, the child should learn to attend to salience, habituate to nonrelevant distractions, tolerate challenge, and exhibit a stress response to threat with recovery back to baseline.

The early stages of "how to do it" involve initiating the appropriate sensorimotor programs to get needs met, learning behavioral sequences, and learning how to manipulate and use objects. The later "how to do it" stages involve learning to inhibit action, increasing working memory span (holding information "on line"), self-correcting and monitoring behavior, planning ahead, engaging in personal and social problem solving, and using hindsight and foresight to inform current plans.

The early stages of "when to do it" emerge with activities that require learning associations, such as anticipation of surprise with peek-a-boo, or

fussing for attention only after hearing that Mom is nearby, which requires some self-regulatory capacity. The later stages of "when to do it"
are more sophisticated and involve inhibiting personal drives when not
appropriate to the social context, engaging in the prosocial behaviors at
the appropriate time, delaying gratification in lieu of a sustained goal,
prioritizing activities, and adjusting plans when circumstances change.

Given its role in establishing an adaptive organization (or cohesion)
for the system as a whole, the executive system has the following overarching goals:

1. *Flexibility*, which allows an optimal balance between activation
   and inhibition, thinking and feeling, positive and negative emotions, distractibility and fixation, rigidity and spontaneity, and
   engagement and disengagement (Clark, 1997, 2003; Mesulam,
   1998, 2002); and
2. *Complexity*, which allows specialization for purposeful and adaptive
   behaviors that is balanced with the capacity for integration of new
   learning and experiences, as well as an internal self-understanding
   and focus that is balanced with an external, other-understanding
   and focus.

When a child is described as having an "executive deficit," hopefully
it is clear that this description, at minimum, warrants further explanation. Once it is more clearly defined, the etiology of the breakdown could
be represented within any system and at any point along the developmental hierarchy. The executive system defies any simple description and
highlights the reality that development is not a distinct process of acquiring one component skill or one competency at a time. From birth to
adulthood, all systems are linked, and each area can reciprocally facilitate
(or impede) the development of others.

APPLYING THE NEURORELATIONAL FRAMEWORK
TO THE CASE OF JOSEPH AND RACHEL

As we reflect on the case of Joseph and Rachel from Chapter 1, the neurorelational framework provides a way to begin to assess their individual
and relational profiles right from the start. The four brain systems described in this chapter provide the template for a comprehensive rather
than segmented (by discipline) process of assessment and intervention
that traditional diagnostic methods do not offer. Here we highlight each
system's contribution to Joseph's and Rachel's difficulties by providing

further information about each of them and their relational patterns, organized according to each brain system.

Regulation System

By understanding regulatory processes, the pediatrician would have noticed right from the start that Joseph had glazed eyes and was not in what is called an "optimal alert processing state of arousal." Both mother's and son's capacity for relating became increasingly limited as they spent more time either shut down (hypoalert) or angry (flooded). As they oscillated between these states of dysregulated arousal, they became further alienated from themselves and each other. Stabilizing the regulatory states of arousal across the sleep–awake cycle is often a primary therapeutic goal because it is so foundational to individual behavioral and interpersonal patterns. In addition, assessing nutritional, feeding, and elimination patterns as part of core regulatory processes are important from a bottom-up perspective. Indeed, commonalities among crying, sleeping, and feeding problems are prevalent (Papoušek, 2008). While these problems may describe normal periods of "disorganization" that resolve into higher maturational levels, or touchpoints (Brazelton, 1992), when they do not resolve with maturation, they can persist or turn into later behavioral problems (Papoušek & von Hofacker, 2008; Wurmser & Papoušek, 2008).

   In the neurorelational framework, we assess the regulation systems of both child and mother and intervene accordingly. Knowing that Joseph and Rachel were in the hypoalert and flooded states (two out of three primary stress response states of arousal) for long periods of time (one of the temporal circumstances that can lead to a load condition), we would further assess by looking at the three other brain systems for clues to potential triggers for emotional dysregulation, and we would consider which strategies would work best in relation to their sensation, relevance, and executive systems. Let's take a look at these other systems, which could contribute to either enhancing regulation or promoting dysregulation in this couple.

Sensory System

Experiences of safety, novelty, and pleasure sustain an alert processing state and support sensory preferences, whereas dangerous, boring, or unpleasant sensory experiences trigger energy upswings, downswings, or both. Joseph's lack of distress response to pain from his shot is a red flag signifying that his sensory responses to pain thresholds are atypically high

or that he has formed a shutdown response to pain for some reason. In either case, a thorough review of his responses to all sensory domains, by a practitioner holding the sensory system in mind, would be advised.

Because relationships provide a primary source of sensory information, all sensory modalities play a crucial role in shaping how we begin to organize our primary relationships. Upon further investigation, it would be noted that both Joseph and Rachel were sensitive to relational sounds and tones of voice, and each one's arousal system reacted differently. Joseph seemed to ignore Rachel's shrill voice, further exasperating her. At the same time, Rachel quickly escalated in response to Joseph's high-pitched tantrums; Joseph usually tuned Mom out, going into a hypoalert state, whereas Mom escalated into a hypervigilant and sometimes flooded state. Joseph's reactions to sensations from his mother and his environment provided immediate information that could be used to help resolve his arousal regulation problems. Not responding to sounds may signify an auditory processing difficulty. Joseph also did not track nonverbal relational cues visually; he was seemingly indifferent to faces and facial expressions and lacked an understanding that faces and body gestures communicate meaningful information (a direct link with the relevance system). In fact, he paid more attention to inanimate objects than to faces, a visual bias that contributed significantly to his consistent lack of eye contact with Rachel early on. Rachel's nonverbal looks, sounds, and gestures went unnoticed. This absence of eye contact began a cascade effect: Rachel felt devalued as a mother, which dysregulated her own states of arousal and skewed the meaning she ascribed to Joseph's relationship with her. Although snippets of these clinical assessments could be garnered from the primary scene described in the pediatrician's office when Joseph was 5 years old, signs of malfunctioning in these systems were present with the first year of life and could have been noted and investigated then.

Relevance System

As sensory processing problems or sensory experiences accumulate through repetition, they form implicit (automatic) bodily memories that are laced with meaning. Unpleasant sensations turn into visceral memories of experiences to dread or avoid, thereby directly affecting states of arousal and motivating actions to move away from the event. In Joseph and Rachel's case, each regularly set off unpleasant responses in the other, creating a vicious cycle of avoidance between them. Chronic conditions of unpleasant, challenging, or threatening experiences set up an expectation of negative experiences as typical. Joseph was primed to take this ongoing expectation

into daily life and to generalize his experience to other relationships. In contrast, pleasant sensations turn into expectations and anticipations for more, thereby directly affecting attention, sustaining the alert processing state, and supporting actions that turn toward the event. We now begin to see another facet of the cascade effect: Joseph and Rachel missed the early phases of falling in love with each other, phases in which relational joy activates the dopamine reward system and turns parent and child toward each other. This missed socioemotional milestone (explained more fully in Chapter 3) now leads, instead, to an avoidance of human contact.

Executive System

Action patterns occur across a continuum of thought and effort, requiring more or less ease depending on the circumstances. By the time Joseph was 5 years old, the action patterns between him and his mother had become rather automatic. At a basic level, the motor system provides reflex responses to a narrow set of stimuli and coordinates movements that are "automatic." These automatic actions are similar to automatic, implicit memory responses in that we don't really have to think about the action sequence (e.g., walking). As emotional patterns from the relevance system became solidified, Rachel and Joseph had developed unhelpful automatic movement patterns, oscillating between seeming indifference (her moving away) and tantrums (his moving against her). Additionally, we saw Joseph's clumsy motor planning, his adherence to repetitive and rigid movements, and his strong preference for predictable routines and repetitive interests. Flexible learning and coordination (allostasis) were not readily observable in Joseph, signaling an at-risk situation that was escalating. At times, Rachel was anxiously hypervigilant, which propelled her to chase him; at other times, she was overwhelmed and flooded with anger, which propelled her first to move against him and, ultimately, move away from him in despair.

Summary of Brain System Involvement

We briefly noted that neither Joseph nor Rachel was well regulated, and neither helped regulate the other. Both seemed to send sensory information to the other that triggered a distinct chase-and-dodge interpersonal pattern. He avoided looking at her eyes, she sounded off in a shrill tone of voice; he ran off, and she chased him down. Neither was providing an experience of satisfying relevance for the other; instead, a perpetual mismatch characterized their interactions. Mom wanted him to look at her; he wanted a predictable routine with no changes. An engaging flow of

conversation with back-and-forth eye contact was missing. Joseph planned ahead but had little flexibility with which to accommodate any real-life changes or to problem-solve. The executive system of his brain worked well only when everyone played his or her part in sustaining the order that he relied upon or demanded. If not, he fell apart and could also escalate very quickly. Rachel's executive problem-solving and planning-ahead skills were hampered by fatigue and emotional defeat (i.e., depression). She took the path of least resistance, which was to allow Joseph to run the show for the most part. This approach paid off in the short run but was costly in the long run. When she had more energy, she worked with time-outs, which escalated into hour-long screaming tantrums and fighting between them. Rachel felt defeated either way.

Given these few scenes, we have gathered a lot of information that allows us to understand that complex variables underlie both Joseph's and Rachel's behavior. There are multiple rather than singular (discipline- or diagnosis-specific) causes. Of course, there is a lot more information that would benefit our understanding. How often is this pattern active in this way? Are there other patterns that are equally rigid and entrenched? What is the relational context and history that Rachel brings to this situation? How have her past experiences influenced her current feeling of futility? Rachel by now has formulated a longstanding appraisal that interprets Joseph's behavior as indicating that he does not love her, stimulating painful feelings that she experiences similarly with her preoccupied husband and her dismissing father.

In applying the neurorelational framework to Joseph and Rachel, we found that they had problems within each system, as summarized in Table 2.3. In the next several chapters, we will see how this type of information helps us target and shape specific interventions for each brain system.

Table 2.3. Identification of Joseph's and Rachel's Neurorelational Difficulties

Four Brain Systems	Joseph	Rachel
Regulation	Oscillates between hypoalert and flooded; exhibits poor sleep pattern	Oscillates between hypoalert and hyperalert; occasionally becomes flooded
Sensory	Does not react to pain; tunes out mom's voice; seems to not process language; does not read nonverbal cues	Is sensitive to sounds; is hypersensitive to visual cues

(Continued)

Table 2.3.   Continued

Four Brain Systems	Joseph	Rachel
Relevance	Does not attend to faces; lacks relational pleasure; attends mostly to objects	Interprets lack of eye contact as rejection; feels Joseph does not love her
Executive	Oscillates between moving away and moving against; exhibits clumsy motor planning; engages in repetitive routines; is reactive and impulsive	Shifts between moving toward, moving away, and moving against; oscillates between being reactive and proactive

One of the ways in which the neurorelational framework identifies and describes individual and dyadic developmental markers is by referring to the socioemotional milestones (ZERO TO THREE, 1994, 2005; Greenspan & Wieder, 1998). In Chapter 3, we explore how the neurorelational framework's four brain systems can be used in conjunction with the socioemotional milestones and three interpersonal modes of *respond*, *direct*, and *reflect* to further illuminate important processes underlying health and problems in parent–child dyads.

NOTE

1. Within this framework and throughout this book, we use the term *behavior* to mean not only observable actions but also thoughts and emotions that are less observable and inferred through actions.

3

Brains in Relationship:
Using the Neurorelational
Framework with Dyads

As noted in Chapter 2, the foundation of the neurorelational framework uses several theories of neuroscience that cover brain function in a global perspective. This framework encompasses two major components: *neuro*, referring to the individual aspect (the brain systems introduced in Chapter 2) and *relational*, referring to the interpersonal aspect of the dyad. In this chapter we consider (1) the socioemotional milestones as a primary way to assess and intervene with dyadic relationships, and (2) three interpersonal modes of behavior that can be used to capture a variety of interpersonal dynamics.

To evaluate the dyad and the quality of the attachment, we use the socioemotional milestones (also referred to as "dyadic" and "interpersonal" milestones in this book) developed by Greenspan and Wieder in the 1980s (Greenspan, 1985, 1992; Greenspan & Lourie, 1981). These were later incorporated into Axis V in the *Diagnostic Classification of Mental Health and Developmental Disorders of Infancy and Early Childhood, Revised* (DC:0–3R) (ZERO TO THREE, 1994, 2005), the system we prefer for triaging and diagnosing children from birth to 5 years old. These milestones include the following:

- Milestone 1—Attention and regulation (birth–3 months)
- Milestone 2—Mutual engagement and attachment (3–6 months)
- Milestone 3—Purposeful, two-way communication (4–10 months)
- Milestone 4—Complex gestures and problem solving (10–18 months)
- Milestone 5—Use of symbols to express thoughts and feelings (18–30 months)

- Milestone 6—Bridges between symbols and emotional themes (30–
  48 months)*

These milestones are assessed in the context of unstructured interactions and play between the parent and child and include different types of toys for which uses and preferences shift according to age ranges: (1) sensory toys (e.g., textured ball, furry puppets, a heavy musical toy with balls on spokes), (2) symbolic toys (e.g., toy telephone, large baby doll, toy cars, toy boat, puppets, dollhouse with furniture), and (3) movement toys (e.g., rotating spinning board, scooter board). As each type of play is observed, the impact of the play equipment on the quality of the parent–child interactions is noted. Some children are much more able to modulate themselves and engage the parent when using certain sensory experiences. Other children are either more unresponsive or overreactive to certain sensory experiences and therefore engage the parent less. Still others are able to make better use of symbolic material. The rating of these socioemotional milestones follows a continuum of capacities outlined by the DC:0–3R, which progresses in the following manner:

- not present at this time;
- barely present, even with support;
- intermittently present, unless special structure or sensorimotor support is available;
- functions immaturely;
- functions at an age-appropriate level but is vulnerable to stress or has a constricted range of affect or both;
- functions at an age-appropriate level even under stress and with a full range of affective states (ZERO TO THREE, 2005, p. 62).†

The behavioral descriptors that accompany each milestone used throughout this chapter come from Greenspan and Wieder's DIR model (Greenspan & Wieder, 1998) and the Functional Emotional Assessment Scale (FEAS; Greenspan, 1996), as well as from the clinical and research versions of the FEAS (Greenspan, DeGangi, & Wieder, 2001).

In the following sections, we present (1) an overview of each socioemotional milestone, (2) the milestones in the context of the neurorelational

---

*From material in the *Diagnostic classification system of mental health and developmental disorders of infancy and early childhood, revised (DC:0–3R)*, by ZERO TO THREE, 2005, Washington, DC: ZERO TO THREE. Used with permission of ZERO TO THREE.
†From material in the *Diagnostic classification system of mental health and developmental disorders of infancy and early childhood, revised (DC:0–3R)*, by ZERO TO THREE, 2005, Washington, DC: ZERO TO THREE. Adapted with permission of ZERO TO THREE.

framework, and (3) the dyadic relationship of Joseph and Rachel discussed in relation to each milestone to exemplify the use of these milestones in a clinical context.

ASSESSING INTERPERSONAL RELATIONSHIPS USING SOCIOEMOTIONAL MILESTONES

Here we describe the socioemotional milestones in a linear, developmental order. As milestones are achieved, they become building blocks for subsequent milestones, so they have the potential to become additive benefits or deficits. Of course, similar to the brain systems, with older children and experienced practitioners, these milestones can also be understood and worked with in nonlinear ways. The parent–child behaviors that are necessary to accomplish these socioemotional milestones are identified for each in accompanying tables.

Because assessing socioemotional milestones is a vital way to identify the degree of health and maturity present in a dyad, experienced infant mental health professionals may simply use these milestones as a stand-alone tool for guiding intervention processes. However, the neurorelational framework provides an additional strategy for identifying and understanding the underlying global brain dynamics that contribute to the success, constriction, or failure of reaching and sustaining these socioemotional milestones. When the milestones are used in the context of the neurorelational framework, they enable clinicians to do the following:

- understand the global causal factors contributing to the breakdown within each partner and, thus, the dyad;
- comprehend the potential contributions of causal factors with increased clarity and precision;
- prioritize where to focus and initiate treatment;
- prioritize the progression of treatment in terms of what might be most valuable for each individual and for the dyad;
- reevaluate other avenues and approaches if progress is not being made in the professional setting;
- increase collaboration and efficiency of a team's service delivery through the use of a common framework.

In the neurorelational framework, the socioemotional milestones are viewed as the product of contributions from all four brain systems, which in turn provide a common language for individual practitioners and team members. Typically, practitioners allocate the evaluation of the socioemotional milestones to mental health clinicians. However, because interpersonal

relationships are central to brain development, they should be the concern of every practitioner who interfaces with infants and young children.

Although these milestones are primarily used for assessing parent–child dyads within the first 4 years of life, they actually describe dynamics that apply to any two individuals in relationship, regardless of age. Thus, these milestones can be used for assessing not only the parent–child dyad but also the parent–parent dyad, the therapist–child dyad, and the therapist–parent dyad. All team members, regardless of discipline, can learn to use them for assessment, intervention, and team discussions. (Additional sources of information regarding the socioemotional milestones are listed later in this chapter.)

Milestone 1: Attention and Regulation

The first socioemotional milestone has a direct parallel with the first brain system, the regulation system, which provides the foundation for all learning and emotional development. Interpersonal development depends on both parties' ability to maintain a regulated state. The term *regulation* is widely used in many early childhood professional circles. In the neurorelational framework, regulation begins with "arousal" regulation (regulation system) and is expanded on within each brain systems. Our use of the term is adapted from the clinical infant research literature (Als, 1982, 1984, 2002; Als & Gibes, 1986; Barnard, 1999; Brazelton, 1973, 1992; Prechtl, 1977) that evaluates regulation in terms of the individual's capacity to sustain optimal health across the 24-hour sleep–awake continuum. This capacity includes (1) an ability to shift into a deep sleep state during the sleep cycle, and (2) an ability to maintain a calm and attentive state (i.e., feeling "just right," the alert processing state) during the awake cycle.

The ability to maintain one's own optimal state of arousal is referred to as "self-regulation." Vulnerable individuals and children (e.g., premature babies, those exposed to toxins, malnutrition, or illness; older adults; mentally or physically ill individuals of all ages) will need more assistance during the sleep and awake cycles from an emotionally connected adult; this assisted process is referred to as "mutual or interactive regulation." Over time, with healthy interactive regulation, a child develops reliable self-regulating abilities.

Our "first language" (NCAST-AVENUW, 2003) of nonverbal communication lasts a lifetime and is universal to all ages across all cultures. Healthy interactive regulation depends on parents' ability to "read" the infant's first language of nonverbal cues. When the reading of cues is successful, the regulation process is stable; when it is not, states of dysregulation may become

typical. Parents' abilities to self-regulate their own states of arousal are crucial for healthy infant development. If the adult (or adults) is dysregulated, the first task is to help him or her enhance the self-ability to maintain healthy state regulation across the sleep–awake cycle. The practitioner's ability to assess all domains of development depends on being able to read both the infant's and parents' nonverbal cues.

Behavioral Markers for Milestone 1

The behavioral markers for attention and regulation (Greenspan, 1996; Greenspan, DeGangi, & Wieder, 2001), listed in Table 3.1, indicate the behaviors needed for the parent and the child to accomplish this first milestone. Although the child's behavioral markers emerge during the age span noted, they generally apply to children of any age. When a certain behavior pertains only to infants, the term *infant* is used.

Table 3.1. Parent–Child Behavioral Markers for Attention and Regulation

Parent	Child (observable between birth and 3 months)
Positive Contributions to Health (Coordination)	
Parent shows sustained interest in his or her child through visual contact, focusing, and reading the child's nonverbal cues (e.g., gestures, vocalizations, eye contact), keeping the child involved in interactive play.	Child is calm and attentive for periods of time (for 2 or more minutes), during which he or she shows interest in and focuses on faces and novel toys.
Parent can follow child's lead in taking needed rest periods (Brazelton, 1973, 1992).	Child can modulate arousal and sustain the alert processing state by taking needed rest periods (Brazelton, 1973, 1992).
Parent interacts calmly with his or her child, able to wait for the child's responses, while showing pleasant and happy affect during playtime.	Child remains calm for periods of time, enjoying touch and movement with the parent, while showing happy, content affect.
Parent is sensitive and responsive to child's need for touch and movement experiences and encourages exploration of the surrounding world.	Child is responsive to parental sensory input through touch and movement, which sustains his or her regulation.
Parent is well modulated in pace and activity level, focusing on child's interest in emotional engagement and object (or objects) of desire.	Child is well modulated in pace and activity level, focusing on a toy or parent for long periods before changing interests.

(Continued)

Table 3.1.   Continued

Parent	Child (observable between birth and 3 months)
Parent facilitates arousal recovery through sensory means at the appropriate level and type of stimulation that soothes infant.	Recovers from distress within 20 minutes with sensory help from parent.

Potential Negative Contributions to Dysregulation (Risk Factors for Load Conditions)

Parent is sluggish or slow-paced but eventually follows child's lead or facilitates engagement.	Child is sluggish or slow-paced but can eventually reach optimal arousal and engagement.
Parent shows flat, somber, or depressed affect.	Child appears sluggish or withdrawn and difficult or slow to engage (underreactive).
Parent becomes more interested in the toys than in the child, ignoring the child.	Child is overly visual, stuck on looking at the toys and not playing with them.
Parent is distracted into other bursts of activity and then returns to playing with child for short periods of time.	Child appears overaroused by toys, environment, or both (overreactive), showing the following behavior: child is moderately active, with occasional burst of changing activity activities, then settling into play with one toy for a short period of time.
Parent is easily and frequently distractible, often walking about the room when interacting with child.	Child appears overaroused by toys, environment, or both (overreactive), showing the following behavior: child is very active, moving from one toy to the next, constantly wandering away from parent and initial points of interest.

Note. From material in "Assessing the Emotional and Social Functioning of Infants and Young Children," by S. I. Greenspan, 1996, in *New Visions for the Developmental Assessment of Infants and Young Children,* by S. J. Meisels and E. Fenichel (Eds.), Washington, DC: ZERO TO THREE. Adapted with permission of ZERO TO THREE. Also from material in *The Functional Emotional Assessment Scale (FEAS) for Infancy and Early Childhood: Clinical and Research Applications* by S. I. Greenspan, G. A. DeGangi, and S. Wieder, 2001, Bethesda, MD: Interdisciplinary Council on Developmental and Learning Disorders. Adapted with permission of Dr. S. I. Greenspan.

Considering Milestone 1 in the Context of the Neurorelational Framework

Although this first socioemotional milestone has a strong connection with the regulatory system, the larger reality is that all brain systems reciprocally influence one another from the beginning. Furthermore, by applying the neurorelational framework to the socioemotional milestones, we can see the degree to which all four brain systems contribute to milestone abilities. In the neurorelational framework, the behavioral markers that we use to

identify the child's and adult's experience of safety are an individual's ability to (1) cycle into deep sleep, (2) maintain an alert processing state, and (3) recover from a stress response. The behavioral markers that we use to identify the experience of challenge or threat are the three primary stress responses of hypoalert, hyperalert, and flooded. Note that these stress responses are not necessarily products of the external environment but may arise in response to internal perceptions. In other words, the experience of safety versus threat may ultimately be a subjective experience. For example, a mobile that triggers crying in one infant would constitute a condition of perceived threat; for the infant who smiles and gurgles, in contrast, it is a condition of safety.

The capacity for arousal regulation is intricately affected by sensory system functioning. The sensory world has alerting, calming, and triggering functions. So when considering regulatory and attentional difficulties, the first place to look for intervention targets, typically, is the sensory system (Dunn, 1997; Williamson & Anzalone, 1997). One way to expand the alert processing state is to engage the baby and help him or her experience joy, which in turn lays the foundation for a healthy relevance system. Finally, the motor system (executive) during early months either supports optimal regulation and attention (e.g., good muscle tone, turning eyes and head to novelty, ability to support head) or contributes to the infant's inability to experience "organized" states of arousal. (See CD-ROM Section 3.1 for a summary table listing the contributions of each brain system to this first socioemotional milestone.)

Now let's apply this information about the first milestone of attention and regulation to Joseph and Rachel, whose relationship was described in Chapter 1 and elaborated in Chapter 2. In particular, we consider how clarifying each system's contribution to regulation problems can help us better organize our intervention strategies for this case.

Joseph and Rachel: Attention and Regulation

Early on, Joseph and Rachel's relationship showed difficulties with this first milestone of attention and regulation. Joseph was underreactive, in a low state of arousal (hypoalert), which, for Rachel, projected an air of indifference. He seemed unresponsive to sensory information when Rachel used her voice, face, and gestures to engage him. Joseph's response to these attempts was either a lack of interest or an active withdrawal from her. From infancy Joseph also underresponded to the pain from the shots he received during visits to the pediatrician's office, so his lack of reactivity was not exclusive to Rachel's sensory input. However, with no one to help her recognize that his lack of response occurred across a variety of sensations, Rachel read these cues as indifference. She was saddened (relevance system) by Joseph's lack of response and felt considerable anxiety about whether to pursue him to coerce a response or to resort to indifference herself.

Rachel's oscillations between intrusive involvement and indifference became a repetitive cycle that lacked flexibility and did not allow for her own recovery into calm, alert states of arousal. As Joseph's oscillations also began shifting from indifference to impulsivity and tantrums (flooded state), his interactions with his mother showed clear signs of risk in this first level of interpersonal functioning. They could not build a solid foundation for vibrant interaction until both of them were able to sustain aligned states of calm. Instead, the sensory exchanges produced from their interactions led to states of distress rather than pleasant, happy experiences.

Where should the practitioner begin? Through the neurorelational framework we know that optimal regulation (through the regulation system) is contingent on the successful processing and the right dose of sensory information (through the sensory system). In turn, this optimal regulation facilitates both the experience of pleasure (through the relevance system) and the ability to pay attention (through the executive system). This knowledge helps narrow down the possibilities of where to start. Joseph's inability to process the sensory information coming from within and outside the relationship contributes to his lack of regulation, lack of joy, and lack of interest in and attention to others. This information could help relieve his mother's sadness as well as give her the courage to begin exploring other possibilities as to the cause of Joseph's difficulties, rather than to perceive them as being only a reflection of her inadequacies. It is possible that with the right practitioner—one who could emotionally support and connect to her early in this process—Rachel might have staved off the eventual downward spiral into an agitated depression.

Understanding the brain systems and how they interact in development and in relationship provides a starting point for the practitioner from which he or she can form a hypothesis and develop a treatment plan. A successful outcome would require a practitioner who knows the socioemotional domain and one who knows the sensory processing domain (or one who knows both domains well) and how these interface with regulation.

Milestone 2: Mutual Engagement and Attachment

Within this second socioemotional milestone, attachment processes incorporate the child's ability to engage in mutual (i.e., with the parent) experiences of joy. Stable attention and regulation (the first milestone) do not guarantee an experience of engagement and high-quality attachments (second milestone), but they are a necessary prerequisite.

Engagement occurs during the alert processing state and involves the ability to (1) mutually focus attention and eye contact while staying calm,

and (2) experience cycles of joy through the unique sensory–motor flow that is created between each parent and child. Because the exchange of non-verbal sensations is the earliest means of establishing a loving attachment, the emphasis on nonverbal aspects of communication is maintained in this milestone. Falling in love with one's partner (regardless of age) is a powerful force that can ignite a motivational surge. The young child's motivation to explore, cooperate, and develop a moral conscience and empathy for others emerges from a healthy, loving attachment. Optimal arousal with playful and positive emotions, or prolonged stress responses with negative affects, create positive or negative associations and expectations within primary re-lationships. These powerful early experiences also affect how parents, in turn, anticipate the emotional experience to unfold with their infant.

Behavioral Markers for Milestone 2

Table 3.2 presents the behavioral markers for mutual engagement and at-tachment (Greenspan, 1996; Greenspan, DeGangi, & Wieder, 2001).

Table 3.2. Parent–Child Behavioral Markers for Mutual Engagement and Attachment

Parent	Child (observable between 3 and 6 months)
Positive Contributions to Health (Coordination)	
Parent shows a relaxed and calm state during interchanges with child.	Child evidences relaxed and calm state and comfort while near parent, showing connection through eye contact.
Parent enjoys warmth of connection but is not overly attentive to child's every move.	Child initiates physical closeness to parent but is not clingy.
Parent initiates engagement and responds with warmth and affection through facial expressions and eye contact.	Child initiates engagement and responds with warmth and smiles through facial expressions and eye contact.
Within cultural variations, parent shows warmth and playful back-and-forth engagement through smiles, joyful looks, inviting gestures, playful movements, and vocalizations.	Child participates in back-and-forth en-gagement with parent through smiles, vocalizations, joyful looks, and gestures.
Parent maintains attention toward child with a verbal or visual connection, signaling an availability, openness, and interest in the child.	Child can focus or pay attention for 30 seconds or more.

(Continued)

Table 3.2.   Continued

Parent	Child (observable between 3 and 6 months)
Parent allows child to move away and explore while staying connected to child through engaging eye contact, pleasant vocalizations, inviting gestures, and warm facial expressions.	If active and away from parent while exploring or playing with toys, the child visually references the parent across space, using gestures or vocalizations to communicate, while staying calm and relaxed.
Parent anticipates playtime interaction with child with curiosity and excitement.	Child anticipates with curiosity and excitement when parent presents an interesting game or toy.
Parent notices child's distress caused by abrupt distraction or unresponsiveness and facilitates repair of rupture (Tronick, 2007).	Child displays signs of discomfort, displeasure, or sadness during engagement if parent becomes unresponsive or distracted from play.
Parent uses the appropriate level and type of stimulation to assist infant's recovery back to baseline.	Child can recover from distress within 15 minutes with sensory help from parent.

Potential Negative Contributions to Dysregulation (Risk Factors for Load Conditions)

Parent is overly anxious, overwhelming child with constant touching, talking, or eye contact.	Child is constantly touching, talking (babbling), or maintaining eye contact without modulation.
Parent is overly vigilant and shows discomfort when relating to child (hyperalert state of arousal).	Child keeps head turned toward parent without modulation of activity through rest periods, appearing hypervigilant with intense staring, wide-open eyes, or taut muscle tone (hyperalert state of arousal).
Parent is overly disengaged toward child, with delayed responses or an indifference in vocal tone, eye contact, and gestures that lack a display of vitality (hypoalert state of arousal).	Child turns head away, averts gaze, moves away, or turns away from parent without visual cuing, back and forth, with parent; appears uninterested, avoidant, detached, or withdrawn from parent (hypoalert state of arousal).
Parent is overly angry toward child, talks intrusively to child, and makes hostile eye contact and gestures.	Child is in prolonged state of distress (flooded), crying for periods greater than 15 minutes without accepting comfort from the parent.

Note. From material in "Assessing the Emotional and Social Functioning of Infants and Young Children," by S. I. Greenspan, 1996, in *New Visions for the Developmental Assessment of Infants and Young Children,* by S. J. Meisels and E. Fenichel (Eds.), Washington, DC: ZERO TO THREE. Adapted with permission of ZERO TO THREE. Also from material in *The Functional Emotional Assessment Scale (FEAS) for Infancy and Early Childhood: Clinical and Research Applications* by S. I. Greenspan, G. A. DeGangi, and S. Wieder, 2001, Bethesda, MD: Interdisciplinary Council on Developmental and Learning Disorders. Adapted with permission of Dr. S. I. Greenspan.

Considering Milestone 2 in the Context of the Neurorelational Framework

The neurorelational framework emphasizes attachment as facilitated by basic conditions of safety, which are defined by the individual infant's state of being—that is, as being able to maintain an alert processing state while awake, recover back to the alert processing state following a stress response, and cycle into deep sleep during the sleep phases. Second, we define behavioral breakdowns that disrupt attachment in terms of stress responses, which are seen as occurring adaptively as well as under conditions of challenge or threat. Third, the exchanges that take place between child and parent are seen as an ongoing feedback loop of sensory–motor transformations that act as the building blocks of either safety or stress responses. Motor expressions from one partner—from the eyes, facial muscles, throat, gestures, and body movements—become sensory information for the other partner. The parent's animated, smiling face (motor expressions) constitutes sensory information that (typically) contributes to the positive valence of the attachment.

During achievement of this second socioemotional milestone, we see again the strong connection between nonverbal sensory–motor experiences and the formation of an intimate relationship. The sensory system is pivotal in its connections to all other brain systems by enhancing the child's ability for optimal regulation and recovery (regulation), providing the means through which engagement occurs (relevance), and facilitating sustained attention (executive). The importance of sensory preferences providing the "bath" in which attachment takes place cannot be underestimated (Perry, 1998). As the dyad builds on the foundation of stable regulation—and assuming (1) that an infant has the ability to tolerate sensations from the parent, and (2) that the parent has the ability to tolerate them from the infant—warm exchanges occur between child and parent when physically close as well as apart.

For the child and parent to experience and tolerate the intense sensory flow of the falling-in-love exchange, they will each need a capacity for modulation. Modulation is the ability to traverse the peaks and valleys of sensory-emotional intensity and stay within the optimal state of arousal while doing so. In operational terms, modulation involves taking a break from sensory stimulation with brief rest periods. These rest periods are not the same as prolonged gaze aversion. If there is too much stimulation and an infant lacks a natural capacity to take a break (e.g., through momentary gaze aversion or turning away), he or she may get stuck in overstimulation. At some point, this overstimulation will interrupt the back-and-forth exchange of emotional closeness by generating a shift in the infant's state of arousal

(regulation system). With continued overstimulation, the infant likely will begin to cry in distress (a flooded state of arousal) or tune out (a hypoalert state of arousal). In both cases, the infant stops responding to playful, nonverbal sensory exchanges, and the pleasant or joyful interchange is interrupted. The challenge for the parent is to notice these shifts and to respond by trying a variety of possibilities: lowering the intensity of stimulation, slowing down the rhythm and taking a break, initiating a different type of sensory stimulation, or removing an offending stimulation in an effort to provide comfort that will calm the infant's distress and bring him or her back from tuning out. Through thoughtful experimentation, parents are involved in a learning process—similar to what a professional would do—of finding the sensory preferences and triggers of his or her unique child.

This description of the engagement process notes how the presence of certain sensations, or lack of other sensations, is crucial to stress recovery. Each one of the three primary stress responses, when accompanied by poor stress recovery back to a calm state of arousal, can become habitual. Anything that is repeated with regularity influences implicit emotional memories (relevance system). The emotional memories that are generated through these three stress responses eventually become linked with patterns of sensations and arousal. These connections form interpersonal styles that can be either adaptive—signifying allostasis (coordination)—or maladaptive—signifying potential allostatic load conditions.

If the infant shows frequent and very quick responses to stress, prolonged stress responses with or without recovery, or the absence of a stress response when one would expect it (e.g., crying in response to a doctor's shot), these become potential contributions to load conditions, signifying the need for intervention (Wurmser, Papoušek, & von Hofacker, 2008). These underlying states of arousal, then, provide important information as to the origins of many diagnostic categories. The age between 3 and 6 months (the time period of this milestone) marks a necessary point of intervention if frequent or prolonged signs of distress or lack of engagement are apparent. The diagnostic categories from the DC:0–3R, that can be considered at this age range include posttraumatic stress disorders, bereavement disorder, regulation disorder of sensory processing, and depression. Some of these diagnostic categories are weighted toward one or two brain systems: (1) regulation disorders are weighted toward the regulation *and* sensory systems in that there may be a vulnerable arousal system in tandem with sensory over- or underreactivity affecting the ability for arousal regulation; (2) bereavement disorders, depression, or both are weighted toward the relevance system (affect); and (3) posttraumatic stress disorders are weighted toward the sensory *and* relevance systems, with emotional memories triggered through one or more sensory experiences

stimulating one or more stress responses. At this point, it is also important to understand that inadequate stress recovery is an indicator of
some problem within the physiology of the child, the parent, or both.
When any of the foregoing circumstances is the case, early intervention
is warranted.

At this juncture, the question becomes, is the attachment pattern between the parent and child gaining in momentum toward (1) experiences
of warmth, comfort, and joy, signifying safety and regulation, and (2) intentional stress recovery, when one or both members of the pair are experiencing any of the three possible stress responses? Or is the attachment
pattern moving toward quicker escalations into the stress responses, signifying more persistent conditions of challenge or threat, accompanied by
prolonged periods of dysregulation and poor stress recovery? (see CD-
ROM Section 3.2 for a summary table listing the contributions of each
brain system to this second socioemotional milestone.)

Joseph and Rachel: Mutual Engagement and Attachment

Joseph and Rachel's foundation for mutual engagement and attachment
was not well established. Having determined earlier that the sensory system plays an important role in engagement and attachment, we can quickly
identify the unique sensory needs of each partner and see why and how
the first and second socioemotional milestones were intensely constricted
right from the start. The mismatch was a recipe for limitations in the first
two dyadic milestones. When Joseph's attention was later engaged, it was
oriented toward mechanical objects and predictable routines, further
alienating Rachel in her attempts at emotional connection. In turn, Rachel's style of communicating was intrusive and overwhelming, both visually and auditorially, to Joseph, even though her behaviors were
maternally relevant and typical among mothers. Nevertheless, Rachel un-
wittingly encouraged Joseph's further avoidance of her because her behavior did not provide him with the kind of sensory information with
which he could naturally engage.

It is important to note that infants such as Joseph require a special
lens through which to interpret their sensory needs—a lens that is not
naturally understood by most parents. Even a highly sensitive and mindful mother could have difficulty understanding how to engage Joseph optimally. This insight expands the common understanding that attachment
depends heavily on the parent's ability to read cues. Although that understanding is true in concept, the co-created nature of attachment means
that vulnerable infants who are extremely difficult to read require the parent to move beyond the commonly understood ways of relating to infants.
This type of reading most often needs professional facilitation. Further-

more, the parent must have the confidence to ask for help, and the professionals responsible must be familiar with the required knowledge.

One way to begin the process of intervention would be to determine Joseph's sensory preferences. Does he respond with calm attention to sensory experiences through any particular type of movement, touch, deep pressure, sights and sounds, or lack of any of these sensations? How can those sensory preferences be used to sustain mutual engagement as long as possible? At which rate, rhythm, and timing does Joseph respond best to the sensory experiences that he does like? All of these questions are answered with the help of a practitioner (or team of practitioners) who can guide the evaluation process through each sensory system while managing Rachel's distress as the story unfolds. Each infant's sensory preferences are unique and cannot be known ahead of time—a fact that can be reassuring to parents in the midst of a crisis brought about by not intuitively knowing how to help their child.

Milestone 3: Purposeful Two-Way Communication

Building on a stable regulatory system with attentional capacities and a sensory–motor flow of pleasurable exchanges, the parent and child now pursue increasingly versatile interactions with each other. The interaction between two people can be referred to as an interpersonal dance; supported in a calm, regulated state, a back-and-forth rhythm can be noted between any two individuals. When the dance goes well, it flows synchronously without interruption. When the dance is awkward, the partners may step on each other's toes or slow down to the point at which the interaction stops. Stepping on each other's toes in a dyadic relationship translates into constant interruptions or intrusions. Not having enough movement within the dance is equivalent to partners not responding to one another, repeatedly giving one-word answers, never keeping the conversation going.

The third socioemotional milestone emphasizes not only the quality and rhythm of the dyadic dance in its back-and-forth movement but also the intentionality involved in how each partner signals for a playful interaction. This signaling builds on previous experiences and is captured by Greenspan and Wieder's (1998) phrase "circles of communication." This term is meant to convey the back-and-forth volleying of a good conversation, whether nonverbal or verbal. Someone starts, the other person responds, and the first person responds in turn. The full circle of communication involves more than only a two-part series, a start with a response; it requires the third piece, the second response, to complete the communication circle (Greenspan & Wieder, 1998). When one person initiates a

conversation but gets only one-word answers in return, the conversation soon grinds to a halt. The circles of communication are a useful tool in observing relationships because the three steps can actually be counted, thus enabling practitioners and dyads to reflect on the flow of information. Early on, the circles of communication between parent and child revolve around falling in love. A coo, a catching of the eye, a smile, a burst of joy, and a back-and-forth rhythm mark the process.

These dynamics are universal concepts that apply not only to parent–child couples who are cooing and babbling with accompanying motherese (a parent's nonsensical, nonverbal conversation with his or her infant) but also to any two adult conversations. What appears to apply to all ages is the comfort zone of being in a mid-range tempo (Beebe & Lachmann, 2002)—not too fast and not too slow. These factors parallel the optimal state of the regulatory process that feels just right during the alert processing state.

Behavioral Markers for Milestone 3

Table 3.3 presents the behavioral markers for purposeful two-way communication (Greenspan 1996; Greenspan, DeGangi, & Wieder, 2001).

Table 3.3.   Parent–Child Behavioral Markers for Purposeful Two-Way Communication

Parent	Child (observable between 4 and 10 months)
Positive Contributions to Health (Coordination)	
Parent makes space available for child to open circles of communication by allowing child to decide on the play topic, initiate play, and show how he or she wants to pursue the play.	Child opens circles of communication with facial play and engagement (e.g., initiating peek-a-boo).
Parent responds to and builds on child's intentions, wishes, and actions.	Child opens circles of communication around objects of interest while also engaging parent through nonverbal means (looks, smiles, gestures, vocalizations).
When opening circles of communication and leading the stimulation, parent paces interaction with child, allowing time for child to respond.	Child participates in opening and closing circles of communication with parent.
Parent avoids over- and understimulating child with sounds or gestures.	Child can handle mid-level range of stimuli from sounds and gestures.

(Continued)

Table 3.3.   Continued

Parent	Child (observable between 4 and 10 months)
Parent allows child the freedom to explore without constrictions, while also providing safety measures and boundaries.	Child initiates purposeful and intentional motor actions (reaching and crawling) to ward objects of desire (toy).
Parent may lead in a way that models a new age-appropriate skill or functions just slightly above child's level (zone of proximal development; Vygotsky, 1978).	Child tolerates and responds with engagement to parent-led interactions or activities.
Parent responds contingently to child by staying with the child's interests most of the time.	Child initiates purposeful and intentional play with faces and toys of interest.
Parent communicates (through gestures, facial muscles, sounds, words, body movement) intentional desire to play or responds to child's desire for play.	Child's play shows intentionality through gestures or other nonverbal means that are consistent with object of interest.
Parent is able to play with toys in a variety of ways.	Child shows variability when playing by engaging in two or more types of different behaviors.
Parent stays attentive and focused on interactive play with child.	Child can pay attention to a person or toy for 1 minute or more.
Parent reads child's gestures and words for help and is responsive.	Child uses gestures and vocalizations to solicit help from parent.
Parent can use distractibility and social engagement to help child recover from stress.	Child can recover from a stress response within 10 minutes by engaging in social interactions.

Potential Negative Contributions to Dysregulation (Risk Factors for Load Conditions)

Parent	Child
Parent's play interactions are aimless, impulsive, or disorganized; parent is unable to build on a theme and take the play to a deeper level.	Child initiates play that is aimless, impulsive, or disorganized, not able to build on parental scaffolding.
Parent does not give clear clues (through gestures or facial cues) that he or she is interested in playing.	Child does not initiate organized or clear gestures for play.
Parent has difficulty getting started in play.	Child needs considerable help to get started in play.
Parent initiates stereotyped, scripted, or repetitive forms of play.	Child initiates play that is stereotyped or repetitive.
Parent fails to close circles of communication by not noticing child's response.	Child fails to close circles of communication by not noticing parent's response.

(Continued)

Table 3.3.   Continued

Parent	Child (observable between 4 and 10 months)
Parent partially or consistently intrudes on the child by doing the opposite of what the child indicates as his or her desire.	Child does not close circles of communication; child notices parent's response and yet does something that has nothing to do with what the parent did.
Parent partially or consistently intrudes on the child by changing activities, once a flow occurs between them, to those of less interest to the child.	Child intrudes on play themes by quickly changing interest.

Note. From material in "Assessing the Emotional and Social Functioning of Infants and Young Children," by S. I. Greenspan, 1996, in *New Visions for the Developmental Assessment of Infants and Young Children,* by S. J. Meisels and E. Fenichel (Eds.), Washington, DC: ZERO TO THREE. Adapted with permission of ZERO TO THREE. Also from material in *The Functional Emotional Assessment Scale (FEAS) for Infancy and Early Childhood: Clinical and Research Applications* by S. I. Greenspan, G. A. DeGangi, and S. Wieder, 2001, Bethesda, MD: Interdisciplinary Council on Developmental and Learning Disorders. Adapted with permission of Dr. S. I. Greenspan.

Considering Milestone 3 in the Context of the Neurorelational Framework

As the interpersonal dance between parent and child becomes routine choreography, with surprises that build flexibility, sensations continue to be a salient means of creating a flow of communication. Playing peek-a-boo, where an established routine is combined with surprises, is a good example of the paradox of stability with flexibility. In this optimal state, the ebb and flow of sensations, from heightened to calm, occur in synchronous movement. As long as regulation, the foundation, is stable and a wide variety of sensations is tolerated, more variety and depth emerge in the communication pattern. With stability comes more chance for flexibility and new experiences.

The flow between the dyadic members relies increasingly on previous patterns and the anticipation of another round of pleasure (engaging the relevance and executive systems). One of the key elements during this milestone is the use of sensations that sustain interpersonal joy, thus creating purposeful rounds of dyadic pleasure that now extend to an active engagement with the world at large. The element of pleasure and excitement generated between the parent–child couple fuels the child's exploration.

Movement, a capacity within the executive system, now can be used with more focused intentionality: the child reaches for toys and crawls to where he or she wants to go. As the motor system matures and evidences new abilities, the child begins to plan and sequence as he or she explores what is interesting in the environment (e.g., using the eyes to scan the larger environment) and decides not only how to get there but also whether help is

needed. Circles of communication that rely on gestures and vocalizations (i.e., grunts) to elicit help begin to emerge during this developmental phase.

With a stable foundation of regulation, sensory, and relevance systems, the executive brain system (through motor) kicks in during this phase. Without a stable foundation of regulation and sensory experiences, patterns of stress arousal and emotional dysregulation are more likely to emerge. Less stable regulation and sensory systems more likely lead toward a pattern of overanxiety, withdrawal, aggression, or some combination of these. A child whose arousal and emotional valence are either underactive or overactive is less likely to plan ahead and more likely to act impulsively. Stable functioning of the first two brain systems (regulation and sensory) enables the other two brain systems (relevance and executive) to mature and expand during this milestone. When the first two brain systems are less stable, a cascading effect begins to occur. More energy goes into states of distress or energy conservation, and less energy is available for observing the surrounding world and planning ahead. (See CD-ROM Section 3.3 for a summary table listing the contributions of each brain system to this third socioemotional milestone.)

Joseph and Rachel: Purposeful, Two-Way Communication

Given that Joseph and Rachel have not successfully assimilated Milestones 1 and 2 (attention and regulation; mutual engagement and attachment), it is not surprising that their pattern of withdrawal and aggression began early, within the first year of Joseph's life. The two have a long history in which the sensations created between them are not pleasurable. What is relevant to Joseph (a toy) does not match what is relevant to Rachel (eyes and faces); consequently, optimal circles of communication have not emerged. Indeed, this dyad's weak foundation supports few circles of communication that contain any pleasure or excitement. In addition, Joseph is not using gestures to communicate (a poorly functioning motor system); he is oriented toward toys he finds interesting, but he does not share them or initiate playful interactions with his mother. When Rachel tries to join him, she plays *next* to him, not *with* him in an interactive manner.

At this point, if intervention were begun, the practitioner team might want to encourage Rachel to build on Joseph's interest in his particular toys with the goal of fostering shared excitement and pleasure. Rachel might play a game that involves bringing objects of interest to Joseph near her own face and eyes and requiring him to reach toward her face for what he wants. In addition, she could be instructed to lower herself to the floor, on her belly, to catch her baby's glance and make eye contact. Both strategies would help Joseph move toward pleasurable engagement (relevance system). When Joseph is frustrated, Rachel could encourage

him to gesture for help, thus guiding him to express his need for something relevant to him while also engaging his mother.

In tracking further details as to what is relevant to Joseph on a sensory level, we find that he is attracted to toys that move or play music. Rachel could engage him by motoring a similar toy alongside his toy and then finding a way to make both motor toys run into each other. Additionally, Rachel and Joseph could exchange musical toys in a back-and-forth rhythm, thereby combining his sensory preferences (sensory system) with his interest in the musical toy box (relevance system).

Milestone 4: Complex Gestures and Problem Solving

The communication aspects of this milestone are dependent on a well-functioning motor system. At this age, arm and leg movements are more organized, enabling pointing, crawling, and then walking; eyes can scan the environment, looking for interesting objects. The child can crawl or walk to those objects or point and grunt for help in getting them—useful ways to engage others and the larger environment. One of the most important aspects of this socioemotional milestone is the types of purposeful movements an infant makes as he or she matures into toddlerhood. Are intentional babbling, gesturing, crawling, and walking taking place? Does the infant-toddler appear to wander without intent?

Another important developmental accomplishment during this phase is the child's ability to point to an object of interest, look at the object while pointing, vocalize, then look back at the parent to see whether the parent's eyes are also tracking the object, and finally resume gazing at the exciting object (this is called *joint attention*). This complex gestural, vocal, and eye-tracking combination is saying, in essence, "Look! This is important to me, and I want to make sure you are tracking what is important to me, and I'm going to check to make sure you share this moment with me." The absence of this form of communication is considered a red flag possibly indicating disorders of social communication along the autistic spectrum.

Simple problem-solving abilities also emerge during this developmental period. In these instances, the circles of communication, achieved through pointing, vocalizing, and referencing eye contact back to the parent, revolve around the daily life problems that need to be solved. In essence, the nonverbal communication conveys messages such as "I need help to get that toy off the shelf that I cannot reach" or "I'm hungry and I want that piece of fruit up on the counter right now" or "I want to find my favorite blanket to cuddle with." As infants and toddlers continue to solve problems, they eventually discover words; then, using gestures and words, parent and child find ways to jointly work through these dilemmas.

Behavioral Markers for Milestone 4

Table 3.4 presents the behavioral markers for complex gestures and problem solving (Greenspan, 1996; Greenspan, DeGangi, & Wieder, 2001).

Table 3.4. Parent–Child Behavioral Markers for Complex Gestures and Problem Solving

Parent	Child (observable between 10 and 18 months)
Positive Contributions to Health (Coordination)	
Parent exposes child to increasingly more intense levels and diverse types of stimulation.	Child tolerates various types of touch (e.g., cuddling, roughhousing, different fabrics, brushing hair and teeth); is comfortable with bright lights, loud sounds, and movement.
Parent uses nonverbal forms of communication through eyes, facial expressions, sounds or vocalizations, gestures, and body movements to promote six or more circles of communication during an interaction.	Child uses nonverbal forms of communication through eyes, facial expressions, sounds, gestures, and body movements to reciprocate and promote six or more circles of communication during an interaction.
Parent tracks child's nonverbal clues that link with appropriate signals for simple problem solving.	Child communicates (through circles of communication involving eyes, facial expressions, vocalizations, gestures, and body movements) an ability to solve simple problems to get needs met (e.g., getting a particular type of food, obtaining a toy that is out of reach, not being able to find a favorite item).
When playing, parent expands on what child is doing while remaining on the child's topic.	Child responds to parental lead toward expansion of a theme or play by creating a new response or different outcome to a familiar aspect to the story.
Parent expansion includes providing a small challenge or interesting twist to the play that requires of the child a slightly different or new response from previous playtimes.	Child imitates or copies something new that parent has initiated.
Parent shows sustained delight and pleasure in however child wishes to play through six or more circles of communication.	Child shows sustained delight and pleasure through six or more playtimes with parent.
Parent allows child to assert self in play.	Child allows parent to take the lead at times during play.
Parent supports play themes of closeness and dependency, assertiveness	Child shows a range of emotional themes during play with parent that span closeness

(Continued)

Table 3.4. Continued

Parent	Child (observable between 10 and 18 months)
and curiosity, aggression, autonomy, or pleasure and excitement by admiring, showing interest, and joining in the child's play or exploration.	and dependency, assertiveness and curiosity, aggression, autonomy, or pleasure and excitement.
Parent sets appropriate limits or redirects the child.	Child responds with cooperation or short protests with recovery to parental setting of limits and redirection.
Parent can pay attention and stay focused on child for as long as child is able to do so.	Child can pay attention or focus for 15 minutes or more.
Parent supports child's own strategies for recovering from distress.	Child can use imitation to deal with, and recover from, distress.

Potential Negative Contributions to Dysregulation (Risk Factors for Load Conditions)

Parent	Child
Parent is rigid or permissive in limit setting, with too much structure, too much chaos, or a lack of involvement.	Child responds to appropriate limit setting with avoidance, aggression, or rote compliance.
Parent is constricted and repetitive in play, using the same themes over and over again (e.g., always wants play to be happy; does not tolerate any aggression or assertiveness during child's play).	Child is repetitive and perseverates with the same constricted themes in play (e.g., only slamming cars into each other or only lining up cars in a row).
Parent is controlling and always takes the lead, using constricted themes of play, and reacting with aggression if play does not go according to parent's desire.	Child insists on always taking the lead and reacts with aggression or distress if play does not exactly follow his or her plan.
Parent is intrusive, randomly changes the emotional play themes, and does not support child's play.	Child impulsively changes emotional themes or activities during play, randomly moving from item to item.
Parent withdraws and does not support a child's play or exploration; participates in a limited number of circles of communication (one to five).	Child opens and closes a limited number circles of communication (one to five), appearing withdrawn.
Parent is anxious or overprotective and does not support the child's play.	Child is anxious and clinging, refusing to engage in play.

Note. From material in "Assessing the Emotional and Social Functioning of Infants and Young Children," by S. I. Greenspan, 1996, in *New Visions for the Developmental Assessment of Infants and Young Children,* by S. J. Meisels and E. Fenichel (Eds.), Washington, DC: ZERO TO THREE. Adapted with permission of ZERO TO THREE. Also from material in *The Functional Emotional Assessment Scale (FEAS) for Infancy and Early Childhood: Clinical and Research Applications* by S. I. Greenspan, G. A. DeGangi, and S. Wieder, 2001, Bethesda, MD: Interdisciplinary Council on Developmental and Learning Disorders. Adapted with permission of Dr. S. I. Greenspan.

Considering Milestone 4 in the Context of the Neurorelational Framework

Under conditions of healthy development, the alert processing window expands for longer periods of time (regulation), making possible more complex circles of communication. If the infant has achieved stable regulation, a tolerance for sensations (sensory), and an ongoing ability to gain pleasure from an intimate relationship with the parent, then that infant's sense of joy becomes an internal factor that motivates purposeful motor movement (executive). The child's ability for initiating purposeful movement (i.e., moving toward what is relevant to him or her) signals the increasing links forming between the relevance and executive systems. For example, the child can experience increasing delight through exploring his or her surroundings and sharing that joy with a parent. In addition, the child can now begin to initiate simple problem-solving actions in response to his or her own distress by signaling the need for a parent's help (an example of early cause–effect reasoning).

A complex interplay now emerges between the relevance and executive systems. Will this infant, who is blossoming into toddlerhood, continue to build on pleasurable experiences of shared joy and the ability to communicate the need for help? Or will this child experience increasingly prominent states of dysregulation, combined with emotional distress, without being able to find ways to engage the parent in recovery and problem solving? If unresolved or unattended vulnerabilities remain within the regulation, sensory, or relevance systems, the motor elements of the executive system will also be affected. Of course, motor elements can bring their own vulnerabilities to the child (e.g., weak muscle tone, postural instability, or poor motor planning skills). (See CD-ROM Section 3.4 for a summary table listing the contributions of each brain system to this fourth socioemotional milestone.)

Joseph and Rachel: Complex Gestures and Problem Solving

Joseph continues to focus on his own world of mechanical toys; increasingly, his relevance system has limited experience with circles of communication and relational joy to reference. His behaviors of either avoiding his mother or protesting her intrusions have become entrenched patterns between the two of them, even at his young age. (What a difference early intervention would have made!) Rachel feels alarmed at being shut out; this feeling resonates with her in significant relationships with men. Strategies of withdrawal and opposition are becoming automatic defensive maneuvers between both of them, precluding the building of warm engagement.

Joseph's gestural and verbal systems are not used for relational problem solving. He cries when frustrated, collapsing into a rage rather than signaling the source of his upset. His lack of trust in his mother around problem-solving issues reflects the absence of pleasurable experiences in the relationship. However, Joseph also brings a weak motor system to this expanding problem, a motor system that does not advance his communication signals. If intervention were to begin during this phase, where would the practitioner or team of practitioners begin? As the child gets older, problems often occur when practitioners start interventions at a developmental level that is beyond the child's current status. Beginning at too advanced a level when earlier socioemotional milestones are so shaky can lead to more frustrations for all parties involved. A better approach is to begin the intervention at the earliest level at which the breakdown began, which the neurorelational framework calls a bottom-up approach. In this case, the first goals of treatment are to build on Joseph's sensory and emotional signals of pleasure and to help Rachel join him there, using his sensory preferences to support his regulation. In turn, pleasurable activities can be used as a reinforcing context in which Joseph can be taught various gesturing signs (e.g., simple sign language).

What sensory experiences enhance Joseph's sense of pleasure and joy and optimize his state of arousal? How can Rachel participate in these experiences, which also provide opportunities for sensory–motor connections between them? We now have another avenue through which to build regulation and engagement. Experimentation takes place; we discover that Joseph loves to swing and that placing him in a swing calms him down. To prevent possible auditory overloads, Rachel does not talk. Not having to defend against the sound of her voice, Joseph has more energy to glance at her face when swinging. They quietly make eye contact, and she smiles. With support from the therapist, Rachel is encouraged simply to make eye contact without initiating any other form of stimulation. A visual connection has begun for brief moments, offering hope that this simple, yet powerful beginning can expand.

Milestone 5: Use of Symbols to Express Thoughts and Feelings

As the rhythm and rate of word production increases, so does the ability to enact everyday life events through playing with toys and dolls. Feeding the baby doll or animal, soothing the baby, putting the baby to sleep, and talking on the phone are daily life activities that are enacted by playing alone or with Mommy or Daddy. As this type of play interaction becomes more sophisticated, the dolls, superheroes, or puppets begin to mirror the

child's emotions—sad or happy or mad—usually through fleeting expressions that may not have a full story to them but that can be "represented" through the child's (or parent's) voice, words, or facial expressions. The ability to put two words together often emerges at about the age of 2 years, when verbalized wishes and intentions, such as "me toy" or "want milk," and feelings, such as "me mad" or "me hurt," debut (Greenspan, 1996).

The emerging ability to connect words to bodily states establishes a link between visceral connections and emotions. As states of arousal are linked with a positive or negative valence, we experience emotions. Identifying bodily states such as hunger and pain (negative experiences) or satiety and pain relief (positive experiences) is the precursor to recognizing and naming emotional states. Again, if the bottom-up experiences of pain, hunger, thirst, and bladder and bowel pressure are not recognized or registered, it may be harder for a child to identify emotions later. During this phase, a range of emotional states and themes is desirable. Ideally, the joy from mutual engagement in the earlier phases has created a solid foundation of attachment. Closeness, dependency, pleasure, and excitement with humor are core themes that practitioners want to observe in the pretend life of the child. However, to have a full emotional range, emotional expressions need to include verbal representations of assertiveness, anger, cautious behavior, boundary enforcement (e.g., pretending to say "no" to a doll), and recovering from distress. These should be included in a similar repertoire of positive expressions.

Behavioral Markers for Milestone 5

Table 3.5 presents the behavioral markers for the use of symbols to express thoughts and feelings as the fifth socioemotional milestone (Greenspan, 1996; Greenspan, DeGangi, & Wieder, 2001).

Table 3.5. Parent–Child Behavioral Markers for Use of Symbols to Express Thoughts and Feelings

Parent	Child (observable between 18 and 30 months)
Positive Contributions to Health (Coordination)	
Parent uses nonverbal and verbal forms of communication through eyes, facial expressions, sounds or verbalizations, gestures, and body movement to promote 10 or more sequential circles of communication in a continuous flow.	Child uses nonverbal and verbal forms of communication through eyes, facial expressions, sounds or verbalizations, gestures, and body movement to reciprocate and promote 10 or more sequential circles of communication in a continuous flow.

(Continued)

Table 3.5. Continued

Parent	Child (observable between 18 and 30 months)
Parent tracks child's nonverbal clues that link with appropriate signals for simple problem solving.	Child tracks parent's cues and participates in simple problem solving.
Parent encourages child's engagement in symbolic play by combining play materials (baby doll, bottle, and bath tub) for that purpose.	Child engages in symbolic play with various toys, going beyond enacting daily life activities of feeding, sleeping, and bathing.
Parent encourages child's engagement in symbolic play by modeling.	Child imitates parental modeling.
Parent shows comfort with make-believe play.	Child enjoys pretend play.
Parent elaborates on child's pretend play by adding complexity to existing theme.	Child can expand play theme.
Parent gives child freedom to express themes of nurturance and dependency without being competitive for nurturance.	Child shows needs for nurturance and dependency and incorporates these needs into play.
Parent sustains pretend play through nonverbal means (e.g., smiling and laughing).	Child shows pleasure through nonverbal means.
Parent sustains pretend play through verbal means (e.g., commenting on how funny something is or what a good idea the child has and by asking questions for elaboration, such as "What happens next?").	Child creates pretend play of two themes that are not logically related or logically connected.
Parent allows child to express themes of assertiveness through pretend play (e.g., putting parent in jail or having parent stay home while child pretends to go to work).	Child uses pretend play to communicate wishes, needs, feelings, and intentions.
Parent supports play themes of closeness and dependency, assertiveness and curiosity, aggression, autonomy, pleasure and excitement, cautiousness or fearfulness, limit setting, and recovery from distress.	Child uses pretend play or words to display at least one idea from any of the following emotional themes during play with parent: closeness or dependency, pleasure and excitement in the context of humor, assertiveness and exploration, cautiousness or fearfulness, anger, limit setting, and recovery from distress.
When playing, parent expands and elaborates on what child is doing while remaining on the child's topic.	Child can focus or pay attention for 30 minutes or more.

(Continued)

Table 3.5   Continued

Parent	Child (observable between 18 and 30 months)
Parent expansion includes providing a challenge or an interesting dimension to the play that requires from the child a slightly different or new response from previous playtimes.	Child uses pretend play and language to respond to a parent's expansion of a theme or play by also creating a new response or different outcome to a familiar aspect to the story.
Parent allows child to assert self in play.	Child uses pretend play to express theme of assertiveness. Child allows parent to take the lead at times during play.
Parent sets appropriate limits or redirects the child.	Child responds to setting of limits and redirection by parent.
Parent allows child to often take the lead during play.	Child allows parent to take the lead at times during play.

Potential Negative Contributions to Dysregulation (Risk Factors for Load Conditions)

Parent	Child
Parent is either permissive without setting up a structure, or overly harsh and punitive with too much rigidity, or oscillates between these extremes (chaos/rigidity: from too permissive/ neglectful to too harsh/abusive).	Child responds to appropriate limit setting with avoidance, aggression, or rote compliance.
Parent only allows certain themes and constricts the play (e.g., always avoiding angry themes).	Child is repetitive and perseverates with the same constricted themes in play (e.g., always showing angry themes).
Parent breaks the flow of playing with child by being intrusive or hostile.	Child insists on always taking the lead and reacts with aggression or distress if play does not exactly follow his or her plan.
Parent breaks the flow of child's play or exploration by withdrawing or does not initiate play (e.g., indifferent).	Child shows indifference to playing with parent.
Parent's anxiety or overprotectiveness breaks the flow of playing with child.	Child is anxious and/or clinging, refusing to engage in play.
Parent breaks the flow of a child's play or exploration by playing at a level far above child's level of competence.	NA
Parent does not show pleasure or excitement in child's play or exploration.	Child does not show any pleasure or delight during playtime with parent.
Parent shows partial pleasure or excitement through a limited number of circles of communication (6–10 circles) during an interaction.	Child opens and closes a limited number of circles of communication (6–10 circles) during an interaction.

(*Continued*)

Table 3.5   Continued

Parent	Child (observable between 18 and 30 months)
Parent is distractible and impulsively interrupts play by randomly introducing new items or themes.	Child impulsively changes emotional themes or activities during play, randomly moving from item to item.

Note. From material in "Assessing the Emotional and Social Functioning of Infants and Young Children," by S. I. Greenspan, 1996, in *New Visions for the Developmental Assessment of Infants and Young Children,* by S. J. Meisels and E. Fenichel (Eds.), Washington, DC: ZERO TO THREE. Adapted with permission of ZERO TO THREE. Also from material in *The Functional Emotional Assessment Scale (FEAS) for Infancy and Early Childhood: Clinical and Research Applications* by S. I. Greenspan, G. A. DeGangi, and S. Wieder, 2001, Bethesda, MD: Interdisciplinary Council on Developmental and Learning Disorders. Adapted with permission of Dr. S. I. Greenspan.

Considering Milestone 5 in the Context of the Neurorelational Framework

At this juncture, we see the emergence of strong connections between bottom-up (regulation and sensation) and top-down (relevance and executive) functions. The interactions involved here focus on organizing meaningful experiences, both positive and negative in valence, into nonverbal (sensory experiences of sounds, sights, touch, etc.) and verbal expressions containing dialogue. The sequential aspects of coordinating emotional themes require executive functions (e.g., cause–effect reasoning, temporal integration) that link the details of past experiences (memory—relevance system) with meaningful emotional themes (emotions—relevance system) in a conversational, two-way flow. Creating sequential events within a simple story line (e.g., baby ate, had a bath, and went to bed feeling happy and safe) demonstrates the capacity for expressing emotional themes through symbolic means.

The emergence of the child's ability to move beyond daily life activities into more active emotional themes is also an important transition. There may be a smooth transition from the daily activity involved in feeding and putting the pretend baby to sleep to expressing closeness and pleasure in that scenario. The expression of closeness and pleasure through symbolic play is a very important feature, just as mutual engagement and attachment were important during the first few months of life. However, it may be more difficult for the child to expand his or her verbal or pretend play into a pretend character who can be angry about not being first or who can be fearful of the fire that comes out of a pretend dragon's mouth. These more negatively valenced themes may be more uncomfortable for either the parent or the child. In fact, at times, the parent may have more difficulty participating comfortably in this type of emotional play than the child.

(Indeed, either partner may have more of a struggle at any one time in one of these socioemotional milestones than the other partner.)

The nonverbal sensory aspects of this type of play are integral to the accurate portrayal of emotional themes (relevance system). Sensory experiences include the nonverbal visual expressions, sounds, and movements that are made as one character creates sounds, words, faces, or movement to match pretend scenarios; for example, crying when hungry, squealing with excitement when splashing in a bath, smiling when rocked to sleep, scowling in anger when being left out, and opening eyes wide in fright when facing a character who looks scary. Here the sensory aspects of emotions are enacted within the play zone. Ideally, emotional occurrences in real life are now reenacted between parent and child during play. Sensory expressions make the play come alive; without them, the characters remain lifeless or inaccurately represent the targeted emotional experience (e.g., representing a character who is sad or mad for being left out by showing a face with no expression does little to communicate what the character is feeling).

Of course, any stress patterns that predominate within a parent–child dyad reduce the likelihood that the pair will be able to create simple emotional themes together in a continuous flow. Instead, the pair's typical stress responses will predominate in the play and be expressed in some way. (See CD-ROM Section 3.5 for a summary table listing the contributions of each brain system to this fifth socioemotional milestone.)

Joseph and Rachel: Use of Symbols to Express Thoughts and Feelings

As time progresses, stress patterns are now typical between Joseph and Rachel. They hardly play together, and Joseph's symbolic play mainly consists of lining up cars or trucks and then banging them into one another in a repetitive mode. He does not fantasize about their having special powers or taking on an emotional theme with the banging. The crashing of the cars holds interest and excitement for him at face value. Rachel does not know how to join in this repetitive and seemingly "utterly boring" play. Things are "okay" at preschool—only a few isolated incidents of aggression out on the playground and a concern that he is not paying as much attention as he needs to have been reported. Nothing is prompting alarm at this point. These complaints are minor and are not consistent enough to warrant further probing by the preschool teacher.

A practitioner who intervenes at this level might have Rachel take a toy car and actually begin crashing it into Joseph's car. If Joseph loves this interaction, then there is all the more reason that this activity may serve as

a point of connection. If all of his collected cars are kept in a box or sack, then Rachel could take them out and hand them one by one to Joseph, facilitating eye contact during this interchange. Over time, perhaps the cars that crash can make sounds together or have a race with each other. Play could gently expand to driving the cars to a joint location and, eventually, taking on passengers who exchange simple verbal conversations. Later on, the car might become tired and need a nap or become hungry and need some gas or get hurt from the crashing and need a doctor to take a look. As passengers take more of a prominent place in the story, they might take on more emotional tones. The slow but steady expansion of symbolic play from repetitive to interactive play would be on its way.

Keep in mind, however, that in our last intervention, we left Joseph in the swing, just beginning to tolerate only eye contact and no other sensory input from Rachel. We need to realize that although the symbolic car play described here may become interactive with enough support and creative experiments in engaging Joseph in his own world of relevance at this age level, we still must attend to the issues with these earlier milestones.

So, back in the swing, we find that Joseph also loves sucking on his pacifier and having blankets piled on top of him. We are slowly discovering his three favorite forms of sensory input: vestibular (swing), oral–motor (pacifier), and deep touch pressure (heavy blankets). Now regulation can occur with rhythmic repetition as he is calmed by swinging, sucking, and deep pressure against his body (sensory system). In addition, mutual engagement and attachment can occur when Rachel narrows her input of sensations to intermittent, playful eye contact with smiles; in this context, Rachel and Joseph might also begin to play peek-a-boo. These earlier milestones cannot be left behind, even if the current milestone is opening up; the earlier relational underpinnings are still weak and must be addressed.

While in the swing, as Joseph is relaxing and beginning to experience warm relational pleasure with his mother, Rachel might eventually add words. Because he loves cars, he may respond to the metaphor of his body being an engine, for example, "Is your tank full? When is your 'engine' running 'just right?'" (Williams & Shellenberger, 1996, pp. 2–6)? "Are you zooming too fast? Can you slow down? Are you going too slow?" Describing his engine as calm and "just right" might offer a way for him to begin to associate words with his relaxed body state. Later on, his verbal capacities can be expanded to include his use of this metaphor ("engine") to express a general bodily state (e.g., running fast, slow, or just right) as well as various emotional valences (e.g., happy, sad, or mad). This type of layering—of working on more than one developmental milestone at a time—is crucial with older children who have multiple constrictions across the milestones.

Milestone 6: Bridging Emotional Themes

With maturity comes movement from simple to more complex story lines that involve a more elaborate range of emotions. Pretend play can be extremely unrealistic, yet very real emotions can be expressed through this medium. During this developmental phase, the reasons behind being sad or happy or mad or scared in the play have a connection to some form of human emotional reality. The dragon puppet is scary because he has a red tongue and his face looks mean; he wants to bite because he is hungry, and he steals a baby to eat. The hero is mad at the mean dragon who took away the baby, and the hero is going to save the day by getting the baby back to his or her parents. Mommy and Daddy are worried and looking for their baby, and the happy ending is that the baby and parents find each other and are reunited with the hero's help. They have a celebration when they are safely reunited. This simple story line has multiple emotional themes within it: danger, meanness, anxiety, fear, safety, kindness, and joy, to name a few. The story has rhyme and reason to it. By asking the "who, why, what, where, and how" questions, the parent or professional can help the child begin to make cause–effect links between the emotions described in the story and the characters' actions. These understandings, in turn, can begin to generalize to real-life situations.

More mature sequences of emotional events are contained in stories encountered during school years, wherein characters are often confronted by an emotional dilemma to solve. Adult versions of this level of emotional development include elaborations of one's complex emotional self, the ability for abstract thinking, and the processing of conflict in intimate relationships.

Behavioral Markers for Milestone 6

Table 3.6 presents the behavioral markers for bridges between symbols and emotional ideas (Greenspan, 1996; Greenspan, DeGangi, & Wieder, 2001).

Considering Milestone 6 in the Context of the Neurorelational Framework

Assuming that regulation and sensory systems are functioning well, a young child can interact with focused attention (regulation and executive systems), using all sensory modalities (i.e., touch, sound, sight, movement, deep-touch pressure) with his or her parent in building emotional stories. For example, the same dragon character might feel bad later for stealing this family's baby and express sadness about how he frightened the family, driven by his impulsive haste while hungry. The dragon apologizes

Table 3.6. Parent–Child Behavioral Markers for Bridging Emotional Themes

Parent	Child (observable between 30 and 48 months)
Positive Contributions to Health (Coordination)	
Parent uses nonverbal and verbal forms of communication through eyes, facial expressions, sounds or words, gestures, and body movement to promote an ongoing flow of circles of communication in the play medium.	Child uses nonverbal and verbal forms of communication through eyes, facial expressions, sounds or verbalizations, gestures, and body movement to reciprocate and promote an ongoing flow of circles of communication in the play medium.
Parent elaborates on child's pretend play, giving depth to the drama by asking who, where, what, how, why, or when questions.	Child shows a planned quality to the story line and can elaborate on when, how, and why questions.
If child strays off topic, parent asks questions to help make bridges back to the pretend play theme (e.g., "What happened to the alligator? He was hungry and going to eat the fish, and now, you are playing with a superhero").	Child allows parent to take the lead at times during play.
Parent assists child in incorporating causality into pretend play themes by asking reality-based questions (e.g., "How come the alligator is so mad now? Did he get his feelings hurt by Superman?").	Child can respond to inquiries by making cause–effect links between events and emotional outcomes.
Parent helps expand and elaborate a wide range of emotional themes, building on others that now include assertiveness, pleasure and excitement, fearfulness, anger, separation and loss, and empathy.	Child can both initiate and build on parent's contribution to an emotional theme. Child uses pretend play or language to communicate two or more emotional themes at a time. Child creates themes of closeness and dependency, pleasure and excitement in the context of humor, and assertiveness. Child's themes expand to include separation and loss, love, and empathy.
Parent supports and guides emotional problem-solving experiences through emotional themes.	Child proposes creative, problem-solving ideas when expressing emotional themes.
Parent is comfortable with a wide range of emotional themes and shows no discomfort or intrusion in the child's expressions.	Child can tolerate exploring vulnerable feelings of shame, embarrassment, jealousy, and envy during playtimes.

(Continued)

Table 3.6. Continued

Parent	Child (observable between 30 and 48 months)
Parent sets appropriate limits or redirects the child.	Child responds to parental setting of limits and redirection by parent.
When child is upset, parent tracks the process, allowing the child space or offering sensory or emotional comfort until recovery to baseline has occurred.	When upset, child can use a combination of self- and interactive regulation strategies to recover back to baseline. Child can set limits for self by reasoning about consequences.

Potential Negative Contributions to Dysregulation (Risk Factors for Load Conditions)

Parent does not show pleasure or delight during playtime with child.	Child does not show pleasure or delight during playtime with parent.
Parent stays within constricted themes, such as primarily expressing positive or negative emotions without the full range.	Child perseverates on the same constricted themes in play (e.g., only playing with the same theme or scripted lines from a story line or movie such as Peter Pan, Cinderella).
Parent intrudes during playtime with child by reacting aggressively or hostilely to child's expressions of an emotional theme.	Child insists on always taking the lead and reacts with aggression or distress if play does not exactly follow his or her plan.
Parent is overly hostile in discipline and punishment of child. Or, parent is overly accommodating of child.	Child responds to appropriate limit setting with avoidance, aggression, or rote compliance.
Parent's anxiety intrudes during playtime with child and diverts attention away from expanding child's theme.	Child is anxious and withdrawn, unable to participate in play.
Parent withdraws or dissociates during playtime with child.	Child is shut down with glazed eyes, not connecting to the parent or play.
Parent impulsively changes emotional themes or activities during play or is easily distracted.	Child impulsively changes emotional themes or activities during play, randomly moving from item to item.

Note. From material in "Assessing the Emotional and Social Functioning of Infants and Young Children," by S. I. Greenspan, 1996, in *New Visions for the Developmental Assessment of Infants and Young Children,* by S. J. Meisels and E. Fenichel (Eds.), Washington, DC: ZERO TO THREE. Adapted with permission of ZERO TO THREE. Also from material in *The Functional Emotional Assessment Scale (FEAS) for Infancy and Early Childhood: Clinical and Research Applications* by S. I. Greenspan, G. A. DeGangi, and S. Wieder, 2001, Bethesda, MD: Interdisciplinary Council on Developmental and Learning Disorders. Adapted with permission of Dr. S. I. Greenspan.

and, over time, joins forces with the hero by flying over the city to help find some bad guys who are trying to rob the same family of its secret jewels. The dragon catches the bad guys, blows fire on them, and the bad guys have to go to hospital jail, where a doctor takes care of their wounds.

Characters can now express more than one meaning and both positive and negative valences.

At this milestone we see a wider range of negative and vulnerable emotional experiences in the stories integrated with a positive baseline: themes of anger, fear, embarrassment, disappointment, loss, and the capacity for empathy are expanded. The emerging ability to elaborate on several emotional themes that link cause and effect (e.g., a new baby is cause for jealous feelings) relies heavily on the overlap between the relevance and executive systems. The sequencing and planning of a story line that holds coherent meaning are akin to the steps involved in motor sequencing, planning, and action. Children who are impulsive in their attention (executive system) or do not make meaningful emotional connections (relevance and executive system) will have trouble creating a coherent story. Helping children structure or sequence the telling or enactment of an emotional story is a top-down strategy. Inherent in any story is a problem or crisis in need of resolution. This is as true for a 3- or 4-year-old's story as it is for adult literature. The problem portrayed in any pretend story offers a key opportunity for intervention: how does the child or parent relate to a character who is sad, mad, happy, jealous, bullying, shy, embarrassed, or frightened by us or with us? Daily life dilemmas among parents, children, siblings, friends, and "bad guys"—even among various aspects within oneself (e.g., the kind self versus the mean self)—have an opportunity to be expressed through the medium of play. A 3-year-old encountering a character who is having a temper tantrum in the story (just like the way the child happens to act at home) has an opportunity, with the help of the therapist or parent, to solve the "problem." This experience can be a pleasurable one that, indeed, enhances self- and interactive regulation; with the parent or therapist's guidance, the child uses words to sequence the steps needed to regulate the character with the tantrum. Encouraging problem-solving skills, which support the further development of the executive system, can become an integrated part of the creative play ("What can this character do next time to not get so upset?") and can help build skills for anticipating distress and managing it via new options in the future.

Notice that nonverbal and sensory aspects (sensory system) of how emotions are communicated (eyes, faces, vocal tone and rhythms, gestures, and movements) remain integral to the child's emerging ability to both express emotions and read them in others (relevance system). The more a parent embraces a full range of emotions within the real parent–child relationship, the more likely the child will be able to rehearse, enact, and experiment with those emotions through play. The more constricted the range of emotional expression in a family system, the more likely it is that the child's expressions of emotions will be constricted during play.

Parents who are uncomfortable with particular emotions will probably bring intrusions or constrictions into the play space. Conversely, children with physiological and learning challenges will likely bring restrictions that will need assistance.

The use of temporal integration (the use of past, present, and future) and sequencing (executive system) allows the child to apply a theme from one story in one week to another theme in the creation of a new story 8 days later. The executive system as a whole supports the child's efforts to elaborate emotional themes into coherent stories that have a beginning, middle, and end. Flexible interaction across all brain systems supports the spontaneous and creative expansion of emotional themes into new and different twists and turns. (See CD-ROM Section 3.6 for a summary table listing the contributions of each brain system to this sixth socioemotional milestone.)

Joseph and Rachel: Bridging Emotional Themes

Interventions that involve Milestone 6 can build on those begun in Milestone 5. As Joseph shifts from crashing cars to tolerating the presence of passengers (Milestone 5), the passengers can begin to develop real-life emotions as the practitioner's and Rachel's characters include a variety of different emotional expressions through facial movements, vocal tones, and gestures. The passengers might share names and end up as neighbors. The characters decide that they are friends and visit each other's home (perhaps made out of blocks or Lincoln Logs). Over time, emotional themes shift from positive to negative to positive valences, or vice versa. Soon, two neighbors become jealous of their neighbor's new car and decide to have a race to see which car runs the fastest. The winner (perhaps Joseph) might have to "help" the other two friends with their sadness or jealousy about not winning. If Joseph doesn't offer any help, the practitioner's character can jump in with empathy to comfort the others, modeling a responsive reaction that facilitates emotional recovery. In these imagined scenarios, we can see the flow of many positive and negative emotional themes (relevance system) being enacted with a beginning, middle, and end sequence that also links cause with effect (executive system). Joseph's interest in cars is now much more involved, and themes of friendship, nurturance, competitiveness, jealousy, disappointment, loss, recovery, and compassion become intertwined with meaning as characters take on real-life emotional reactions through the ebb and flow of play (more on emotional themes in the relevance system).

However, without that sort of intervention, by the time Joseph matures through this developmental period and approaches the age of 5 years, he has accumulated a cascading array of difficulties that now extend into his daily school life. Gone are the days of intermittent concerns during

the earlier years at preschool. Alarms are going off on all levels. Teachers complain that he does not listen or pay attention when he is not interested in the subject matter, and he is either combative or isolating himself on the playground.

Rachel's attempts to respond appropriately to Joseph have failed. Now, confronted with his vicious temper tantrums, she tries to implement a behavioral modification plan she has seen on a popular television show, instituting time-outs. Over time, however, Joseph's behavior does not improve with time-outs. Instead, he becomes more cruel and then violent toward his siblings. Having a lay person's limited understanding of negative reinforcement, Rachel slowly increases his time-outs to where they last up to 1 hour at a time. His continued defiance and lack of regulation control provoke Rachel to revoke further privileges from him, including dinner. His rageful and violent behavior causes Rachel to lock her son in his room during these episodes to prevent dangerous outcomes, such as breaking fragile objects and leaving shards of cut glass everywhere.

When Joseph gets into treatment at this age, he uses pretend play to put his therapist into time-outs every session, locking the door and throwing away the key. He screams and yells at the therapist that she has to stay in there "for a long, long time." Every time she asks whether she can come out, he ragefully insists that she must remain in her room without dinner or dessert. The therapist's first assessment and working hypothesis is that of a traumatic-type response because Joseph demonstrates the type of constrictive and repetitive play scenario that often accompanies traumatized children's reenactment of their experiences. Rachel admits that things have been out of control, but she explains that had she not enforced the behavioral measures she learned on television, Joseph would have harmed himself, her, or his siblings. Using a strength-based therapeutic approach (Bernstein, Hans, & Percansky, 1991; McDonough, 1995, 2000, 2004) the therapist supports Rachel's need to protect herself and the other siblings from Joseph's rages; she also explains that this is a critical situation that needs immediate attention and that they can experiment together to find new ways to help Joseph. Rachel is more than willing to learn and take direction, and she and the therapist establish a learning relationship where they share their observations. Slowly, with a bottom-up approach, Rachel and the therapist begin to find (1) sensory ways to soothe and engage Joseph, (2) words for his emotions, (3) alternate ways for him to express his rage, and (4) ways for him to begin to care for himself and others.

Chapter 1 listed a range of possible diagnostic categories that a practitioner might identify for Joseph and Rachel:

- a possible trauma response for Joseph, related to a poor connection with his mother;

- regulatory and sensorimotor processing problems for Joseph;
- a mood component of anxiety, depression, and anger for both Joseph and Rachel;
- an attentional, executive problem for Joseph;
- an autistic spectrum disorder or Asperger syndrome for Joseph;
- a lack of proper parenting skills;
- a painful relational history for Rachel, highlighting disappointment and loss;
- a relational/attachment problem (in the parent–child dyad);
- a marital problem (for the couple).

In fact, Joseph and Rachel now suffer from every one of these diagnostic categories; his primary diagnosis is listed as Asperger syndrome. As the treatment unfolds and the therapist begins to work through the turmoil both Joseph and Rachel have endured and stimulated within each other—albeit through well-meaning intentions and the common wisdom within our parenting culture—each one of these diagnostic labels becomes clinically relevant. Although holding in mind multiple diagnostic categories is certainly an option for organizing one's clinical judgment, seeing the underlying contributions from the four brain systems to each diagnosis may provide greater clinical clarity.

The discussion in this chapter points to the salient need for early intervention, well within Joseph's first year of life, as a viable way to have minimized the repercussions of his early symptoms and conditions. For example, even given his Asperger syndrome, Joseph could have made much more progress developmentally, and Rachel's frustration and sadness could have been greatly diminished. The clinical discussion in Chapter 2 focused on the four neurorelational brain systems as they applied to Joseph and Rachel. The integration of those brain systems and intervention strategies within the six socioemotional milestones presented in this chapter allow us to see the power of using a brain-based approach to assessment and intervention right from the start.

Additional resources on socioemotional milestones include the following texts:

- Axis V in DC:0–3R (ZERO TO THREE, 2005);
- Greenspan's (1996) chapter, "Assessing the Emotional and Social Functioning of Infants and Young Children," in *New Visions for the Assessment of Infants and Young Children;*
- Greenspan (1999), *Building Healthy Minds;*
- Greenspan and Wieder (1998), *The Child With Special Needs;*

- Greenspan, DeGangi, and Wieder's (2001) clinical and research versions of the FEAS, in *The Functional Emotional Assessment Scale (FEAS) for Infancy and Early Childhood: Clinical and Research Applications;*
- Interdisciplinary Council of Developmental and Learning Disorders (ICDL) Web site: www.icdl.com

THE USE OF INTERPERSONAL MODES IN THE NEURORELATIONAL FRAMEWORK

During the 1970s, the emotional styles of behavior emerged as a personality theory from the Family Studies department at Michigan State University. Three simple yet intuitively meaningful styles were presented as the "head, heart, and hand" rubric, in which individual and interpersonal ways of relating could be classified. The *heart* is oriented toward the use of emotions and feeling, the *hand* is oriented toward the use of actions and doing, and the *head* is oriented toward the use of thoughts and thinking. The predecessors of this heuristic can be found in the three philosophical traditions of humanism (heart), empiricism (hand), and rationalism (head) that can also be seen as underlying three predominant trends in psychological theories: humanistic, behavioral, and cognitive (Dobbs, 2000). This heuristic has shown up in many formats over the centuries. Its components are not new; if anything, they keep reappearing in new formats,[1] but are deeply rooted in how we understand ourselves and our relationships with others.

One more recent format comes in the form of an empirically based research instrument—the Strength Deployment Inventory (SDI)—used to investigate the motivational styles of 516 interdisciplinary health care professionals over a 10-year period. The researchers measured the fluctuations between three personality constructs of altruistic-nurturing (which we correlate with heart), assertive-directive (hand), and analytic-autonomizing (head) designed "to help individuals identify their motives in relating to others under two kinds of conditions: when everything is going well in their relationships and when they are in conflict with others" (Drinka, Miller, & Goodman, 1996, p. 51). Similarly, we use this heuristic to help individuals and professionals identify their interpersonal modes under conditions of safety, challenge, and threat.

The neurorelational framework views the head, heart, and hand metaphor as applicable to multiple contexts: from individual ways of being in the world, to parenting modes that promote development, to varying therapeutic approaches to children and families, and to interdisciplinary team dynamics. Within each of these contexts, the healthy versions of this

triad support coordination, whereas the unhealthy versions support conditions of load. To convey added nuances of relational characteristics, we use the terms of *respond* (heart), *direct* (hand), and *reflect* (head) to differentiate the coordination versions of the triad, and we use the terms *overaccommodate, demand,* and *detach* to convey the potential load versions of these three interpersonal modes of relating.

We begin with the underlying premise that there is "purpose or motive behind all behavior" (Drinka et al., 1996, p. 51), and we emphasize the powerful early linkages between the emotional (relevance) and motor (executive) systems. When newborns move their eyes and head, as they turn toward or away from others, they are expressing emotional-action tendencies. As development of the motor system progresses into crawling and walking, these emotional-action tendencies become even more pronounced (during socioemotional Milestone 4) and gradually develop into interpersonal modes of relating (Horney, 1945, 1950).

The neurorelational framework emphasizes the early beginnings of three modes of interpersonal behavior that are healthy and become automatic with repetition (see Figure 3.1).

Practitioners might ask the following assessment questions:

- Does an infant-toddler naturally move toward others, initiating emotional connections even when upset?
- When upset with others, does the infant-toddler "stand up to them" by crying or protesting vocally?
- Does the infant-toddler physically and emotionally withdraw from others when upset for a short period of time, wanting to be left alone?

In older children, adolescents, and adults, when these interactional modes become rigid (overused) or chaotic, they can become maladaptive, as indicated in Figure 3.2. These more extreme behaviors are discussed in later chapters.

The following paragraphs introduce the coordination version of the respond, direct, and reflect modes of interpersonal behavior as they relate to the clinical context in the neurorelational framework. Interventions can be seen as promoting different types of learning as exemplified in the interpersonal modes of behavior. The neurorelational framework makes equal use of all three modes. The respond approach to intervention values learning through emotions, which includes any type of engaging and nurturing (Ammen & Limberg, 2005; Jernberg & Booth, 1999); mirroring and empathy (for building a positive therapeutic alliance, McDonough, 2000; for transforming internal representations, Lieberman,

Emotionally engages with others	Emotionally stands up to others	Emotionally withdraws from others

Figure 3.1. Precursors to the respond, direct, and reflect interpersonal modes that support coordination.

Overly accommodates and relies on others or anxiously controls others	Overly opposes and demands from others	Overly detached from others

Figure 3.2. Three interpersonal modes of behavior that can contribute to conditions of load.

1991; Lieberman, Silverman, & Pawl, 2000; Lieberman, Weston, & Pawl, 1991; and for building connections and collaboration, Downing, 2008); and validation or active listening (Faber & Mazlish, 2002) one gives to an individual or family. When these skills are modeled and demonstrated, they can be learned through imitation. The neurorelational framework emphasizes the importance of establishing a strong therapeutic alliance as the basis for connecting with families. Such an alliance is maintained throughout the course of treatment with both child and parents. Someone whose personality orientation is based on the responsive approach would be comfortable expressing warmth and empathy and would prefer compromising in conflict; in general, he or she would prefer to seek harmonizing relationships in responding to everyday situations in life (Dobbs, 2000).

The direct approach values learning through doing or action and includes any procedure one applies to the child and family, including structuring and challenging (Ammen & Limberg, 2005; Jernberg & Booth, 1999); coaching (Wieder & Greenspan, 2005); directing, dramatic play, role-play, social skills (Mesibov, 1984; Rogers, 2000); and context and skill-building remediation (Hinckley, Patterson, & Carr, 2001; Johnson, 2004). Often, remediation techniques for learning speech and language, motor, social, relational skills, and so on, follow a continuum: At one end they can be process oriented, interactive, and following the child's personal interests (constructivist remediation); at the other end they can be teacher-led, product-oriented, noninteractive, and highly prearranged (instructionist remediation) (Johnson, 2004). This range within types of interventions can also include approaches to medical procedures. The phrase "the action is in the interaction" (Shahmoon-Shanok, 2000, p. 333) captures the emphasis of the neurorelational framework on learning through experiences. If the parents have the flexibility to learn through coaching or modeling, then the interpersonal domain, via play, can be used as the active relational medium through which change is fostered. "Doing" in

the form of "playing" is a child's language (Frost, Wortham, & Reifel, 2001), regardless of the skill being learned (e.g., motor, sensory, emotional, educational capacities), and it is the medium through which constricted interpersonal modes can also be altered (Greenspan & Wieder, 1998). By having the parent present and working within the context of the dyad, the professional can help parent and child shift interpersonal patterns at the same time important functional skills are being learned (e.g., speech and language, motor, reading). Someone whose personality orientation is toward the directive approach would be comfortable with setting boundaries, supporting autonomy (Downing, 2008), initiating action, giving instructions, and tolerating conflict; he or she would prefer to press for results and measurable outcomes in responding to everyday situations in life (Dobbs, 2000).

The reflect approach values learning through thinking and the use of the mind, which includes any type of education one teaches to a family. In addition, some clinical traditions highlight the importance of gaining insight through self-reflection on the past, insight-oriented interpretation (Lieberman et al., 1991), understanding the meaning of one's behavior, self-observation, and awareness in-the-moment (Siegel, 2007a, 2007b; Siegel & Hartzell, 2003; Stern, 2004), and analysis of beliefs (Sigel, McGillicuddy-De Lisi, & Goodnow, 1992). In addition to insight and self-reflective capacities, this interpersonal approach can facilitate relational negotiations (Downing, 2008) and collaborative problem solving (Greene, 2001; Greene, Ablon, & Goring, 2003; Greene et al., 2004), and metacognitive skills (Schraw, 1998). Often these skills have to be taught to a child and scaffolded by an adult to be learned. These strategies are emphasized in the relevance and executive systems as reflections on personal meanings (referred to as "representations" in infant mental health; Maltese, 2005), increasing self- and other-awareness, and problem-solving abilities emerge. Someone whose personality orientation is based on a reflective approach would be comfortable with gathering knowledge, using logical analysis, appealing to rules and facts, and using insight; he or she would prefer self-reliance in responding to everyday life situations (Dobbs, 2000).

In actuality, there are many ways in which these three respond, direct, and reflect orientations to learning can play out in practice, in personalities, and in interpersonal dynamics in families and on an interdisciplinary team. In the experience of one of the authors (CL), the process of treatment draws on these three modes initially in an unfolding, sequential manner. First, the professional works to establish the therapeutic alliance (responsive mode), then moves onto specific action-based interventions (direct mode), and culminates in a feedback process (reflect mode). As the

treatment progresses, these modes are used in an increasingly dynamic manner. The relevance system chapters further elaborates these three orientations as essential parenting modes to the development of a child's self in relationship to others. When we use the term *relationship-based approaches*, we are referring to intervention approaches that rely on the context of relationships as central to the focus of intervention (Stern, 1995; Weston, Ivins, Heffron, & Sweet, 1997), recognizing that relationships organize development and shape and facilitate learning. Some clinical models and personalities may be weighted strongly toward one of the three orientations; others may function in a variety of ways, yet still maintaining particular strengths. For example, Susan McDonough's Interactive Guidance (1995, 2000, 2004) clinical approach blends a strong responsive purpose (engaging resistant parents by means of therapeutic alliance) with a reflective element that remains empathetic and strength-based (viewing and discussing with parents videotaped replay of their live parent–child interactions). Thus, although there is an integration here of responsive and reflective orientations, a particular strength of Interactive Guidance is its responsive emphasis on how to engage, build, and maintain a strong alliance with difficult families who might otherwise be viewed as noncompliant or oppositional.

In terms of personal emotional styles, in addition to blending two or three elements, a person might shift between them. These shifts can be productive (shifting from a smiling face to a firm "no" when a child goes near an electrical outlet), but they can also be unproductive. For example, a parent could oscillate between being firm and directive about no treats before dinner and giving in quickly to a whining child by changing the rules to "okay, just one cookie" (an oscillation from direct to respond), creating a situation with unclear limits.

The neurorelational framework encourages the ongoing and long-term goal of developing the ability to integrate and productively shift among the respond, direct, and reflect ways of learning and relating, according to the context. For practitioners,[2] the first challenge is to increase one's self-reflection, considering whether one is more affectively oriented (responsive), action-oriented (directive), cognitively/insight-oriented (reflect), or some type of blend. Through this exercise, practitioners can become more aware of the strengths and limitations of each of these orientations, and this knowledge can guide their continual journey toward maturation and growth.

The global introduction to the neurorelational framework of Part I now prepares us for Part II, in which we provide detailed explorations of each brain system, with an emphasis on pertinent behaviors to observe, along with assessment and intervention principles and strategies.

NOTES

1. Karen Horney's (1945, 1950) work within the interpersonal perspective of psychoanalysis also provides a parallel triad of moving toward, against, and away, offering another foundation for the triadic emotional and interpersonal modes of interactions that will be discussed throughout this book

2. Any number of disciplines can use the neurorelational framework. We use the terms *therapist*, *practitioner*, and *professional* interchangeably to imply any person who works with infants, children, and their families.

II

The Brain Systems

4

Functions and Behaviors of the Regulation System

The regulation system provides the foundation for a child's physical, socioemotional, and educational growth and development. Regulatory capacities set the stage for the quality with which both developmental and socioemotional milestones emerge. In the case example that follows, Danny's regulation system functioned poorly from birth, and he lagged far behind his well-regulated twin brother in meeting socioemotional and developmental milestones. The parents' eventual understanding of the regulation system allowed them to reframe their son's problematic behavior and became the point of entry for alleviating Danny's stress responses.

Kenny and Danny were premature twins but not at all alike. Roly-poly Kenny, who had been overfed in utero, transitioned easily between sleep and awake cycles, smiled and giggled frequently, and was easy to soothe. Danny, who had suffered from fetal malnutrition, also referred to as intrauterine growth retardation (IUGR), and the reason for the twins' premature births, spent most of his time crying. Just after delivery, Danny was rushed to the neonatal intensive care unit (NICU), where he remained for 3 weeks. The NICU policy prohibited Barbara and Bill from even holding Danny, telling them that being held would expend precious calories. The forced separation was very painful for the parents. Barbara, befriending a night nurse, visited the NICU at midnight each night so that she could hold Danny for a few minutes as he was brought out of his isolette to be weighed. These cherished moments helped her cope with the losses.

Danny was initially fed through a feeding tube, again as a way to conserve energy until his weak suck grew strong enough that he could use a preemie nipple for bottle feedings. Unfortunately, the feeding problems persisted after Danny came home. Due to his suck-swallow-breathe coordination problems, the fast flow of liquid from the bottle or the breast would choke him. Within a few

months' time, Danny began to associate the breast or bottle nipple with fear. At feeding time, he would scream, turn beet red, arch his back, flail his arms and legs, and splay his fingers—all signals of great distress. How was feeding to become a safe experience when it was associated with threat?

Moreover, Danny started to have trouble getting to sleep and staying asleep. He would awaken in the middle of the night several times a week, screaming in a high-pitched cry. The only thing that soothed him was the rapid motion of a portable bouncer. His parents wondered why holding him, walking him, or rocking him would not work. Should they let him cry it out when he was capable of screaming for 2 hours at a time? What would happen when Danny outgrew the bouncer? Barbara and Bill needed help to learn how to soothe Danny and calm his chaotic responses during all of the daily routines and transitions. In time, their support would help him acquire his own self-regulatory capacities. However, that journey was tumultuous. Danny was inconsolable for the first few years of life and, during this time, his parents had far more questions than answers.

Kenny, on the other hand, was thriving. His sleeping and feeding patterns were stable early on, and he was fully capable of playful engagements full of joy and circles of communication (socioemotional Milestones 1, 2, and 3) well within the appropriate time frame. Danny, however, struggled with the basics of daily life. By the time he was 1 year old, Barbara and Bill were stressed and exhausted. They had begun the parenting process with robust regulation systems, but were now showing signs of disarray from chronic sleep deprivation and the huge energy expenditure that it took to care for Danny during this turbulent beginning. Crying, feeding, and sleeping problems are three very common concerns that propel parents to seek help from professionals (Papoušek, 2008). Who would they turn to and what would be done to help them?

In this chapter, we review the critical components of a well-functioning regulation system and the behavioral components of states of arousal. We also emphasize the dual capacity of stress responses as healthy and adaptive, contributing to coordination, as well as unhealthy, contributing to load conditions. Considering these dual capacities, professionals can enhance the functioning of the child's and adults' regulatory system as a way to bolster both individual and relational health and well-being. The extreme and chronic stress responses that Danny experienced, if left untreated, would likely have led to any number of childhood developmental delays, mental health diagnoses, adult disease processes, or all the above. In time, this situation also may even have led to child abuse.

THE FUNCTION OF THE REGULATION SYSTEM

The functioning of the regulation system is central to health and learning. A poorly functioning regulation system can have a dramatic impact on

one's physical and mental health: poor stress recovery has been implicated in childhood and adult-onset conditions, such as diabetes, asthma, cardiovascular disease, autoimmune diseases, depression, and anxiety (Kaltsas & Chrousos, 2007; McEwen, 2002). Whereas *health* is often defined according to separate domains, such as mental health, physical health, and academic health, the construct of optimal regulation is viewed as the underpinning to health across domains.

States of Arousal: Informants of the Regulation System

A *state of arousal* is defined as a cluster of physiological and behavioral signals (sensory–motor transformations) that regularly occur together and reflect the degree and type of response to internal and external sensory stimuli (adapted from Barnard, 1999). Recall that in Chapter 2 we described arousal as a distributed property across brain systems, which means that all brain systems can influence and be influenced by arousal in such a way that contributes to either coordination or potential load behaviors. We further define regulation as the process by which the brain manages the flow of energy (expends, conserves, restores) to support the adaptive functioning of the body. Although we cannot *see* energy, we can see its expression in behavior. The states of arousal reflect a continuum from low to high energy expression:

LOW → sleep ↔ drowsy ↔ hypoalert ↔ alert processing ↔ hyperalert ↔ flooded ← HIGH

Two predominant states of arousal characterize self-regulation: cycling into deep sleep and the alert processing state. The capacity for these two salient states, one while asleep and one while awake, creates an individual's experience of safety in the world. The alert processing state, characterized by both calmness and alertness at the same time, reflects the maintenance of physiological balance that allows one to expend energy by attending, engaging, and learning; the sleep states are necessary for replenishing and conserving energy. When the regulation system is compromised, a person will not sleep well and will not be able to sustain an alert processing state (Pivik, 2007). Optimal regulation also involves the capacity to make both gradual and rapid state changes across the arousal continuum (that are appropriate to context), recover back to baseline, and modulate the highs and lows of energy within a given state. For example, when an external challenge or threat to survival is present, it is both efficient and adaptive to rapidly shift to a flooded state to support fight or flight and then gradually

return to baseline once the challenge or threat subsides. At the other end of the continuum, it is optimal to make gradual transitions from lower to higher arousal states when transitioning from sleep into wakefulness. A baby who awakens with an abrupt shift to a flooded state (e.g., on feeling wetness in his or her diaper) exemplifies a costly energy expenditure.

A well-functioning regulation system is manifest through the following:

- the capacity for deep sleep cycling;
- the capacity for alert processing;
- the capacity for the adaptive expression of all stress responses;
- the capacity for distinct states of arousal and smooth transitions between them;
- the capacity for connection to visceral cues; and
- the capacity for efficient stress recovery.

The degree to which one can sustain or recover back to an alert processing state often determines whether coordination or load conditions dominate. Adaptive stress responses are appropriate to the context and include an ability to recover back to baseline in an efficient manner. Load conditions (patterns) are characterized by any one or more of the following: (1) too frequent stress responses to real or perceived stressors; (2) an inability to adjust (habituate) to challenges that are no longer threatening; (3) a prolonged stress response or one where "the stress response gets stuck in the 'on' position" after the stressor is removed (McEwen, 2002, p. 200); and (4) inadequate stress recovery back to baseline health (McEwen, 2002; see also Cacioppo & Berntson, 2007). Load conditions mean that wear and tear is occurring within the body on an ongoing basis. The notion that health problems begin at the onset of the actual disease presentation is incorrect. In fact, "the processes that produce chronic as well as acute health problems can be in place long before the disease manifests" (Cacioppo, 2000, p. 18). The work of McEwen (2002) presents four allostatic load conditions and examines the activating and inhibiting nervous system processes involved. Table 4.1 summarizes these four load patterns, the underlying mechanisms of activation and inhibition accompanying each pattern, and the potential consequences to health with these patterns.

Self- and Interactive Regulation

Self-regulation and interactive regulation are overlapping and dynamic processes. In any interaction, there is a flow between the regulation systems of "self" and "other." The behavior and physiology of the individual (child and

Table 4.1. Stress Patterns and Associated Health Issues

Allostatic Load Patterns	Neurophysiological Activation and Inhibition Patterns	Potential Associated Health Issues
1. Too frequent stress responses to real or perceived stressors (e.g., poverty, child abuse, caregiver for someone with a chronic illness).	Full activation (SNS) and inhibition (via the HPA) cycle that occurs too frequently.	*Overproduction of adrenaline:* • Increase in heart attack and stroke (too much adrenaline = surge in blood pressure = damage to vessels of the heart and brain or lesions where plaque builds and restricts blood flow ["hardening of the arteries"]) • Hypertension
2. Inability to adjust (habituate) to initial challenges that, over time, should no longer be threatening (e.g., public speaking, daily commute).	Full activation (SNS) and inhibition (HPA) cycle when it is not necessary.	*Overproduction of cortisol:* • Melancholic depression • Obsessive compulsive disorder • Panic disorder • Alcoholism • Lowered immune systems • Decrease in memory functions • Increase in anxiety • Diabetes • Malnutrition • Hyperthyroidism • Functional gastrointestinal disease
3. Prolonged stress response after stressor is removed (e.g., remaining activated after an argument, elevated blood pressure hours following a test).	Both activation (SNS) and inhibition (HPA) return to baseline more slowly or do not shut off when stressor is no longer present.	

(Continued)

Table 4.1. Continued

Allostatic Load Patterns	Neurophysiological Activation and Inhibition Patterns	Potential Associated Health Issues
All the above load conditions involve long-term overexposure to adrenaline and cortisol		
4. Inadequate stress recovery back to baseline.	Decreased inhibition (HPA) to restore balance and promote stress recovery; other systems then compensate and stay activated.	*Underproduction of cortisol:* Allergies Asthma Autoimmune diseases Chronic fatigue syndrome Rashes Rheumatoid arthritis PTSD
In the above load condition there is long-term overexposure to inflammatory cytokines		

Note. From *The End of Stress As We Know It*, by Bruce McEwen, © 2002, Washington, DC: National Academy of Sciences. Adapted with permission of The National Academies Press and Bruce McEwen.

adult) supports or perturbs self-regulation; at the same time, that physiology is being continuously influenced by the changing behavior and physiology of the other (interactive regulation), as well as stimulation in the environment (adapted from Fogel, 1993, p. 29). Each partner's regulatory system will influence how the dyad manages the flow of energy and information. Ideally, interactions support coordination for both participants, but they can also move one or both into a condition of load. The degree to which the relationship supports the adaptive capacity to expend, conserve, and restore energy determines whether the relationship supports coordination. It is likely no accident that mothers essentially fall in love with their newborns, which gives them a steady energy dose to help offset the energy drains of sleep deprivation, changes in routine, and multiple other new energy expenditures. The energy that comes from falling in love helps protect the mother's self-regulatory capacities and gives her more fuel for interactive regulation. During the first year of an infant's life, the parent–child relationship usually requires the parent to expend more energy to achieve coordination for his or her child. In turn, the parents' efforts in regulating their child during this first year, when successful, can provide stress buffering so that their child is less intensely reactive to stressful events (i.e., shots at the doctor's office) (Gunnar & Fisher and the Early Experience, Stress, and Prevention Science Network, 2006, p. 659).

Self-regulation problems can occur (1) if one can self-regulate but has trouble staying regulated in certain relationships, or (2) if one has few self-regulation capacities (i.e., only through eating) and can stay regulated only with the help of certain others. The child who requires a high degree of interactive regulation to achieve coordination likely does not have functional self-regulatory capacities. For the child in possible load conditions from a variety of risk factors (e.g., a premature infant, an infant with fetal malnutrition, a baby in a home with chronic domestic violence), growth and development are potentially disrupted. In fact, chronic stress not only contributes to disease and disorders through wear and tear on bodily organs but disrupts brain regions predominantly responsible for coping and self regulation (Compas, 2006).

What about the parent of a baby with a compromised regulation system from the very start (e.g., a very low birth weight baby, a baby exposed to substances in utero, a baby with a severe genetic disorder)? This baby demands much more interactive regulation from the parent, and the demand may be relentless, without breaks, and eventually depleting. What if the baby's capacity for alert processing is so narrow that there is no eye contact, no cooing? Here, the parent not only has an accumulating energy debt but is also deprived of the replenishing, falling-in-love energy flow. What if the child, like Danny in our case example, primarily

screams and cries, rejects the breast, recoils to touch, and arches and stiff-
ens to an embrace? Now we can add the energy depletion of intense grief,
disappointment, and maybe even guilt to the mix. This stressed parent is
experiencing energy depletion with no offset and is almost certain to be
in a load condition.

Visceral Self

The initial connections to a visceral self (primary sensors, or interorecep-
tors that connect to the bodily organs in the internal milieu; Dworkin,
2007) begin with the development of a feedback loop between parent and
child. There are two primary aspects to the communications between parent and child that have to come together: (1) an infant's experiences of
distress and comfort are linked to the visceral organs to support accurate
behavioral signals, and (2) the strength and accuracy of both the signal
being sent by the child and the reading of the signal by the parent. The
baby should be able to display signals that reflect a range of positive and
negative associations, such as a sense of satisfaction in response to satiation of hunger, relief after a diaper change, or alleviation of pain. The signals that are communicated may be similar but indicate very different
messages, such as varying types of cry. A hungry cry may sound different
from a "wet" cry, which in turn is different from a pain cry or an overstimulated cry. For example, Brazelton describes "(1) a piercing, painful-
sounding cry; (2) a demanding, urgent cry; (3) a bored, hollow cry;" and
(4) a fussy, rhythmic, but not urgent cry that occurs when a baby is tired
or overloaded with too many stimuli, common between 3 and 12 weeks of
age (Brazelton, 1992, p. 60). Brazelton notes that this last pattern (often referred to as "colic") occurs in about 85% of babies and that often following
this type of crying infants "slept better and longer and more effectively"
(Brazelton, 1992, p. 63). (Note that this is an example in which temporary
behavioral disorganization can lead to further organization—what Brazelton calls a "touchpoint.") However, if the cry is either a weak or a difficult
signal to read (e.g., similar type of cry for each of these conditions or excessive crying), the parent may have difficulty interpreting the meaning of
the signal. A misread cue can create other difficulties. For example, a parent who misses a cue in the child signaling fatigue may soon encounter a
full-blown tantrum as the child becomes overtired. Cultural meanings are
also involved in the reading of infant's signals. For example, some cultures
value overfeeding an infant; in other words, plump babies are considered
happy babies. In this situation, the signals of satiation are not in the vocabulary of the parent and, therefore, may not be read, potentially leading

to disruptions in the establishment of accurate links between bodily states and relational events (a cause–effect relationship).

The ability to respond to visceral cues as an adult is critical to an individual's capacity to manage (regulate) the flow of energy and information. The autonomic nervous system (ANS), through its connections from brain to bodily organs, communicates the state of affairs within the viscera—what we refer to as the visceral self. These connections are always busy, but only rarely, relatively speaking, do they send signals to the conscious brain that alerts one to some discrete aspect of the visceral self (e.g., feeling hungry, feeling bowel pressure, feeling pain). If we are awake and alert, then it is adaptive for hunger pangs to begin to harness our attention. Awakening in the middle of the night to hunger pangs is efficient for an infant; it is not at all efficient for an adult. Most important, the visceral connections lay the foundation for the recognition of emotional states. Connections to one's own bodily cues, including pain, are a prerequisite for having an awareness of others' emotional states, so these cues can be considered the early origins of empathy (Moriguchi et al., 2007).

Physiological Underpinnings of the Regulation System

In the regulation system, we focus mainly upon the mechanisms that sustain and coordinate organ functioning, specifically the ANS. Although physiology is often described and studied according to a number of separate systems (e.g., autonomic, endocrine, immune, cardiovascular), these systems actually overlap as well as integrate by means of chemical and electrical communication (Silverthorn, 2006). In addition, it has become increasingly clear that physiology and behavior are also overlapping and integrated. In other words, one's physiology is not somehow separate from one's behavior and relationships. Nature does not respect the artificial distinctions that are typically made between the social/behavioral and the physiological levels (Berntson, Cacioppo, & Sarter, 2003; Berntson, Sarter, & Cacioppo, 2003b; Cacioppo & Berntson, 2002). With this integrated view in mind, we focus on the mechanisms of the ANS to elaborate the physiological underpinnings that regulate activation and inhibition. These two processes are fundamental aspects of functioning regardless of the level of analysis, be it physiology or social behavior, and provide a way to organize the multiple overlapping processes involved in a healthy regulation system.

Two general processes—activation and inhibition—are mediated by the nervous and endocrine (chemical messengers) systems. Working together, they provide the effect of a gas pedal and a brake pedal, which in

turn modulate the body's processes. Hence, they speed up, slow down, and modulate behaviors of energy expression. We define modulation in the regulation system as the process of balancing the activation and inhibition of energy through changes in dimensions of intensity, duration, and rhythm. The ANS coordinates the range of energy expression and is divided into two branches: the sympathetic nervous system (SNS) and the parasympathetic nervous system (PNS), which are connected with organs, smooth muscles, and glands throughout the body and brain. The sympathetic branch is primarily responsible for the activating energy (gas pedal) expressions of arousal (e.g., a flooded state), whereas the parasympathetic side is primarily responsible for the inhibiting energy (brake pedal) expressions of arousal (e.g., hypoalert awake state and deep sleep). Speeding up, slowing down, or modulating the action of these muscles and organs is an internal form of sensory–motor transformation that becomes organized into general and discrete states of arousal—from very high inhibition to very high activation and everything in between.

In these processes, chemical messengers (hormones and neurotransmitters) communicate with the SNS and PNS to direct the actions of target areas, including eyes, facial muscles, and internal organs—the larynx, heart, lungs, stomach, intestines, kidneys, and genitals. Thus, the external behaviors that we learn to read as states of arousal (in the next section) have direct connections with internal muscles and organs, emerging from the effect that chemical messengers have on influencing the gas and brake pedals of our nervous system. These physiological systems continually respond to the individual's perceptions of safety, challenge, or threat that emerge from interactions with others and the environment. Studies of loneliness and its relationship to disease provide an excellent example of how social behaviors, perceptions, and physiological levels interact. Social isolation has been found to be causally related to biological compromise. Summarizing House, Landis, and Umberson's (1988) work, Kiecolt-Glaser, Glaser, Cacioppo, and Malarkey (1998, p. 661) note: "Data from large, well-controlled epidemiological studies suggest that poor personal relationships constitute a major risk factor for morbidity and mortality, with statistical effect sizes comparable to those of such well-established health risk factors as smoking, blood pressure, blood lipids, obesity, and physical activity" (see also Cacioppo, Ernst, et al., 2002).

The most typical hormonal response to stress is one in which the adrenal glands first release adrenaline for a quick burst of energy to allow the body to respond and subsequently release cortisol, which serves to down-regulate the effect of the fight/flight (flooded) reaction (Gunnar & Quevedo, 2007; Kaltsas & Chrousos, 2007; McEwen, 2002).

Although the adrenal glands are involved in both the up and down regulation processes, adrenaline release is supported by the sympathetic-adrenomedullary system (SAM) and cortisol release is supported by the hypothalamic-pituitary-adrenocortical system (HPA). Research shows that cortisol plays a complex role in stress responses and both under- and overproduction of cortisol can lead to health problems. Low levels of cortisol secretion at the time of a stressor (referred to as an HPA sluggish response [McEwen, 2002]; or a suppressed response [Yehuda, 2000, 2001]) have been "implicated not only in asthma but also arthritis, fibromyalgia, chronic fatigue syndrome, and the skin rash known as dermatitis" (2002, p. 100). This pattern has also been associated with posttraumatic stress disorder (PTSD) (Gunnar & Quevedo, 2008). At the other extreme, prolonged high levels of cortisol secretion have been associated with depression (Gunnar & Quevedo, 2007). Gunnar and Quevedo state that "the brain is a major target organ for the steroid hormones produced by the HPA axis" (2007, p. 152), and areas of the brain involved in memory have been shown to be particularly vulnerable to the damaging effects of high cortisol.

Activation and Inhibition

Activation and inhibition are global processes that are inherent to all four brain systems and thus are discussed in each brain system chapter. The ability to modulate one's arousal states, particularly the arousal states related to stress responses, requires a sound brake system interacting with a good acceleration system—much like using the gas pedal and the brake pedal alternately when driving a car around town. The 10th cranial nerve, known as the vagus nerve, constitutes the PNS—which has two branches—the ventral vagal system and the dorsal vagal system. Each branch contributes to the support of certain functions, depending on the individual's perception of safety, challenge, or threat.

During the alert processing state, under conditions of perceived safety, a well-functioning ventral vagal branch acts as a fast-acting brake that allows for slowing down or speeding up (by releasing the brake) the energy needed to sustain conversation or engage in a learning task. The quality of this nerve's functioning, or vagal tone, is central to the modulation of arousal energy (Porges, 1995, 2001; Sahar, Shalev, & Porges, 2001). Schore quotes Field, Pickens, Fox, Nawrocki, and Gonzalez (1995) in defining vagal tone as " 'the amount of inhibitory influence on the heart by the parasympathetic nervous system' (Field, Pickens, Fox, Nawrocki, & Gonzalez, 1995, p. 227) and although it is present at birth it evolves in an

experience-dependent manner over the first two years" (Schore, 2003a, p. 167). Porges's polyvagal theory posits that "good" vagal tone affects multiple functions—everything from the suck, swallow, breathe capacities involved in feeding to coordinating vocalizations, pitch, prosody, and intonation involved in speech and language communication to skills involved in socioemotional expression through facial features (Porges, 2003, 2004). However, as Berntson, Cacioppo, and Grossman (2007) note, there is still much to be learned about how to precisely define and operationalize vagal tone. Specifically, "If we begin to think about . . . vagal activity in terms of multivariate, correlated antecedents and consequences, in light of contextual specificity and generality, then we are more likely to be able to see where the connections/associations are real and where they are absent or spurious" (p. 299).

The modulatory biological rhythms provided through the sleep-wake cycles, vagal tone, a newborn's orienting response, and arousal modulation are considered precursors (antecedents) to mother–infant synchrony. In other words, the research suggests that the quality of these early physiological processes in the infant lays a foundation for the infant's capacity to participate in interpersonal, social dialogue (Feldman, 2006, 2007). With respect to the sleep-wake cycle, there are natural energy oscillations that reliably occur across the 24-hour day-night cycle, known as circadian rhythms. The rise and fall of energy levels that mark these rhythms are regulated by the hypothalamus (Moore & Eichler, 1972; Stephan & Zucker, 1972). The hypothalamus, often referred to as the master regulator, not only regulates circadian rhythms but also acts as the control center for the endocrine and autonomic nervous systems (Carlson, 2001). Thus, the hypothalamus plays a central role in mediating coordination for the regulation system.

Risk Factors, Strengths, and Resources

In the neurorelational framework, risk factors are viewed as any context that increases the possibility of conditions for load. Conversely, the absence of primary risk factors is regarded as a strength or resource. In other words, good prenatal care, full-term birth, low maternal stress, and adequate financial resources are all strengths. When assessing the regulation system, professionals must consider such risk factors as genetic disorders, fetal malnutrition, in utero toxins, maternal stress, prematurity, multiple births, and poor living conditions—basically, any internal and external condition that may disrupt the child's physiology. The degree to which natural biological rhythms and needs are disrupted will exacerbate load

conditions. A birth that is characterized by risk factors for load conditions will intensify the need for interactive regulation from an adult who can (1) learn to read the important signals provided by the infant's states of arousal and (2) understand the capacities that emerge from these biological rhythms. Professionals across all disciplines must teach and empower parents to promote these biological rhythms when they are disrupted.

As already noted, an infant's physiology has a crucial affect on the capacity for social engagement (Feldman, 2006). A link most certainly exists between early in utero complications (i.e., disruptions to early biological rhythms) and poor outcomes for parent and child relationships as well as health factors. For example, within the United States foster care system, nearly 80% of the children were exposed to substances in utero, and 40% were born either at low birth weight or prematurely (Dicker & Gordon, 2000, 2002). Infants born with physiological disruptions to biological rhythms are more difficult to care for, which increases the risk that these infants will be passed from caregiver to caregiver. The problem is further compounded when parents have regulatory difficulties of their own (e.g., substance abuse, grief, depression, domestic violence) because they will naturally have fewer resources to harness for interactive regulation and learning how to support the disrupted biological rhythms. The interaction effect of multiple load conditions often leads parents (including foster parents; Lindhiem & Dozier, 2007) to make weak commitments to their child. Most often, both the parent and child need interventions that help stabilize and promote their regulation systems. (Unfortunately, in the United States, the number of children under the age of 5 in the foster care system is increasing, representing about 30% of all children in foster care [Dicker, Gordon, & Knitzer, 2001]. Therefore, understanding the links among physical, developmental, emotional, and academic health is imperative for such a vulnerable population.)

For the child, the presence of biological vulnerabilities within a context of unstable or absent emotional care takes a serious toll on the immune system, as reflected in the following figures:

- Eighty percent of children in foster care have at least one chronic health condition (Dicker & Gordon, 2002).
- Twenty-five percent of children in the foster care system have three or more chronic health problems, which is three to seven times greater than that found among other children living in poverty (Dicker & Gordon, 2002).
- More than half of the children in foster care have developmental delays (e.g., speech and language development delays, motor development problems, hearing and vision problems, and growth

retardation), which is four to five times that found among children in the general population (Dicker & Gordon, 2000, 2002; Dicker, Gordon, & Knitzer, 2001; Oser & Cohen, 2003).

- The hormone cortisol (important to stress response recovery and immune functioning) was measured in foster care children and a control group over a 3-day period. The control group showed the expected peak in cortisol in the mornings with a decline at each time point throughout the day. In contrast, the foster care children showed atypical cortisol levels and patterns. For example, most had low cortisol levels in the mornings, although some showed extremely high cortisol levels at this time. "Even after 2 or 3 years in a foster home, children continued to show unusual levels of cortisol production" (Dozier, Dozier, & Manni, 2002, p. 10).

So what behaviors do we need to see with respect to optimal regulation? When do those behaviors represent coordination or load conditions? How can the states of arousal structure the meanings that we give to the behaviors observed in infants, children, and their parents? The following section addresses these questions.

CLINICALLY RELEVANT BEHAVIORS OF THE REGULATION SYSTEM

In this section, we focus on describing the states of arousal as they are evidenced by infants and children, however, these states are exhibited across the lifespan. In the neurorelational framework, the states of arousal provide one of the baseline rubrics that organize assessment and intervention. Viewing behavior according to states of arousal gives insight into capacities for self-regulation and interactive regulation. States of arousal (also referred to as states of consciousness)—sleep, drowsy, hypoalert, alert processing, hyperalert, and flooded (Als, 1984, 2002; Als & Gibes, 1986; Barnard, 1999; Brazelton, 1973, 1984, 1992; Browne, MacLeod, & Smith-Sharp, 1999; Prechtl, 1977)—form the core of our assessment of the regulation system and set the course for intervention strategies. We use the states of arousal as the starting point for assessment because they help us organize behaviors along a continuum of variations in activation and inhibition. Under normative conditions, activation and inhibition organize into coordinated patterns that form discrete states of arousal. By understanding the behaviors that reflect these states, we are able to begin decoding the quality of energy use that is taking place within the regulation system. Considered the father of infant research, Louis Sander (1988)

describes the recurrence of states of arousal in their interactional context as providing the organization that governs the quality of inner experience, undergirding the development of the structure we call the self. (For an overview of Sander's contributions, see Nahum, 2000.)

Three adaptive stress responses—hypoalert, hyperalert, and flooded—are embedded within the optimal sleep-awake cycle of physiological rhythms. In other words, in their adaptive expressions, stress responses contribute to the optimal functioning of the regulation system. All three of the stress responses are adaptive, but the extreme flooded state, which enables the most activation of energy, is the one most commonly cited in the literature. Despite receiving a lot of attention, a full-blown fight–flight response is actually rare (hopefully). Thus, the flooded state is also intended to reflect increasing levels of activation but without the full-on adrenaline surge. In fact, during all stress response states, varying degrees of SNS and PNS activity (gas and brake) are possible.

In the neurorelational framework, the hyperalert state reflects the most complexity in terms of potential blends of varying degrees of activation (gas) alongside varying degrees of inhibition (brake); the flooded state is dominated by activation; the hypoalert state is dominated by inhibition. The specific SNS/PNS parameters that correspond directly to each behavioral arousal state are not yet completely known. What is known is that rather than simple connections, there are multiple SNS/PNS patterns that contribute to stress reactivity and behavior in general (Berntson, Boysen, & Cacioppo, 1991; Bernston, Cacioppo, & Quigley, 1991; Berntson, Cacioppo, Quigley, & Fabro, 1994). Recall that in Chapter 2 we introduced the reciprocal, uncoupled, and coupled patterns of autonomic control; some of these patterns have a broader range of energy expressions than others (some have a more restricted range), and we know more about the SNS/PNS processes that underlie the energy extremes (fight-flight, sleep) (Cannon, 1927; McEwen, 2002). (For further discussion of our proposed links between Berntson and Cacioppo's patterns of autonomic control and behavioral concomitants to the states of arousal, see CD-ROM Section 4.1.) During sleep states, the PNS inhibits the activity of the heart and other internal organs to promote rest and also activates processes that restore energy and promote digestion, especially during deep sleep states. In awake states, the parasympathetic branch calms the body's response to an emergency (i.e., a flooded state) and modulates degrees of activation within the alert processing state (Porges, 2004).

Each state of arousal produces a cluster of nonverbal signals that we read as behaviors and that indicate varying aspects of regulation. Once these indicators of regulation are viewed in relation to contextual factors and behavioral dimensions, they become meaningful messages about degrees of coordination or potential load conditions. Professionals learning

to decode the meaning of the messages must learn to understand the individual child's first language (NCAST-AVENUW, 2003) of nonverbal signals and cues. Although we tend to speak less loudly with our first language as we mature, it continues to speak for life and often remains an amazingly accurate, powerful, and meaningful form of expression.

Sleep States of Arousal

The total amount of time spent sleeping decreases with age. Newborns sleep an average of 12–16 hours, 6-month-olds about 10–14 hours (Barnard, 1999), young children about 10–12 hours, and adults an average of 7–8.5 hours (Rechtschaffen & Siegel, 2000) per day. The distribution of sleep across the 24-hour cycle also shifts with age. Most infants sleep 10–12 hours at night with awakenings for feeding. Bottle-fed infants sleep in longer time frames (3–4 hours) than breastfed infants (about 2 hours) because formula requires more time to digest. The term *sleep segments* refers to the number of times an infant shifts from sleep to awake and back to sleep again during a 24-hour period. Sleep segments are most frequent during the first month after birth, an average of six segments (even more frequent with breastfed infants), then shifting to five segments from 2–5 months of age, and decreasing to four segments from 6–12 months of age (Barnard, 1999).

Sleeping throughout the night (8 hours) without awakenings is achieved by about 70% of American 3-month-olds, 83% by 6 months, and 90% by 12-month-olds (Brazelton, 1992). The negative effects of inadequate sleep cycling have been implicated in neurocognitive and cardiovascular functioning, metabolic factors, socioeconomic status, loneliness, and longevity (Pivik, 2007).

Deep Sleep State

Behavioral cues of deep sleep are closed, still eyes, relaxed facial and body muscles (with occasional shifts or twitches), and a smooth and regular breathing pattern (see Figure 4.1). During deep sleep, the thresholds to sensory stimulation are very high, such that even loud noises, bright lights, touch, or passive movements may not cause an awakening (Barnard, 1999; Blackburn, 1986a, 1986b). For example, sleeping through a mild earthquake or a home burglary is indeed possible during deep sleep. In deep sleep, sympathetic activity decreases and heart rate and blood pressure decline; metabolic rate, brain temperature, and brain activity are at their lowest. Conversely, parasympathetic activity increases, stimulating digestive motility and restorative processes, while muscle tone and reflexes remain intact (Baharav et al.,

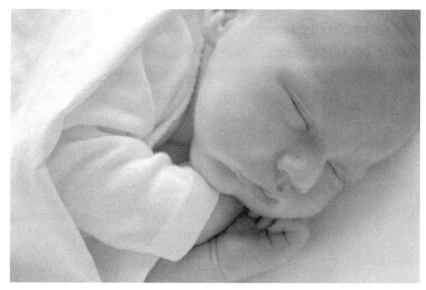

Figure 4.1. Deep sleep state.

1995; Carlson, 2001). The importance of deep sleep is that it is a restorative processes, including cellular repair, and it supports general health. Column 2 of Table 4.2 summarizes the behavioral cues of the deep sleep state.

Active Sleep State

During active sleep, breathing is irregular and rapid, heart rate and blood pressure increase, and brain temperature and metabolic rate increase. In infants, dreaming occurs during this light state of sleep (Brazelton, 1992); in adults, however, dreaming is not restricted to one particular sleep stage (Kleitman, 1963; Pivik, 2007). As Figure 4.2 suggests, behavioral cues include rapid eye movements (REM) and, in infants only, a variety of facial and body movements such as grimacing, twitching, and moving body parts (McNamara, Lijowska, & Thach, 2002) (see Table 4.2, column 3). During active sleep, thresholds to sensory stimulation are lower than with deep sleep, and thus not much external (e.g., noise) or internal stimulation (e.g., hunger) is required to increase arousal to wakefulness. If one has not achieved enough rest, the stimulation may produce a brief arousal with a return to sleep (Barnard, 1999; Blackburn, 1986a, 1986b).

During one sleep cycle, lasting 60–90 minutes, a newborn will cycle from active sleep to deep sleep and back to active sleep. In this cycle, the newborn actually spends more time in active (light) sleep than deep (quiet) sleep (Barnard, 1999). Thus, because newborns spend less time in

Table 4.2. Behavioral Cues Associated with Deep Sleep, Active Sleep, and States of Drowsiness

Target Muscles and Organs	Deep Sleep Behaviors	Active Sleep Behaviors	Drowsy Behaviors
Eyes	Closed and still	Rapid eye movements; fluttering beneath closed lids	May be open or closed; open eyes may be dull or glossy; may be excessive blinking, fluttering, or "heavy" eyelids
Facial expression	Relaxed, no movement	Potentially a variety of brief smiles, grimaces (in infants)	Facial muscles are re-laxed, without move ment; with occasional grimaces or twitches or jaw dropping
Heart and lungs	Smooth and regular respirations; slow and steady heart rate; pink coloring (e.g., in nailbeds, inner lips, indicating healthy blood flow)	Irregular, rapid, and shallow breathing patterns; increase in heart rate and blood pressure	Breathing and heart rates become irregular
Tone of voice	None	Fussing or crying sounds in infants	May include weak sounds or groans
Muscle movement	Very still, relaxed muscle tone; occasional spontaneous startle or twitch; motor reflexes remain intact; in the gut, there is relaxed and smooth motor movement with peristalsis	Irregular atonia (muscle twitches) and arm-leg extensions in infants; males have penile erections, clitoral engorgement in females; atonia (lack of muscle tension and tone) in adults	Head and body move ments are irregular or labile, such as twitches, or mild startle responses, reflecting relaxing muscle tone
Rhythm and rate of interaction	None	None	Slow to no response to others

deep sleep, their ability to cycle into deep sleep is important. With matu-ration, the sleep cycle differentiates into five sleep stages (stages I–IV and REM sleep). Sleep stages III and IV are considered deep sleep stages in adults. Adults who are stressed often do not experience these two stages,

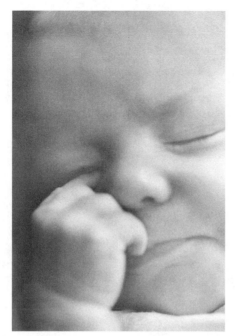

Figure 4.2.   Active sleep state.

and thus do not have the restorative support that deep sleep provides (Hall et al., 2004; Neylan et al., 2003).

Drowsy State

The drowsy state is a transitional state wherein one is neither fully awake nor asleep (see Figure 4.3). Behavioral cues include heavy eyelids, glossed eyes, irregular breathing, relaxed muscle tone, and irregular movements with occasional twitches or startles (see Table 4.2, column 4). In a drowsy state, the child's energy level may decrease or increase, moving him or her into either sleep or a temporary hypoalert state. Drowsy is a transitional state, and what is important to consider is reading whether the infant needs to slowly shift into sleep, thereby decreasing sensory stimulation to facilitate that, or whether it's appropriate to wake up, in which case more stimulation can be provided. In either case, a most important point for parents is to support a smooth rhythm of transition involving—either a gradual, slow descent into slumber or a gradual, slow ascent into wakefulness (Als, 1984; Browne et al., 1999). In the drowsy state, responses to stimulation may be absent, may be delayed, lull one to sleep, or produce a

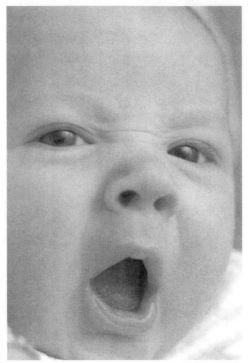

Figure 4.3.   Drowsy state.

startle response (often in reaction to a novel or intense stimulus) (Barnard, 1999; Blackburn, 1986a, 1986b). For example, the noise on a crowded bus may lull a child to sleep, but the sirens of a fire truck racing by may startle him or her to alertness. Frequent drowsy states during the day usually indicate disruptions to sleep during the night.

Table 4.2 details the behavioral cues associated with deep sleep, active sleep, and states of drowsiness. The sensory–motor transformations that take place in the target muscles and organs noted in column 1 contribute to the cluster of behaviors and physiological changes that organize states of arousal.

Awake States of Arousal

A person can experience at least four awake states: hypoalert, alert processing, hyperalert, and flooded. As noted, the alert processing state is the ideal waking state because it supports and facilitates optimal functioning, processing of information, and development due to its high degree of receptivity to many types of information. The hypoalert, hyperalert, and

flooded states reflect healthy, typical stress response states when expressed with the appropriate frequency, duration, intensity, and rhythm and in the appropriate contexts. Stress responses that are too frequent or repetitive, have a prolonged stress response (especially when one would expect habituation to the sensory trigger or the stressor no longer exists), lack recovery, or occur out of context signal that coordination within the regulation system has begun to falter and the person is experiencing a load condition (Berntson & Cacioppo, 2007; McEwen, 2002). Risk factors for conditions of load include poor clarity of states, abrupt or chaotic state transitions, and poor or absent modulation capacities (Als, 1982, 1984, 2002; Als & Gibes, 1986). In general, a load condition can be assumed when one or more of the three stress response states—hypoalert, hyperalert, flooded—dominate the landscape. With chronic persistence of maladaptive responses, these states become traits (Perry, Pollard, Blakely, Baker, & Vigilante, 1995). In a description similar to that of McEwen, Porges states, "the duration of the response is an important feature that distinguishes between adaptive and maladaptive reactions" (Porges, 2003, p. 40). He also aligns with McEwen's concept that the physiological mechanisms that support a response to stress have adaptive functions in the short term but "can be damaging if employed for long periods when it is no longer needed" (Porges, 2003, p. 40). In addition to the dimensions of duration, the frequency and intensity issues are addressed by the nature and degree of stress-reactivity (Cacioppo, 2000; Cacioppo et al., 1998). The same stressor, Cacioppo states, "can have profoundly different effects on physiological activation across individuals or in individuals across different life circumstances even when comparable levels of coping, performance, and perceived stress are expressed" (Cacioppo et al., 1998, p. 671).

As already noted, the stress response states can potentially reflect a number of SNS/PNS patterns that express a broad range of activation–inhibition patterns. Within this range, some behavioral responses are more commonly associated with an adaptive stress response (e.g., daydreaming in the hypoalert state), and others are more associated with a maladaptive stress response (e.g., depressed or dissociated in the hypoalert state). Many people tend to drift into a preferred stress response or pattern among stress responses; however, we suggest that during intervention practitioners foster the development and expression of all three stress responses, especially in their modulated and adaptive forms. Table 4.3 provides behavioral cues associated with the four awake states.

Hypoalert State

On waking and preparing for sleep, the hypoalert state appears as a brief period of daydreaming or "spacing out" that usually signals a lack of

Table 4.3. Behavioral Markers Distinguishing Adaptive and Load Versions of Stress Responses

Stress Responses	Hypoalert	Hyperalert	Flooded
Adaptive level	Daydreaming (e.g., temporarily tunes out to take a break from sustained mental effort)	Increased anxiety in anticipation of a previous negative experience (e.g., getting a shot at the doctor's office; taking a test)	Robust crying or upset (e.g., from sudden pain, hunger, or startling sound) accompanied by stress recovery
	Disengages to "take a breather" (e.g., when someone is annoying him or her, when a challenge feels too great)	Excited anticipation (e.g., the guest of honor is arriving for the surprise party)	Appropriate anger (e.g., from an injustice or mean-spirited attack) accompanied by stress recovery
Load level	Prolonged or too frequent periods of glazed eyes, looking through rather than at other, vacuous eye contact (e.g., dissociated, disconnected)	Prolonged or too frequent periods of wide-eyed staring (hypervigilant gaze) or darting eyes; inability to stop engaging with person or object; perseveration; prolonged clinging	Prolonged or too frequent periods of crying, screaming, tantrums, raging, or being hyperexcited

engagement with the environment and with others (see Figure 4.4). In a hypoalert state, one can look dazed, self-absorbed, and feel "turned inward." Adaptive hypoalert states occur multiple times per day as a means of conserving or restoring energy, for example, before gearing up for the next task or activity. With infants and young children, a tuning-out break can facilitate energy conservation, whereas novel stimulation can bring them back to an alert processing state. The hypoalert state can also be strengthened or provoked by the situation, for example, when the environment lacks relevance or novelty (i.e., boredom). It is also important to note that the hypoalert state had an evolutionary advantage for young children and females in that to be quiet and still was safer than being seen and heard under conditions of danger. In contrast, the flooded state with its shot of adrenaline held an evolutionary advantage for adolescent and adult males, catalyzing them to fight or flee under conditions of danger (Perry et al., 1995).

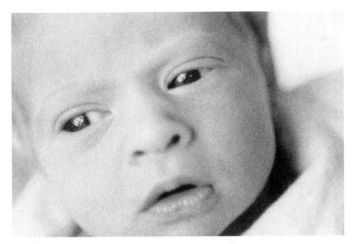

Figure 4.4.   Hypoalert state.

Behavioral cues for the hypoalert state are encompassed broadly by slowed and reduced movement within the context of wakeful muscle tone (see Table 4.4, column 2). One may have a fixed gaze and appear to be "looking through" rather than "looking at" something; the face typically shows muscle tone but lacks expression; the voice may be flat or monotone; the body is relatively still and not engaged in much movement, purposeful or otherwise; responses to stimuli may be slow or delayed (Als, 1984, 2002; Als & Gibes, 1986; Browne et al., 1998; Schore, 2003a). Within the hypoalert state, thresholds to stimulation vary depending on the intensity and relevance of the stimulus. With low-intensity stimuli that have little relevance, irregular rhythms or increasing intensity may be required to produce an orienting response, and the response, although occurring, may be sluggish. Conversely, with high-intensity or relevant stimulation, the orienting response out of the hypoalert state should be swift.

In a load condition, however, the hypoalert state may be dominant throughout the day. In such cases, the increasing inhibition moves into maladaptive response patterns of depression and, more severe, dissociation—a split from awareness of self and others (Schore, 2001). For infants with potential conditions for load (e.g., premature babies), an already compromised regulation system may predispose them to a hypoalert state during most waking hours. To the trained eye, these infants are seen as underresponsive and disconnected, but many mistakenly describe them as good babies because they do not "make a fuss." For this reason, hypoalert infants are often underrecognized and thereby miss out on opportunities for intervention. The hypoalert state can also become dominant when a cry for help goes unanswered. For example, the infant in the crib at the orphanage may cry

Table 4.4. Behavioral Cues Associated with Hypoalert, Alert Processing, Hyperalert, and Flooded States

Target Muscles and Organs	Hypoalert Behaviors	Alert Processing Behaviors	Hyperalert Behaviors	Flooded Behaviors
Eyes	Glazed; looking through you rather than at you; prolonged gaze aversion; staring off into space; dull or distant look	Bright and shiny with focused attention, processing information from faces and objects	Wide open; staring or darting; possible appearance of vigilance, fear, or panic; may or may not be combined with glazed eyes	Tightly closed or wide open; piercing with dilated pupils
Attention	Eyes do not scan room looking for interests; may prefer to stare at objects for long periods of time; exhibits a lack of information processing; may get "stuck" on something	Focused attention requires modulatory capacities with quick rest periods through shifting eyes or turning head	Intense focus, steadfast gaze or fixation on sensory stimulus, unable to break gaze or modulate	Either intense, narrow focus or continual roving with scattered attention; in either case, information is poorly processed or not processed at all
Facial expression	Flat and expressionless; no smiles	Neutral, smiles and joy, increasing range of modulated positive and negative affect with maturation	Raised eyebrows, especially with inside corners turned up; mouth wide open and staring (startle); may have trembling lips or mouth, grimace, or furrowed brow	Grimaced; clenched jaw or teeth; wide, open mouth; dry mouth
Heart and lungs	Heart rate and breathing rate are slowed; shallow breathing may be present (inhibitory energy may be supported by the	Breathing and heart rate are regular and rhythmic, with variability (the modulatory capacities to quickly speed up	Increased breathing and heart rate or very slowed breathing as if forgetting to take a breath; varying degrees of activation and inhibition result in a wide range of possible	Irregular and increased breathing pattern; increased heart and breathing rate

	dorsal vagal system; Schore, 2003a, 2003b; McEwen, 2002)	and slow down during engagement is likely provided by the ventral vagal system, with a balance of activating and inhibiting energy)	combinations and degrees of vigilance and dissociation (based on a coupled pattern) (this coupled energy may be supported by both sympathetic and dorsal vagal systems)	
Tone of voice	Weak, flat, monotone, sad, or some combination; lacks a musical quality; may be silent	Melodic and fluctuating with modulation	High-pitched, nasal "sing-song" voice; moaning or groaning indicating pain; elevated tone; quivering or fluctuating rapidly or whimpering	High-pitched, loud, hostile, gruff, shrill, or piercing
Muscle movement	Slumped posture with low muscle tone, lacking initiative or purposeful movement; aimless wandering without focus; slow, labored moving; in the gut, loss of bladder and bowel control (through increased motility and contractions; may occur from intense activation of the dorsal vagal branch of the parasympathetic system)	Stable, balanced, and coordinated with staying in the midline position; engaged but relaxed muscle tone; gestures are coordinated movements, fluctuating with the up and down flow of engagement; the gut is regulated, with smooth digestion and elimination (supported by the dorsal vagal system)	Tense or rigid body postures showing stiffness, or there may be rapid, repetitive body movements (rocking); gestures may show flailing with finger splays or wringing of hands; trembling, grabbing, clinging, or cowering; in the gut, there may be motor movement such as churning, butterflies, spit-up, hiccoughs, and diarrhea	Active and tense; may include arching, finger splays, increased tension in face and posture; sudden and abrupt arm or leg movements; gestures may be forceful or threatening; in the gut, there is often a lack of appetite and constipation (the sympathetic system slows and stops stomach digestion and peristalsis—the intestinal movement and contractions)
Rhythm and rate of interaction	Slow and delayed	Midrange in tempo	Fast and jerky, or withdrawn	Fast, erratic, and impulsive

relentlessly for weeks (flooded state), but when no help comes, she may slip into and remain in a dissociated state. An infant or young child victimized by abuse may shut down and remain in a depressed or dissociative state. The second branch of the PNS, the dorsal vagal system, is associated with the prolonged periods of dissociation, shutdown, and immobilization that occur within this hypoalert continuum (Porges, 2003, 2004; Schore, 2003a, 2003b). A hypoalert state may also participate in a chaotic pattern of stress response expressions, such as the child that alternates unpredictably between anxious hypervigilance and depression. In all of these situations, the hypoalert state is an expression of a condition of allodynamic load. When this becomes the primary way of being in the world, a child or adult will be characterized as having a high degree of avoidance or detachment (similar to Horney's [1945, 1950] interpersonal strategy of "moving away" from others).

Alert Processing State

The alert processing state encompasses a variable and flexible range of experiences and behaviors that balance internal needs with external circumstances (e.g., from engagement with a book to cooing with an infant to socializing at a party; see Figure 4.5). It is synonymous with an ability to pay attention—a task that ultimately has contributions from all four brain systems and that, in its mature state, demonstrates important maturational markers within all brain systems. Alert processing sustains smooth functioning within the body, awareness of internal and external stimuli, attention to relevant information, a capacity for abrupt shifts or

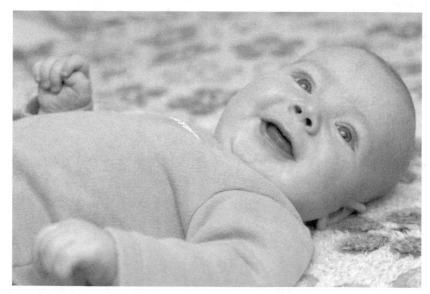

Figure 4.5.   Alert processing state.

gradual changes of energy and emotion, and the capacity for interpersonal engagement with expressions of joy. This state is the hallmark of awake regulation because it provides the optimal baseline for learning, relating, emotional experience, sensory processing, and behavioral adaptability. This arousal state is often described as a comfort zone, a feeling that is "just right," and a "window of opportunity."

The behaviors that characterize this state can be defined broadly as those that reflect a smooth modulation of engagement between the internal self and external world (see Table 4.4, column 3). Specific behavioral indices include (1) eyes that are bright and shiny; that orient, track, and affix; and that shift toward and away from the object of focus; (2) facial expressions that change smoothly and flexibly, as appropriate to context (including expressions of sadness and joy); (3) regular breathing; (4) tone of voice that fluctuates relative to content and exhibits a range of prosody; and (5) coordinated muscle movements. The most important features of an alert processing state are a rhythm and quality of engagement and interaction that are adaptable and flexible enough to remain in sync with the prevailing context.

This adaptability and flexibility are provided by modulation capacities, which in turn are supported by vagal tone. Chewing and sucking, amplifying/filtering sensory stimulation (e.g., listening to Mom's voice in a noisy room), motor orienting/head turning in response to the human voice, and vocalizations (Porges, 2003, 2004) are all important functions that occur within the alert processing state, and all are directly affected by vagal tone. Thus, the alert processing state, supported by vagal modulation, is the sine qua non of the emergence of oral-motor capacities, speech and language communication, affect expression and regulation, and arousal regulation.

Hyperalert State

The hyperalert state reflects increasing activation with varying degrees of inhibition. A hyperalert state is typically marked by increased activation and may occur in response to circumstances that require a longer-than-usual energy expenditure but not a full-blown surge of energy. For example, a child who is trying to finish homework so he can watch a favorite show before bedtime, but is running out of time, may begin to get restless, speed the tempo of his decision making, and begin to "think out loud" to stay focused and be more efficient.

Behavioral cues that reflect the hyperalert state (see Figure 4.6) include widened eyes that are fixed or hypervigilant, tightening facial muscles, flushed skin color, tensing body muscles, rigid or repetitive movements and postures, and sometimes visceral discomfort, such as a stomachache

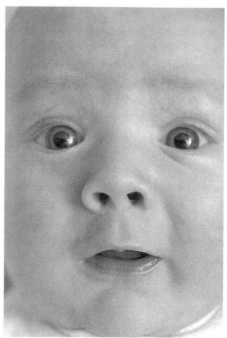

Figure 4.6. Hyperalert state.

or "butterflies" (see Table 4.4, column 4). During this state, one may be highly sensitive to stimulation in the environment, scanning relevant features in anticipation of some potential challenge or threat, such as a potential verbal reprimand or fight. Should a full-blown energy expenditure be required, the body has been readied to move into action, and the mind has also had some extra time to consider alternative responses, which increases the likelihood that the most adaptive and efficient action will be taken. One's ability to accurately anticipate the amount of energy that will be needed is a highly important adaptive capacity. For example, consider a job applicant who needs extra energy and alertness to prepare and perform well for a stressful interview. Optimally, increased energy was expended prior to the actual interview to gather and review materials, and time was spent mentally rehearsing or walking through possible scenarios. This anticipatory preparation is an adaptive and efficient skill to the extent that it allows one to modulate the appropriate degrees of activation and inhibition during the event itself.

A hyperalert child with increasing activation may show chronic anxiety behaviors, accompanied by clinging to a familiar or desired caregiver. For example, if a child is afraid of his teacher at school, he may not want to go to school, getting progressively more activated when it's time to leave the house or separate from Mom to go to class. Another scenario

might include a child with high anxiety who aims to please all the adults in her environment for fear of being scolded or reprimanded. When this style of coping predominates for prolonged periods of time, this child or adult will likely be characterized as having a high degree of compliance (similar to Horney's [1945, 1950] interpersonal strategy of "moving toward" others).

However, a hyperalert state can also involve a combination of increased activation alongside increased inhibition, such as when a child feels fearful and wants to retreat or withdraw from a challenging situation. For example, a child who does not like to be put on the spot in front of her classmates may feel agitated or anxious but has learned that staying still and quiet protects her from being called on by the teacher. In another situation, a child may exhibit more and more inhibition (while also being internally activated) in response to fear that motivates him or her to pull away from a challenging or threatening situation. For example, a child who witnesses his parents escalate into domestic violence may find over time that withdrawal protects him from becoming a part of the cycle of physical abuse. Even though his heart is pounding and his eyes are vigilant, he may appear to be quietly curled up in a dark corner. In an even more intense example, the child may display more "frozen" and rigid signs of anxiety, such as wide-eyed staring, a tense type of stillness, and withdrawal behaviors. "Behaviorally this is like 'riding the gas and the brake at the same time,' and the simultaneous activation of hyperexcitation and hyperinhibition results in the 'freeze response'" (Schore, 2001, p. 231; see also Berntson, Boysen, & Cacioppo, 1991, and Berntson, Cacioppo, & Quigley, 1991, for a discussion on the coupled pattern; Levine, 1997). Practitioners, then, can learn to distinguish through observation when a reduction in movement and activity is due to muscle tension (increased inhibition alongside activation) versus muscle relaxation (increased inhibition without activation—a more discrete hypoalert state).

Prolonged conditions of coupled activation and inhibition patterns are quite taxing to the nervous system and hold a range of load condition possibilities. When both energies are oscillating or equally engaged under challenge or threat, a child may be in a chronic pattern of alternating or coupling vigilance with dissociation (Schore, 2001). Such a child may go unnoticed, again because of being quiet, particularly in a school setting. He or she may be reprimanded for not paying attention or may be labeled as uncooperative. Unable to fully process information, the child may not "hear" his or her name being called or may be missing large chunks of information that leave him or her feeling disoriented to the task at hand. If that child is disciplined for a lack of responsiveness, the combination of dissociation and vigilance can increase (Perry & Szalavitz, 2006).

Flooded State

The flooded state involves the greatest energy expenditure and thus is optimal only when it is the most efficient and adaptive strategy given the circumstances. For example, if you find yourself in harm's way, you must decide on (or unconsciously react with) your most adaptive strategy—fight, flight (flooded states), or freeze (coupled hypo- and hyperalert state). If you are in a state of intense grief and sorrow, then being flooded with tears could be the most adaptive behavior. For infants and children, the flooded state may emerge as a result of fatigue, hunger, discomfort, pain, fear, or some type of sensory overload (Barnard, 1999; Blackburn, 1986a, 1986b). The capacity for either avoiding this state or knowing when this state is adaptive reflects developing maturity in the regulation system. An infant's experience of the flooded state (of course, when not prolonged) may even be good exercise for building flexibility across the arousal range and may reflect a need to release built-up energy (Brazelton, 1992). It may take time for a 2-year-old to learn that throwing a tantrum when denied a want either is a waste or serves only to bring further discomfort. In general, whether it is adaptive to move into this state depends on the situation, namely, the biological needs involved (e.g., hunger, thirst, elimination), the type of stimuli present, and the timing of the response.

Behavioral cues that reflect a flooded state (see Figure 4.7) include either wide or piercing eyes, dilated pupils, rigid muscles, fast and abrupt movements, impulsive speech or movements, flailing or lack of coordination, narrow or erratic focus, and an inability to process information (see Table 4.4, column 5). During a flooded state, one may be either amazingly unresponsive to internal or external stimuli (e.g., a severe injury may go unnoticed until the immediate threat is over) or extremely reactive to stimulation perceived as unpleasant (e.g., someone's tone of voice or a television set at an everyday volume may become the trigger that escalates rage).

Danny is an example of a child who spent much of his time shifting into a flooded state. This state of arousal is most likely to get the most attention due to the sheer "noise" levels inherent with this type of energy, thus, the potential for intervention occurring sooner rather than later. However, the flooded state is also most likely to be quickly labeled as oppositional or intentionally defiant behavior. Media coverage has heightened public awareness of very young children being kicked out of preschools due to flooded states. When this becomes a chronic pattern of behavior, a child or adult will likely be characterized as having high *defiance* (similar to Horney's [1945, 1950] interpersonal strategy of "moving against" others).

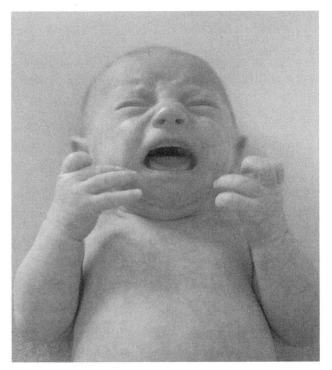

Figure 4.7. Flooded state.

Table 4.4 summarizes the behavioral cues associated with hypoalert, alert processing, hyperalert, and flooded states of arousal. The sensory–motor transformations that take place in the target muscles and organs (noted in column 1) contribute to the cluster of behaviors and physiological changes that organize states of arousal.

Barbara and her 1-year-old twins, Kenny and Danny, demonstrated very different stress responses in the same context. During an emergency, Barbara's intense facial, vocal, and gestural motor expressions stimulated different stress responses in her infants. While driving in the fast lane on the freeway with the twins strapped into car seats in the backseat, she had to stop abruptly when one of her tires suddenly blew out. As she turned back to look at her twin boys and saw cars fast approaching from the rear, her face showed an expression of fear, her tone of voice expressed panic, and her gestures expressed frantic tension (hyperalert and flooded state; a coupled pattern). Kenny began to cry in distress as he saw and felt his mother's terror. Danny, whom we described as "inconsolable" in his first few years of life, responded by shutting down, glazing over in some gradation of mild dissociation. The tension mounted over the next few minutes as Barbara frantically called 911 on her cell phone. Some relief occurred as cars did manage

to stop behind her, thus averting a multicar pileup. A police car soon came and stopped the flow of traffic, allowing Barbara to drive to the opposite side of the freeway, onto the shoulder.

Then, under much safer conditions, Barbara called for help to get her tire changed. Now her facial and vocal tone and slower speaking and gestures showed relief mixed with lingering fears from the recent terror. She used her tone of voice and a calmed facial expression to reassure her boys that everything was all right. She put on some soothing and familiar music they both liked to listen to while driving around. Soon, Kenny, who had been crying (expending energy), tuned out the other sounds on the freeway and fell asleep. Danny, who had shut down (conserving energy), became more alert and shifted to the alert processing state, enjoying the music. Although the intense effects of fear remained within Barbara's viscera for the rest of that day and as a memory for a long time to come, her external sensorimotor features in her face and voice had begun to calm down because the cortisol her body had produced was now taking effect some 25 minutes later (Gunnar & Quevedo, 2007), helping reduce the energy rush from adrenaline.

How can we use the behaviors explored in this section to determine assessment and intervention priorities when working with troubled dyads? We now turn to how behaviors that reflect states of arousal are organized into regulation system capacities that either support coordination or lead to load conditions.

5

Assessment and Intervention Principles, Priorities, and Strategies for the Regulation System

During the process of assessment and intervention, the initial priority for the professional is to decode the language of the regulation system. As mentioned, although we cannot see energy, we can see its expression in behavior. In the various professional fields, disciplines tend to focus on discrete bits and pieces of this nonverbal language of the arousal states. For example, mental health professionals tend to look at faces, speech and language professionals tend to listen to the production of vocal sounds, occupational therapy professionals look at motor planning and sensory thresholds, physical therapists see motor stability or instability as well as execution, and medical professionals focus on symptoms of illness (e.g., stomachache) from internal organs (viscera). In actuality, all of these bits and pieces—these clusters of behaviors and physiology from target muscles and organs—create a complete expression of the states of arousal. Consequently, it is important for professionals in each discipline to consider what they see in relation to this gestalt. In this chapter, we first identify the brain–behavior capacities that support optimal functioning or contribute to potential load conditions. Then, in the assessment and intervention strategies section, we consider the child's and adult's individual behaviors in relation to these clinical priorities.

ASSESSMENT AND INTERVENTION PRINCIPLES AND PRIORITIES FOR THE REGULATION SYSTEM

Keep in mind that coordination is supported by the capacities for deep sleep cycling, alert processing, clarity of states and smooth transitions,

connection to visceral cues, expression of adaptive stress responses, and efficient stress recovery. When any capacity is not present, is limited, or is even inconsistent, the child or adult can be at risk for load conditions.

Capacity for Deep Sleep Cycling

The capacity to cycle into deep sleep is a top priority given that good sleep is so supportive of optimal functioning across systems, and conversely, poor sleep can create such widespread disruption across systems. In terms of assessment, if a child is not sleeping well, it will be difficult to determine whether there is another level of meaning to observed behaviors that goes beyond the effects of poor sleep. In terms of intervention, establishing good-quality sleep can change the landscape of daytime behaviors.

Good-quality sleep is critical to the efficient and adaptive use of energy. The body needs this period of slowing down to replenish and conserve energy. In addition, it is thought that neurons within the brain undergo chemical processes that promote consolidation of memories during sleep. For example, studies indicate that increased mental activity during the day (e.g., studying for exams) increases the amount of deep sleep that occurs the next night, presumably because of the increased demand for consolidation of new learning (Backhaus, Hoeckesfeld, Born, Hohagen, & Junghanns, 2008; Gais, Lucas, & Born, 2006). Sleep is critical to allodynamic coordination. It provides both restoration and protection so that we have the resources to function optimally while awake.

Capacity for Alert Processing

As noted, the alert processing state is the optimal zone for taking in the greatest amount of information about the self, others, and the environment. The capacity to achieve an optimal alert processing state is supported by three factors: (1) high-quality sleep (Als, 2002; Moore, Adler, Williams, & Jackson, 2002; Pivik, 2007), (2) the perception of safety (Perry et al., 1995), and (3) the ability to modulate gradations in arousal levels. The importance of high-quality sleep was discussed in the preceding section. The perception of safety is a necessary condition for optimal regulation. When a child does not achieve an alert state that is appropriate to his or her age, when there is a prolonged stress response, or when there is a poor capacity for recovery back to baseline, then it becomes important to consider the child's perception of challenge or threat. The source of a perceived threat may be obvious, as in known abuse situations; it may be

subtle, as in avoidance of activities that tap into an underlying weakness; or it may be covert, as with physical discomfort or when a child has strong reactions "for no reason" (sometimes due to sensory defensiveness). Discovering the source of a perceived threat may sometimes be complicated and time-consuming, yet once discovered, the payoff is likely to be substantial.

Flexible and adaptive modulation enables one to maintain an alert processing state. It is an important developmental task facilitated by caretakers who accurately read the infant's cues and scaffold his or her modulatory abilities. An infant who takes periodic breaks from eye contact demonstrates a maturing ability for down-modulation (i.e., pressing the vagal brake). Similarly, an infant engaged in stimulating play, with accompanying excitement and joy, should be able to withdraw, become calm, and stabilize. Conversely, an infant who shifts from daydreaming to orienting toward a face, making eye contact, and smiling demonstrates an ability for up-modulation (i.e., releasing the vagal brake) to promote engagement with the external world. A caretaker who recognizes these cues and respects the modulatory flow is scaffolding the infant's modulatory abilities. A caretaker who provides opposing rather than complementary energy, such as repeatedly stimulating an infant during down-regulation or repeatedly ignoring an infant's curiosity, undermines the development of modulatory abilities.

As an infant matures into childhood, he or she should show the capacity to sustain alert processing for increasing periods of time. A child with a narrow window for alert processing will require more interactive regulation to support recovery back to baseline and expand that window, thus allowing a more solid foundation for future development and learning. The same principle holds true for adults.

Capacity for Clarity of States and Smooth Transitions Between States

Clear arousal states indicate a coalescing of regulatory mechanisms to support organized behavior. Smooth transitions between states are an aspect of modulation capacities and are evidence of an organized nervous system (Als, 1982, 1984, 2002; D'Apolito, 1991). For example, we observe optimal clarity and transitions in an infant as she gradually moves from being asleep to drowsy to hypoalert and then to alert. Perhaps she becomes fussy due to hunger (hyperalert) but then down-modulates to being calm and relaxed (hypoalert) once feeding begins. During feeding, she begins to move and make eye contact (alert), then tunes out for a few

minutes, then resumes eye contact and maybe some visual exploration. Once feeding is complete, she up-modulates to a more active alert state, wiggling more robustly and engaging with Mom's gaze and then her own toes and back to Mom's eyes again. In this example, the behavior feels purposeful (adaptive), and the balance of activation and inhibition appears to flow efficiently with an absence of abrupt shifts and surprises. However, the infant who exhibits clear states but abrupt transitions—for example, shifting from sleep to crying and screaming (flooded) in an instant—demonstrates a costly use of energy (maladaptive) and poor communication through behavior.

Poor clarity of states is often associated with less organization within immature or disrupted autonomic mechanisms (Als, 1982, 1984, 2002; D'Apolito, 1991). For example, an indistinct mix between hypoalert and drowsy states, such as staring eyes alongside muscle twitches (with loss of muscle tone), may reflect a sleep problem or an immature capacity for modulation of energy. The use of language here can be tricky. States of arousal associated with stress responses, while considered conditions of dysregulation, can actually portray quite organized behavior that enhances clarity. The robust cry of a hungry infant is an example of an organized condition of being flooded; a perturbed adult who can articulately argue for his or her case in front of another adult who holds authority over him or her may also be in an organized flooded state even though activation runs high. Less organized behavior—and thus less clarity within a state—is seen in an infant who is flailing while screaming in a high-pitched tone that does not communicate clearly the difference between hunger or distress or an adult who is kicking and yelling obscenities without any indication of what is distressing him or her.

Assisting the infant through interactive regulation can support developing capacities and increase clarity of states. Dimming the lights for an infant who gives unclear signals between hypoalert and drowsy states would reduce the available visual stimulation and facilitate closing of the eyes (assisting toward a clear drowsy state). In contrast, touching and movement would increase external stimulation and facilitate more active muscle movement (assisting toward a clear hypoalert state or perhaps shifting to an alert processing state).

Capacity for Connection to Visceral Cues

As noted, the quality of our connection to our bodies exerts a major influence on our capacity for efficient and adaptive energy use, providing the foundation for the emergent visceral self. Visceral cues lay the foundation

for an emerging connection with conscious and unconscious "somatic markers" (Damasio, 1996), which guide our intuitive understanding of safety and danger, thereby predisposing the development of an emotional self (relevance system) in one direction (safety) or another (danger). In extreme cases, there are those who are cut off from or who have very limited connection to bodily signals (e.g., anorexia nervosa). Not surprisingly, this extreme is characterized by a lack of emotional awareness, a general restriction of emotional experience, and can be accompanied by a lack of empathy for others (a.k.a. alexithymia; Moriguchi et al., 2007). At the other extreme are those who are overconnected or too broadly influenced by bodily signals (e.g., a somatic disorder, anxiety disorder). This often means that while one is connected to bodily signals, there is an inability to modulate the intensity of these cues, with an overreliance on emotional states that lacks integrating emotions with thoughts. In these examples, it is clear that the disruption of visceral signals in either direction has the potential to create widespread effects from the regulation system to all other systems and thus to disrupt overall coordination.

When clear signals from the child are accurately interpreted and understood by the parents, an ongoing feedback loop is created in which the first layer of meaning is laid down for established bodily connections. In other words, adaptive responses from others and the associated behavioral routines become linked with visceral experiences. As words are acquired and integrated, adults help expand and enhance meanings by assigning various verbal labels to bodily needs (e.g., "Are you hungry?" and "Do you have to go to the bathroom?") and the meeting of those needs (e.g., "Let's eat" and "Let's go potty"). Infants with immature physiology (e.g., due to prematurity) may receive signals that are out of balance such that some signals have much greater strength than others. Thus, a child who is overly sensitive to temperature may frequently feel hot or cold—experiences that create distress and also overshadow other bodily cues. Such imbalances prompt us to consider what potential impact they may have on the maturing physiological processes and how that impact shapes self-awareness. How well can a child develop and expand bodily awareness if he or she is in frequent discomfort? Furthermore, when the full range of bodily events is not registered in awareness, what might be the impact on the learning of adaptive behaviors? For example, if feeding produces pain due to severe gastroesophageal reflux, such an experience will probably shape the child's learning around feeding events. This infant, who has learned to associate eating with discomfort, may begin to tense up (become vigilant and stay hyperalert) any time he or she eats. In this example, the experience of pain has overridden the experience of pleasure that usually comes with eating experiences.

At each level of this assessment, it is important to explore whether the child is giving strong, clear signals and whether the parent is accurately interpreting and appropriately responding to the child's expression of his or her bodily cues. When a child has some type of physiological disruption (e.g., very low birth weight, prematurity, medical condition), the parent does not have the luxury of relying on common meanings or intuition to accurately interpret the visceral cues that underlie the behaviors. For example, the parent "tries everything" to engage, but the child remains unresponsive, or "tries everything" to soothe, but the child remains inconsolable, as in the case example of Danny. In this case, parents need to be taught how to make sense of often very subtle cues with the help of a professional. In some situations, the child exhibits appropriate behaviors to represent his or her bodily cues, but the parent's past experience skews his or her interpretation (e.g., "She's just trying to manipulate me"). In fact, "in a study to determine the 'goodness-of-fit' between infant cry characteristics and the mother's perception of the cry" it was found that "matches and mismatches between infant cry characteristics at 1 month and the mother's perception of the cry are related to cognitive and language outcome at 18 months in term and preterm infants" (Lester et al., 1995, p. 516). Whether the weakness lies with the child, the parent, or both, an otherwise healthy visceral connection may become compromised over time. Table 5.1 presents examples of effective versus ineffective infant cuing and parent reading/response behaviors.

Table 5.1. Examples of Strengths and Weaknesses in Child or Parent in Creating Visceral Feedback Loops Within the Child

Infant Cuing Examples		Parent Reading and Response Examples	
Strong Signals	Weak Signals or Problems	Strong Reading Ability	Weak Connections or Problems
Robust cry when hungry and can eat	Robust cry when hungry but too flooded to eat	Recognizes a cry as a symbol of distress	Views infant crying as manipulative behavior
Clear signals when tired and falls asleep with minimal assistance	Most of time spent in hypoalert state with weak signals indicating awake versus asleep states	Responds to tired signals in infant by facilitating sleep	Misreads the signal (e.g., keeps stimulating infant through play or loud environmental noises when infant needs a nap)

(Continued)

Table 5.1.   Continued

Infant Cuing Examples		Parent Reading and Response Examples	
Strong Signals	Weak Signals or Problems	Strong Reading Ability	Weak Connections or Problems
Clear differences in cries between being upset from wet diapers versus being in pain	Weak signals for hunger, pain, or diaper wetness exist (for older children it might be hunger, bowel/ bladder pressure, thirst, satiety), which may be the result of chronic hypoalert state with poor registration of bodily cues	Differentiates the types of cries infant makes	Assumes under- standing of the signal before investigating the signal (e.g., usu- ally assumes all crying is from being hungry)
Continues to send cues when parent misreads	Lacks differentia- tion of cries (e.g., all cries sound the same with high-intensity distress), which may be the result of chronic hyper- alert or flooded state with too many painful in- ternal sensations	Has difficulty read- ing because cues are unclear or lack differentia- tion and reaches out for profes- sional help	Has difficulty read- ing because cues are unclear or lack differentiation from infant and gives up

Capacity for Expression of Adaptive Stress Responses

An important aspect of coordination is the capacity to modulate flexibly across a broad range of energy expressions. A flexible and adaptive regu- lation system is seen in the capacity to express all stress response states (hypoalert, hyperalert, flooded) in a way that is appropriate to the context and includes a recovery back to baseline in a timely manner. In other words, one must gauge the best use of energy according to the circumstances—the right amount of energy, in the right place, and at the right time. To do this, a person needs to be a good judge of the circumstances that call for him or her to either conserve or expend energy.

It is sometimes difficult to bear in mind that appropriate stress re- sponses are healthy. The process of learning how to handle discomfort,

such as conflict and grief, is certainly painful and stressful but very important. Such stressful experiences might feel bad for the child and be hard for the parent to watch, but they begin the process of learning about the self and others and thus begin to equip the child to better manage self and others. A parent who rushes to comfort and calm the child at the slightest sign of stress, despite the situation, is actually depriving the child's growing brain of the opportunity develop needed coping skills.

Capacity for Efficient Stress Recovery

When one shifts into a stress response, the story is not over until there is a recovery back to baseline. If a stress response occurs during wakefulness, then adequate recovery is defined by movement into an alert processing state. If a stress response occurs during sleep, then adequate recovery is defined by movement back into sleep. Stress recovery can be facilitated (or hindered) by self or others. For an infant, self-facilitated recovery may involve sucking a thumb, babbling, periodic movements, or breaking eye contact (Brazelton, 1992). Interactive stress recovery for the infant may involve the parent's voice, rocking or bouncing, or gazing into each other's eyes (see Worksheet 5.2 at the end of this chapter). For a young child, self-facilitated recovery may involve retreating from the situation, distraction, or problem solving. Interactive stress recovery for a young child may involve removing the child from the situation, providing a distraction, or assisting with problem solving. In the examples noted in the previous section, a healthy stress response is a good thing when it is followed by stress recovery and appropriate to the context.

When stress responses turn into load conditions, then a child, dyad, and family likely need some form of intervention. If the family is not able to maintain a stable rhythm of recovery from stressful experiences, stress responses can become prolonged, possibly leading to rigid interpersonal relationships within the family system, or the stress responses can become too frequent, leading to chaotic interpersonal relationships.

We use these capacities as benchmarks for assessing coordination and conditions of load. By tracking the details of each capacity, we gain a deeper understanding of what may be undeveloped or breaking down within a child or dyad. Identifying parts of a brain system that are not working well can help guide treatment strategies.

ASSESSMENT AND INTERVENTION STRATEGIES

As mentioned in Chapter 4, Danny's feeding and sleeping capacities were disrupted from the start. Moving into his second year, other routines of daily life

activities also became disrupted, much to his parents' dismay. Even though Danny was sleeping through the night, he would scream at the top of his lungs within 30 seconds of awakening. Morning routines, such as getting him changed, dressed, and fed, would take several hours, with much of the time being spent in a flooded state while struggling to get one activity accomplished after another. Diaper changes were followed by prolonged screaming and thrashing, which could last up to 2 hours. Routines such as changing clothes, whether in the morning or in the evening, were fraught with defiance and refusals to cooperate.

Grandparents and friends of Barbara and Bill advised them more than once that they were too permissive and that Danny "got away with too much." They recommended solutions supporting a strong hands-on approach, such as spankings, firm discipline with negative consequences, and medication for obsessiveness. However, suggestions from books and other family members leaned toward a hands-off approach that involved ignoring his tantrums and refusing to engage with Danny until he calmed down and was willing to be cooperative, claiming that he needed to do this "on his own." To whom should they listen?

Assessment and intervention strategies can be characterized broadly as emphasizing hands-on versus hands-off approaches or as emphasizing self-regulation versus interactive regulation. As seen in the case example of Danny, major debates occur among professionals and parents about how to regulate a child's energy expenditures (e.g., prevent tantrums), how to help a child conserve energy (e.g., get a child to go to sleep or stay asleep), and how to help a child restore energy (e.g., how to feed an infant or recover from tantrums as a toddler). The two primary approaches of a hands-on or hands-off philosophy to child development tend to dominate such debates, although each advises very different activities. In the case of Danny, neither side was searching for the *meaning* behind his extreme behaviors; rather, the emphasis was on how to get him to stop screaming in the most expedient manner. As this section unfolds, we learn what interventions proved to be effective for this individual case, and we also see how effective intervention goes hand in hand with understanding the meaning of behaviors. (Further discussion of the variables in this case also occurs in Chapter 12.)

The hands-on/hands-off controversy sometimes centers on how much self- versus interactive regulation should be expected with children. It is important to be mindful of cultural issues in this area when providing assessment and intervention. Cultural values tend to judge certain interventions in terms of whether they support independence or dependence. For example, those who advocate that infants and young children sleep on their own (Ferber, 1985) value independence (and implicitly, an infant's self-regulation), and those who advocate co-sleeping (McKenna, 1986, 1993) support family values that rely on dependence (and implicitly, interactive regulation). A similar controversy exists as to

how much stimulation a medically vulnerable (e.g., low birth weight) infant should receive. Some advocate minimal contact—as in the case of Danny's NICU experience—where the concern is overstimulating a vulnerable nervous system to expend too much energy. However, others advocate providing optimal levels of touch, visual, and auditory information to stimulate an underaroused infant (Resnick, Eyler, Nelon, Eitzman, & Bucciarelli, 1987). To make matters more confusing, some research has shown that both approaches have yielded beneficial outcomes (Feldman & Eidelman, 2003). The neurorelational framework advocates an individualized approach to stimulation that tracks the degree of challenge or threat to the infant, based on reading arousal cues, to avoid an unhelpful amount of sensory information in either direction (understimulation or overstimulation).

Self- and Interactive Intervention Guidelines

From the perspective of the neurorelational framework, there is no one-size-fits-all answer as to how much, how little, or what type of intervention is needed due to the dynamic nature of physiology, behavior, and relationships. However, we find several guidelines to be useful. First, it is valuable for parents and professionals to have an understanding of the developmental process of self- and interactive regulation. All infants need consistent interactive regulation, which can recede as self-regulation expands with age. Second, self- and interactive regulation ebb and flow across the life span. One does not grow out of the need for interactive regulation but can become more skilled at using both self- and interactive regulatory strategies.

Third, the greater the vulnerability of the child's regulation system, and the younger the child is, the greater the need for interactive regulation. However, an adult must also support the child's capacity for self-regulation, which means discovering the ways a child is able to self-regulate, and then help him or her build on those strategies. Worksheet 5.2 (at the end of the chapter) provides suggestions for how a child can use his or her own strategies (self-regulation) or those provided by a parent or parent figure (interactive regulation).

Fourth, although self- and interactive regulatory guidelines that emerge from research, theory, and other sources may be important to consider, they cannot be applied without first considering the values and needs of the child and family. We suggest that the most important guideline to follow is that of respecting what the child's cues tell us about the three core regulation benchmarks—a capacity for deep sleep cycling, a

capacity for the alert processing state, and a capacity for stress recovery. These three benchmarks are used to shape approaches to addressing problems across all brain systems:

- support healthy sleep cycles;
- promote and expand the alert processing state; and
- enhance efficient stress recovery.

Fifth, the parents' capacities for interactive regulation must be assessed. It is more difficult for a mother to help her infant regulate when she herself is not regulated, so it may be important for the parents to provide interactive regulation for each other (e.g., taking turns, making sure at least one of them gets a good night's sleep) so they can better support their infant. Furthermore, a professional cannot assume that all parents will read and respond to cues in the same way. Some mothers may hear an infant's cry as a scream or interpret hyporesponsiveness as being relaxed. In every case, it is important to consider the parent's needs as well as the child's and then consider how to make best use of potential resources and limitations.

Sixth, the child's needs must be weighed against the cultural values the family holds toward self- and interactive regulation. For example, the American Academy of Pediatrics advocates against co-sleeping as unsafe (Ostfeld et al., 2006; Task Force on Sudden Infant Death Syndrome, 2005). If a family that immigrated from a part of the world where co-sleeping is an accepted routine, the parents will have no reservations about the practice. A professional working with this family may be worried about the co-sleeping arrangement and believe that it is not healthy, especially considering research and pediatric guidelines. Perhaps unbeknownst to this professional, research (from a cultural anthropology perspective) exists citing the biological benefits of co-sleeping as long as the parents are not using substances or involved in destructive behaviors (McKenna, 1986, 1993; McKenna & McDade, 2005; Sunderland, 2006). Furthermore, where is the baby's physiology in all of this? Often long forgotten. If the infant is in fact sleeping well under the co-sleeping arrangement, perhaps with a breastfeeding mother, and the parents are well equipped to provide safety, then the professional's values need to be reconsidered in relation to evidence of the child's healthy sleep cycling and the family's social and ethnic values. However, if the infant has inherent vulnerabilities (e.g., is premature) and is touch sensitive, then that infant may be overstimulated and not able to cycle into deep sleep. The issue then becomes holding the tension between the infant's physiology in relation to individual family and cultural values, the professional's experience, and existing research

controversies (recall that the definition of "evidence-based" is a process wherein research is held in tension with family and professional wisdom and values; Buysse & Wesley, 2006). (See Brazelton, 1992, and Sunderland, 2006, for further discussion regarding co-sleeping versus sleeping alone.)

As mentioned, crying, feeding, and sleeping problems are typically the driving force behind families coming for help during the first year of their infant's life. Feeding and sleeping problems are last to rule out on the triage list of the *Diagnostic Classification 0–3R* (ZERO TO THREE, 2005, pp. 66–67). These are the last to "rule-out" because arousal regulation disruptions are the first to show up with distress of any kind and they underlie *all* diagnostic categories. With any type of distress—physical or emotional—among the first things altered are sleeping and eating patterns, as well as emotional states (crying), or any combination among these three. Papoušek (2008) voices concern about the potential artificial distinctions made between "regulatory disorders" (as primarily arousal, sensory, and sensorimotor driven) and the separate categories of feeding, sleeping, and affective disorders. In fact, clinical research has found that early excessive crying preceded the manifestation of later regulatory disorders in more than 70% of the clients (Maldonado-Duran & Sandera-Garcia, 1996). As professionals gain experience working together in an interdisciplinary context, it is likely that early "regulatory" problems will be understood as underlying many diagnostic categories, including medical, developmental, mental, and academic health.

Tracking the Dimensions of Behavior

When assessing an individual's behavior, the sensorimotor dimensions of duration, intensity, and rhythm help us analyze the quality of actions and reactions that occur in real time for the individual and the dyad. In intervention, these dimensions help us track progress toward the therapeutic goal:

- Duration: the long and the short of the behavior;
- Intensity: the high and the low of the behavior;
- Rhythm: the slow and the fast of the behavior.

These dimensions offer up clues as to the underlying meanings for behaviors. For example, a change in intensity signals that something occurred around the time of the change, a tantrum of shorter duration tells us that something about this tantrum was probably not as severe, and so on. (See

also infant researcher's use of these dimensions: Beebe & Lachman, 2002; Beebe, Stern, & Jaffe, 1979; Sander, 1988; Stern, 1971, 1982; Tronick, 2007). When determining priorities and charting a course for intervention, we need to consider that variations in behavioral expression occur over time and across settings. This point is likely familiar. A child who appears anxious and distractible in one setting (such as school) may appear relaxed and focused in another setting, such as home. A child who appears irritable and agitated in the mornings may be much more easygoing in the evenings. A more intricate (and less familiar) point is that variations in the duration, intensity, and rhythms involved in the same situation might influence the behavioral response. Using these behavioral dimensions helps us better understand behavior, better understand the context, implement intervention strategies, and monitor change with intervention. In addition, each individual and dyad (mother, father, teacher, therapist, grandparents) co-create varying behavioral dimensions that can potentially expose developmental vulnerabilities and resiliencies within different relationships.

Assessment and Intervention Steps

Ongoing assessment is inherent in the intervention process. Hence, some of the following steps include both an assessment and intervention component. Once developmental gaps and specific needs are clarified, intervention often proceeds as a bottom-up process (first regulation, then sensory, and so on), especially for younger children. For an older child or parent, a top-down approach (first executive, then relevance, etc.) may be more appropriate as long as the bottom-up issues are being addressed in tandem. The age, the need of the child, and the parent's capacities determine the method. In the following material, steps 1 through 3 are general assessment steps, and steps 5 through 9 apply the assessment and intervention priorities.

Step 1: Assess Developmental and Socioemotional Milestones

Greenspan and Meisels (1996) have provided several useful assessment guidelines for those working with infants and young children. Although space does not permit a full review here, we highlight a few practices to include and a few to avoid.

1. Always use multiple sources of information: "Assessment must be based on an integrated developmental model; involves multiple

sources of information and multiple components" (Greenspan & Meisels, 1996, p. 17); "formal tests or tools should not be the cornerstone of the assessment of an infant or young child" (Greenspan & Meisels, 1996, p. 24).

2. The child's primary relationship is the cornerstone of an assessment: "The child's relationships and interactions with his or her most trusted caregiver should form the cornerstone of an assessment" (Greenspan & Meisels, 1996, p. 19).

3. Do not separate child from parents: "Young children should never be challenged during assessment by separation from their parents or familiar caregivers" (Greenspan & Meisels, 1996, p. 23).

4. The examiner should know the child: "Young children should never be assessed by a strange examiner" (Greenspan & Meisels, 1996, p. 24).

Several screeners and tools are available to assist in the data-gathering process. A screener is a process that is used to evaluate the strengths and potential red flags to determine if further assessment or follow-up is indicated. Screeners are often filled out by parents or may be completed during an interview with the parents. The process provides insights for the parents and wonderful teaching moments for professionals when there is open discussion. For developmental milestones, examples of recommended screeners are as follows:

- Ages & Stages Questionnaires (ASQ) (Bricker & Squires, 1999), ages 4 months through 60 months, available in Spanish, French, and Korean (usually parent completed; can also be used in a professional interview format);
- Child Development Inventory (CDI) (Ireton, 1992), ages 15 months to 6 years (parent completed, can also include professional interview and observation of child);
- Parents' Evaluation of Developmental Status (PEDS) (Glascoe, 1997) and the PEDS: Developmental Milestones (PEDS:DM) (Glascoe & Robertshaw, 2006), ages 0 through 8 years, English and Spanish (parent completed);
- Communication and Symbolic Behavior Scales Developmental Profile (CSBS-DP) (Wetherby & Prizant, 2002), functional ages 6–25 months, chronological ages 6 months to 6 years (specific to development of both verbal and nonverbal communication) (parent completed, can be administered with professional interview; if concerns, includes a more extensive parent-completed questionnaire and professional behavior sample/interaction).

For socioemotional milestones, examples of recommended screeners are as follows:

- Ages & Stages Questionnaires: Social-Emotional (ASQ:SE) (Squires, Bricker, & Twombly, 2002), ages 6–60 months (usually parent completed; can also be used in a professional interview format);
- Social-Emotional Scale in the Bayley Scales of Infant and Toddler Development, 3rd ed. (Greenspan, 2005) includes a sensory section at the beginning that assesses the child's use of environmental and relational stimuli for birth to 42-months;
- Vineland Social-Emotional Early Childhood Scale (SEEC) (Sparrow, Balla, & Cicchetti, 1998), ages birth to 5 years, 11 months (professional interview with parent/caretaker).

For screeners and scales more directly dedicated to assessing aspects of the regulation system in terms of arousal, sleeping, feeding, interactions, and reading infant's cues, see the following:

- The Infant-Toddler Symptom Checklist (7–30 months) (DeGangi, Poisson, Sickel, & Wiener, 1995). This screener directly assesses sensory and regulatory disorders.
- Parent-Child Interaction (PCI) Feeding Scales (birth to 12 months) (Barnard, 1979; Kelly & Barnard, 2000).
- Parent-Child Interaction (PCI) Teaching Scales (birth to 36 month) (Barnard, 1979; Kelly & Barnard, 2000).
- Beginning Rhythms Manual and Sleep Activity Record (birth to 12 months) (Barnard, 1999).
- *BabyCues: A Child's First Language* (birth to young children) (NCAST-AVENUW, 2003). This is a great tool for learning how to read infant cues; cards with infant and toddler facial pictures are on the front with an accurate description of the emotion on the back.
- *Promoting Maternal Mental Health During Pregnancy* (pregnant mothers) (Solchany, 2001). This material is designed to move beyond the physical changes during pregnancy and early motherhood to discuss the emotional challenges of parenting. Typical socioemotional development (e.g., early brain development, attachment) and atypical disruptions (e.g., postpartum depression, unresolved grief) that will affect the parent–child interactions are highlighted.

When significant delays, problem indicators, or both exist, an assessment is often indicated as the next step, which usually consists of

administered tests, structured observations, or both. The goals of the assessment involve looking for the child's and family's strengths as well as concerns; establishing a baseline of where, when, how often, and with what intensity and duration the problems occur; evaluating the developmental age in relation to chronological age; discovering contextual stressors at home and school that may be impacting functional behaviors; and deciphering what contexts bring out the best and the worst in the child (Kranowitz, 1998). Administering the structured assessments, often a standardized protocol, usually requires specialized training (Finello, 2005; administering a formal test instrument in the context of the real-time needs of infants and toddlers can be a rigorous undertaking, as is the need to track the meaning of nonverbal cues between parent and child, while pacing the degree of intrusiveness a test may be imposing on a family's cultural context). One example of a standardized assessment tool for infants that assesses for developmental delays is the *Bayley Scales of Infant and Toddler Development*, 3rd edition (Bayley, 2005) and for early socioemotional delays is the *Functional Emotional Assessment Scale, Research Version* (Greenspan, DeGangi, & Wieder, 2001). Other resources that evaluate testing materials for early intervention can be found in Bagnato, Neisworth, and Munson, (1997) and in Buros Institute (2007), which evaluates over 2,200 commercially available tests across a wide range of ages and categories, including developmental, personality, intelligence and aptitude, neuropsychological, educational, speech and language, hearing, and sensorimotor domains.

Step 2: Assess the Contributions of the Regulation System to Developmental and Socioemotional Milestone Delays

Regulation cuts across all domains of development (National Research Council & Institute of Medicine, 2000) and as such can potentially impact the functioning of all brain systems and all behavior. One question a professional can ask to begin the part-to-whole assessment process is, "Are the problems or delays I am seeing at least partly due to the influence of the regulation system?"

For example, milestone delays in a child who is undergoing frequent medical procedures may be due to the fact that organ systems cannot stabilize into regular patterns and the context of disruption does not support the emergence of skills. The same scenario could underlie milestone delays for an abused infant due to chronic stress. For some children, disruptions to regulation such as following poor sleep, during a stress response, or a poor ability to modulate alert processing in particular settings or with specific people, may cause emerging developmental abilities (i.e., not yet "automatic") to become compromised.

Any problems in the regulation brain system will of course be re-flected in socioemotional/regulation milestone delay. Given that the first socioemotional milestone is about the child's capacity for regulation and the first milestone is the foundation for all subsequent social-emotional milestones, any delay here is clearly significant.

In addition to developmental and socioemotional milestones, T. Berry Brazelton's *Touchpoints* (1992) offers important emotional and behavioral guidelines that are based on an important shift from viewing development in a linear fashion, to recognizing the strengths and clarity that develop-ment, indeed, unfolds in nonlinear ways. Brazelton's life's work points to many and varied touchpoints that are essential to understand as a profes-sional in the clinical field of child development (www.touchpoints.org). It is very important to understand the difference between temporary setbacks in development, or regressions, and a child's delays that are red flags. As stated, all stress responses are normative and actually necessary. During times of typical developmental disruptions, stress responses within the child and likely the family will escalate. Differentiating typical regressions from delays may not always be crystal clear. We believe that this is an ex-ample of how understanding load conditions and tracking the dimensions of intensity, duration, and rhythm as a baseline (is the problem getting better or worse over a few week's time?) can bring further clarity in delin-eating whether this is a temporary setback for the child and actually an opportunity for the family system to grow together, or becoming an acute condition that needs more immediate attention and follow-through.

Step 3: Assess Risk, Strengths, and Resources of Child and Parent

During this part of the assessment process, one weighs the risk factors for both the child and parent in relation to (1) the potential needs the child will have for interactive regulation, and (2) the adult's ability to provide for those needs and also sustain self-regulation. The greater the number of vulnerabilities in both child and or parent, the more the practitioner will need to regulate the parent as well. Greater risks in combination with fewer strengths and protective factors are associated with chronic, long-term problems (Campbell, 2002). The imbalances and need for self and interac-tive regulation can begin to determine which professionals will be needed to work on a team as well as the intensity and duration of intervention.

Given that low birth weight and premature infants are born with a more vulnerable nervous system, the greatest risk factor for a poor regu-latory system comes from premature births. Indeed, premature births are a major public health concern in the United States due to our high rate of preterm deliveries (11% of all births, which is high compared to other

developed nations; Mancuso, Schetter, Rini, Roesch, & Hobel, 2004). Three factors—maternal prenatal anxiety (anxiety specific to pregnancy; Roesch, Schetter, Woo, & Hobel, 2004), corticotrophin-releasing hormone (CRH; a hormone released as part of the HPA axis; Hobel, Arora, & Korst, 1999), and premature births—have been linked with each other (Mancuso et al., 2004). These provide another window into the connections between psychosocial and neuroendocrine factors.

The current understanding is that the placenta itself secretes CRH, so a bidirectional relationship occurs between the placenta and the HPA axis, which may affect or even amplify both fetal and maternal HPA responsiveness to stress (Mancuso et al., 2004). Findings indicated that "women who delivered preterm had significantly higher rates of CRH at both 18 to 20 weeks gestation and 28 to 30 weeks gestation compared with women who delivered term" (Mancuso et al., 2004, p. 762).

Besides maternal stress and premature births, risk factors that are most likely to affect the regulation system of the infant include any developmental disruptions (e.g., genetic disorders such as autism, Down syndrome, fragile X syndrome, Williams syndrome; Bellugi, Litchenberger, Jones, Lai, & St. George, 2001; Hagerman, 1996; Rubenstein, Lotspeich, & Ciaranello, 1990; Rutter, Bailey, Bolton, & LeCouteur, 1993) or toxic insults to the in utero and external environment (e.g., smoking [Abel, 1980], alcohol [Olson, Streissguth, Bookstein, Barr, & Sampson, 1994], maternal substance use [Dalterio & Fried, 1992; Singer, Arendt, et al., 1997; Singer, Yamashita, et al., 1997], lead [Bellinger, Titlebaum, Hu, & Needleman, 1994; Leftwich & Collins, 1994], and mercury [Pearson & Dietrich, 1985]). For a comprehensive overview of genetic and environmental disruptions, see Wachs (2000).

Another potent risk factor, fetal malnutrition, also referred to as intrauterine growth retardation (IUGR), occurs when the fetus is malnourished due to insufficient blood flow (which deprives the fetus not only of nutrients but also of oxygen) and results in low birth weight infants. The perception of the function of the placenta has shifted from being viewed as a passive conduit to being an active regulator of the transfer of nutrients to the fetus (Sibley et al., 2005). Even more impressive, the incidence of adult-onset diabetes, hypertension, metabolic disorders, and cardiovascular disease has been "strongly related to growth before birth" (Sibley et al., 2005, p. 827), referred to as "fetal programming" (Barker, 1995; Coe & Lubach, 2008), and specifically linked to the functioning of the placenta organ itself (Sibley et al., 2005). Research is being conducted to identify placental phenotypes during pregnancy so that at-risk in utero situations can be identified and distinguished from small fetuses that are not at risk (Sibley et al., 2005). Poor nutrition, both prenatally and postnatally, has serious developmental effects (e.g., iron-deficiency anemia is associated with attentional difficulties, affect regulation, and social problems [Lozoff et al., 1998; Lozoff, Jimenez,

Hagen, Mollen, & Wolf, 2000; Poulsen, 2005]); malnutrition can affect central nervous system processes in permanent ways (e.g., reductions in cortical volume and synapses; Levitsky & Strupp, 1995) as well as interfere with developmental processes, such as myelination (Ballabriga, 1990).

Perhaps one of the most global risk factors in the regulation system is poor vagal tone, which implies poor inhibition. Studies have shown that those with poor vagal tone, whether preterm or full-term births, are less able to regulate the vagal brake, potentially contributing to emotional and behavioral problems that are associated with diagnostic categories from posttraumatic stress disorder to autism to heart disease (McEwen, 2002; Porges, 2003, 2004). For the parent, risk factors include low maternal education (American Association on Intellectual and Developmental Disabilities, 2008), inadequate food, shelter, or clothing, substance abuse, and chronic medical or psychiatric conditions (see Worksheet 5.1; a complete History Worksheet for all four brain systems is available on the CD-ROM, Section 12.2).

Worksheet 5.1. History Worksheet for the Regulation System

Parental Risk Factors That Can Compromise a Parent's Ability to Provide Interactive Regulation	Global Questions That Assess the Overall Functioning of the Regulation System	Child Risk Factors That Can Decrease Self-Regulation and Increase Need for Interactive Regulation
☐ Significant prenatal stressors ☐ No or poor prenatal care ☐ History of or current substance abuse, smoking ☐ Teenage pregnancy ☐ Poor nutrition ☐ Premature labor ☐ Multiple births ☐ Genetic disorder(s) ☐ Chronic medical condition(s) ☐ Chronic allergies ☐ Sleep difficulties ☐ Rigid or chaotic pattern of arousal energy that is entrenched (hypoalert, hyperalert, flooded) ☐ Low maternal education ☐ Few financial resources ☐ Inadequate food, shelter, or clothing ☐ Limited community resources	• Are stress responses adaptive? That is, does a person show adequate recovery? • Is the person's use of energy efficient and flexible or rigid and chaotic? • How does the person conserve energy?	☐ Prenatal maternal stress ☐ No or poor prenatal care ☐ Intrauterine growth retardation or fetal malnutrition ☐ Toxins in utero ☐ Premature birth ☐ Genetic disorder(s) ☐ Infant medical condition(s) ☐ Chronic allergies ☐ Feeding problems ☐ Poor suck, swallow, and breath coordination ☐ Poor nutrition ☐ Sleep difficulties ☐ Rigid or chaotic pattern of arousal energy that is entrenched (hypoalert, hyperalert, flooded

Step 5: Support Capacity for Deep Sleep Cycling

When sleep is disrupted, restoring it becomes one of the first intervention goals. First, identify the problems in the child's sleep and then consider how the parent's behaviors related to bedtime rituals might be affecting those cycles. Table 5.2 can be used to determine the behavioral dimensions of problematic sleep patterns, such as a child sleeping too much or too little, parents having a difficult time soothing a child to sleep, or a child's sleep problems creating sleep problems for the parent. Noting the intensity, duration, and rhythm dimensions of a child's sleep behavior can both assist the professional in flagging difficulties as well as provide clues about the therapeutic goals for improving this brain system's capacities.

After the need is clearly profiled in terms of the target behaviors (supporting sleep), the following intervention sequence can be used.

1. *Rule out a disease or physical process.* Although this step is a baseline priority for any presenting problem, fairly common medical conditions can contribute to poor sleep and can be overlooked. Digestive problems, allergies, or enlarged tonsils and adenoids can cause discomfort or breathing problems and result in sleep disruption (Léger et al., 2006; Sperber & Tarasiuk, 2007; Wei, Mayo, Smith, Reese, & Weatherly, 2007). Breathing problems during sleep cause decreased oxygen intake and subsequent stimulation of the sympathetic nervous system and brain arousal

Table 5.2.   Behavioral Dimensions of Problematic Sleep Patterns

Duration	Intensity	Rhythm
Individual: The cumulative sleep time of the infant, child, or adult across a 24-hour period goes over or under the following typical parameters (cumulative averages of sleep): Newborns: 16 hours 6-month-olds: 15 hours Young children: 10–12 hours Adults: 7–8 hours	*Individual:* It takes more than 20 minutes for an infant, child, or adult to relax into a sleep cycle on his or her own	*Individual:* The infant, child, or adult has jerky or abrupt transitions from the sleep states to the drowsy state to the awake state, or vice versa
	Dyad: It takes more than 20 minutes for the parent to help the child relax into a sleep cycle	*Individual:* The child or adult does not cycle into deep sleep states
	Dyad: The child's or parent's poor state regulation is interfering with adequate sleep cycling	*Dyad:* Either the parent's or the child's sleep patterns frequently disrupt the other's sleep cycle

(Baylor, Mouton, Shamoon, & Goebel, 1995). Children with atypical craniofacial features, primarily atypical jaw bones, tongue, and associated structures, often have breathing difficulties during sleep (Zucconi et al., 1999). In some cases, a sleep study can provide further information.

We recommend that medication support be low on the list of options when it comes to sleep problems. However, there are important exceptions to this rule of thumb: (1) when there is an underlying disease process or condition that disrupts sleep, and quality sleep cannot be restored through other means; or (2) when the child or family is in a load condition and the need to gain sleep stabilization is urgent. Melatonin is a sleep hormone secreted by the pineal gland in the brain that assists in regulating circadian rhythms; it is stimulated with darkness at nightfall and assists in inducing sleep. Although continued research is necessary, melatonin as a supplement before bedtime shows promise as a safe and effective option for children (Ivanenko, McLaughlin Crabtree, & Tauman, 2003) and adults (Chase & Gidal, 1997) with chronic insomnia and sleep disturbances. As with any supplement, this should be used only under the supervision of a knowledgeable health care provider well versed in the possible interactional or harmful effects of such substances with his or her particular child.

2. *Use regulation strategies.* For preverbal children, the parent takes careful notice of the child's natural sleep cycle and supports any cues toward drowsiness and sleep states. The parent should abide by the child's natural movement into the awake state and not wake the child out of a sleep cycle to bathe or feed. Another helpful strategy is to make sure the child is not hungry when entering the sleep cycle or is not likely to dip into hunger during the sleep cycling. Often, feeding and sleeping issues work in tandem to create difficulties.

From birth, Danny had regulatory problems that were evidenced with both feeding and sleeping patterns. During the first year of life, his feeding difficulties likely stemmed from his poor suck-swallow-breathe coordination. The pediatrician advised Barbara and Bill to add cereal to Danny's pumped breast milk. By having more of a "paste" consistency, Danny had more control over the rate of the flow of the liquid. This intervention made his feeding routines much less frantic and full of panic and thus gradually resolved his stress response to a nipple.

In addition, Barbara began to suspect that Danny shifted abruptly from an alert processing state to a flooded state when hungry. She began to look more closely for any signs that Danny was hungry *before* he made the state change and soon noticed that sucking his thumb and subtle rooting movements were hunger cues. She began to feed him at the first sign of these cues, before he began to cry, and Danny was then able to remain in the alert processing state during feedings. This had an immediate impact on his sleep patterns, as well. Previously, his

flooded state left him unable to eat and he would "collapse" into sleep from sheer exhaustion, only to awaken again in a flooded state due to hunger. At a later age (2 years), another feeding issue emerged; Danny would wake up and start screaming within 30 seconds. Another pediatrician with whom they consulted suspected that Danny may not have sufficient energy reserves to get through the night without waking up hungry. Getting a nutritional consultation and feeding Danny later at night so that he had enough calories to sustain him was a helpful contribution toward eliminating the quick escalation into a flooded state on awakening.

For older children with verbal abilities (in the clinical experience of one of the authors [CL], at least 3 years of age), one can teach deep breathing and muscle relaxation exercises (such as tension–release) (Kendall & Hedtke, 2006). In addition, making dietary changes (e.g., reduce or prohibit sugar intake 3 hours before bed) may promote better sleep patterns (Consumer Reports Health, 2006). Note that for preverbal children or those with significant developmental breakdowns, sensory strategies (which follow) are particularly applicable and effective.

3. *Use sensory strategies.* Promote sleep by using the child's sensory preferences for calming, soothing, and gradually reducing arousal to help create a regular routine for relaxation into sleep. For example, to enter a drowsy state, one child may prefer being rocked or listening to a familiar lullaby (interactive regulation), whereas another may prefer sucking his or her thumb or cuddling a soft blanket (self-regulation) (see Worksheet 5.2). Massage for infants and across all ages may enhance down-regulating arousal into sleep cycles. Keep in mind that whether a child or adult experiences a particular sensation as pleasant or unpleasant is a purely subjective matter; that is, "sensory safety" is a unique, individual experience (safety is in the "senses" of the beholder). Furthermore, sensory preferences cannot be discovered without exploration and experimentation. The behavioral dimensions of intensity, duration, and rhythm guide your exploration to discover the "just right" sensory combinations that support relaxation to sleep. Also, track responses to sensory information to ensure that they are not inadvertently causing reactions other than relaxation (e.g., a rocking motion actually activates or creates discomfort for the baby). In general, low intensity and slow, regular rhythms are typically used in our culture for facilitating sleep cycling. As always, however, the child has the last word as to what level of rhythm, intensity, and duration facilitate his or her optimal state changes.

Danny's flooded states in his early months were characterized by extreme dimensions of high intensity, long duration, and fast rhythms. After trying many interventions, his parents found a counterintuitive solution to calm him by matching the intensity of Danny's crying with the fast rhythm of a bouncer. However, it

was the only intervention that was effective. Barbara learned early that she could not soothe him by holding him, touching him, or rocking him; indeed, these attempts only escalated his stress response. She was not able to include other strategies until she began working with an occupational therapist when Danny was 12 months old. Within a couple of months, as a result of this work, she was able to rock Danny in a chair, wherein this motion became soothing rather than disruptive to him. Though some of his tactile sensitivities were also addressed at this time, it wasn't until Danny was 2 years old that the meaning and severity of his extreme reactions to his diaper changes were revealed. One of Danny's first words (at 25 months, he also had a speech delay) was "towel." When saying this word, he pointed to his bottom. Barbara quickly responded and dried his bottom with a towel. Realizing that this was comforting for him, she immediately began this ritual with every diaper change, and the prolonged flooded states from a diaper change stopped. This was the first time she was able to realize the extreme distress that the sensation of wetness gave him; before she had thought it was a temperature issue and tried using warm wipes and keeping his body warm during changes. When these did not soothe him, she was left feeling confused as to the cause of the flooded response to a diaper change.

The experience of sensory preferences and sensory threat is highly unique to each individual. Once sensory preferences are identified, it then becomes important to identify the right "dose" for the child. One must titrate (decrease/increase the dose in incremental amounts to find the right intensity, rhythm, and duration) sensory information according the child's ability to relax into a drowsy or sleep state. When titrating upward, start from the least intrusive (e.g., parent's voice) to the most engaging (e.g., cuddling, rocking) (Brazelton, 1992; see Worksheet 5.2 at the end of this chapter). Slowing down the rate and rhythm of how a parent provides attempts to soothe through various sensory modalities not only helps the parent learn more about his or her baby's sensory preferences, it can also facilitate the infant's ability to self-regulate.

Applying the behavioral dimensions to the sensory system in a step-by-step way can be a useful method to get rapid and profound changes in regulation problems (problems are usually expressed through dimensions that are occurring in extremes), whether in sleep or awake cycles. One may apply these dimensions in two ways: by (1) matching—by mirroring or replicating the intensity and rhythm the child is displaying (Beebe & Lachmann, 2002) (fast/fast; slow/slow; high/high; low/low) or by (2) countering—by providing the opposite dimension that the child is displaying (e.g., if fast/then slow; if high/then low; if short/then long and vice versa) (adapted concept from Dunn, 2004). The duration dimension is determined by the child's arousal response to the intensity–rhythm intervention; for this reason, Table 5.3 addresses experimenting with only the

two variables of intensity and rhythm. The table provides an overview of possible ways, via relational or environmental means, to both match and counter dimensions related to sensory and motor domains across the sleep and awake cycles. Using low intensity and slow, regular rhythm combinations would seem most intuitive for assisting the sleep cycle. However, as we saw with Danny, this is not always the case. To soothe him into sleep, his high-intensity and fast rhythm crying needed to be matched with high-intensity and fast rhythm movement—a counterintuitive strategy. "The goal is to provide just the right amount of just the right kind of sensory information for both the baby and the caregiver so that their relationship becomes positive and generative of more interactions" (Dunn, 2004, p. 179) during the awake states and facilitates relaxation into sleep states when appropriate. When experimenting, the best strategy to prevent overstimulation is to begin with the "low and slow" dimensions for facilitating sleep and move to midrange dimensions, and gradually shifting to "high and fast" dimensions in small increments if the current levels are unsuccessful in assisting state regulation. Experimentation with these dimensions is useful in addressing all three intervention markers: (1) supporting the sleep cycle, (2) promoting and expanding the alert processing state, and (3) enhancing efficient stress recovery. Table 5.3 provides examples of experimenting with various ways and means of regulating arousal.

Table 5.3. Experimenting with Matching and Countering Sensory-Based Dimensions for Arousal Regulation

| Sensory Domains | Child with High-Intensity, Fast Rhythm | | Child with Low-Intensity, Slow Rhythm | |
	Matching the Child	Countering the Child	Matching the Child	Countering the Child
Vision	*Environmental:* Fast-moving mobile with bright colors	*Environmental:* Turn down or turn off lights	*Environmental:* Turn down or turn off lights	*Environmental:* Fast-moving toy with bright colors
	Relational: Exaggerated facial expressions	*Relational:* Do not make eye contact to decrease visual input	*Relational:* Only make eye contact, with no other type of sensory input (no sounds, touch, or movement)	*Relational:* Play a fast-moving interactive game, such as peek-a-boo or "I'm going to get you!"

(Continued)

Table 5.3.   Continued

	Child with High-Intensity, Fast Rhythm		Child with Low-Intensity, Slow Rhythm	
Sensory Domains	Matching the Child	Countering the Child	Matching the Child	Countering the Child
Hearing	*Environmental:* Play music that is loud and fast	*Relational:* Sing music that is soft and slow	*Environmental:* Reduce or eliminate sounds and volume; play slow-paced music	*Environmental:* Play music with high tones and fast rhythm (such as Mozart)
	Relational: Sing songs that are loud and fast	*Environmental:* Turn off all sounds from TV, radio, DVD	*Relational:* Speak in a low tone and a slow, regular rhythm	*Relational:* Talk or sing in a high-pitched tone and fast-paced rhythm
Touch and touch pressure	*Relational:* Hold tightly	*Relational:* Hold gently	*Environmental:* Loosely place blankets on infant	*Environmental:* Position infant with feet pressed firmly up against the side of crib
			Relational: Touch lightly	*Relational:* Swaddle firmly; massage with deep pressure
Smell	*Relational:* Provide/offer intense, alerting smell (smell of fresh orange or scented flower)	*Relational:* Familiar smell, such as smell of parent	*Relational:* Offer scent that is loved or a strong preference	*Relational:* Offer scent that is arousing— lemon
Taste	*Relational:* Provide/offer alerting taste, such as something sour	*Relational:* Provide/offer soothing taste, such as preference for a particular sweet	*Environmental:* Tastes that are preferences	*Environmental:* Taste that is tart
Movement	*Environmental:* Drive car on the freeway	*Environmental:* Drive slowly on side streets	*Environmental:* Place in an automatic slow swing	*Environmental:* Place in automatic swing on fast pace

(Continued)

Table 5.3.   Continued

Sensory Domains	Child with High-Intensity, Fast Rhythm		Child with Low-Intensity, Slow Rhythm	
	Matching the Child	Countering the Child	Matching the Child	Countering the Child
	Relational: Rock rapidly to match the rhythm of infant's crying	*Relational:* Rock slowly	*Relational:* Swing slowly	*Relational:* Move up into the air with wide range of motion
Motor	*Relational:* Adjust position to see if increased flexion is helpful	*Relational:* Adjust position to see if decreased flexion is helpful	*Relational:* Do not move child or oneself; only adjust one part of the body at a time (adjust head or extremities slowly)	*Relational:* Pick up and reposition with more stability (hold trunk firmly) or provide better body support through pillows, chair

4. *Use relevance strategies.* If sleep dysregulation continues, move to the relevance system to see whether contributions from trauma, nighttime domestic violence, flashback dreams, the birth of a new sibling, adjustments to a move, new experiences of separation, or other anxiety triggers are disrupting sleep. Establishing emotional safety is critical for healthy sleep cycling to occur (Dahl, 1998). Emotional safety may be communicated through sensory means. As just mentioned, Table 5.3 can be used as a resource for exploring comforting sensory experiences for a child. Establishing emotional safety, of course, means taking steps to remove overt and obvious threats to safety as well as working with parents to stabilize their own regulation patterns so that they can create a nurturing emotional climate for the child. In a context of marital discord, just seeing the parents together in a calm state as they share in the bedtime routine may be so soothing for the child that he or she falls to sleep. However, the degree of parental conflict may require private sessions for the couple. Parental expectations as to the degree of closeness/dependency and separateness/autonomy may be the source of conflicts surrounding bedtime rituals and routines. Furthermore, individual therapy may help a parent who is anxious about separation or is assuming pejorative meanings in response to his or her infant/child's sleep routines. Unresolved grief and loss or traumatic memories may be the unrecognized source. (For further discussion on sleep disorders see Schieche, Rupprecht, & Papoušek, 2008.)

5. *Use executive strategies.* If sleep dysregulation continues, consider the executive system contributions, for example, any motor problems that may interfere with the child's comfort. Ensure comfortable positions for sleep, such as alignment of the body, comfortable flexion of limbs, and support of muscles (a back roll or neck roll). At the same time, too much movement can disrupt the child's relaxation and arouse a drowsy child. Importantly, providing consistent bedtime routines develops a procedural memory in the child for state changes and help initiate and support the down-regulation sequence. Consistent routines and rhythms also help the child anticipate familiar sensory patterns and interactions, and this regularity and predictability have a down-regulating and soothing effect (i.e., as opposed to irregularity and unpredictability). Older children can participate in planning for the sleep routines (e.g., choosing what book they want read to them or which stuffed animal will kiss everyone goodnight) as well as choosing his or her sensory preferences (e.g., lowering the lights, picking out the calming music, touching a favorite fabric).

Step 5: Promote and Expand Capacity for Alert Processing

As noted, the alert processing state establishes the baseline for all learning, for the achievement of socioemotional milestones within relationships, and for physiological health that supports coordination. Any risk factors for load conditions may affect the quality and the ability to sustain the alert processing state. For vulnerable infants, such as preemies, the timing of interventions is crucial for sustaining the alert processing state. Table 5.4 provides profiles of problematic alert processing states in terms of behavioral dimensions—that is, alert processing states that are too short (duration) or are not sustained due to over up- or down-modulation (intensity) or unpaced and chaotic (rhythm) state changes.

It is important to determine the nature of the disruptions to alert processing, such as a propensity to be overaroused or underaroused, the predominance of a particular stress response, or poor modulation within the alert processing state. To establish or further support the alert processing state, try the following intervention suggestions, which draw on the various brain systems.

1. *Use regulation strategies.* Feed at regular intervals to support energy levels and avoid an unnecessary state change (for an infant, as soon as he or she gets fussy; for an older child, as soon as he or she gets cranky). Ideally, the parent can plan ahead and always have healthy snacks in the car or carry-along bag. Do not awaken the child, because this undermines the child's capacity for maintaining a quality alert processing state when awake. When the child is ill, in pain, or not feeling well, respect his or her need for extra sleep and rest (as opposed to "toughing it out"). Support modulation

Table 5.4.   Behavioral Dimensions of Problematic Alert Processing Patterns

Duration	Intensity	Rhythm
Individual: The infant, child, or adult is unable to sustain an active alert processing state within the following lengths of time (typical capacities to focus or pay attention; Greenspan, 1996): 3–6 months: 30 seconds or longer 5–10 months: (on toy or person) 1 minute or longer 10–13 months: (while playing on own) 5 or more minutes 13–18 months: (focused play on own) 15 or more minutes 18–25 months: 30 minutes or more Age 2 and up: (sustain the alert processing state) lengthy periods of time depending on the context and the task at hand	*Individual:* The infant, child, or adult is unable to modulate within the alert processing state (e.g., does not break gaze, shift vocal tone up or down, stretch and move around)	*Individual:* The infant, child, or adult is unable to pace his or her interest in dyadic engagement
Dyad: The child and the adult are unable to be in the alert processing state together at the same time	*Individual:* The infant, child, or adult is unable to up-modulate arousal so as to shift out of a hypoalert state into an alert processing state (e.g., does not respond to new sounds, notice an interesting toy, return to playing a game)	*Dyad:* The adult is unable to pace activities to match the infant/child's rhythms in a way that support the maintenance of the alert processing state (e.g., the parent of a low-energy child does not slow down his or her own transitions when indicated)
	Individual: The infant, child, or adult is unable to down-modulate arousal so as to shift out of a hyperalert/flooded state into an alert processing state (e.g., does not use rest periods, gaze aversion, or self-soothing measures such as sucking	

(Continued)

Table 5.4.   Continued

Duration	Intensity	Rhythm
	thumb or pacifier; older—chewing gum, drinking a cup of hot chocolate)	
	Dyad: The adult is unable to modulate self in ways (up or down) that support his or her child's capacity to maintain an alert processing state	

by taking short breaks. Encourage activities that assist with the coordination of breathing, heart rate, and sustaining breath control (e.g., deep breathing, swimming, playing a wind instrument for older children) because they may naturally support the healthy use of vagal tone, which promotes calm, relaxation, and modulation. Diet, such as an excess of carbohydrates or snacks that cause surges in blood sugar, disrupts the energy regulation needed for alert processing. Families with children who are either malnourished or have excessive weight gain may need to work with a nutritionist to help them change their dietary habits. A lack of exercise may also be the culprit.

2. *Use sensory strategies.* In supporting and expanding the alert processing state, the timing of sensory information from the relationship is critical. Being able to use a wide range of intensity (from low to high) that supports engagement during the alert processing state is valuable and must be tailored to the child and context. Assist with down-modulation of high-arousal emotion within the alert processing state (e.g., joy) by slowing down one's voice, lowering eyes, and breaking gaze. Using a wide range of rhythms that are individually tailored to the child and context is essential in promoting and expanding the alert processing state. As a beginning way to teach the infant/child ways to sustain the alert processing state, surround him or her with sensory preferences that cross a variety of modalities: sounds, sights, touch, touch pressure, taste, movement, and smell (see Table 5.3). Again, the emphasis is on preferences rather than overloading the child with as many opportunities as possible.

3. *Use relevance strategies.* Novelty and interest support alert processing. Notice what types of things in the environment keep a child curious, intrigued, and wanting to explore and use this motivation when a mild degree of up-regulation is desired. If down-regulation is the goal, then

minimize exposure to things that appeal to the child's interest. Make sure that emotional warmth is communicated. Build on previous experiences that have been positive and enjoyable. Consider the possibility that something in the relationship or the environment may be triggering a sense of challenge or threat (that might be disrupting the alert processing state). Parents themselves who are in load conditions of depression, anxiety, or hostility often have trouble following their child's lead. In addition, they may disrupt the flow of engagement. In either case, individual sessions with the parent(s) may be warranted to further explore these dynamics.

4. *Use executive strategies.* Make certain the task or activity at hand is not too challenging. If so, go back to an earlier point of success to sustain alert processing. Once engaged again, slowly increase the difficulty level and provide scaffolding and support as needed. For some older children, structured physical activities, such as baseball or martial arts, may expand focused attention as well as sequencing and planning abilities.

Step 6: Support Capacity for Adaptive Expression of All Stress Responses

Because all stress responses are adaptive, one wants to see that both adult and child can express all three states in a flexible manner. This requires that one be able to modulate shifts into higher or lower states of arousal and then back again. In Table 5.5, we provide profiles of problematic stress responses in terms of behavioral dimensions—that is, stress responses that are too long or short (duration), overly intense or lax (intensity), or unpaced and chaotic (rhythm).

The issue of developing a capacity to express all three stress responses often leads us into the cultural domain, where the therapist's desire to promote and expand the child's physiological responses may contrast with the parent's culturally shaped comfort zone. What is typical in one family (e.g., high-intensity yelling matches with quick recovery) is considered highly inappropriate in another. Thus, in some circumstances, it is important to respect the choices of parents, who may have strong cultural prohibitions against expression of particular stress responses. Provide an education about adaptive stress responses to these parents, but also try to find ways to elicit greater variation in the range of arousal without provoking a threat to their values. Ideally, one wants versatile stress response capacities. For parents who are open and willing to expand their child's repertoire of adaptive stress responses, we suggest specific approaches for the high-arousal child and for the low-arousal child.

1. *Down-regulating stress responses in children (toddler and older).* Parents can promote down-regulation using the sensory, relevance, and executive systems. Using the sensory systems, parents can help their child release

Table 5.5. Behavioral Dimensions of Problematic Stress Responses

Duration	Intensity	Rhythm
Individual: The infant, child, or adult cannot express adaptive stress responses for an appropriate length of time in relation to the context	*Individual:* The infant, child, or adult is unable to move "up" into higher states of arousal when appropriate (hyperalert or flooded)	*Individual:* The infant, child, or adult is unable to shift from fast into slow rhythms (from flooded or hyperalert into alert processing or to hypoalert), or vice versa, when appropriate to the context
	Individual: The infant, child, or adult is unable to move "down" into lower states of arousal (hypoalert) with disappointment, loss, or when appropriate (taking time to tune out and daydream)	
	Dyad: The parent cannot remain calm while a child shifts into either low or high arousal states	

high energy by guiding the child to jump up and down, push up against a wall, push up against the parent with pillows (with the parent pushing back), pound a pillow, crash into the couch, and so on. Once the child has discharged most of the flooded response state, the parent can attempt to mirror the child's experience or help the child find his or her own words (if the child is old enough) to describe the experience. Once the parent mirrors accurately or the child has been able to identify the feelings that provoked the flooded state, the parent can soothe or sit quietly with the child as he or she gradually shifts into a lower arousal state. Some children may need to shift into a lower-energy arousal state before they will be able to tolerate mirroring or talking about the experience. Using this approach, the parent is accessing both relevance and executive strategies. The relevance strategy involves using a responsive parenting approach with a child during the extremes of a stress response (i.e., mirroring, empathy), and the executive reflective strategy involves the promotion of the child's self-reflection, insight, and problem solving in anticipation of future events.

2. *Up-regulating stress responses in children (toddler and older).* For children who seem unable or unwilling to display stress responses, professionals can promote a healthy expression of high arousal states (e.g., anger, frustration, disappointment, or anxiety) by using a combination of sensory and relevance systems. In the context of a play session in which one is

following the child's lead, the practitioner looks for opportunities to promote up-regulation and model healthy expression of emotion. This can be done in a number of ways. For example, the professional can co-create with the child and the parent a story in real time in which one of the characters becomes increasingly upset and angry. In a slightly different format, the practitioner can use role playing to accomplish a similar goal: the child enacts emotions with which he or she is uncomfortable. Yet another version is to enact a dramatic play, complete with costumes, that involves high-intensity, fast rhythm of emotion. Especially important in this process is the practitioner's use of nonverbal cues from facial expressions, vocal tones, and gestures (Greenspan & Wieder, 1998). These sensory components are typically linked with the child's avoidance of the particular emotional expression. The practitioner titrates the sensory components of the emotional expressions to allow the child to develop comfort and familiarity with them. The titration principle is discussed in Chapter 7.

Step 7: Support Clarity of States and Transitions Between States

The movement across arousal states is optimal when accomplished with clarity and smoothness. A lack of state clarity is an indication of a nervous system vulnerability that precludes optimal integration of arousal, sensory information, emotional expression, and motor activity. An absence of smooth transitions between states indicates poor self-modulation, which may again be related to a compromised nervous system (Als, 1984; D'Apolito, 1991). To evaluate this capacity, we assess the duration of stress responses, the clarity of intensity within a state of arousal, and the smoothness and responsiveness of rhythm dimensions. Table 5.6 provides profiles of unclear states and irregular transitions in terms of the behavioral dimensions of duration, intensity, and rhythm.

The following strategies are useful for all children and are particularly salient for those with a compromised nervous system (e.g., due to exposure to toxins in utero, fetal malnutrition, lack of oxygen at birth).

1. *Use regulation strategies.* The parent is taught to remain aware of the child's level of arousal on a regular basis. When there is a state transition (e.g., getting ready for bed), the parent tracks whether the child is moving up or down the arousal curve. Whenever possible, interactions and caregiving routines are timed to correspond with a child's alert processing state.

2. *Use sensory strategies.* The child is helped to transition from one arousal state to another through careful handling, positioning, and interactions that support slow transitions rather than abrupt ones. If a bath causes a flooded state, then the child may be sponge-bathed one arm and leg at a time while continuing to be wrapped and posturally supported. Such types of developmental care principles are promoted by NIDCAP

Table 5.6.   Behavioral Dimensions of Unclear States and Irregular Transitions

Duration	Intensity	Rhythm
Individual: The infant, child, or adult stays in a prolonged stress response (more than 20–25 minutes) and does not make a smooth transition back to baseline (Greenspan, 1996; Gunnar & Quevedo, 2007)	*Individual:* The infant, child, or adult displays mixed signals. For example, glazed eyes (hypoalert) simultaneously with flailing arms (flooded)	*Individual:* The infant, child, or adult does not transition through the states of arousal in a smooth sequence that is appropriate to timing and context
		Individual: When a sudden change occurs in the environment, the stress response state appears chaotic and disorganized or rigid and inflexible

(Als, 2002) trained professionals and the FIRST training (Family Infant Relationship Support Training Program; Browne, MacLeod, & Smith-Sharp, 1999) for professionals and parents.

   3. *Use relevance strategies.* When the child is able to smoothly self-regulate, even for a very brief period of time, the parent notices and praises in a way that promotes pleasure for the child.

   4. *Use executive strategies.* Again, predictable and consistent routines help a child handle transitions without needing to defend against them.

Step 8: Support Connection to Visceral Cues

To assess the development of a child's visceral self—that is, his or her capacity to connect to visceral cues—we can explore whether a child's behavior reflects the registration of bodily signals and whether the parent can read these signals accurately. The most basic bodily signals include feelings of hunger/fullness, tired/alert, wet/dry, pain/pleasure, and bladder and bowel pressure/elimination of pressure. For a smooth feedback loop of communication to form between the child and parent, the child's behavior must reflect the registration of bodily cues, and the parent must be able to accurately decode the meaning of those cues. Using Table 5.1, one can begin to assess the cues involved in the expression of bodily signals. How strong are the child's signals? How well does the parent read the signals?

   There are many behavioral cues that can facilitate the parent's ability to read what is occurring in the infant. For example, is there a grimace or smile when defecating? Do the eyebrows furrow before spitting up? Is the face relaxed when feeding? An assessment that involves observation of a

182   Infant/Child Mental Health

dyad during feeding routines can be performed using the NCAST Feeding Scale (Barnard, 1979). The scale assesses the quality of the interaction, the states of arousal, and many of the cues discussed in this chapter.

What do all of these cues say about similar expressions in other situations? For a toddler, we can begin to read the bodily cues expressed during various emotional experiences. For example, is there a rigidity or a broad range of emotional expression? Do bodily cues reflect enjoyment of activities expected to be pleasurable, such as with singing or looking through a picture book? With verbal children, we can enlist feedback to better understand a child's bodily experience of emotions. For example, when observing an emotional expression, you may ask, "What do you feel in your body . . . in your tummy . . . in your chest . . . in your throat . . . in your face?"

1. *Use regulation strategies.* Educate the parents about the continuum of visceral signals that reflects subtle, moderate, or severe distress (see Table 5.7). A premature infant may struggle to stay engaged with a parent, but the energy expenditure may be too great and cause him or her to have a bowel movement in response (Als, 1984, 2002; Als & Gibes, 1986; Browne et al., 1996). Subtler cues prior to this may have been missed—for example, the infant hiccoughed earlier during the interaction. The message in the hiccoughs was, "I need a break and do not know how to down-regulate on my own." With help decoding these types of cues, a parent can become the external modulation that reduces the intensity, slows the rhythm, or shortens the duration of distress. The importance of expressing more severe signals of autonomic and visceral distress cannot be overemphasized. For example, a child's death occurred (Candace Newmaker, April 2000) when practitioners intentionally ignored physiological cues of distress that were verbalized or heard—for example, statements to the effect that she couldn't breathe, felt sick, was throwing up, was dying,

Table 5.7.   Range of Visceral Cues Signaling Degree of Regulation Distress

Subtle Visceral Cues	Moderate Visceral Cues	Severe Visceral Cues
Yawning	Spitting up	Gagging
Sighing	Hiccoughing	Choking
	Heartburn	Vomiting
	Stomachache	Reflux
	Bowels churning	Ulcers
	Passing gas	Intestinal bleeds
		Bowel movement
		Diarrhea
		Fecal/urinary incontinence

needed to defecate (Mercer, 2001, 2002; Mercer, Sarner & Rosa, 2003), with sounds of the child's agonal respirations (breathing pattern and sounds often heard during the dying process) (personal communication, Linda Rosa, January 31, 2008). The practitioners involved grossly misinterpreted these behavioral cues as resistance to surrendering to the attachment figure in charge (Mercer et al., 2003).

At times, support and education from a professional may not help a parent accurately read an infant or child's cues. In these cases, individual treatment may be warranted to explore potential assumptions or projections that may be distorting the message in the child's signals.

Deep breathing and relaxation exercises can be used to help determine the degree of visceral disconnection for an older child, and also used to enhance the registration of weak visceral cues. For example, a 5-year-old boy rapidly jiggling his leg may answer "no" when asked if he needs to go to the bathroom. However, after slowing him down with deep breathing, he may be able to feel the sensation of pressure in his bladder.

2. *Use sensory strategies.* A strategy to facilitate visceral connections, especially for anxious reactions, is to use sensory preferences to enhance comfort. Certain smells may be relaxing (e.g., lavender), favorite blankets and textures provide comfort through touch, and swinging motions can provide kinesthetic soothing. Whatever enables sensory comfort for a child is a primary tool the practitioner can use to mirror the child's visceral state of pleasure, which can establish a baseline to expand into other visceral sensations. This process can then assist parents in learning how to mirror visceral cues as they observe the child's responses.

3. *Use of the relevance system.* For the infant, feeding and diaper changes are repeated rhythmic experiences that create procedural memories of an emerging need (e.g., hunger) and the meeting of that need (e.g., sated). Using the responsive interpersonal mode, parents can use sounds and facial expressions (sensory system) to mirror the child's experience, which helps link that experience with meaning (relevance system). However, it is important that this mirroring accurately reflect the meaning of the child's cues or the link will reinforce a mismatch. In other words, if the child is satiated and the parent misreads cues as hunger, then the parent's mirroring and response (e.g., feeding) will not match the child's actual visceral signals. Accurately interpreting and responding to distress cues teaches the child that emotional signals are "seen" (mirrored) and responded to, thereby laying the foundation for the later emergence of empathy.

4. *Use of the executive system.* Parents need to be able to anticipate these visceral connections from the start and, as the child matures, begin to teach him or her how to anticipate them as well. Therapists can model

for parents how to check in with the child regarding hunger, fullness, thirst, and pressure in bowels or bladder.

Step 9: Enhance Capacity for Efficient Stress Recovery

At this point, we assess for individual and dyadic load patterns. The dimensions below help identify load versions of stress responses and further illuminate the treatment priorities for enhancing stress recovery abilities (see Table 5.8).

1. *Use regulation strategies.* Stress recovery can occur through interactive regulation (e.g., parent provides soothing with voice, facial expression,

Table 5.8. Behavioral Dimensions of Problematic Stress Response Patterns

Duration	Intensity	Rhythm
Individual: The infant, child, or adult typically stays in a stress response longer than is typical Typical durations: Birth–3 months: greater than 20 minutes (Greenspan, 1996) 3–6 months: greater than 15 minutes (Greenspan, 1996) 5–10 months: greater than 10 minutes (Greenspan, 1996) During toddler years when it is age-appropriate for temper outbursts, recovery occurs within 20 minutes	*Dyad:* When in a stress response state, parents must exert a high degree of energy to assist the child's recovery back to the alert processing state	*Individual:* The infant, child, or adult makes abrupt and rapid shifts in states of arousal from one extreme to another or, conversely, sluggish and slow responses
Dyad: The child and parent stay in prolonged stress responses at the same time	*Individual:* The infant, child, or adult has a narrow range of self-regulation strategies (e.g., sucking thumb only) (see Worksheet 5.1)	*Individual:* The infant, child, or adult oscillates between any two of the three stress response states
	Individual: The infant, child, or adult has a narrow range of interactive regulation strategies to assist recovery	*Individual:* The infant, child, or adult rigidly uses only stress response

(Continued)

Table 5.8.   Continued

Duration	Intensity	Rhythm
	Dyad: The child and the parent both exhibit high-intensity stress responses (hyperalert, flooded) or low-intensity stress responses (hypoalert)	*Individual:* The infant, child, or adult exhibits aspects of two stress responses simultaneously in a coupled pattern (e.g., simultaneous hypoalert [dissociation] with hypervigilance)
		Dyad: The dyadic pattern rapidly oscillates from one stress pattern into another as a couple (also see co-occurring patterns discussed in Chapter 12)

or movement) or through self-regulation (e.g., child sucking thumb, taking a visual break) (see Worksheet 5.2 at the end of this chapter). A child with a limited ability to be soothed, either through self- or interactive regulation, often warrants a referral to a specialist—for example, a maternal-child nurse specialist, an occupational therapist, or an infant mental health specialist—to help promote and expand the repertoire of soothing sensory experiences for the child. Also, time of day and context can alter a child's sensory preferences (i.e., what is soothing in the morning may not work in the evening), so parents must be flexible in offering potential means to stress recovery. Ideally, the professional works with the child and parent together so that the parent's abilities grow alongside the child's abilities.

2. *Use sensory strategies.* Experiment with using both matching and countering dimensions to promote stress recovery (use Table 5.3). If the child is nervous, is agitated, or has been crying for a prolonged period of time, then attempt to calm by countering the dimensions, slowing everything down, and finding the sensations that soothe (see suggestions from Table 5.3, column 3). However, as we saw with Danny, sometimes matching the high intensity and fast rhythm of stress response with the same intensity and rhythm of sensory information is more soothing (see suggestions from Table 5.3, column 2). If the child is flat and tuned out for prolonged periods of time, then engage either by first matching the stress response with low intensity and slow rhythm of sensory input (see suggestions from Table 5.3, column 4) or by gradually countering with high intensity and fast rhythm of sensory input (see suggestions from Table 5.3, column 5). Recall that slow, low-intensity rhythms are a good place to

start, titrating slowly upward into midrange, followed by faster, higher-intensity rhythms as long as child does not shift into a different stress response.

3. *Use relevance strategies.* Once the child has been soothed into a calm state, parents can assist with processing the cause of the upset by mirroring the child's emotional tone ("Oh! You are so mad!"). If the child is verbal, the parent can add a verbal component of helping him or her "unpack" the narrative sequence ("Jake took your toy; that's not fair!"). Professionals need to understand the meanings that parents and family members (including extended family) assign to their child's behaviors. For instance, with Danny, many family and friends had characterized him as being an oppositional, defiant child, recommending harsh discipline as the "answer" that left Barbara and Bill confused. When the presenting problem is a child's stress response, professionals must first educate parents about the body's physiological responses to stress and how these correlate with the three primary stress response states or blends. This information begins to neutralize the emotional charge around prior negative labels and also begins to shift appraisals about the potential meanings of the child's behavior. Parents who attribute negative valences to their child's stress responses need private sessions to process the origin of their assumptions, developmental expectations, and personal distress that is evoked from the interaction.

4. *Use executive strategies.* During the early phase of intervention, one can begin by asking parents to observe patterns of problem behaviors. One suggestion for tracking the targeted stress response behaviors is to create an activity chart that records the activity level, target state of arousal that is problematic, what the parent thought the cause was, what was done about it, all foods eaten, and all sleep patterns (see sample chart on the CD-ROM, Section 5.1). Experimentation and learning are key in trying to understand the origins of the child's distress and finding different routes to recovery. To preempt a stress response in verbal children, review with them memories of previous stressful experiences and co-create strategies to avoid the intensity of the emotional reaction. A parent's consistency in maintaining routines, daily rhythms, and limits can provide a soothing atmosphere for a child. By observing them, the professional can assess the parents' executive capacities for participating in their child's therapy.

When Danny was 2 years old, another professional (a developmental pediatrician) suggested that Barbara and Bill keep a journal for at least 1 week to document activities, times of day, and reactions (similar to the suggested format for a chart on the CD-ROM, Section 5.1). Within a few days, Barbara began to see clusters of prolonged stress responses during the long morning rituals marked by

a series of flooded states. With help, the parents began to put the pieces of the puzzle together. First, Danny was waking up hungry. Second, Barbara was changing his diaper and clothes before feeding him, and both activities exploited his tactile hypersensitivities and provoked a threat response. It was no wonder that basic routines took up an entire morning! When the parents changed the routine and fed him late at night, he awoke in the morning hungry but not in a flooded state (they suspected that too long a time between feedings was causing a flooded state on awakening due to a drop in blood sugar). Next, Danny was guided straight from bed to the breakfast table, without Barbara engaging him (another form of overstimulation). After he was fed, then the diaper and clothes could be changed. Of course, drying his bottom helped tremendously with the diaper change, and clothes were often changed very slowly or not at all due to his over-reactivity to the tactile stimulation. By following his visceral needs and his unique sensory preferences and threats, Danny's alert processing window gradually began to expand. For the first time, soon after Danny's second birthday, Barbara and Bill were no longer just surviving, but actually falling in love with their son.

Table 5.9 summarizes the various causes and solutions of the regulation problems experienced by Danny across the four brain systems.

SUMMARY POINTS FOR PRACTITIONERS: REGULATION

Clinicians can consider their cases and identify whether any of the behaviors they observe might have contributions from the regulation system. These contributions may be identified from any of the following points:

- There are historical factors that increase the vulnerability toward arousal regulation problems and conditions of load.
- The child or parent does not regulate arousal well on his or her own.
- The child or parent cannot regulate even with interactive regulation.
- The child or parent does not recognize bodily signals (pain, hunger, fullness, thirst, tiredness) and appropriately respond to them.
- Parents are unable to read infant/child cues.

Furthermore, professionals can make note of the disciplines weighted in this brain system and begin to create professional networks that can be used for referrals when necessary. Disciplines weighted in the regulation system include the following:

- medical practitioners (including obstetricians, labor and delivery nurses, NICU nurses, midwives, lactation consultants, maternal–child nurses, gynecologists, pediatricians, pediatric nurses, nurse practitioners, psychiatrists, neurologists, allergists, endocrinologists);

Table 5.9. Distributed Causes of Danny's Regulation Problems

Brain System	First Year		Second Year	
	Problem	Solution	Problem	Solution
Regulation	1. Potentially poor vagal tone with compromises in suck, swallow, breathe coordination and unstable state regulation pattern	1. Thick cereal paste combined with milk helps control rate of flow	1. Abrupt state transitions from a sleep state to a flooded state within seconds	1. Feeding late at night before going to sleep to keep blood sugar levels up during transition to awake states
	2. Unable to eat, falling asleep when hungry from exhausted crying	2. Feeding during alert processing state, following subtler cues of hunger, allows him to fall asleep when fed and stay asleep, thus increasing quality of sleep	2. Danny's stress pattern is to stay flooded for long periods of time	2. Efforts to figure out all the contributions to the stress pattern
Sensory	1. Only one source of sensory comfort, the bouncer	1. Occupational therapist helps expand sensory experiences of safety and reduce challenge or threat	1. Hypersensitive to wetness on his skin and tactile sensations from changing clothes	1. Danny's own first use of words to communicate his distress and desire to have his bottom dried
	2. Hypersensitive to tactile sensations, including touch, sounds, and some forms of movement	2. Occupational therapist helps expand vestibular options so that the rocking sensation is soothing		

Relevance	1. Feeding associated with threat from choking episodes 2. Sensations such as touch, sounds, and movement are experienced as threat	1. Having a way to control the flow of milk diminishes threat to self 2. Occupational therapist helps reduce hypersensitivities so Danny can find more sensory safety	1. Danny's preverbal experiences of sensory threat presumably provoke extremely negative meanings 2. Wetness on skin and changing clothes is sensory threat	1. Danny's ability to use words to communicate his experience of threat are revealed and responded to by parents 2. Experience of threat is decreased by involving Danny in the process of changing clothes
Executive	1. Anticipating threatening feeding experiences 2. Current routines keep Danny in load versions of stress response patterns	1. Thickening the milk to eliminate choking during feedings 2. Threat is reduced by increasing types of movement that Danny can tolerate 3. Parents notice subtle cues as to when to feed so feedings can occur prior to a stress response	1. Current routines keep Danny in load versions of stress responses, wherein he seems to experience the world as threatening	1. Parents keep a chart for 1 week, tracking every activity and Danny's stress responses 2. Parents change routine by feeding first, before changing diaper or clothes 3. Parents slow down all transitions, which helps Danny tolerate changes

- nutritionists;
- feeding specialists (speech and language therapists and occupational therapists);
- occupational therapists who can help identify triggers and preferences for arousal regulation;
- infant mental health specialists.

In terms of intervention, parents can play an important role. In particular, involving them in the following strategies can be beneficial:

- Use states of arousal as a way to guide interactive regulation.
- Use sensory preferences for alerting, comfort, relaxation, and stress recovery.
- Make conscious links to the visceral (body) self.
- Use relaxation techniques for both parents and older children.

In addition, all practitioners can consider the following possible strategies for assessment and intervention:

- Observe and support the parents' learning to read nonverbal cues of states of arousal and to understand the meaning of stress and stress recovery.
- Collaborate with an occupational therapist to help identify triggers and preferences.
- Learn to teach relaxation techniques, such as deep breathing, to parents and older children.
- Learn to teach how to regulate arousal and create shared joy by incorporating sensory preferences and identifying sensory triggers.
- Observe the infant's communication of visceral cues and the parents' reading of these cues.

Worksheet 5.2 summarizes the regulation concepts and can also be used to assess (often with the assistance of parents) the regulation system in infants, children, and parents. This worksheet is also available on the CD-ROM, Section 5.2.

Whereas the priority of the regulation system is modulating the flow of energy, the main concern of the sensory system is processing and modulating the flow of information. We turn to learning more about the sensory system, which shapes our perceptions and experiences of self, others, and the world.

Worksheet 5.2. Assessment of the Regulation System in the Infant, Child, and Parent

Resources and Strengths Toward Allodynamic Coordination	Risk Factors for Conditions of Allodynamic Load
Check whatever applies to the child, and circle what applies to the parent (including the parent's developmental history).	*Check whatever applies to the child, and circle what applies to the parent (including the parent's developmental history).*

Resources and Strengths Toward Allodynamic Coordination	Risk Factors for Conditions of Allodynamic Load
☐ Clarity of states of arousal	☐ Lack of clarity of states of arousal

☐ Smooth transitions between states of arousal, moving up and down the arousal ladder from low to high to midline levels of arousal	☐ Disturbed sleep
	    ☐ Difficulty going to sleep
	    ☐ Difficulty staying asleep
	    ☐ Primarily restless sleep without deep sleep

☐ Deep sleep cycling	
☐ Adequate cumulative sleep	☐ Not enough cumulative sleep
☐ Adequate alert processing state window	☐ Narrow alert processing state window

☐ Shows variety of stress responses in context:
    ☐ Hypoalert
    ☐ Hyperalert
    ☐ Flooded
	☐ Poor modulation within the alert processing state
	☐ Prolonged stress response(s) (check all that apply)
	    ☐ Hypoalert
	    ☐ Hyperalert
	    ☐ Flooded

☐ Adequate stress recovery within time parameters	
☐ Modulates within the alert processing state	☐ Rapid shifts into a stress response(s)

☐ Stress recovery can occur on *own* through a variety of means:
    ☐ Sucking
    ☐ Breaking eye contact
    ☐ Visual stimulation (mobile)
    ☐ Sounds (favorite music)
    ☐ Swaddling
    ☐ Rolling over
    ☐ Other
	☐ Intensity of stress response
	    ☐ Too high
	    ☐ Too low
	☐ Rigid use of one primary stress response
	☐ Rapid oscillations from one stress response to another
	☐ Co-occurring pattern (two stress states at once)

☐ Stress recovery can occur efficiently through *relationship* across a variety of means:
    ☐ Sound of parent's voice, singing
    ☐ Presence of primary parent, such as standing by bedside
    ☐ Gazing into each other's face
    ☐ Placing hand on stomach
    ☐ Holding snugly
    ☐ Rocking or gliding or bouncing
    ☐ Breast or bottle feeding when hungry
    ☐ Other
	☐ Interactive stress recovery for infants is limited to one or two means of soothing (such as only through feeding or rocking)
	☐ Interactive stress recovery for adults is limited to one or two means of soothing (such as only through sexual contact)
	☐ Nonresponsive to pain internally or externally
	☐ Poor suck, swallow, and breathing coordination (poor vagal tone indicator)

☐ Strong suck, swallow, breathe capacities in infant (good vagal tone indicator)	

6

Functions and Behaviors of the Sensory System

The sensory system allows us to experience our bodies and the world around us, and relationships provide a primary medium through which the flow of sensory information exchange occurs. The task of the sensory system is to integrate the raw data of impinging sensory signals in a way that gives us an accurate picture of sensory events, as well as to modulate those signals in a way that is most adaptive to the situation at hand. The ingredients that make up the sensory experience come from (1) the type of information from the environment, including relationships; (2) the brain's innate capacities to process sensory data; and (3) the degree to which these innate capacities are (or are not) facilitated by the sensory environment. Whether a child achieves coordination or slips into load conditions depends on the dynamic interaction among these ingredients and influences from the other brain systems.

Genetic factors in interaction with in utero events set the baseline for a child's sensory capacities. This baseline will greatly influence, *but not determine*, the quality of emerging developmental and socioemotional milestones. For example, "Maternal behavior can effectively change gene-controlled patterns of stress responsivity" (Gunnar & Quevedo, 2007, p. 164). From birth, one's relationships and environment provide the sensory data that shape subsequent development. An infant's relationships provide the primary means of sensory information exchange. As the major players in the sensory world, parents have the capacity to influence many of the sensory dimensions of that world, including the quality and rhythm of their own behaviors. As such, "caregivers are by far the most powerful sources of stress and the most effective defense against harmful stressors" (Gunnar & Quevedo, 2007, p. 164). In an impoverished sensory

environment, especially one that lacks a consistent caretaker, even the most robust brain can wither; conversely, a rich sensory environment can strengthen a vulnerable brain. But it is not quite that clear-cut. Sometimes a child will not benefit from a rich sensory environment because it might be too overstimulating. Indeed, the pathways from sensory signals to sensory experience are as unique to the individual as fingerprints are, meaning that each child has a unique composition of sensory preferences and triggers.

The degree of sensory match or mismatch between the child and the environment (and perhaps especially the parents) will determine the degree to which a child's sensory processing capacities are supported and enhanced as well as the degree that a child's preferences and triggers either enhance or diminish the quality of development. A goodness-of-fit match (Chess & Thomas, 1999; Lester et al., 1995; Resch, 2008) exists when (1) the parents and environment provide enough quality sensory data to promote optimal sensory processing (e.g., conversation, books, opportunities for exploratory activities), and (2) sensory triggers are scarce enough, sensory preferences are plentiful enough, and preferences are consistently used for pleasure, stress recovery, and settling into sleep. A mismatch exists when (1) the available sensory data in the relationship and environment are impoverished or of poor quality, and (2) triggers are plentiful, preferences are scarce, and preferences are rarely used for pleasure, stress recovery, and relaxation into sleep cycles.

The primary constructs discussed within this chapter include (1) how the developing sensory system works and develops in the context of relationships and the environment, (2) how disruptions to sensory processing and modulation may be demonstrated in behavior, and (3) how the professional can assess and intervene with the child, parents, and environment to optimize a child's sensory functioning and development.

Laura's case example will help us understand the sensory system and how we can use this information to unravel the complexity of behavior. A victim of severe neglect from birth, Laura's sensory world was impoverished. She received little sensory input to spark her curiosity, engage her joy, or drive her exploration. As a consequence, her innate sensory processing capacities lay dormant, and her sensory preferences were scarce. A victim of abuse, her sensory world was also dangerous, wrought with stimuli that led to fear and pain. By the time she reached treatment, her sensory triggers dominated the clinical picture, and she had learned to anticipate most sensory events as potentially harmful. For Laura, pleasure was not defined by the usual sensory preferences, such as a mother's happy eyes, melodic voice, and warm embrace; rather, her only pleasure was relief—from threat, fear, and boredom.

Laura's mother abused a variety of drugs, and her father was a drug dealer. At the age of 15 months, she was taken from her parents after reports of severe neglect and abuse. She was found hungry, dirty, and living out of a car with her parents. As is often the case in these situations, very little was revealed about the details of her history due to the confidentiality requirements within the child welfare system. Laura's first foster placement was with a busy mother who was already caring for four other foster children and her own 9-year-old daughter. During Laura's stay, the foster mother complained that she resisted parental limits, ignored directives, was often aggressive, had chronic diarrhea, and refused to toilet train. Due to the mounting complaints, the social worker requested an evaluation with an early intervention assessment team. The team concluded that Laura had mental retardation, reactive attachment disorder, and oppositional-defiant disorder.

This foster mother had no plans to adopt Laura so, at age 2 and a half, she was placed with Juan and Mary, an eager young foster–adopt couple who were willing to work with her despite the diagnoses and delays. Juan and Mary made several 2-hour visits with Laura in her first foster placement and saw that she alternated between wandering aimlessly and screaming. She received very little attention from her foster mother, although the 9-year-old made occasional attempts to engage her. Even then, Laura was not very responsive to these attempts and spoke only one or two words. Juan and Mary also noticed that the foster family did not seem to have regular routines, and they even watched Laura go without eating and fall asleep on the floor.

The new social worker on the case, who had been trained in the neurorelational framework, began to explore the underpinnings of Laura's behaviors. She wondered whether her diagnoses stemmed from (1) an inability to hear well, (2) an inability to understand words, (3) the absence of sensory comfort and pleasure in the relationships and environment, (4) trauma-induced flooded states versus defiance, or (5) some combination of these factors. The social worker wondered if experiences of sensory pleasure with her new foster parents would begin to promote progress across developmental and socioemotional milestones. She asked Juan and Mary to journal Laura's behaviors and pay special attention to what brought her comfort (her preferences) and what led to a stress response (her triggers).

During the first week, Laura primarily cried, had tantrums, barely spoke, hoarded food under her bed, had persistent diarrhea, refused to sleep in her room alone, and showed no stranger anxiety. Curiously, she did not seem to register pain. For example, when she fell down, she would smile instead of showing any distress. Juan and Mary were good observers and very patient with Laura. They noticed that she exhibited more stress response states when the house was bustling and was more often calm and easier to soothe when things were quiet. Thus, Juan and Mary began to work at maintaining a quiet environment, slowing down the pace of activities in the house, and slowing down the pace of words and gestures used with Laura. They established more daily routines and limited visitors; Juan took time off of work to be more available. Suspecting a history of food deprivation, they placed food in the lower kitchen cupboards within easy reach so that Laura could access it and eat without restrictions.

Within 2 weeks, the couple reported that Laura's tantrums had decreased and she had begun to use two-word phrases such as "go outside" and "play ball." Superdawg, the family dog, became a constant companion and profound source of comfort for Laura. She loved to stroke, hug, and sleep with her new best friend. Although odd behaviors around food persisted (e.g., hiding food underneath her bed), within a month she began eating with Juan and Mary at the table. After 2 months, she began talking nonstop and seemed to be using new words each day, although she was still difficult to understand. Her tantrums decreased to protests as she became better able to use words and gestures to get her needs met. Laura also began to show appropriate stranger anxiety with unfamiliar people, clinging and hovering behind Mary's legs. At Laura's last visit with the pediatrician, the couple's suspicion of a food allergy was confirmed, and a new diet stopped the diarrhea. Juan, Mary, and the social worker were thrilled with Laura's progress.

THE FUNCTION OF THE SENSORY BRAIN SYSTEM

The quality of functioning within the sensory system shapes the quality of emerging developmental and socioemotional milestones. Indeed, all learning is sensory based. Sensory experiences build sensory–motor memories which are at the root of perception (Roley, 2006). Thus, to support ongoing development, learning, and relational connections, the optimal functioning of the sensory system becomes a primary goal for assessment and intervention. "Optimal functioning" means that the sensory system represents the sensory events occurring in the body and the world in a way that is accurate (processing) and appropriate to context (modulation). Here we take a closer look at the mechanisms of processing and modulation—their physiological underpinnings and the sensory self that emerges from them.

Sensory Capacities

The flow of sensory signals in the body and the world must progress through a series of changes before becoming a sensory experience. The sensory components that make up experience include sights, sounds, touch, pain, taste, smell, balance (vestibular), and body position (proprioception). In general, sensory processing is the transduction of different types of energy in the environment into signals that combine to become sensory information. Sensory processing involves modality-specific perceptions (e.g., color, pitch, tickle) as well as multimodal perceptual elaborations (e.g., a fireworks display, verbal and gestural communication).

Sensory modulation is the process of balancing the flow of sensory signals so that the information that takes center stage is relevant and appropriate to the context. Sensory modulation involves amodal properties (i.e., properties not specific to any single modality, conveyed simultaneously by several modalities), such as intensity, rate, duration, and rhythm.

Although processing and modulation are integrated processes, this dual rubric is useful because each tends to have different implications for assessment and intervention that also tend to be weighted toward different disciplinary specialties. A well-functioning sensory system is manifest through the following capacities:

- the capacity to receive, translate, associate, and elaborate sensory signals within and across sensory modalities in a developmentally appropriate way (*sensory processing*);
- the capacity to balance the flow of sensory signals in a way that is appropriate to context (*sensory modulation*).

These two capacities share similarities with the concept of sensory integration. Jean Ayres, a pioneer in the field of occupational therapy, defined sensory integration as:

> the neurological process that organizes sensation from one's own body and from the environment and makes it possible to use the body effectively within the environment. The spatial and temporal aspects of inputs from different sensory modalities are interpreted, associated, and unified. Sensory integration is information processing. (Ayres, 1989, p. 11)

Contemporary occupational therapists use the phrase "sensory processing" as the more expansive term containing several parts, of which sensory integration and sensory modulation are two components (Miller & Lane, 2000). In contrast, the neurorelational framework highlights processing and modulation, as already defined, as processes that have differing physiological underpinnings. This rubric reflects our perspective of the neuroscience research.

Physiological Underpinnings of the Sensory System

The sensory system can contribute to coordination or load conditions based on the quality of processing and modulation within and across sensory modalities. Recall from the information in Chapter 2 that the

term *sensory modality* refers to the general class or type of sensory information conveyed (e.g., vision, hearing, taste). Each sensory modality travels an independent path at the entry level (e.g., retinas in the eyes, cochlea in the ears, tastebuds on the tongue) but soon associates with other sensory modalities to form the perception of a unified sensory experience. The current knowledge base contains varying views of how each sensory modality contributes to behavior and development.

Each sensory modality conveys the following common properties of information: (1) where in space or on the body that the sensory signal is experienced (location); (2) the strength, force, or concentration of the sensory signal (intensity); and (3) the temporal nature of the sensory signal (duration, rhythm) (Gardner & Martin, 2000). We distinguish sensory processing and sensory modulation according to these physiological underpinnings:

- Processing is weighted toward the modality and location attributes of the sensory information (what is it, where is it?).
- Modulation is weighted toward the intensity and timing attributes of the sensory information (how much of it, how fast is it, how long does it last?).

The primary areas that translate visual, auditory, and somatosensory data are more fully formed at birth than other areas of the cortex. The primary areas create "maps" of the sensory field onto the cortex, forming *cortical maps* (Kandel, 2000). Cortical maps contain point-to-point projections from specific areas of the receptor sense organs (e.g., retinas, cochlea, cutaneous receptors) to specific areas of the primary cortex (banks of the calcarine fissure for vision, Heschel's gyrus for hearing, postcentral gyrus for body representation) (Saper, Iversen, & Frakowiak, 2000). These areas are the cortical entry points for transforming auditory data into words and music, visual data into people and objects, and cutaneous data into a perception of touch and heat. The motor areas complete the sensory–motor loop: movement is a response to sensory information but also initiates the "selection" of sensory data; these processes are reciprocal and integrated and determined by the particular perception-action context. Sensory and motor systems connect across multiple levels in the brain to form ongoing and reciprocal interacting loops (Kandel, 2000). Sensory and motor systems are also integrated at the neural level via multimodal neurons. For example, the premotor areas in the brain contain neurons that integrate motor, visual, somatosensory, and auditory information about objects/events in close personal space (Fogassi et al., 1996; Gentilucci,

Scandolara, Pigarev, & Rizzolatti, 1983; Graziano, Reiss, & Gross, 1999; Rizzolatti, Fogassi, & Gallese, 2000, 2002; Rizzolatti, Scandolara, Matelli, & Gentilucci, 1981). These sensory–motor processes create a cohesive internal experience and also connect us with the experiences of others and events in the environment in real time. As we engage with others through our movements, we become their sensory data; as we act on and modify the environment, our "marks" become sensory data for others. We create sensory experiences for others, and others create sensory experiences for us, experiences that take on various meanings relative according to the context.

Cortical maps represent the elementary properties of stimuli (e.g., the perception of lines and edges), but as these data are passed on to subsequent synaptic levels (the point where one neuron connects with another), they become associated with other sense properties and elaborated to form meaningful representations of the world (e.g., the line of a horizon, the smile on a face) (Amaral, 2000). Given this organization, disruptions at an elemental level may complicate processing at a higher one. A mild disruption may result in a milestone delay that is subtle initially but eventually leads to significant complications in achieving a particular competency. For example, a child's difficulties in discriminating the phonemes of spoken language—a very early emerging ability—can pave the way for a learning disability in reading—a later emerging ability (Liberman, Shankweiler, & Liberman, 1989). A severe disruption may completely eliminate the ability to create a representation of a sensory modality and thereby disrupt all potential competencies associated with that modality. For example, a congenital or acquired condition causing total deafness at birth would disrupt any competency associated with hearing (e.g., sound localization, speech, playing an instrument). At the same time, having multiple synaptic levels as well as multimodal neurons at various levels means that there is built-in flexibility, and disruptions may be modified or compensated through learning (Huttenlocher, 2002). For example, with appropriate intervention, a reading disabled child learns to discriminate phonemes using other sensory routes (e.g., Lindamood & Lindamood, 1984; Torgesen, Wagner, Rashotte, Alexander, & Conway, 1997), or reading comprehension is enhanced using sensorimotor enactments and imagination (Glenberg, Gutierrez, Levin, Japuntich, & Kaschak, 2004), or a child who is congenitally deaf naturally develops enhanced detection of vibration (Levanen & Hamdorf, 2001). These benefits to learning exploit the neural underpinnings of sensory–motor plasticity.

The sensory modalities can be organized according to their structural and functional properties. Mesulam (1998, 2000b) presented an organization based on anatomical, physiological, and behavioral features, whereby the sensory modalities are differentiated, some modalities more

than others. For the more differentiated senses located in the higher cortical areas, which include visual, auditory, and somatosensory modes, the
modality-specific processing is greatly enhanced and elaborated. For example, in the visual modality, the entry-level neurons (the first to receive
information from the sensory organ) respond to highly specific properties of the visual signal, such as line orientation or contrast. As the visual
signal travels, it becomes more defined (e.g., color, movement) and elaborated (e.g., object, face, action) as it merges and integrates with other sensory signals, a process that yields meaning based on personal, relational,
and environmental context. Consistent with the "what"/"where" definition of sensory processing, these modalities segregate according to "what"
and "where" processing streams—the "what" streams convey identity, and
the "where" streams convey position and motion. For example, the dorsal
visual stream tracks movement and the ventral visual stream identifies
objects (Mishkin, Ungerleider, & Macko, 1983). A similar organization for
auditory and somatosensory has been demonstrated more recently
(Rauschecker & Tian, 2000; Reed, Klatzky, & Halgren, 2005; Sestieri et al.,
2006; Tian, Reser, Durham, Kustov, & Rauschecker, 2001). A great deal of
real estate in the brain is devoted to processing within and across the visual, auditory, and somatosensory modalities.

For the less differentiated senses, which include olfactory (smell),
gustatory (taste), and vestibular (balance), there is much less fidelity of the
sensory signals (Mesulam, 2000b). For those senses, the response properties of neurons at the entry level are less specific, and less real estate in the
brain is devoted to processing within those modalities. For example, in the
primary vestibular area, neurons are not specialized to respond only to
various properties of the vestibular sense. To the contrary, the majority of
neurons in the primary vestibular area are multisensory (i.e., they respond
to more than one sense modality; Brandt & Dieterich, 1999).

Structurally, the primary areas of the differentiated senses are more
removed from the brain regions that are affiliated with bodily states, emotions, and memories, as compared with the primary areas of the less differentiated senses (Mesulam, 1998, 2000b). Functionally, the more highly
differentiated modalities are oriented toward representing the external
world or sensory events in the surround (e.g., sights, sounds), whereas the
less differentiated modalities are oriented toward representing the internal world or sensory events more closely associated with the body (the
uniqueness of the somatosenses will be addressed shortly). The external
senses lend themselves to greater objectivity and a more precise, detailed
description of perceptual variations; the internal senses are more subjective and often lack the same descriptive clarity (i.e., their qualities are
vaguer or more abstract).

The somatosenses are unique because aspects of bodily perceptions have contributions from both the highly differentiated and less differentiated regions. The highly differentiated pathways represent (1) the proprioceptive senses that arise from joint and muscle signals in relation to the body's movement and position and (2) the cutaneous sense of touch pressure (Gardner, Martin, & Jessell, 2000). The less differentiated pathways represent (1) broad stroke touch and light touch, (2) temperature and pain, and (3) the visceral senses (Gardner & Kandel, 2000; Snell, 2006). The perceptions represented by the more diffuse pathways are considered to be more directly related to survival. They intersect with limbic (older) brain regions and have direct access to brain regions that facilitate alerting and arousal reactions (versus indirect access of the differentiated sensory modalities).

Sensory Processing

Sensory processing can be thought of as a parts-to-whole sequence, with the parts representing the individual sensory modalities and the whole being the unified sensory experience. Once energy in the world is received by sensory receptors, it travels a nerve path to specialized neurons in the brain that pass on raw sensory data through a series of progressive levels. Early in the journey, the sensory information represented is more general, and it becomes increasingly specific as it evolves to a highly specific end. For example, the car stereo turns on, sound waves enter the ear, travel the auditory nerve, and reach the auditory cortex to become volume and pitch, then melody and rhythm, then music, then a particular song, then a song that floods the mind with associated memories, with only the latter stages of processing being available to conscious experience.

As sensory data feed forward in the parts-to-whole sequence, we cannot predict the exact course of their journey because along the way sensory signals become increasingly intermingled in a complex web of associated back-and-forth connections from all regions of the brain and thus open to vast and variable influences. One could never play a song and presume to predict the memories that flood a child's mind. However, one could make other reasonable predictions and observations. What if a child does not respond at all to the music? What if a child seems to be singing along but is completely out of sync with the rhythm? What if a child's tone is on key but the words are off? What if a child covers her ears and runs screaming from the room? What if a child brightens and approaches to dance with you? These responses are all potentially meaningful; for assessment, each hints at a different point in the parts-to-whole sequence, and each has the potential to provide a key to intervention.

As with any neuroanatomical description of behavior, there is no one-to-one correspondence between the hierarchy of sensory processing in the brain and the behavior we observe in the world. However, the sensory hierarchy can serve as a heuristic guide for investigating the potential disruptions to accuracy within and across sensory modalities, thereby leading to more informed hypotheses and intervention strategies. Adapted from Mesulam's (1998) discussion of sensory processing, this hierarchy involves four levels: entry, elemental, association, and elaboration. Sensory processing begins when receptors of a sensory organ pick up a form of energy that is converted to an electrical impulse and transported to the brain (entry level). These signals enter awareness only if they reach the brain, so, for example, if the nerves in the cochlea are damaged, sound waves may not stimulate them to send signals to the auditory nerve. As already noted, sensory modalities in primary cortical areas form very precise maps of the stimulus range or field (in visual, auditory, and somatosensory regions). Within these maps, individual neurons specialize to represent specific aspects along the continuum of a general stimulus such as light-to-dark contrast, vertical-to-horizontal line orientations, and low-to-high frequencies. From here, point-to-point projections to secondary areas combine these elements to represent the more rudimentary attributes of the sensory modalities (e.g., elemental levels including speech sounds and patterns, melody and rhythm, depth and motion). The information is passed on to association areas that more fully merge sensory modalities to support perceptions such as objects, faces, words, music, spatial locations, and complex movement (association level). At this level, meaning begins to take shape. Finally, at the highest level, the elaboration level, association areas combine in transmodal areas, where the brain translates faces into recognition and identification, words into meaningful communication, events into personal experiences, and spatial locations into venues for exploration and pursuit of goals. Within any sensory modality, a disruption at the entry or elemental levels may shut down the entire sensory system (e.g., deafness, blindness). In general, disruptions at lower levels affect the optimal functioning of the higher levels.

The transformation of sensory processes into meaningful experience takes on greater complexity and specificity at higher levels and nearly always implies learning. For example, at the association level, meaning is a series of sounds that represent a known word or a visual image that represents an object for a specific use. At the elaboration level, meaning is in the context of personal experience, for example, the word refers to your deceased father's profession, or the object is your wedding band, or the purpose of the object depends upon the action being performed.

From the womb, brain development follows the progressive sequence as the sensory hierarchy just described. Entry levels reach maturity in the womb, elemental levels are mature by the end of the first year, and brain areas that support association and elaboration mature throughout adolescence and into early adulthood (Huttenlocher, 1990; Huttenlocher & Dabholkar, 1997). This developmental sequence means that *age of disruption* as well as *level of disruption* are highly salient factors. In general, disruption to more than one sensory modality at a lower level (closer to the primary area) suggests a more complicated clinical picture. Conversely, disruption that affects a single sensory modality at a midlevel suggests a more specific and more treatable issue. The most important factors for outcome are related to the severity and chronicity of the disruption, for example, extreme sensory deprivation, such as that in an orphanage (especially for children adopted after 2 years or more) (Gunnar & Fisher and the Early Experience, Stress, and Prevention Science Network, 2006; Gunnar, Van Dulmen, & The International Adoption Project Team, 2007; Parker & Nelson and The Bucharest Early Intervention Project Core Group, 2005; Zeanah et al., 2003).

Here, we have presented sensory processing in a modality-specific way, whereby the sensory modalities become increasingly integrated at higher synaptic levels because, when working with children with developmental delays, this lends to deconstructing functional capacities according to (1) the potential sources of disruption via sensory modality and (2) the general point in the developmental timeline that the disruption altered the functional trajectory. Both of these factors have direct translation to questions of treatment: (1) what sensory domain should take focus in intervention, and (2) how far back do we go to shore up the developmental building blocks needed for current and future optimal functioning? However, as noted, neurons across several regions of the brain, including motor areas, are multisensory, meaning that they respond to more than one sensory parameter. This feature of sensory–motor processing is important in understanding the varied nature of perception and action relative to context in real time. In other words, perceptions take on very different meanings depending on the context and relevant potential actions, such as proximity to self or the purpose or goal of a particular action (e.g., a child observing an angry adult yelling at another child in the store calls up a very different behavioral response than a child looking at an angry parent yelling at him or her at home). This integrated, real-time view of sensory–motor brain processes (the embodied cognition view) will likely become much more prominent in future research, especially in the context of intervention, as it highlights how higher-level cognitive functions such as language comprehension and memory can be enhanced through an appreciation

of the integrated ("meshed") nature of perception and action in context (Dijkstra, Kaschak, & Swaan, 2007; Kaschak et al., 2005).

Sensory Modulation

Sensory modulation involves the intensity, duration, and rhythm attributes of sensory stimuli (how much, how long, and how fast) (Miller & Lane, 2000). The chemical processes that coordinate activation and inhibition within sensory modalities are part of the physiological underpinnings to modulation. In the regulation system, we referred to *modulation* as the balancing of energy because it affects overall arousal levels (e.g., deep sleep as the dominance of inhibition, flooded as the dominance of activation). In the sensory system, *modulation* refers to activation and inhibition of sensory signals—processes that determine the sensory information that will ultimately influence behavior—what will be "taken in" and what will be "screened out." There is an immense amount of sensory information in the body and the world that is not so important to behavior and should not dominate, for example, vibrations from the heart beating or the flicker of a leaf. Ultimately, the goal of sensory modulation is to represent incoming information in a way that best guides behavior as appropriate to context.

Our bodies and brains are preset to give greater weight to what matters most for survival, thus managing the dominance of sensory signals (to some extent) without the help of modulation. For example, we have a greater concentration of sensory receptors on our fingertips than we have on our backs, with a similar biased allocation of brain tissue for fingers versus the back (Gardner & Kandel, 2000). Beyond this preset bias, sensory modulation takes on the role of negotiating the real-time flow of ever-changing sensory signals. Ideally, what matters most rises above the sensory mix and is accurately represented in its strength and temporal charactcristics. In this way, we are equipped to attend to and track sensory information and guide behavior in a manner that is appropriate to the situation at hand (Amaral, 2000).

A structure near the center of the brain, the thalamus, is the hub for sensory processing and modulation. The thalamus acts as a gateway for the flow of information, emphasizing some signals and muting others. In other words, not all signals have equal status. For cxamplc, during the deepest stage of sleep, the thalamus acts like a bouncer at the velvet rope, allowing only the most important neural messages to enter the cortex. When we are awake, the bouncer still shows favoritism but is far more flexible. If a sensory event has high information content (i.e., importance), then the sensory signals must "organize a loud, commanding neuronal shout" to recruit the attention of the appropriate sensory motor processes from the masses

(Pfaff, 2006). Sensory events that tend to activate are those that are novel, unexpected, irregular in rhythm, and so forth; sensory events that tend to inhibit are those that are familiar, predictable, regular in rhythm, and so on.

The sensory data that either gain entry or are turned away influence ongoing learning and memory. The quality of modulation plays a central role in the quality of learning. In general, most learning occurs at the midrange alert processing state, when activation and inhibition are in balance. A loss of balance in either direction—too much activation or too much inhibition—typically tends to reduce learning. For example, increasing activation lends to increased scanning and distractibility, whereas increasing inhibition lends to decreased scanning and inattention. Either of these responses is desirable if appropriate to context, but not a good thing if a child is taking in too much unimportant information or screening out too much important information.

All sensory modalities (except smell) must connect through the thalamus as they make their way to their respective locations in the brain. Once they reach this point, multiple paths navigate the sensory hierarchy. As mentioned in Chapter 2, a "quick and dirty" response (LeDoux, 1996, 2002) is associated with a subcortical bottom-up pathway, wherein there are direct connections between the thalamus and the amygdala. These links are more efficient in rapidly eliciting an emotional response (unconsciously), but they are limited in their representation of the stimulus and therefore may be less accurate. A longer and slower pathway travels through the entire information-processing hierarchy before reaching the amygdala, thus it is much more accurate in its representation of the sensory stimulus; this is called the thalamo-cortical-amygdala pathway (LeDoux, 1996, 2002). In this way, both bottom-up and top-down properties of sensory events can be emphasized and maintained. Sensory modulation shapes what we learn, and through these reciprocal connections, what we learn shapes modulation.

Two of the most basic and common forms of learning are *habituation* and *sensitization*, processes that in general determine whether a sensory event will be screened out or taken in. Shorthand definitions of these two terms follow:

- *Habituation*: a decrease in responsiveness on repeated exposure to a stimulus.
- *Sensitization*: an increase in responsiveness on repeated exposure to a stimulus.

Eric Kandel (see Kandel, 2007, for a review), through his lab's work with the sea slug *aplysia* (which earned him and his colleagues a Nobel Prize in

Physiology and Medicine in 2000), showed that repeated exposures to a benign stimulus induced chemical changes that coincided with reduced behavioral reactivity with each stimulus delivery. In other words, with a stimulus posing no real threat to life (but not limb, in this case), the sea slug got used to it. This fundamental and highly adaptive process of habituation appears strikingly similar in humans. *Habituation* supports coordination in the sense that it allows us to settle down and feel safe in a sometimes capricious sensory world. Without this adaptive capacity, benign sensory events would repeatedly set off a stress response and eventually lead to load conditions. For example, a child who is repeatedly triggered by sensory events that overwhelm him or her may attempt to cope by blocking out or withdrawing, both variations of a hypoalert load state. In addition, a person who habituates too quickly may have tendencies toward a chronic hypoalert state wherein novel stimulation regularly goes unnoticed.

On the flip side, the sea slug's exposure to a threatening stimulus induced chemical changes that coincided with an enhanced behavioral reactivity, known as *sensitization*. A robust increase in behavioral reactivity can occur following a single stimulus presentation. This process is also highly adaptive, intended to alert us to danger and get us out of harm's way. However, this process can go awry in two ways that may induce a load condition. First, the stimuli that produced the activating response may have been an actual threat at first, but then experience showed that it was not so bad after all, or quite safe. If this higher level of learning, gleaned from experience, does not eventually usurp the knee-jerk activation, constant overreactivity, which may even generalize to associated stimuli, may be the result. Second, the stimuli that produced the activating response may actually *be* a threat, as is the case for a child with extreme sensitivity to noise or a child who is a victim of abuse. If sensory signals precede the sensory event, and these preceding signals provoke a stress response, then the child has reached another level of learning that allows him or her to *anticipate* the threatening event. This is adaptive, on one hand, but also places a heavy load on all four brain systems in a situation of repeated stressors.

As we can see, there are strong connections between behavioral reactions to sensory information and arousal, emotions, and attention. Many professionals have "seen" and documented this clinical phenomenon (Baranek, David, Poe, Stone, & Watson, 2006; DeGangi, 2000; DeGangi, DiPietro, Greenspan, & Porges, 1991; Miller, Reisman, McIntosh, & Simon, 2001; Miller & Summers, 2001; Williamson & Anzalone, 2001), which may be why, in parallel tracks, the infant mental health field defines these phenomenon in the DC:0–3R (ZERO TO THREE, 1994, 2005) under the

category of regulatory disorders; similarly, the early intervention field in
the occupational therapy discipline has developed a taxonomy of sensory
integration dysfunction (Fisher & Murray, 1991) that includes "sensory
modulation dysfunction" (Miller & Lane, 2000; Miller, Robinson, & Moulton, 2004). In addition, in a recent study of diagnostic judgments, when
occupational therapists and psychologists were both presented with two
toddler cases (one designed to present a general anxiety disorder and another designed to present sensory overresponsivity),

> more occupational therapists diagnosed as sensory-over responsive, while
> more psychologists diagnosed with a general anxiety disorder. The overlap
> in judgments of sensory over-responsivity and anxiety supports the notion
> that these constructs in part reflect different professionals' perspectives upon
> behaviors as well as the difficulty in distinguishing these constructs in tod-
> dlers. (Ben-Sasson, Cermak, Orsmond, Carter, & Fogg, 2007, p. 526)

This confusion speaks to the problem of not having a common language across disciplines; it also provides an example of why dimensional
perspectives to understanding behavior (Chapter 2) can be so useful when
phenomenon span the arousal, sensory, emotional, and attentional domains. It is helpful to note that preliminary data from empirical research
are emerging that examine sensory responses in conjunction with physiological measures, beginning to validate the behaviors of modulation disorders for diagnostic purposes and document the physiology that guides
our understanding of the underlying challenges. For example, in pilot
data collected on children identified as having sensory modulation dysfunction, associations among sensation, arousal (electrodermal activity),
emotions, and attention were found (Miller et al., 2004). This finding
lends support to the importance of assessing symptom expressions across
all four brain systems at the same time.

In another set of comparison pilot studies between children with particular identified diagnosis or dysfunction and a control group, physiological measures (electrodermal activity) revealed that children diagnosed with
fragile X syndrome differed from the control group by "demonstrating
greater magnitude, more responses per stimulation, responses on a greater
proportion of trails, and lower rates of habituation" (Miller et al., 1999, p.
268). Children diagnosed with ADHD showed "greater abnormalities in
sensory modulation" on physiological measures and "displayed more variability" in their responses (Mangeot et al., 2001, p. 399). Some children
identified with sensory-modulation disruptions showed no electrodermal
responses (EDRs; all control children did respond), whereas the majority
"showed more and larger EDR than control children" (McIntosh, Miller,
Shyu, & Hagerman, 1999, p. 608). In a review of lessons learned from over

a decade of conducting pilot studies, Miller et al. (2007) noted that it is common that the same children display combinations of under- and over-responsiveness, often to differing sensory modalities.

While electrodermal responses index sympathetic nervous system (SNS) activation and anxiety (Dawson, Schell, & Filion, 2007), suggesting that the SNS is creating the heightened arousal, pilot studies have also begun investigating the role of the parasympathetic nervous system (PNS) through vagal tone. Children with sensory modulation disturbances "had significantly lower vagal tone than the typically developing sample" (Schaaf, Miller, Seawell, & O'Keefe, 2003, p. 442), suggesting that low vagal tone may also contribute to the rise in activation (due to poor inhibition). Decreased and disorganized vagal tone has also been implicated in premature infants who had poorer clinical outcomes than those with higher PNS activity (DiPietro & Porges, 1991). Thus, future studies are recommended that combine indexes for both SNS and PNS to investigate the role of these systems' activity in sensory modulation difficulties (Miller et al., 2007). In fact, stress researchers studying the effects of trauma maltreatment are also now suggesting that using one physiological marker alone, such as cortisol, is not sufficient to provide enough insight into the impact of maltreatment, due to the variety of hypo- and hyperresponsiveness to threatening stimuli. Gunnar and Fisher (2006) recommend combined measures that can look at the relationship and changes between the SNS (activating) and hypothalamic-pituitary-adrenocortical (HPA) axis (inhibiting) dynamics. In conclusion, research contributions from genetic, temperament, and environmental arenas are indicating the importance of recognizing and incorporating the interrelated dynamics of activation and inhibition for both assessment and intervention paradigms across diagnostic criteria.

Self- and Interactive Regulation

The process of communicating and relating is a sensory experience. Professionals across disciplines are not necessarily trained to think of interactions as sensory in their origins. Nevertheless, smell, touch, facial expressions, vocal sounds, tone, rhythms, gestures, and movements are all raw data that will be organized into perceptions and meaning by the other brain systems. For an infant or child, the parent relationship provides the greatest source of sensory information. The reverse is also true—the infant or child often provides the greatest source of sensory information for the parent.

The sensory system provides the means by which developing brains learn about the things they like and do not like. This process of getting to know the sensory self (more on this topic in the following section) sets

the stage for how a child learns to recognize, respond to, and anticipate sensory events in the body, relationships, and the world that are likely to represent three basic conditions: safety, challenge, or threat. Typically, sensory preferences tend to support the experience of safety, and sensory triggers tend to promote experiences of challenge or threat. Perceptions of safety, challenge, and threat are most adaptive when they occur within the context of supportive and nurturing interactive regulation.

In typical situations, an infant or child exhibits behaviors that adequately communicate his or her sensory preferences and triggers to others. A *sensory trigger*, whether coming from a person or the surroundings, provokes a response of dislike or distress; a *sensory preference* provokes a response of pleasure, enjoyment, or calm, thereby naturally promoting self-regulation. Through these behaviors, the parent becomes acquainted with the child's unique sensory profile and, often without even being conscious of it, will adjust the environment and his or her behavior to create a better fit with the child's sensory self (note that we did not say "a perfect fit"). An infant may be able to self-soothe while sucking a thumb or pacifier, relax after pushing her feet up against the crib, brighten or fuss when the house is bustling, laugh or cry when Daddy sings, or turn toward or away from an approaching stranger. The parent who allows, anticipates, or responds to these cues in a supportive way is engaging in interactive regulation. Over time, this interactive regulation in essence teaches the child to pay attention to what makes him or her feel good—or not. A child, for example, develops an ability to say "no" to an invitation to play on a merry-go-round when prior experience has been scary or uncomfortable for him or her. The sensory preferences and triggers described thus far are typical, but they become a problem when they repeatedly induce a stress response and thereby increase the risk for a load condition.

When sensory events too often induce stress responses (sensitization), then a more thorough investigation of preferences and triggers is in order. As noted in the previous chapter, the younger and the more vulnerable a child is, the more interactive regulation he or she will need. The fundamental goal is to use the relationship as a means of increasing sensory preferences that enhance safety (signaled by deep sleep and alert processing states) and decreasing sensory triggers that promote challenge and threat (stress response states). This process supports coordination.

Sensory Self

In the last chapter, we noted that connection to the visceral self (i.e., the ability to experience and modulate the feelings related to the body's organs)

not only orients one to basic physical needs but also provides crucial information for guiding many aspects of behavior, including emotions and decisions. The sensory self contains and expands on the visceral self to reflect the full range of information exchange as the body interacts in relationships and the world. The sensory self reflects one's capacities to integrate internal and external sensory information in a way that fosters contextually accurate perceptions of self, others, and the world.

Even an infant has a rudimentary sensory self; for example, a baby who conveys feeling discomfort (internal information) and is soothed by the parent's touch, holding, and vocal expressions (external information). The sensory self reflects the unique sensory makeup of the individual and is always changing. As a person interacts with his or her world, the sensory self influences ongoing experience (e.g., what is sought and avoided) and is influenced by ongoing experience (e.g., discovery or validation of a trigger), which can then influence future sensory opportunities.

In general, a coordinated sensory self is defined by a balance between stability and flexibility in sensory preferences and triggers. It is optimal to have a good idea of what we like and dislike, and it is also optimal to know when it is adaptive to be tolerant, open to discovery, or daring. A sensory self in a load condition is defined by a loss of balance that moves toward severe rigidity (e.g., a child whose preferences and triggers are so fixed that behavior is almost obsessively repetitive and any novelty produces a stress response) or severe variability (e.g., a child whose preferences and triggers are so erratic that it is difficult to even define the sensory self and difficult to intervene through this system).

When we left Juan and Mary, they were feeling pleased with how well Laura seemed to be doing, but then an unexpected event occurred.

Before the adoption process concluded, Laura's birth mother resurfaced and asked for reunification. Because she was participating in a drug treatment program, and to mobilize a rapid reunification process, she was quickly granted full-weekend visits on a weekly basis. After the first weekend, Laura returned to Juan and Mary unable to sleep at night and either screaming or staring vacuously during the day. After the second weekend, her language diminished and she regressed to babbling. However, after each visit, Laura gradually returned to her previous level of functioning, and she never lost her affection for Superdawg. After the third weekend, Laura did not return to baseline. Her diarrhea returned, and her aggressive behaviors reemerged. She screamed every time she was not in control, ran around the house yelling "bitch" repeatedly, began pulling out her own and Mary's eyelashes, and tore the hair off all her dolls. In other words, Laura's stress responses steadily and severely increased (sensitization) following visits with her birth mother.

Juan and Mary were frightened and dejected. They felt powerless to stop what was happening. At their request for more help, the social worker referred them to

me (CL). I reviewed the social worker's observations, Laura's history, and the foster–adopt parents' logs and made the following hypothesis and functional observations. It seemed clear that Laura's serious decline was related to the weekend visits with her biological mother. For the sake of her future placement, it was important to clearly define my interpretation of her decline to the court. First, Laura's initial foster home placement presented her with a combination of over- and understimulation that probably affected her development to the point where she had appeared mentally retarded. The overstimulation came in the form of the sheer number of children in the house and the chaotic mismanagement that resulted. The understimulation arose from the depleted foster mother's inability to provide any kind of nurturance and strong commitment to a very traumatized child.

In my initial interactions with Laura, I perceived more capacities than perhaps earlier testing had documented. She easily entered into puppet play and made up stories that had basic cause-and-effect scenes in them; she spontaneously picked up building materials and began creating simple structures; and she had evidenced a language burst after her first few weeks with Juan and Mary. These behaviors indicated a good brain that needed safety, nurturance, and engagement. I perceived that she had a speech and language delay that needed further attention from a speech and language specialist. Second, in the care of Juan and Mary, Laura's defiant behaviors had also shifted to healthy forms of protests with attempts to communicate her needs. To me, this shift indicated that she could sustain an alert processing state wherein she could not only recognize her needs but also begin to communicate them accurately. Third, her reactive attachment diagnosis (approaching others without caution) was already resolved with Juan and Mary, so much so that Laura had shown appropriate anxiety toward strangers. This shift suggested to me that Laura, having experienced warm and safe relationships, now allowed herself to register appropriate anxiety that was previously blocked as part of her trauma response. Fourth, her inability to feel pain was likely the result of prolonged, severe stress resulting in a blunted perception of pain occurring simultaneously with heightened awareness of sensory stimuli. In fact, sustained stressors can produce blunted pain responses even as they increase the acuity of certain forms of sensory functioning (Sapolsky, 1994).

It seemed clear that Laura's serious decline was directly related to the weekend reunification visits, and her reactions were now perhaps intensified because she had begun to experience sensory safety and comfort in her new home. The weekend visits exposed Laura to intermittent sources of relational threat that destabilized her slowly growing sense of safety and created sensitized responses. Moreover, Laura began communicating her experience of sensory threat in anticipation of the visits by protesting the weekend visits with crying and fearful questioning. When her bags were packed for the overnight stay, she would anxiously ask "night? night?" thus communicating her concerns about staying overnight.

Laura was now in chronic state of load day and night—tantamount to a 911 situation. I wrote an emergency letter to the court, detailing the sequence of events as well as my understanding of their meaning, and suggested a temporary

but immediate cessation to the reunification visits. Moreover, I asserted that this cycle of movement between safety and threat was an assault to Laura's mental health, setting up an even more damaging and grave situation whereby she would begin to link the forced reunification visits with the mother to Juan and Mary. This linkage would erode the perceptions of trust and safety that she had begun to feel with them and reintroduce a frightening loss of control (Sapolsky, 1994). I explained that it was critical for Laura to return to her most recent baseline of healthy functioning with Juan and Mary, because at this point she had lost all the progress she had made and was in jeopardy of not being able to regain it. Finally, I recommended to the courts that once Laura returned to her baseline functioning, she be carefully evaluated with each set of parents, and the evaluation should be conducted by someone qualified to do dyadic infant mental health assessments.

CLINICALLY RELEVANT BEHAVIORS OF THE SENSORY SYSTEM

In this section, we provide baseline descriptors of clinically relevant behaviors, both typical and atypical, weighted toward the various sensory modalities. The examples provided are intended to represent a range of developmental and socioemotional benchmarks but not to be comprehensive or exhaustive. This sampling of behaviors, as viewed through a sensory lens, is intended to help professionals (and parents working with professionals) begin to develop a template to guide thinking about assessment and intervention. As with all atypical behaviors, it is important to consider the meaning of those behaviors. They might (1) relate to the child's physiology and a particular sensory modality, (2) relate to the child's environment (a lack of, or too much, sensory stimulation), or (3) indicate a mismatch between the child's innate physiology and the environment (including relationships). Please note that the following modalities of hearing, sight, touch, taste, and smell are oriented toward the *external* milieu.

Hearing

Recall that Joseph (Chapters 1–3) responded slowly or not at all to his mother's voice. Laura was essentially mute during the first 3 years of her life. Once she began to talk, her articulation was poor and her language remained delayed. Table 6.1 shows coordinated and atypical auditory behaviors.

Table 6.1. Typical (Coordinated) and Atypical (Potential for Load Condition) Auditory Behaviors

Typical (Coordinated) for Infant, Child, or Adult	Atypical (Potential for Load Condition) for Infant, Child, or Adult
Turns toward the sound of a voice or a novel noise	Responds slowly or not at all to sounds and voices
Tolerates multiple ambient sounds at the same time (e.g., rain, TV, people talking)	Avoids noisy environments; covers ears for protection; does not react to auditory "chaos"
Takes delight in novel sounds	Shows no interest or startles in response to novel sounds
Coos and babbles in early infancy; imitates sounds and "plays with" sound sequences in infancy	Exhibits delayed cooing and babbling; does not imitate sounds and sound sequences; random sounds
Links up sound sequences to objects and intent; forms words	Does not connect sounds and words to objects, intent, or both
Discriminates and tolerates a variety of sounds from low to high ranges in pitch and tone	Cannot discriminate among sounds or between foreground and background noise; selectively responds to certain sounds or frequencies; cannot tolerate noises that are loud, sudden, or high-pitched
Accurately discriminates between sounds that are similar (phonetic awareness); "hears" and enjoys rhymes	Cannot hear the difference between similar sounds (such as *b* or *d*); does not "hear" rhymes
With optimal conditions, can understand a question and can follow simple directions, multistep directions, or both	Easily confused by questions, instructions, or both; unable to follow simple directions
Age-appropriate reading skills, able to express thoughts in written and verbal formats	Has trouble reading and verbalizing or writing thoughts

Vision

Early on, Joseph showed a lack of interest in faces and was drawn toward objects; as he developed, he did not accurately "read" nonverbal cues from others. Danny (presented in the regulation system chapters), a premature infant, would often become fixated on watching his father's or mother's face, enthralled, but unable to modulate his visual system by averting his gaze for natural rest periods. Laura, when finally engaged with nurturing parents, would sustain attention in observing their faces but was unable to imitate their facial expressions for quite some time. Table 6.2 shows coordinated and atypical visual behaviors.

Table 6.2.   Typical (Coordinated) and Atypical (Potential for Load Condition) Visual Behaviors

Typical (Coordinated) for Infant, Child, or Adult	Atypical (Potential for Load Condition) for Infant, Child, or Adult
Notices a happy face and smiles in response	Does not respond to a smile with a smile
Shows ability to make and sustain eye contact with brief visual breaks (modulation)	Exhibits perpetual side glancing; exhibits continual gaze aversion
Has bright, shiny eyes indicating engagement, interest, or curiosity; shows an interest in novel, eye-catching patterns and colors in the environment	Exhibits glazed eyes
Shows ability to fixate on faces or objects, alternating with ability to shift focus (modulation)	Cannot alternate between fixation on faces or objects and shifting focus to modulate visual tracking
Moves eyes together in a coordinated manner	Shows uncoordinated movement of both eyes (e.g., lazy eye)
With eyes, tracks the movement of a face or an object of interest	Shows poor tracking of moving objects of interest
In addition to imitating sounds from cooing and babbling, imitates facial and oral–motor expressions	In addition to the lack of imitative cooing and babbling sounds, does not imitate facial and oral–motor expressions
Discriminates between pictures, words, symbols, and objects that look alike and those that are different	Poorly discriminates between pictures, words, symbols, and objects that look alike and those that are distinctly different (Kranowitz, 1998)
Shows ability to coordinate visual information with fine motor movement, gross motor movement, or both (e.g., can look at blackboard and copy a letter of the alphabet; can catch a ball or throw a ball)	Exhibits poor visual–motor coordination (commonly related to learning disabilities; e.g., difficulty keeping track of space while reading; trouble keeping columns and lines while doing math; poor use of space on a page when writing; unable to dodge obstacles when running; frequently bumps into things)
Accurately reads nonverbal cues from others	Inaccurately reads nonverbal cues from others
Accurately sees letters and words while reading and writing; understands spatial dimensions such as up/down, right/left, before/after	Reversals occur in a variety of ways, including reversing letters (b/d), words (god/dog), or directions (right/left or up/down) (Kranowitz, 1998)
Visualizes while reading; able to create mental images of people, places, and things	Unable to visualize what one is reading; difficult to call up mental images of people, places, and things (Kranowitz, 1998)

Touch

There are two different types of touch: light stroking and deep pressure touch. Danny was overly reactive to the ordinary daily routines and to his parents' touches. Laura was at first indiscriminating; she would go to just about anyone for touch. Later, she became more discriminating and actually preferred to touch and be touched by the family dog—who became her steady source of sensory comfort through the tactile system. Table 6.3 shows coordinated and atypical tactile behaviors.

Table 6.3. Typical (Coordinated) and Atypical (Potential for Load Condition) Tactile Behaviors

Typical (Coordinated) for Infant, Child, or Adult	Atypical (Potential for Load Condition) for Infant, Child, or Adult
Displays comfort through cuddling, molding into parent's body, hugging, or massage (deep touch pressure); if a sensory preference, this type of touch is calming or alerting	Resists the deep pressure involved in cuddling, hugging, and massage
Displays comfort level with a range of human touch, from light touch or stroking to discrete touch from attachment figures; avoids close contact with strangers	Becomes distressed by touch from attachment figures (e.g., kisses) or is indiscriminate about who touches him or her
Is comfortable with different clothing textures (e.g., starchy cloth, tags on shirts) and textures (e.g., grass, sand, hardwood floors)	Becomes distressed by certain types of clothing, footwear, or textures
Is comfortable with daily hygienic procedures (e.g., changing diapers, taking bath, washing hair, hair brushing, wiping nose or face, trimming nails)	Becomes distressed by certain daily life hygienic routines
Is nonreactive to light touch and responds with glee when tickled by parent or in anticipation of a tickling game	Responds with distress, as if in pain, with light touch, in anticipation of light touch, or when tickled by parent, even when parent is gentle
Can locate specific point of touch	Cannot locate specific point of touch
Tolerates changing clothes, changing diapers, or both	Becomes distressed by changing clothes or diapers
Tolerates a wide variety of food textures and temperatures	Known as a picky eater, consistently refusing certain food textures (e.g., soft, hard, lumpy, crunchy) or temperatures (e.g., hot or cold)

Taste and Smell

Smell and taste have strong interconnections that can contribute to typical experiences of sensory aversion. Kenny, Danny's twin brother (Chapter 4 case example), had an unpleasant experience with eating a rotten egg and refused to eat eggs after that. Seeing eggs could induce a memory of the rotten taste in his mouth; he would gag and spit as if tasting the egg all over again. In addition to the taste of eggs becoming aversive, Kenny was also repulsed by the smell of cooked eggs from this point on. For quite some time following his unpleasant experience, Kenny's visceral response to the smell of eggs prompted a feeling of wanting to throw up. Years later, he still refused to eat them.

Two populations that are especially vulnerable to taste and smell aversions are children born prematurely and those with autistic spectrum disorders. Preemies may be aversive to tastes and smells across the board, having an easy gag reflex due to tube feedings that sets up a defensive reaction to the feeding process. Children with autistic spectrum disorders may be very picky eaters who are hypersensitive to food textures (listed under touch sensations), tastes, and smells. Table 6.4 shows coordinated and atypical taste and smell behaviors.

Table 6.4. Typical (Coordinated) and Atypical (Potential for Load Condition) Taste and Smell Behaviors

Typical (Coordinated) for Infant, Child, or Adult	Atypical (Potential for Load Condition) for Infant, Child, or Adult
Taste Behaviors	
Has ability to enjoy eating through bottle or breastfeeding (infant or child)	Is aversive to tastes through bottle or breastfeeding (infant or child)
Demonstrates a normal range of exploring common foods	Has strong aversion to common foods or lacks pleasure in eating
With maturation, explores and tolerates a variety of tastes	Strong aversion to exploration of new tastes or seems to always place things in mouth (e.g., licks toys, wants to taste Play-Doh)
Smell Behaviors	
Orients to parent's body scent (infant or child)	Has a strong aversive response to parent's body scent (infant or child)
Enjoys scents that are associated with parents, loved ones, or pleasurable foods	Has strong aversive responses to common smells, or never notices or enjoys smells
With maturation, explores and tolerates a variety of smells	Shows strong aversion to the exploration of new or unusual smells, or has little awareness of smells

Please note that the following modalities of proprioception, vestibular, and pain (which also includes visceral connections) are oriented toward the *internal* milieu.

Proprioception

As noted, Joseph's awareness of his body through proprioceptive means was consistently off. On one hand, he would bump into table corners and lunge toward objects rather than reach for them. On the other hand, he would jump on couches and beds, seemingly seeking a certain type of

Table 6.5.   Typical (Coordinated) and Atypical (Potential for Load Condition) Proprioceptive Behaviors

Typical (Coordinated) for Infant, Child, or Adult	Atypical (Potential for Load Condition) for Infant, Child, or Adult
Can adjust body posture in response to an uncomfortable position	Does not notice that body is out of alignment or in an uncomfortable or awkward position
Has an "internal" body map—can accurately locate all parts of body and understands body in relation to others	Cannot locate parts of own body or tell impact of own body on others (e.g., running into, smashing into, crashing into others clumsily or being too close to others; breaks toys easily)
Is able to adjust to location of body up against bed, floor, or chair	Is unable to adjust to location of body up against bed, floor, or chair (e.g., might fall out of chair because of lack of awareness of seated positioning)
Adequately adjusts body to avoid intentional bumping or crashing, yet is not overly distressed if it occurs	Clumsily bumps, trips, or falls into objects or people on a consistent basis
If this is a sensory preference, there may be extra intensity and active resistance used with joints, ligaments, and muscles in different parts of the body (e.g., such as force used when walking, frequent rubbing of hands together, chewing on clothes), or an overall intense use of joints and muscles (e.g., loves jumping jacks, wrestling, playing football, drumming) that helps organize, calm, or alert the individual	Extreme use of this sensory input may include behaviors that typically identify the individual as aggressive with a propensity for hitting, biting, pushing, hurling, banging, or crashing self or others (Blanche & Schaaf, 2001); discomfort with this sensory modality may include anxiety or distress with joints being moved, when objects are approaching, or one is asked to perform weight-bearing activities (carrying or pushing an object) (Blanche & Schaaf, 2001)

proprioceptive stimulation. Table 6.5 shows coordinated and atypical proprioceptive behaviors.

Vestibular (Balance)

As noted, Danny was only able to be soothed at first through one particular bouncing motion. In occupational therapy, one goal became to expand his repertoire of other vestibular movements; this was successful, so much so that after a few weeks of therapy, Danny was able to be soothed by being rocked in a rocking chair. One detail that was not included in the case of Laura is that she responded very positively to her foster–adopt father picking her up and swinging her in the air. This movement became a sensory preference that alerted her to emotional engagement when she was in a hypoalert state of arousal. Balance is most often associated with the vestibular sensory modality; however, visual and proprioception also contribute to it (Gordon, Chilardi, & Ghez, 1995; Interdisciplinary Council on Developmental and Learning Disorders–Diagnostic Manual for Infancy and Early Childhood Work Groups, 2005). Table 6.6 shows coordinated and atypical vestibular behaviors.

Table 6.6. Typical (Coordinated) and Atypical (Potential for Load Condition) Vestibular Behaviors

Typical (Coordinated) for Infant, Child, or Adult	Atypical (Potential for Load Condition) for Infant, Child, or Adult
Shows enjoyment when parents move infant through various motions (e.g., swinging up, down, around in space)	Cries in distress when parents move infant through various motions (e.g., swinging up, down, around in space)
Can maintain balance and posture	Is clumsy because he or she does not know how to regulate movement in space
Engages in play or daily activities that require movement, without dizziness or nausea	Is susceptible to motion sickness of any kind (e.g., from riding in cars, to swings, to boats)
Demonstrates a typical range of balance	Easily becomes dizzy when turning or walking in a circle; rarely becomes dizzy when spinning
Maintains good balance on playground equipment (e.g., swings, monkey bars, merry-go-rounds)	Shows poor balance on playground equipment
Is at ease with heights	Is prone to vertigo

Table 6.7. Typical (Coordinated) and Atypical (Potential for Load Condition) Pain Behaviors

Typical (Coordinated) for Infant, Child, or Adult	Atypical (Potential for Load Condition) for Infant, Child, or Adult
Has an accurate awareness of painful stimuli (e.g., cries when getting a shot)	Is under- or overresponsive to pain (e.g., does not respond to a shot; responds with increasing distress to shots)
Shows appropriate responses to pain from external events that are environmental or relational in nature (e.g., shots, falling down, a slap from a parent)	Has strong reactions, sensitized reactions, or both to pain or shows little to no awareness to pain, whether environmental or relational
Shows appropriate responses to pain from internal events (e.g., sore throat, teething, headache, visceral pain)	Shows strong reactions, sensitized reactions, or both to internal sensory events, or shows little to no awareness of these events
With maturation, shows increasing awareness of internal bodily cues, such as bowel and bladder pressure, hunger, and thirst cues	With maturation, shows little to no awareness or ignores internal bodily cues, such as bowel and bladder pressure, hunger, and thirst cues

Pain

Pain is not a sensory modality per se, but it is a crucial sensory experience that is survival oriented. In clinical terms, pain is a fundamental indicator of basic sensory functioning that is distributed across all sensory systems. It acts as a monitor of the child's perception of both internal and external sources of sensory discomfort. Joseph was unresponsive to pain right from infancy, suggesting a basic processing problem in pain-mediating mechanisms. Laura was also unresponsive to pain when she first came to her foster–adopt parents' home. Later, as we shall see, she did begin to have strong reactions to pain, accompanied by flashbacks from previous injuries, indicating that her original insensitivity to pain was a defensive response to trauma and not a processing problem. Table 6.7 shows coordinated and atypical pain behaviors.

We now look at how behaviors that reflect sensory processing and modulation are organized into sensory system capacities that either support coordination or potentially contribute to load conditions.

7

Assessment and Intervention Principles, Priorities, and Strategies for the Sensory System

In the neurorelational framework, the focus of assessment is on *functional behavior in context*, with the goal of identifying not only the contributions to load conditions but also the resources for coordination. Diagnostic labels are not enough, but they are also not disregarded. Rather, they are used to the extent that they provide guidance and direction for intervention, further assessment, or both. In the sensory system, the professional organizes assessment according to the processing and modulatory capacities of the child. To assist professionals in gaining an overview of a child's or parent's sensory functioning in a most general way, one can use processing and modulation worksheets (located at the end of this chapter and on the CD-ROM). These worksheets identify functional aspects of the sensory system, helping the professional target both strengths and weaknesses. Many times, a referral to a specialist in a particular sensory area will be warranted; additional formal assessment tools are listed later in this chapter.

ASSESSMENT AND INTERVENTION PRINCIPLES AND PRIORITIES FOR THE SENSORY SYSTEM

Assessment and intervention for sensory processing and modulation issues tend to have different priorities and goals. For processing issues, assessment is weighted toward investigating and isolating disruptions to accuracy within and across modalities, and intervention is weighted toward remediation of specific skills and abilities. For modulation issues, assessment is weighted toward investigating and isolating the sensory

components that set off a stress response (i.e., triggers); intervention is weighted toward altering the intensity and timing dimensions in accordance with sensory preferences as well as desensitizing modalities that produce stress responses. Our first capacity reflects the emphasis on sensory processing issues and the second capacity on sensory modulation issues. Recall that the sensory processing capacity is defined as the ability to receive, translate, associate, and elaborate sensory signals within and across sensory modalities in a developmentally appropriate way.

The Capacity for Sensory Processing

The emergence of all milestones—developmental and socioemotional—is based on the capacity to receive, translate, associate, and elaborate sensory signals in an accurate and efficient manner, relative to one's age and context. In a typical situation, this capacity develops naturally; a child does not "choose" whether to cooperate with sensory development. That is, a child exhibiting a delay in reaching a milestone is much more likely to have a disruption within this capacity than a lack of interest or motivation. A delay might mean that a given milestone is (1) out of the typical range for age, or (2) discrepant relative to other milestones. Either way, the cause of the disruption may originate from the sensory system itself or the environment. This section deals with disruptions to the sensory system itself.

Behavior is always a reflection of a bidirectional influence within sensory modalities (feed-forward and feedback connections within a modality) as well as a commingling across sensory modalities (lateral influence from neural neighborhood and extended community). From the very start, for example, the capacity to integrate sources of sensory information lays the foundation for speech and language, which, as noted in Chapter 2, are distributed properties with important contributions from all brain systems. The proto-linguistic communication skills of cooing and babbling back and forth between a parent and baby require multiple co-occurring processes. For example, first, the baby has to have the receptive capacity to hear and process the mother's sounds coming from her motherese. Second, the infant needs to have the oral–motor strength to express cooing sounds back to the mother. Poor oral–motor functioning can lead to feeding problems that lead to speech and articulation problems. Third, both members of the dyad have to have the capacity to engage visually in affective interactions of back-and-forth cooing and babbling conversations (relates to the second and third socioemotional milestones). This is an example of an intersection point where socioemotional milestones and learning capacities come together.

A problem behavior may be weighted toward (1) a particular sensory modality, for example, poor listening ability and the auditory modality; or (2) the influence of another commingled modality, for example, trouble getting visual cues from mouth movements when listening. No behavior represents a singular sensory modality. So, to understand the sensory modalities that may contribute to a particular problem, we must do our best to deconstruct the behavior into its component sensory parts. This process can begin with knowledge of the various sensory modalities (e.g., seeing, hearing, touch) and the dimensions that pertain to them (e.g., intensity, location, temporal aspects).

Bear in mind that the current knowledge base regarding how each sensory modality contributes to behavior and development varies. When fine-tuning our hypotheses in practice, this knowledge imbalance means that (1) we have more detailed and reliable assessment information available to us for some senses than others, and (2) we have more assessment tools at our disposal for some senses than others. For example, we know a lot about how disruptions within the auditory and visual modalities can lead to a learning disability in reading, but we have much less detailed knowledge about how sensory modalities lead to a learning disability in math or how a hypersensitivity to noise might play a role in a learning disability. We are gaining knowledge about the visceral senses and the influence on emotions and behavior, for example, social behavior (Cacioppo, Hawkley, & Berntson, 2003) and decision making (Bechara & Damasio, 2005; Bechara, Damasio, Tranel, & Damasio, 2005), but we know little about how multisensory integration contributes to behavior (Wallace, 2004). Nonetheless, the senses, the presenting problems about which there is little research, or both should not be ignored. All sensory modalities should be considered with any presenting problem. We do not have mounds of evidence-based research for every child's profile, but we do have evidence-based guideposts (studies that provide some versus no information) alongside general neuroscience principles. Together, these can keep us from doing harm as we attempt to help.

A well-functioning sensory processing system helps a child generate a complete picture of self, others, and the world across time. When sensory information is accurately and efficiently processed, it allows the child to build perceptions from both internal and external sources that are stable and trustworthy. Subtle, moderate, or severe disruptions in the processing hierarchy can distort the quality of sensory information in a variety of ways, leading to "incomplete pictures" or inconsistent perceptions, directly affecting the quality of ongoing learning and relationships. For example, disruptions within the auditory modality may affect the clarity of sound perception or expression and then restrict or confuse the

flow of communication between a parent and child. A disruption in the visual modality may affect the security a child feels moving around in the world and may lend to restricted movement and reduced opportunities for exploration. These are just two examples from an infinite number of possibilities.

In deconstructing a particular behavior, recall that we need to consider the behavior *in context* and with the goal of discovering contributions to load conditions as well as resources for coordination. The first question to ask is whether the behavior is weighted toward the processing or modulation arena. Processing problems are hinted at when a child seems to miss or lack an expected behavior, often related to a skill or ability, such as navigating space, language, academics (e.g., reading, writing, arithmetic), and memory. A more obvious example would be a child who cannot name the letters of the alphabet in first grade. A less obvious example would be a child who "understood the material just fine" one day but failed a test the next day. Processing problems are also suspected when a child exhibits a disproportionate focus on details, poor looking and listening skills, an inability to "get the gist," and an inability to understand the importance of context.

Once a processing problem is suspected, the professional should explore (1) whether there are developmental events in the history that might be related to the presenting problem (e.g., a history of ear infections may be related to language delays); (2) which sensory modality is likely the primary culprit; (3) the degree of developmental gap with respect to age; (4) the degree of developmental gap with respect to other milestones; (5) the level in the sensory hierarchy from which problems or inaccuracies seem to emerge; and (6) whether the problem changes with contextual or relational factors. The ongoing exploration involves honing in on the disruption, teasing out the precise conditions in which the errors occur (both within task and within context), determining how consistently they occur, and, most important, at what point accuracy and automaticity (fast and 100% accurate functioning; this concept is discussed more in depth in a later section) emerge. This exploration process involves both slowing down and breaking down the behavior—focusing attention on smaller increments of the behavior in efforts to understand it more completely and going back to earlier developmental levels—attempting to identify the point at which the child demonstrates automatic and complete accuracy. It is also important to consider how a disruption might contribute to other milestones and social interactions. For example, a child who cannot comprehend language accurately and efficiently for his or her age may be shy or withdrawn with peers or may appear disinterested or inattentive in the classroom.

Deconstructing behavior according to its sensory contributions may often involve direct assessment (e.g., neuropsychology, speech and language); however, the professional should be exploring potential sensory disruptions well before making referrals for testing. Observations of behavior according to context (i.e., history of the behavior, environment in which it occurs, dimension variations that affect the behavior, state of arousal during the behavior) can help guide questions, generate hypotheses, and fine-tune hypotheses such that a referral for direct assessment is accompanied by well-informed questions and options to consider.

Any sensory processing disruption, from mild to severe, can throw off the quality of the sensory information and thereby directly affect the quality of relationships and learning. A problem in one domain—learning or relationships—will affect the other domain. Thus, if a child has a problem learning in school, that problem will probably have an origin in the sensory system, and the disruption may also affect the relationship domain. Because of this domino effect, assessment must go beyond the problem under focus. Too often, a problem is viewed as isolated in that its relational effects are not treated in a parallel process. The professional must always return to the big picture and consider the connections across domains—not just other sensory modalities or processing problems but also relationships and learning.

The Capacity for Sensory Modulation

When sensory modulation is working well, the sensory information that is most important to the context will take center stage, whether it initiates activation or not, and the less important sensory information will get screened out. A modulation issue is suspected with a child who exhibits rapid changes or large swings in states of arousal or excessive reactivity, avoidance, or withdrawal in response to seemingly typical situations (e.g., birthday parties, going to the movies) or, conversely, a child who does *not* exhibit rapid or large arousal shifts where appropriate. For suspected modulation issues, the initial step in assessment is to investigate and isolate the sensory components that set off a stress response (i.e., triggers) and those that reflect sensory preferences.

Sensory modulation implies a balance of activation and inhibition in the flow of sensory information. Two distinct conditions support modulation:

- Fluctuations in activation, inhibition, or both are appropriate to context.
- The "sensory selves" in dyadic relationship are well matched.

Condition One: Fluctuations in Activation, Inhibition, or Both Are Appropriate to Context

The capacity for sensory modulation involves adjusting or varying the flow of sensory information through changes in the dimensions of intensity, duration, and rhythm of sensory data. Modulation occurs in response to the amount of the sensory information from internal (bodily) and external (world) sources in relation to the goals of the particular time and place. For example, if the goal is sleep, optimal modulation would involve inhibition of sensory information. A general way to think about what is appropriate to context is to consider the dimensions for the various types of sensory information that best facilitate (1) sleep; (2) the promotion, maintenance, and expansion of the alert processing state; and (3) stress recovery. For example, a toddler with a tummy ache (internal sensory source) will need more sensory signals from the parent to convey soothing and restore comfort in the child and thereby facilitate relaxation into sleep. A child in a war-torn area of the world may have to habituate to the distant sounds of artillery fire (external sensory source) to relax into sleep, which could be accomplished more efficiently with help from a parent to create the illusion of safety. *An important rule of thumb:* All children, especially younger ones, will need help from a parent to manage real or perceived perceptions of sensory threat, recover from a stress response, and achieve a perception of safety (Levine & Kline, 2008).

Accurate perceptions of safety, challenge, and threat allow the child to take in important sensory information (be aware and involved) and screen out unimportant information (be relaxed and focused). It is important that a child be able to recognize and learn about all three conditions of safety, challenge, and threat within his or her environment. For example, a child who always notices danger cannot experience as much pleasure and relax; a child who never notices danger is at greater risk for harm.

Under typical conditions, we learn the most from sensory information when in the alert processing state. Within this state, the potential fluctuations in activation and inhibition are expansive. For example, if the goal is socializing, more sensory information needs to come in; however, if the goal is studying, distracting sensory information needs to be screened out. The unconscious process of habituation supports this ability to sharpen focus because it allows us to get used to benign ambient sensory signals. For example, a child can habituate to the hardness of a wooden chair against his or her rear or the sound of a faulty air conditioner in the classroom. Some children are quite capable of tuning out even irregular high-intensity stimuli such as the sound of a jackhammer,

whereas others can become increasingly sensitized to it, at first annoyed and eventually compelled to leave or cover their ears. These inherent physiological abilities to take in or screen out sensory information are unique to each individual and are typical up to the point that they do not regularly disrupt functioning and development. For example, the child who covers his or her ears daily to block out the faulty air conditioner in the classroom can no longer function well as a student or further develop abilities within that setting.

A child's ability to modulate different types of sensory information within a typical range is reflected by the degree of positive (engaging), neutral, or negative responses he or she displays. For example, an infant in an alert processing state should remain comfortable and engaged when exposed to multiple sources of benign sensory stimulation. At younger ages and for those with vulnerable physiologies, there is much less ability for what we would consider intentional or active inhibition to sustain balance. With maturity, a child has the increasing ability for volitional activation and inhibition—for example, crawling toward or away from a noisy object, walking around or lying down, speeding up or slowing down speech, looking away from or continuing to stare at a child who is behaving in a provoking manner.

A child with a poor ability to habituate or with a propensity to become sensitized is at constant risk for a stress response. In general, taking in too much sensory information leads to overactivation (and hyperalert or flooded arousal states), whereas not taking in enough sensory information leads to overinhibition (and a hypoaroused state). For example, a preemie with poor vagal tone (unable to inhibit) is likely to be overactivated (flooded) by the typical range and level of sensory information. Similar to the classic learned helplessness experiments (Finkelstein & Ramey, 1977; Seligman, 1975; Seligman & Maier, 1967), this infant may shift from flooded to shut down in a chronic hypoalert state. For a child who is too often in a hypoalert state, it is very important to distinguish a modulation problem from a processing problem. For example, a disruption at the entrance level of the visual modality (e.g., cataracts) will prevent visual signals from being processed accurately and will likely dampen reactivity to this type of sensory information. As with arousal levels that can combine varying degrees of both inhibition and activation, individual sensory profiles can vary. Whereas some individuals may consistently show sensitized/activation reactions, and others may consistently show too much habituation/inhibition, others will consistently show both activated and inhibited responses to sensory information. Variations can occur during different parts of the day in relation to degrees of tiredness and circadian rhythms, or they can occur within the same sensory modality

on a regular basis (e.g., child is overreactive to sounds and at the same time does not respond to his or her name being called). In one research study, both hyper- and hyporesponsiveness was evident *simultaneously* in about 38% of the children with a diagnosis of autism (Baranek, David, Poe, Stone, & Watson, 2006). This may be a behavioral representation of the coactive autonomic pattern (autonomic modes of control; Berntson, Cacioppo, & Quigley, 1991).

Sensory signals perceived as harmful or even painful (i.e., threats, triggers), even if considered typical by others, can produce a more intense stress response with each presentation. This type of sensitization can quickly lead to a load condition. Although a more intense response may be adaptive given the context (i.e., situations of abuse or neglect), even a highly adaptive stress response can shift into a load condition when the sensory trigger occurs too frequently. When there are many types of sensory triggers or triggers that are too frequent, a child will need much more help from an adult (interactive regulation) to recover and achieve optimal regulation.

We distinguish between sensory events that can be considered traumatic and those that produce symptoms of posttraumatic stress disorder (PTSD). In general, traditional diagnostic approaches (*DSM-IV-TR*, American Psychiatric Association, 1994; DC:0–3R, ZERO TO THREE, 2005) define the source of PTSD as witnessing or experiencing violence or bodily harm. We use the phrase "traumatic experience" because it allows for a less discrete, more dimensional view of sensory events that can be considered sources of triggers for threat on a continuum. For example, Danny experienced an intense and prolonged stress response with each feeding experience (until he gained control of his swallowing) and diaper change (until his skin was dried after a clean-up). For him, these responses contributed to load conditions that included traumatic experience (e.g., choking episodes while feeding, extremely sensitized aversion to wetness). On the other hand, Laura's traumatic experiences of witnessing domestic violence as well as personally experiencing bodily harm (as we will later learn), met criteria for PTSD and could certainly be considered more severe. The four conditions that define load provide additional guidelines and discrete parameters for understanding and interpreting infants' and young children's traumatic experiences that may not qualify as PTSD. From the neurorelational perspective, however, the general principles and priorities for assessment and intervention are the same.

Table 7.1 summarizes what healthy modulation of sensory information might look like in terms of activation and inhibition according to the

Table 7.1. Adaptive and Load Versions of Primary Stress Responses Correlated with Sensory Modulation Processes of Activation and Inhibition

	Hypoalert (high habituation)	Hyperalert (blends of habituation–sensitization)	Flooded (overly sensitized)
Adaptive level	Screens out nonthreatening sensory information that is no longer novel	Is engrossed in (staring at) novel or curious stimuli and responds appropriately to alarming sensory information	Reacts to sudden levels of intense information
Load condition level	Is underreactive to novel or painful stimulation	Is unable to stop engaging with persons or objects in response to typical levels of sensory information; perseveres	Overreacts (has exaggerated or frequent stressful responses) to typical levels of sensory information

three primary stress responses (adaptive level) as well as how disruptions in modulation might appear in each of the stress response states (on a load condition level).

Condition Two: The "Sensory Selves" in Dyadic Relationship Are Well Matched

In relationships, interactions that are characterized by the presence of a predominance of sensory preferences of both individuals promote feelings of pleasure and safety. For children and adults, the pleasure and safety that come with basic sensory preferences provide the gateway to falling in love and a sense of security. In general, dyadic sensory patterns can tip the dyad toward coordination or load conditions. In well-matched dyads, the parent and child mirror (or match) one another in their pleasurable responses to various sensory modalities. Mirroring is discussed in more detail in Chapters 8 and 9 (the relevance brain system), but simply put, in Winnicott's words, "The precursor of the mirror is the mother's face. What does the infant see when he looks at his mother? He sees himself" (1967, p. 131). Gestures, vocal pitch, tone, and so on, can also be matched in addition to facial expressions. Many now believe that mirroring is a bidirectional process by the age of 3 or 4 months (e.g., Beebe & Lachmann, 2002). In these complementary matches, differences in sensory preferences do not disrupt the ongoing flow of interactions.

In chronically mismatched dyads, however, the sensory signals from parent or child disrupt smooth interaction and trigger the other into a stress response that turns into a load condition. It is especially important to understand how the parent affects the infant's sensory system and vice versa. For example, a mother's loud, high-pitched voice might overwhelm her baby. Conversely, the baby may reach a high pitch in his or her cry that is a sensory trigger for the mother. Tronick's (2007) research indicates that adaptive levels of mismatch and their concomitant stress are indeed quite common and in fact can build resilience by means of repeated successful repairs. We are concerned with those patterns of mismatch that become a chronic source of maladaptive stress.

Members of dyads who experience a lot of sensory triggers can easily associate one another with threat. The child's arousal states and expressions of displeasure may reveal perceived conditions of challenge or threat. Perceptions of challenge or threat can arise from two primary sources: (1) typical caretaking activities and environmental activity (for a child such as Danny in Chapter 4, who over- or underreacts to typical levels of sensory information), and (2) a mismatched sensory dyad, whereby the dimensions of the interactions (intensity, rhythm, and duration) provoke stress responses (e.g., the father does not stop tickling when the child is distressed; a depressed mother's chronic lack of vitality leaves a child in a shut-down state). A mismatch in the sensory dyad can also influence the appraisals (meanings) that are made in these relationships (relevance). If the parent's natural style elicits displeasure in the child, the parent may feel inadequate or rejected. For example, a mother whose child withdraws from her stroking of his or her skin may take it personally and draw conclusions that will disrupt the relational bond. The mothers of both Joseph and Danny each felt, at some point, that her child disliked or did not love her. A mother who carries these negative appraisals is under tremendous stress, making it much more difficult for her to take a step back and figure out a different strategy.

The judge responded to my (CL) recommendation letter by temporarily stopping Laura's visits with her birth mother and ordering dyadic assessments with the birth mother, as well as with Juan and Mary, once Laura had recovered her developmental gains. When Laura was observed with her birth mother, the mother appeared unable to connect with, comfort, or set limits with her daughter. When Laura initiated aggressive play, the mother responded with glee, showing pleasure with the "duels" as well as dominating Laura so she (the mother) could "win." The mother also bit Laura's neck and appeared to genuinely perceive this sadistic behavior as typical and playful. The evaluator noted a disorganized and ambivalent attachment pattern and warned that this type of play was fostering sociopathic traits. In contrast, when Laura was observed with Juan and Mary, the interactions

were rich with tender gestures and words. They recognized opportunities for connection and respectfully joined her play. When Laura "attacked" them, their play characters exhibited distress and made pleas for kindness and friendship. When Laura was angry, they were able to provide comfort and show affection, eventually calming her so she could accept being held. The evaluator noted a secure attachment, made a strong recommendation for the adoption process to proceed, and the court agreed.

With the adoption moving forward, Juan and Mary asked me to work with Laura; I agreed to do so in the context of a dyadic therapy model, where one parent was always present in the sessions. Abuse was a common theme in Laura's play. She always took the role of the aggressor who tormented a baby. She would speak in a low, gruff tone of voice and make sadistic-sounding laughs while pulling the baby's hair and limbs and biting the baby. The parents shared that Laura would often become more aggressive for no reason during play at home. As Juan and Mary reflected with me about her play, they began to realize how certain tones and playful gestures that they considered benign might actually trigger threat for Laura. They also realized that Laura had a difficult time taking in sensory comfort, especially because she was so easily triggered for threat, which led her to become aggressive instead. With renewed empathy, Juan and Mary paid much closer attention to the subtle shifts in Laura's behavior that might give them clues about the sensory signals that were her triggers for threat. Although they did not know exactly why, they understood that they needed to be especially cautious about how they treated her, especially her hair and limbs, during caretaking routines and in play.

In addition, Laura went for a speech and language evaluation. The tests verified that her hearing was fine and she had dramatically increased her vocabulary in the prior 6 months. However, there were still problems. Laura had poor articulation, likely stemming from weak oral–motor muscles. She used mostly nouns and verbs without articles and connectors, she did not sequence words well, she sometimes confused pronouns, and she rarely used emotional words (e.g., happy, sad, mad, scared). These delays represented processing problems; her constricted range of emotional words also reflected the level of emotional neglect she had experienced.

ASSESSMENT AND INTERVENTION STRATEGIES

Parents come to the practitioner with presenting problems that usually fall into one or two categories: (1) the child is not exhibiting some expected behavior (e.g., "My child is not talking"), or (2) the child is exhibiting an undesired or atypical behavior (e.g., "My child is constantly throwing tantrums"). Regardless of diagnostic label or presenting problem, the absence of an expected behavior or the presence of an undesirable behavior may have some etiological basis in the sensory system. This basis is readily

apparent with problems related to language and learning, but less so with problems related to attention, emotions, and relationships. Yet consider that all the brain systems are reliant on the sensory system to deliver good data to them, which means that any presenting problem may have sensory components. Accurately isolating those sensory components enables intervention to be targeted appropriately.

Less than optimal or misguided interventions can occur when assumptions are made about the etiology of a particular behavior and the sensory system is overlooked. For example, one child with social problems and a high-functioning autism diagnosis actually had a significant disruption in the visual modality, which created difficulties with reading faces and gestures accurately. This etiology was missed due to a faulty assumption that the autism diagnosis provided all the necessary information. Similarly, an assessment approach that evaluates for a particular disorder is inadequate at best and often does harm. For example, an assessment for ADHD may be positive for all diagnostic criteria but completely misses a potential sensory etiology, such as inattention because of disruptions in comprehension of language. Such narrow assessments lead to similarly narrow interventions that, if wrong or incomplete, only compound or complicate the problem and waste valuable time. In early intervention, time is a child's greatest ally—the sooner we get it right, the better.

Two fundamental principles—titration and automaticity—are especially important for sensory system interventions. Titration is a guide for the ongoing process of intervention. Automaticity is a goal for gauging the progress of intervention.

Titration: Maintaining the Balance

Titration is critical to successful intervention, no matter what the specifics of the problem. Simply put, it means "not too little, not too much." Titration involves giving the "right dose" of sensory information so that the child is challenged but not overwhelmed. To determine the right dose, the professional must have a keen understanding of the child's stress response cues. In general, as cues emerge, the professional or parent alters the intervention until the alert processing state is reestablished. How this is achieved depends on the child—it might mean backing off; switching to a different activity; adjusting dimensions of intensity, duration, and rhythm; or all of these. How one alters the intervention and for how long depend on the child's capacity to recover from stress. Another important aspect of titration is that of building tolerance for greater intensity of challenge (Tronick, 2007). Initially, it is best to learn all the ways to reestablish alert

processing with a child because those skills become a professional's or parent's toolbox for stress recovery. With time, it is just as important to expand the child's tolerance for challenge. Being able to tolerate challenge is a useful ability for all of us to have, and it is especially necessary for a child in intervention. Children with sensory processing problems need to tolerate challenge, given that intervention becomes such a central part of their life for a time. For a child with sensory modulation problems, expanding the capacity to tolerate dimensional (intensity, duration, rhythm) variations is the staple of multiple types of interventions. In every intervention session (whether in a clinic, private practice, or a school setting) the child should be challenged, and at the end of that session, the child should leave feeling successful. Proper titration is key.

Another aspect of titration is that of sequencing the emphasis on preferences and strengths as well as triggers and problems for the family. Often, parents bring a high degree of urgency for relief and an equally high degree of pressure to focus on the problems. In response to these parental states, the practitioner might first assess for any potential triggers underlying the child's problematic behaviors and later shift the focus to his or her strengths. At the same time, a strengths-based approach emphasizes what the child and parents are doing right from the first encounter forward. However, some anxious parents may find an early emphasis on strengths to be even more anxiety-producing, so their state of mind has to be considered. In intervention one always has to find and use preferences that convey a sense of safety to all involved to establish a secure relationship in a safe and playful haven.

Automaticity: Mastery Matters

Automaticity is critical to successful intervention. It means that a particular skill or milestone has been learned to the point of mastery—that is, the skill or milestone can be performed accurately and quickly (or "automatically") all of the time. This gold standard is applied to any fundamental or building block ability. If another skill is layered on a fundamental ability, then that fundamental ability must be automatic. For example, being able to identify or name letters of the alphabet with 80% mastery is not good enough, even though it is often considered adequate in school settings. That precursor skill is so fundamental to later skills that it must be 100% accurate *and* fast. When a precursor skill is not mastered to the point of automaticity, then it will continue to contribute to breakdowns downstream. For example, recognition and enjoyment of rhymes is expected at about the age of 3–4 years, but if not exhibited, it is most often

overlooked. However, at the age of 5 or 6, when the same child struggles with phonics, the phonics problem, which has its roots in the rhyming deficit, gains the attention of teachers and parents. In intervention, if the approach skips over the earlier level of breakdown, then the child may still learn to read with compensatory skills, but there is no guarantee that the earlier level of breakdown will not continue to have long-term effects. The impact of a weak foundation may show up through mediocre progress, either in the present or down the road when the child can no longer compensate when challenged with more advanced material. The automaticity guideline is also important in evaluating intervention progress. All too often, an ability exhibited is considered an ability learned, and the focus of intervention moves on to the next goal. Even more concerning is the tendency to consider an ability exhibited with support as an ability learned, despite the fact that it has not been demonstrated independently. In each of these examples, no automaticity standard was assessed or expected.

As I worked with Laura and her new parents, the aggression and sadism in her play gradually diminished, and she was increasingly able to create family and relationship themes that involved pleasure and joy. In addition to the dyadic therapy, Juan and Mary wanted Laura to attend a preschool and begin speech and language therapy. Because of budget limitations, the family faced a difficult choice. They could afford for Laura to do only two of those three activities. They opted for preschool as well as speech and language therapy because Laura was demonstrating more typical behavior without sadistic violence in her play. I agreed to consult with Juan and Mary on an as-needed basis to manage Laura's ongoing developmental challenges. Her language continued to improve with intervention, and although there were still modulation problems (sensory overload, intermittent difficulty with staying asleep), things went relatively well for a time. However, when Laura entered preschool, she began to display aggressive behavior again, and the severity escalated quickly. Within 2 weeks, she was losing bladder and bowel control (which, incidentally, continued for an entire year—a powerful effect of threat) and was biting not only other children but also her teacher, all of whom she liked. At home, she began having intense nightmares. In one, her "old daddy" cut off her arm while she was playing in a park, and she subsequently became terrified that "old daddy" would kidnap her from preschool. Significantly, she also awoke during the night crying in pain, rubbing her leg, and asking her parents to rub her leg. The request was an indication of her increasing health: Laura was probably allowing herself to feel some of the original, previously dissociated pain from her early experiences. Though this behavior indicated that she had begun to feel even safer with her new parents, Juan and Mary were alarmed by the obvious building stress, so they reinstated therapy sessions with me.

Similar to the request to the judge to stop maternal visitations until recovery of her previous level of functioning resumed, I first recommended that Laura

stop attending preschool until she could recover, once again, to her previous baseline typical behaviors. Her current school offered numerous learning stations and activities, but something about the open space, the many sounds, and the number of people presented a strong threat for Laura. Maybe this setting was too similar to the noisy, open park in her dream where her father had cut off her arm. I suspected that the teacher's disciplinary style was triggering Laura's memory of duels where she was dominated and bitten, and perhaps she was biting others in reaction to the perceived attack. In addition, I explained to Juan and Mary that Laura was showing classic signs of PTSD. Her nightmares, awakening with pain in her leg, and new expressions about "old daddy" were clues to the sensory experiences that had occurred earlier in her life.

During this phase of intervention, Laura became fixated on having either her mother or me playing the role of "old daddy," at whom she would repeatedly roar as a means of scaring him away. Although her attempts to control her fear had productive intent, the means by which she was trying to achieve this goal were similar to her previous aggressive behavior. When Laura played the abuser and roared, her mother and I alternated victim–protector roles by coming to the rescue of the victim, stopping the abuser, and then providing comfort and empathy. The new goals of dyadic therapy were to enable Laura to experience fear and pain (sensory processing at the entrance level), accept sensory comfort and empathy (sensory modulation), and eventually be able to "take control" and clearly articulate a command to stop the activity (sensory processing at the association-elaboration level). As these were modeled for her, she began to learn, through imitation, ways to experience the role of the victim and protector, expanding her singular, rigid identification with the role of the aggressor (more on these roles in Chapter 9).

Fortunately, the speech and language therapy was able to continue during this period. The language therapist and I agreed to work closely with each other. She shifted her goals to focus on increasing Laura's emotional vocabulary, incorporating story themes that involved safety, challenge, and threat and teaching Laura how to use her language to negotiate interactions that felt threatening. The speech and language therapist also suggested that I ask Laura to repeat my words when I asked her to do something; to slow down my speech with her, draw her attention to my mouth, clearly articulate consonant and vowels, and insert small breaks between phrases. The bidirectional collaboration provided a rich synthesis of both processing and modulation treatment goals.

Assessment and Intervention Steps

For sensory system interventions, we stress the importance of using consistent, repeated strategies to effect change, which, for practical reasons, will usually necessitate parent involvement in direct intervention. If a child engages in a remedial or learning activity only once per week, without spaced repetition or rehearsal at home (e.g., "distributed practice"; Cepeda, Pashler, Vul, Wixted, & Rohrer, 2006; Rohrer & Pashler, 2007), then this

approach does not take advantage of well-established strategies to improve learning (Greene, 1989). Therefore, we recommend giving parents assignments in which they are trained and coached to conduct specific activities or tasks to address the child's processing or modulation problem. Our position, consistent with the research on the effectiveness of early intervention (Guralnick, 1996; Majnemer, 1998), is that remedial efforts toward durable and lasting change require an approach that includes parent involvement, is individualized to the child's and family's needs, is clearly defined in terms of objectives and strategies, and provides the right intensity and frequency of intervention.

Step 1: Review Developmental and Socioemotional Milestones and Consider the Potential Contributions of the Sensory System to the Presenting Problem (or Problems)

Sensory processing problems, modulation problems, or both may be implicated in any developmental or socioemotional delay. For example, a 4-year-old child who cannot follow more than one simple instruction at a time from his or her parent may have an auditory processing problem. A child who is tactilely defensive may avoid and turn away from a parent's embrace. Identifying the sensory system contribution allows the practitioner to pinpoint necessary remediation and intervention strategies as well as identify potential team members.

In addition, in reviewing developmental and socioemotional milestones, one can consider any place along the milestones where automaticity is lacking. Regardless of a child's age or presenting problem, go back in time to review the quality and automaticity of each developmental and socioemotional milestone, noting any glitches in the developmental sequence and whether or how they resolved. In addition, clearly define the presenting problem, placing greater emphasis on areas that have roots to prior developmental issues. If the behavior is performed weakly or poorly in some contexts but well in others, then the behavior is not yet automatic. A behavior that is present with support does *not* mean that the child has mastered the skill or the milestone. The next section provides some suggestions for specific sensory screeners and assessment tools.

Step 2: Assess Risk, Strengths, and Resources of Child and Parent

Risk factors are those existing internal and external vulnerabilities for both the child and the adult. The family history, in utero history, and medical

and developmental history provide data about the severity and pervasiveness of presenting problems.

Tools for getting started in data gathering include (1) the history worksheet in Worksheet 7.1 (a complete History Worksheet for all four brain systems is available for use in Section 12.2 on the CD-ROM); (2) descriptions of risk factors for sensory processing disorders (see Worksheet 7.2 at the end of the chapter; also on the CD-ROM Section 7.1); and (3) asking parents questions about how typical sensations affect arousal (see Worksheet 7.3 at the end of this chapter; also CD-ROM Section 7.2).

In addition, there are several research-based screeners and assessment instruments that produce data that can be used in an individualized sensory profile. Because many parents and professionals are unfamiliar with thinking about behavior in sensory terms, it is often useful for these adults just to observe the child with such a profile in hand for a week or so before actually filling it out. Examples of parental report sensory screeners include the following:

- The Infant-Toddler Symptom Checklist (7–30 months) (DeGangi, Poisson, Sickel, & Wiener, 1995).
- The Sensorimotor History Questionnaire for Preschoolers (3–4 years) (DeGangi & Blazer-Martin, 2000, Appendix C).

Worksheet 7.1.   History Worksheet for the Sensory System

Parental Risk Factors That Can Compromise a Parent's Ability to Provide Interactive Support	Global Questions That Assess the Overall Functioning of the Sensory System	Child Risk Factors That Can Decrease Self-Regulation and Increase the Need for Interactive Regulation
☐ Loss of hearing or vision ☐ Inaccurate processing of information ☐ Slow processing of information ☐ Speech abnormality ☐ Learning disorder(s) ☐ Overreactive, under-reactive, or both to sensory information	• How quickly and efficiently does the child/adult process sensory information? • How reactive is the child/adult to sensory information from relationships? • Is the child/adult leaning toward types of sensory information that are considered safe as opposed to those that are threatening?	☐ Loss of hearing or vision ☐ Inaccurate processing of information ☐ Slow processing of information ☐ Speech delay ☐ Learning disorder(s) ☐ Overreactive, underreactive, or both to sensory information ☐ Institutional care or neglect without adequate sensory information

- Social-Emotional Scale in the *Bayley Scales of Infant and Toddler Development* (Greenspan, 2005) includes a sensory section at the beginning that assesses the child's use of environmental and relational stimuli for birth to 42 months.

The following parent-reported sensory profiles for infants and children, and self-reported for adolescents and adults, organize reactions to various sensory modalities into diagnostic-like categories:

- Infant/Toddler Sensory Profile (birth–6 months; 7–36 months) in English and Spanish (Dunn & Daniels, 2002; Dunn, 2002);
- Sensory Profile (ages 3–10 years, also in Spanish) (Dunn, 1999);
- Adolescent/Adult Sensory Profile (self-questionnaire) (Brown & Dunn, 2002).

Practitioners can also use more formal assessment instruments that are based on direct clinical observations of the child, including the following:

- Test of Sensory Function in Infants (TSFI) (4–18 months) (De-Gangi & Greenspan, 1989) offers a systematic method of assessing each sensory modality's reactivity.
- Sensory Integration and Praxis Test (SIPT) (4–8 years, 11 months) (Ayres, 1989) most often used by occupational therapists trained in sensory integration.

Step 3: Support the Capacity to Receive, Translate, Associate, and Elaborate Sensory Signals Within and Across Sensory Modalities in a Developmentally Appropriate Way

First, determine the external contextual conditions that have a positive or negative influence on the problem. With support, does the missing behavior "show up" or the problem behavior "go away?" What kind of support is helpful—prompting to think ahead; choices; changing dimensions of intensity, duration, and rhythm? Is the behavior consistent across settings and relationships?

Next, determine the internal contextual conditions that have a positive or negative influence on the problem. When the problem behavior is or is not expressed, is the child tired, alert, feeling successful, depressed, anxious, angry?

Now, begin to think about the sensory modalities and levels of processing that may be involved in the problem. Every ability or skill is made up of component parts that are probably weighted toward a modality. Consider whether the task can be manipulated in a way that teases out sensory modalities, for example, by changing or supporting the way an activity is presented, how responses are provided, or both.

Finally, consider the precursor skills or building blocks for the desired behavior. Every skill is made up of precursors, and it can be highly informative to find out whether they are in place. For example, decades of research on literacy and reading disorders has yielded a very specific set of foundational skills that are needed for a child to become a fluent reader (Brown, Palincsar, & Purcell, 1986; Ehri, 1998; Schwanenflugel, Hamilton, Kuhn, Wisenbaker, & Stahl, 2004; Torgesen, 1999; Torgesen, Rashotte, & Alexander, 2001). In kindergarten, the red flags for an emerging disability are apparent in weak phonological skills: poor phonemic awareness (i.e., ability to hear, distinguish, and blend individual sounds), weak knowledge of letter names, and poor ability to match sound to print. Lacking in critical foundational skills, these children struggle to decode words (letters-to-sounds in the right sequence), and word reading becomes slow, labored, and inaccurate. Thus, sight word reading, the next building block in the reading hierarchy, becomes dislodged. The budding combination of poor decoding with lack of sight word acquisition leads to poor fluency and poor spelling, which then leads to poor reading vocabulary and poor reading comprehension. By the third or fourth grade, this child presents with a severe learning disability. However, when detected early and addressed with appropriate intervention, the iterative effects of the downward spiral can be eliminated or minimized.

This level of detailed analysis is not available for every academic skill, and there are still many important and robust indicators for emerging learning problems. Thus, always consider the child's history alongside presenting problems. With processing disruptions, it is almost inevitable that there were hints of an emerging difficulty; thus, it is usually necessary to obtain knowledge about the relevant precursor skills. Sometimes a review of relevant literature is enough to guide the next step in intervention; other times, a consultation or a referral for additional assessment is warranted. In making these decisions, bear in mind that a learning disability is remediated most efficiently early on, before the downward spiral is set in motion. In fact, several studies have shown that poor readers at the end of first grade rarely close the gap (Francis, Shaywitz, Stuebing, Shaywitz, & Fletcher, 1996; Juel, 1988; Shaywitz et al.,

1999; Torgesen & Burgess, 1998). The following Web sites are useful sources of information:

- National Center for Learning Disabilities (www.ncld.org)—Excellent source of information on learning disabilities and other developmental disorders; site for parents and teachers that is geared toward advocacy, communicating research findings, and simple, easy-to-use information guides (e.g., LD checklist for teachers).
- National Dissemination Center for Children with Disabilities (www.nichcy.org)—Dissemination center for children with developmental disabilities; excellent briefing papers for professionals.
- OSEP Ideas that Work (osepideasthatwork.org)—Sponsored by the U.S. Department of Education, Office of Special Education Programs, and geared toward teachers and parents; helpful information for professionals wanting to collaborate with teachers; provides information on special education assessment, interventions, and accommodations, as well as relevant research on literacy. Most documents are available in English and Spanish.
- SharpBrains (www.sharpbrains.com)—Mission is to provide information on the brain fitness market; includes a wealth of quality information on learning, education, and memory; easy-to-digest neuroscience.
- BrainConnection (www.brainconnection.com)—Neuroscience site with a focus on learning and education: Education Connection and Library section includes education topics and clinical topics.

At this point in the process, you may be making a referral. For the practitioner or teacher making a referral, the focus is on having a solid base of information about the problem and asking specific, relevant questions. The referring practitioner or teacher should also ask for suggestions that would be useful for all team members, regardless of discipline. The primary or lead provider should take a coordinating role so that all team members and parents are on the same page, working toward the same goals with complementary approaches, and updating those goals on a regular basis.

Regulation strategies. A child with a sensory processing problem is likely to have regulation difficulties, although those difficulties may be subtle with processing issues of lesser severity. Many times, children with learning disorders must call on more resources and expend greater energy to complete a task compared with their peers. Thus, they may become fatigued more easily or quickly than expected (shift into a hypoalert state)

or may become busier or more anxious than expected (shift into a hyper-alert state). In a learning or challenge context, a child typically cannot remain in either of these states for long without becoming increasingly stressed (moving further along the continuum of a stress response) and slipping further behind in school. Consequently, the initial goal of treatment is to learn about the child's stress response cues and the preferences that assist him or her in returning to alert processing.

An alert processing state is a necessary prerequisite for building automaticity. It is critical to keep this fact in mind when planning, referring, or engaging in a particular treatment approach. There are a multitude of remedial programs designed to address sensory processing problems. For many of these interventions, especially those that do not have a built-in motivational component (e.g., the use of colorful manipulatives or interesting stories), the repetitive nature of the stimuli (e.g., "skill and drill" activities) does not encourage arousal activation, meaning that the child may be able to complete the task but in a hypoalert state. Even programs that purport to enhance motivation (our interpretation: increase arousal) may use sensory pathways that do not have the activating effect for the individual child being treated. In addition, a child who spends too much time in a stress response with too little recovery may simply not be ready for an intervention of this type. When this is the case, the onus falls on those providing treatment (and the parents) to consult with the appropriate specialist so that techniques and strategies can be incorporated into ongoing activities that will still address the problem in some way.

For example, consider a child with severe mood swings and a reading disorder. He may benefit from a Fast ForWord program (Scientific Learning Corporation [n.d.]; What Works Clearinghouse [2007]), a computer-based intensive program that can strengthen language and reading skills, but knowing that this intervention requires a significant amount of sustained focus, we can anticipate that this child would be out of control in 5 minutes. In this situation, the priority becomes increasing the child's capacity for alert processing so that he or she *can* soon participate in intervention. Practitioners and parents would want to avoid moving too fast and scurrying the child into the program to prevent having the desired intervention itself become a sensory trigger. As a supplement, the treatment team could consult with an educational or reading specialist or neuropsychologist to determine what activities could be incorporated into ongoing treatments that would help to build component skills for reading.

Sensory strategies. As common sense would have it, sensory strategies are the primary entree for addressing sensory processing disruptions. At this point, the professional has already (a) clearly defined the presenting

problem (in terms of history and milestones); (b) identified the internal and external dimensions that seem to influence the problem (either positively or negatively); (c) at least begun to think about the sensory modalities and levels that might be involved in the problem; (d) at least begun to consider the precursor skills that support the desired behavior; and (e) looked for strengths in other sensory modalities that can be used as compensatory resources to assist the weak sensory modality (e.g., utilizing visual–spatial strength to help compensate for an auditory–verbal processing weakness). The use of the following sensory strategies assumes that the professional is armed with this information.

By using sensory strategies, we can engage in an intervention and simultaneously continue to explore sensory modalities and precursor skills in an effort to further clarify the sensory culprits. The following sequence and sampling of strategies is in no way exhaustive but is intended to stimulate ideas and creativity.

If a child exhibits a skill sometimes, try to determine what supports the expression by altering the sensory modalities or conditions and watch for change. Does the child do better in a hard or soft chair, with a full stomach or a little hungry, with white noise or silence, alone or with peers? Once the ideal conditions are known (e.g., the child is relaxed and looking forward to a reward, the environment is quiet with a few peers nearby), the goal is to expand the range in which the skill is exhibited by titrating internal and external conditions from the body and environment. As new skills are acquired, vary the context to build and ensure automaticity.

Use both internal and external factors (e.g., allowing a low-to-moderate level of anxiety, completing a task within a certain amount of time) to ramp up the level of perceived challenge. Explore lower to higher level abilities within a sensory modality for a particular task by altering the way sensory information is presented. For example, consider a child who stumbles over words when reading a sentence or story book, but reads a vertical list of words just fine. If you wanted to begin exploring the visual modality, then you might experiment with the following, looking for any changes that result. Enlarge the whole page of the story book, put more space between the words, cover the surround, ask questions to see whether the pictures distract or confuse rather than support, change the font or case, shorten sentences into phrases, determine whether the child reads the words but no longer understands meaning (so begins to stumble), and so forth. Return to the precursor skills for a particular problem area until the level of automaticity is found. Once that level is determined, start there and draw from sensory modalities known to be strengths to build the skill at small increments. Think about the internal and external factors that will enhance the learning process.

In addition to the strategies just described, also consider the following:

- Make a referral to a specialist to determine where the sensory processing breakdown is occurring through challenge tests. Assessment specialists can provide the best feedback when the referral is accompanied by your review of history and milestones, the findings from your sensory explorations, the findings from your review of internal and external conditions that influence the problems and, most important, the specific questions to be answered.
- For those conducting assessments (e.g., speech and language, psychoeducational, neuropsychological, occupational therapist professionals), findings should be accompanied by strategies not only for further assessment but also for addressing the problem in ways that are applicable to all members of the treatment team.
- Many professionals tend to relegate motor problems to the occupational or physical therapist, assuming that such issues have little bearing on their work with the child. However, there is often a sensory side to motor problems that may be overlooked that can be addressed by a wide range of professionals. Sensory issues may hinder motor development (e.g., reduced exploration). For example, a child's poor discrimination of words in the presence of noise may lead to sluggish or absent orienting; a child who has trouble localizing the source of sound may orient inaccurately; a child may not understand the importance of particular sounds and does not respond to them; poor visual perception may impact visually guided motor movements; and problems with touch and pressure may impact the ease of manipulating objects in the hand.

Relevance strategies. Relevance strategies are the key to promoting an alert processing state for the individual child. Whether your goal is assessment or intervention, you should look for answers to the following questions. What matters most to this child? What is he or she interested in? How does he or she like to spend free time? What makes this child feel good? If you are not sure, watch what the child does, where he or she directs attention, or what you say that creates a spark of interest. Does the child like rewards? If so, what type—praise and tickles or stickers and jelly beans? Some kids become clingy and dependent with a parent in the room, some become stellar performers. These are all clues about how to keep a particular child engaged.

For example, Morel was a boy considered "untestable" due to his noncompliance, lack of respect for authority, apparent pleasure at provoking others, and complete indifference to consequences. Through his parents,

one of the authors (JT) learned that one thing Morel really cared about was being viewed as smart—he loved nothing more than being told how smart he was. I used this relevance-based strategy in countless variants to engage his best effort and sustain compliance: "This one's too easy . . . this one might be too hard . . . don't feel bad if you don't get this, this is MIT stuff . . . this is for really big kids"; interspersed with, "Wow, look how smart you are! . . . I can't believe you got that one!" and so on.

A different relevance strategy is needed for the child who shuts down because "everything is hard." This child might need to be let "off the hook" by being told he or she is not *expected* to be able to perform a certain activity because it is "too hard . . . for older kids . . . something not taught yet," and so forth. Ultimately, you do not want the child to link the challenge of working with you to shame or embarrassment, and it is a rare child who will say, "I'm ashamed . . . I'm embarrassed." More likely, the child will "shrivel" or "act out."

Children with more serious emotional disorders will probably require a different type of sensitivity. For example, if a child with bipolar disorder enters your office in a rage, and it takes the entire session to achieve stress recovery, it is still important to avoid shame, even if no work was completed. The professional conducting tests sometimes has to let go of his or her initial agenda and adopt a new one: help the child recover and stay associated with safety. The goal is to use what is relevant to the child to sustain alert processing, titrate challenge, and leave the child walking out the door with a sense of pride and accomplishment.

Executive strategies. Executive strategies are important for everyone involved in the child's life. They can be taught and practiced daily, even integrated into daily routines. The executive system helps the child both remediate and compensate for sensory processing problems and, importantly, helps the child help him- or herself. Executive strategies involve things like planning ahead, trying different ways of learning something, using memory strategies, categorizing information, linking new learning to something well known so it is easier to remember, learning top-down ways to inhibit impulses (e.g., self-talk, focused breathing), and so on. These are typically thought of as strategies for older children, but there are many that can be used even with toddlers (e.g., using a rhyme to remember where something is).

If a child learns even one internal or external condition that promotes learning and then uses that strategy independently, he or she is using an executive strategy. The child has also taken an important step toward building one of his or her most valuable assets—insight. Insight is very important because it is the gateway to all sorts of executive strategies. A child with insight can always move a step closer to a more efficient and

more adaptive way of doing things. A child with insight is less likely to get stuck—knowing weaknesses and strengths provides options to go through, go around, or get help.

One of the more important executive strategies is *anticipation.* In most situations, just a little bit of forward thinking can go a long way toward preventing problems and hampering progress. A child who anticipates that he or she will need help eliminates the element of surprise and readies the regulation system for when that time comes. When a parent anticipates that a spelling test will be a big challenge for the child, he or she can ask the teacher for the spelling words ahead of time and come up with a few creative ideas for study. When a teacher anticipates a child's embarrassment, he or she can avoid exposing the fact that the child cannot write his or her name yet. When a therapist anticipates a child's need for success, he or she can save for last the activity that allows the child to "show off."

It is especially important for the professional to teach parents how to use *their* executive system to anticipate the child's needs for support and to best titrate degrees of challenge to expand a particular ability or skill. For example, if a child's weakness is to use gestures and resist using words, a parent could anticipate ways to encourage the use of words. The next time the child is hungry, the parent might use playful obstruction—pretend that he or she does not know what the child wants or offer the wrong thing—so that the child is more motivated to use words to express a need (Greenspan & Wieder, 1998). In this example, the child is presented with a challenge (the parent's "confusion") and has the increased motivation (hunger) to initiate problem solving.

Even though we have plenty of theoretical history to support the idea that *doing* enhances learning (e.g., Piaget), as of yet, there is little empirical research with children to advance an embodied cognition view of intervention. The work that has been done shows considerable promise. To enhance reading comprehension and memory, a series of studies had children manipulate objects to simulate actions described in the text and also imagine the same actions. When compared to rereading, both strategies resulted in markedly better comprehension of and memory for the material in the text (Glenberg, Gutierrez, Levin, Japuntich, & Kaschak, 2004).

Step 4: Expand the Capacity to Balance the Flow of Sensory Signals in a Way That Is Appropriate to the Context

Modulation is best achieved by using sensory preferences because those preferences support the optimal cycle between sleep and alert processing

and assist with stress recovery. Issues with sensory modulation can present in many behaviors and alongside many diagnostic labels. Children with a diagnosis of ADHD will likely have enormous difficulty modulating fluctuations between activation and inhibition and are often unable to sustain an alert processing state. They are likely to perceive threat in benign situations and often exhibit quick and robust shifts into activation or inhibition (Miller, Reisman, McIntosh, & Simon, 2001). Children with learning disorders may experience associated shame or anxiety at school or home that disrupts the alert processing state. Members of dyads who exhibit mismatched interactions may experience so many sensory triggers from the other that they begin to associate the relationship with threat.

We suggest creating a profile of preferences and triggers for each child, adult, and dyad. You can use your own observation of neutral, positive, and stressed responses or you can use the material in Section 7.3 on the CD-ROM for a systematic approach to tracking sensory preferences and triggers. The Individualized Sensory Profile Worksheet in Section 7.3 on the CD-ROM is an observation-based tool that can be used on its own or in conjunction with testing materials. (Also see the tools listed in step 2 for how to develop an individual sensory profile.)

Intervention involves the ongoing analysis and modification of the individual child's sensory profile, and it may begin from three different vantage points: (1) a focus on facilitating dyadic change; (2) remediation for the problematic sensory modalities; or (3) facilitating compensatory support from other sensory modalities (e.g., language therapy, educational therapy). The following sections provide intervention strategies for modulation problems using the lens of each brain system.

Regulation strategies. The first goal is to tip the scale toward safe experiences; as you decrease perceptions/experiences of threat, you also need to increase perceptions/experiences of safety. This process involves not only the ongoing gathering of information but also modeling for the parents how to act on it. This process can begin very early in the treatment by simply decreasing one sensory trigger and enhancing one sensory preference. The practitioner needs to educate the parent about preferences and triggers; one very effective way to do this is to have the parent begin to identify his or her own sensory profile, for example, by using Dunn's Sensory Profile for adults (Dunn & Daniels, 2002) or the Sensory-Motor Preference Checklist (Williams & Shellenberger, 1996). Parents should also gain an understanding of the relationship between sensory signals and regulation. In general, sensory stimuli that are prolonged, unchanging, familiar, expected, and slow tend to be unarousing or calming (inhibitory), whereas sensory stimuli that are brief, changing, novel, unexpected, and rapid tend to be arousing or stimulating (excitatory) (Pfaff, 2006, p. 20).

Depending on the individual and the context, a slow, familiar, and expected type of stimulation may facilitate sleep or restore calm following a flooded state. For example, when a child has experienced a sensory threat, it is advisable to first begin with slow rhythms and low-intensity stimuli that are familiar and repetitive. For Laura, reducing the stimulation at home, following routines, and playing with or simply being with the family dog provided stabilizing sensory experiences. Conversely, a rapid, changing, novel, and unexpected type of stimulation may help engage and sustain an alert processing state. For Jack, a 1-year-old preemie, being gently lifted up and down (vestibular) shifted him out of a hypoalert state into alert, pleasurable engagement. This simple intervention was the jump-start for eye–face gazing and for he and his mother to fall in love. At the same time, arousing rhythms may be frightening or overstimulating for some children, triggering stress responses (such as Laura's response to preschool). For still others, sensory events that elicit combinations of inhibition and activation provide the right mixture. When children shift too quickly and easily into a stress response as a reaction to daily routines, referral to a specialist (e.g., occupational therapist) is warranted to explore the sensory signals, identify a "daily diet" of preferences, and help the child learn how to tolerate triggers (often referred to as a sensory diet) (Williamson & Anzalone, 1997).

Sensory strategies. All professionals and parents can learn to apply basic intervention strategies to address sensory modulation problems. With a child's profile of preferences and triggers as a baseline, the goal becomes to gradually adjust the intensity, duration, and rhythm dimensions of sensory modalities, events, or both until the child can tolerate, take in, or make use of the sensory input. For example, for the hyperalert/ flooded child, one could start by slowing down the rhythm, decreasing the intensity, and shortening the duration of a stimulus within a particular sensory modality (making use of the titration guideline) and note changes in the child's behavior. Conversely, for the hypoalert child, intensity and rhythm dimensions could be increased and duration lengthened. Note that these are starting points, and most children will have mixed profiles. For example, Danny loved the fast rhythm of the bouncer but cried in response to most other types of vestibular motion. Thus, he had to learn to tolerate other vestibular variations. Starting with a very short duration and a slow rhythm, he gradually learned to adjust to the gentle movement of a rocking chair.

As a general rule of thumb, the professional common wisdom (a part of the process involved in evidence-based decision making; Buysee & Wesley, 2006) includes that proprioceptive and deep-touch pressure input are calming and modulating to the nervous system, helping shift stress

response states into the alert processing state. The effect of proprioception on arousal state, specifically by calming and organizing an individual
who is experiencing over-arousal, is key and as such, proprioception is
seen as a pivotal factor in a therapeutic program (Blanche & Schaaf, 2001).
Proprioceptive interventions can include working the muscles and joints
by having the child push up against pillows held by the parent, the child
pushing against a wall with both arms, or the child pulling him- or herself
up a ramp with a rope. The use of yoga provides self-initiated proprioceptive input. In a preliminary study with adults with sensory defensiveness, participation in six 90-minute sessions of Kripalu yoga significantly
improved baseline vagal tone, and state and anxiety inventory scores
decreased (Mollo, Schaaf, & Benevides, 2007).

Deep pressure touch includes massage (Hernandez-Reif, Diego, &
Field, 2007), skin-to-skin "kangaroo care" (Feldman & Eidelman, 2003),
and Grandin's (1992) development of the "squeeze machine" (Edelson,
Edelson, Kerr, & Grandin, 1999). Early phases of research show promising
results for deep pressure touch interventions. They (1) reduced overarousal
and anxiety in children with autistic spectrum disorders (Edelson et al.,
1999); (2) reduced stress responses and increased weight gain and greater
gastric motility associated with an increase in vagal activity (the parasympathetic nervous system's improvement of inhibition) in preterm infants
(Diego, Field, & Hernandez-Reif, 2006); (3) reduced cortisol levels in both
infants (Field et al., 1996) and preterm infants (Acolet et al., 1993); (4)
decreased anxiety in adults (Field, Diego, & Hernandez-Reif, 2007); and
(5) reduced anxiety and highly aggressive behaviors in a adult with autism (Blairs & Slater, 2007).

The child who is triggered by sensory signals coming from people,
objects, and surroundings is likely to have not only a more pervasive sensory modulation problem but also a sensory processing problem. For example, a child who is easily triggered by sounds from all sources—voices,
toys, activity in the surround, ambient noise, and so on—likely has a sensitivity in the auditory modality where all sound is too intense, too fast,
too long, or some combination thereof. That child may also have (or is at
risk for) an accompanying sensory processing problem. In addition to
adjusting sensory dimensions, this child's profile warrants referral to an
audiologist or neuropsychologist and potentially a speech–language therapist, and his or her sensory environments need to be carefully considered. For example, this child would probably have trouble at a birthday
party and increased problems in a highly active, less structured preschool
with a large number of children in the classroom.

The child who is triggered by sensory signals coming from isolated
sources may present a less complicated profile. However, depending on

the nature of the trigger, you may need to consider trauma-related factors. For example, an internationally adopted child with whom I (CL) worked was frequently in a hypoalert (shut-down) state. Her mother spoke rapidly (her typical pace) and occasionally with an exasperated facial expression and frustrated vocal tone. The mother's style was not abusive in any way but nevertheless appeared to be associated with the girl's frequent shut-downs. The mother learned to slowly alter one dimension at a time—a calm tone of voice, then warmer or more neutral facial expressions, then a slower pace of speech, then shorter sentences—and the child's hypoalert stress responses diminished within a few months. Once the mother grew accustomed to her new sensory dimensions, she noticed that her husband's typical vocal tones and rhythms seemed to be too loud and too fast!

Relevance strategies. The sensory system is the portal for parent–infant bonding and attachment. The falling-in-love experience (the relevance system) is mediated by taste (breast milk), smell, eye contact, touch, voice, and so on. We are wired to make contact through the visual system, especially face-to-face and eye contact. Indeed, if the child demonstrates a strong preference for nonrelational visual sources of information that engage him or her, then such a preference may be a red flag that eye contact is overstimulating. An aversion to eye contact may indicate the possible presence of autism, Asperger syndrome, a nonverbal learning disorder, or a vulnerability due to premature birth. In any of these cases, other sources of sensory communication can take on greater importance for sustaining an emotional bond with others. For example, augmented communication techniques are being used with autistic adolescents who are unable to communicate with spoken language (Koenig, 2007). Skin-to-skin contact, also known as "kangaroo care," first used with premature infants in Bogotá, Colombia, as an alternative to incubators (due to a shortage), is now being used with premature infants in a variety of Western neonatal intensive care units (Feldman, Weller, Sirota, & Eidelman, 2003). Feldman and Edelman (2003) reported that preemies with this tactile contact showed more rapid improvement across a variety of neurodevelopmental features— from vagal tone maturity, to improvement in state organization with longer periods in deep sleep and the alert processing state, to improved habituation and orientation capacities compared with similar premature infants. In addition, in a matched comparison study, results suggested that each parent's relationship (mother and father) with her or his child was "characterized by higher sensitivity, lower intrusiveness, higher parent–infant reciprocity, and lower infant negative emotionality" (Feldman et al., 2003, p. 103). Massage with children with disabilities such as autism may also greatly improve the parents' capacity to feel physically and emotionally close. In one study, the parents' emotional baseline before learning

how to massage their children was distress. Following the intervention parents reported they were able to feel close to their children, and the children were able to express a range of cues to initiate massage (Cullen-Powell, Barlow, & Cushway, 2005).

Parents often need help accepting that their own natural inclinations and behaviors could serve as a sensory trigger or experience of threat for their child. One can first help a parent identify his or her own sensitivities (e.g., use of sensory screeners for adults that identify their unique preferences and triggers), which then generally leads to the emergence of empathy for the child's particular unique sensitivities and aversions. By emphasizing that all relationships are the product of the flow of sensory information, one can provide a more neutral perspective that can help parents step beyond a sense of shame or guilt. In a sense, then, it is not their fault and, more important, there *is* something they can do about it. It is a positive prognostic indicator when parents demonstrate the flexibility to alter their sensory style; they show the ability to both self-reflect and take in external feedback. However, if parents reject the message or respond with hostile statements directed at the child (e.g., "Why should I do anything differently, he's the one who has to change. He's just being a spoiled brat!"), these are poor prognostic indicators and usually warrant individual parent intervention as a priority or in tandem with dyadic play-based sessions. Often, such hostile comments are red flags that the parent may have an abusive history; this history presents an even more critical situation when the child is experienced as the aggressor, as abusing or hurting the parent. These appraisals are addressed further in the relevance system (see Chapters 8 and 9).

Executive strategies. Just as parents plan ahead for their child's regulatory needs (e.g., mealtimes, having snacks in the car), it is also important to plan ahead for their sensory needs. As already noted, anticipation of needs and triggers can prevent many repetitive problems. Separations serve as a good example because they often provoke problems. For a child going to Grandma's house for the weekend, a parent could plan ahead by first making a mental list of the child's sensory preferences. Then, to prime the child for the transition, ask her what she would like to have with her, suggest her preferences, and ask what would help her feel better if she misses Mommy. Make up a list of games to play with Grandma, set up a schedule of "phone hug" times with Mommy, and arrange a nighttime routine. All of these ideas have the same general purpose: to give the child an easily accessible source of comfort. At the same time, the child is being taught how to self-regulate and use executive strategies independently. In some cases, such as with preverbal children, the adult must be able to accurately assess the child's needs and preferences to plan ahead.

For example, in Laura's case, the social worker suggested that she take two of her favorite toys and a stuffed dog (resembling Superdawg) to sleep with her at night when she was at her birth mother's house. While these did not eliminate her sense of threat, they were important sensory preferences that she could use for self-soothing.

Professionals and parents also need to investigate and anticipate the sensory triggers that occur outside the home, for example, at school. One young preschool girl got upset every morning when her friends greeted her with a hug, but she was fine with being hugged when they said good-bye in the afternoon. Once the parents figured out this pattern, they approached the teacher with a solution. The teacher agreed and explained to the girl's friends that although she liked them a lot, she needed "morning space" but loved their hugs in the afternoon. The girls agreed, and one girl asked permission to give "double hugs" when she said goodbye.

As children mature, they should gradually develop the ability to plan ahead for their own sensory triggers and preferences. A parent who provides this support when the child is young helps lay the foundation for the child to internalize and independently use these strategies later.

Laura's treatment with me ended when the family moved out of state to be closer to family support. In concert with Juan and Mary's sensitivities to Laura, they packed up all of her belongings and placed them in tow, so that she would have immediate access to familiar things she loved in a strange, new place. And, of course, Superdawg rode in the back seat as they traveled across the country. Mary called after they arrived to report Laura's initial reaction to the new house. She ran through the house, checking each room, and then proclaimed with a huge smile, "No old daddy in this house!" We were pleased that Laura had taken the initiative to visually investigate the potential for challenge or threat (sensory triggers), trusted her own perception of safety, and provided a robust, integrated verbal and emotional response.

Following Laura's official adoption, court reports were sent to Mary and Juan that revealed the horror of Laura's prior abuse inflicted by her father. She had witnessed her father severely beating her mother, had been hit by flying objects that were intended for the mother, had been bitten by her father on multiple occasions, and at least once had been held at knife point by her father. The mother had never protested or intervened to protect her daughter. Records showed that the father had a long history of sadistic behavior, which included torture with knives and a prior conviction of willful cruelty to a child. In retrospect, it was striking to us just how clearly Laura was communicating her story through her sensory triggers and play themes, not to mention how well she responded when others were able to listen and follow her arousal, sensory, and emotional cues.

After the family was settled a bit in their new home, I helped Juan and Mary transfer to another infant mental health therapist. Later, I checked in with the

therapist, and she commented that she would never have guessed that Laura's early life had been so traumatic because she showed no residual signs of trauma in her play activities. Indeed, she seemed to be well on her way to a safer, pleasure-filled life.

Laura's case demonstrates an approach in which sensory modulation and processing took center stage in treatment goals. After a history of experiencing severe triggers and threat, Laura was finally able to experience preferences and safety through her relationships with Juan, Mary, and her therapists. In this process, the speech and language therapist and I shared the same goals to improve Laura's ability to both process and modulate sensory information. I was able to make more progress because I had guidance from the speech and language therapist as to how best to accommodate Laura's processing and articulation issues. Conversely, with guidance from me, the speech and language therapist was able to better sustain Laura's alert processing state in the sessions and build her language abilities in a way that was relevant to her need for a range of words to help her accurately describe her world as she experienced varying degrees of challenge, threat, and finally safety.

SUMMARY POINTS FOR PRACTITIONERS: SENSORY

Professionals can consider their cases and identify whether any of the behaviors they observe might have contributions from the sensory system. These contributions may be identified from any of the following broad points:

- The child evidences difficulty in a sensory processing level.
- The child shows uneven skills in processing sensory information.
- The child has narrow sensory preferences, frequent sensory triggers, or both that stimulate stress responses.
- The parent is having trouble modulating sensory information for him- or herself (Heller, 2002), for his or her child (Kranowitz, 1998; Miller, 2007), or both.

In addition, professionals can make note of the disciplines weighted in this brain system and begin to create professional networks that can be used for referrals, if necessary. Disciplines weighted in the sensory system include the following:

- neuropsychologists and psychologists (testing, partial or global);
- occupational therapists (somatosensory and vestibular sensations; oral–motor functions, visual–motor processes);

- developmental optometrists (visual processing);
- audiologists (auditory processing);
- speech and language therapists (auditory, oral–motor);
- educational therapists (visual and auditory processing);
- cognitive psychologists who specialize in processing difficulties.

In terms of intervention, parents can play an important role. In particular, involving them in the following strategies can be beneficial:

- Support auditory skills by speaking slowly.
- Support the creation of internal visual pictures and images during activities.
- Slow down interactions to assist tracking of sensory information.
- Minimize sensory triggers of threat and begin to build capacity to tolerate through titration, always oscillating back to safety.

In addition, all practitioners can consider the following possible strategies for assessment and intervention:

- Begin to support the use of sensory awareness and tracking (what do you hear, see, smell?).
- Begin to notice whether matching or countering sensory behavioral dimensions are more soothing.
- Use titration and automaticity principles.

Worksheets 7.2 and 7.3 can be used (often with the assistance of parents) to assess sensory processing and modulation in infants, children, and parents. These worksheets are also available in Sections 7.1 and 7.2 on the CD-ROM.

Because sensations directly affect arousal, they also directly affect the positive and negative valence of emotions, the development of memories, and the meanings that are both private and shared. Next we explore the relevance system's integration of emotions, memories, and meanings.

Worksheet 7.2. Assessment of Sensory Processing in the Infant, Child, and Parent

Resources and Strengths Toward Allodynamic Coordination	Risk Factors for Processing Problems and Conditions of Allodynamic Load
Check whatever applies to the child, and circle what applies to the parent (including the parent's developmental history).	*Check whatever applies to the child, and circle what applies to the parent (including the parent's developmental history).*

Visual:

- ☐ "Reads" facial expressions and discriminates the nuances of facial expressions
- ☐ "Reads" body gestures and discriminates nuances in gestures
- ☐ "Reads" emotion through a combination of these visual cues
- ☐ Can navigate an environment independently with sufficient exposure
- ☐ Can recall places, people, etc.
- ☐ Can manage visual learning materials, can "see" visual relationships

Visual:

- ☐ Does not appear to react to emotional expression, shows limited reciprocity in facial expression, seems unaware that the other is angry, worried, sad, etc.
- ☐ Does not appear to pick up gestural cues that convey another's feelings/intents, for example, ready to go—looking at the clock, worried; fidgeting, bored—listless, yawning
- ☐ Only seems to pick up others emotions when there is an explicit verbal expression; only seems to pick up on others' emotions when the facial expressions and gestures are dramatic/extreme; seems often caught off guard by others' emotional expression, as though lacking awareness of the emotional escalation
- ☐ Is often lost; takes a very long time to learn the map of a new environment
- ☐ Does not recognize faces, does not remember a place or the route, does not notice when something very obvious is different or has been changed; sometimes, there is a hyperfocus on certain visual elements with unawareness of others, (e.g., hyperfocus on faces)
- ☐ Struggles with visual materials (e.g., puzzles, blocks, math, science); judges distance or size poorly

Auditory:

- ☐ Identifies tones of voice and nuances of tone; distinguishes foreground sounds from background noise
- ☐ Enjoys rhymes, such as nursery rhymes and songs; shows appreciation for the rhythm

Auditory:

- ☐ Does not hear nuances in tone (e.g., escalating frustration); does not discriminate one sound (e.g., of a telephone) from background noise (e.g., on the radio)
- ☐ Shows no particular pleasure in rhyming or "playing with" rhymes; appears confused/

(Continued)

Worksheet 7.2. Continued

Resources and Strengths Toward Allodynamic Coordination	Risk Factors for Processing Problems and Conditions of Allodynamic Load
☐ Begins to generate rhymes with made up words and real words	disinterested in story rhymes and nursery rhymes
☐ Accurately interprets the words he or she hears and can understand words presented in phrases/sentences	☐ Cannot generate rhymes at all or only with made-up words; when given a word, has a hard time coming up with a rhyming word
☐ Can identify beginning sounds and ending sounds, can determine the phonemes that make up a blend, such as *bl* and *st*	☐ Does not discriminate words accurately, "mishears," does not discriminate similar sounds such as words beginning with a *b* and *d* or a *p* and *t*.
☐ Exhibits age-appropriate development in speech and language milestones	☐ Does not "hear" the sounds in words or cannot arrange them in the right sequence
	☐ Shows "lags" or delays, seems to lose speech/language skills when tired or under stress; seems to have "gaps" in development

Touch:

Touch:

☐ Discriminates types of tactile/cutaneous stimulation (temperature, pain, pressure) and localizes source of touch	☐ Has difficulty identifying what is touching him or her (ICDL-DMIC, 2005) or where on the body the touch is located
	☐ When eyes are occluded, may not be able to identify what type of sensory input is being received

Smell:

Smell:

☐ Accurately identifies smells and their distinctions	☐ Does not notice pungent odors, will eat something that has gone bad, may not distinguish the difference between dad's body odor and mother's perfume

Taste:

Taste:

☐ Accurately identifies tastes and their distinctions	☐ Does not distinguish between distinct tastes, such as sour, sweet, and bitter

Proprioception:

Proprioception:

☐ Perceives body in space as well as direction and force of body in motion	☐ Has difficulty judging timing, force and distance (e.g., may hold a pencil too tightly or too loosely, does not use enough pressure when using utensils to cut up food, kicks a ball with too much or too little force) (ICDL-DMIC, 2005)

(Continued)

Worksheet 7.2.   Continued

Resources and Strengths Toward Allodynamic Coordination	Risk Factors for Processing Problems and Conditions of Allodynamic Load
Vestibular:	*Vestibular:*
☐ Sustains balance and with both passive and active motion	☐ Has difficulty sensing speed of movements or sense of direction of movement with eyes closed (ICDL-DMIC, 2005) ☐ "Poor righting and equilibrium reactions" (ICDL-DMIC, 2005, p. 93) ☐ Poor trunk stability and rotation of trunk ☐ Falls/topples easily; avoidance of moving up and down a staircase; avoidance of walking on any raised surface; avoidance of heights
Pain:	*Pain:*
☐ Discriminates pain from all senses and can localize the source	☐ Has difficulty identifying exactly where the pain is coming from (e.g., feels uncomfortable, but does not know whether it is in stomach or gut or chest) or what type of pain it is (e.g., sharp, dull, throbbing, intermittent, or constant) or the initiation of pain (e.g., does not notice pain with skinned knee)

Worksheet 7.3.   Assessment of Sensory Modulation in the Infant, Child, and Parent

Resources and Strengths Toward Allodynamic Coordination	Risk Factors for Conditions of Allodynamic Load
Check whatever applies to the child, and circle what applies to the parent (including the parent's developmental history).	*Check whatever applies to the child, and circle what applies to the parent (including the parent's developmental history).*
☐ Has strong oral–motor strength as exhibited by action of tongue, lips, and cheeks for chewing and biting as protolinguistic movements ☐ Responsive to internal pain (gut, stomach) and surface pain (skinned knee) ☐ Can recognize a tight chest, tight throat, or changes in breathing as accompanied by strong feelings	☐ Loss of hearing ☐ Loss of sight ☐ Poor oral–motor structure (such as excessive drooling, cleft palate, prefers only soft foods) ☐ Overresponsive to sensory information (needs low-intensity, short duration, and/ or slow rhythm of sensory stimulation to respond to the experience) ☐ Underresponsive to sensory information (needs high-intensity, long duration, and/ or fast rhythm of sensory stimulation respond to the experience)

(Continued)

Worksheet 7.3.   Continued

Resources and Strengths Toward Allodynamic Coordination	Risk Factors for Conditions of Allodynamic Load
Sensory Experiences That Constitute Preferences *In the following list, circle whether the sensory modalities help the child or the parent (depending on whom you are evaluating), calm down, help become alert and engaged, or seem to have no effect.*	☐ Has a narrow range of preferences (two or fewer modalities) for calming or alerting ☐ Poor modulation of sensory information (cannot regulate intensity [high/low] or duration [long/short] or rhythm [fast/slow] of sensory information) ☐ Prefers sensory information coming from inanimate objects rather than through relationships ☐ Sensory triggers that create prolonged (load condition) stress responses, as per the following

Sight (e.g., looks at face/toy)

    Calms   Alerts   No Effect

Hearing (e.g., turns to voice/music)

    Calms   Alerts   No Effect

Touch (e.g., enjoys being held, touching blanket)

    Calms   Alerts   No Effect

Smell (e.g., sniffs skin/clothing)

    Calms   Alerts   No Effect

Taste (e.g., mint calms, sour alerts)

    Calms   Alerts   No Effect

Proprioception (e.g., jumping, chewing)

    Calms   Alerts   No Effect

Vestibular (e.g., swinging, rocking)

    Calms   Alerts   No Effect

Multiple (Enjoys sensory information from multiple sources within environment and relationships)

    Calms   Alerts   No Effect

Sensory Experiences That Trigger Adaptive Stress Responses	*Sensory Experiences That Trigger Load Conditions of Stress Responses*
As you observe the child or parent or record their narratives, jot down sensory events in he appropriate modalities that result in **adaptive stress responses.** *Also check the appropriate items to identify the specific type(s) of stress response(s) (e.g., the child cries, but only briefly, after the doctor puts a cold stethoscope on his or her chest; therapist jots event in tactile modality and circles the third stress response—flooded).*	*As you observe the child or parent or record their narratives, jot down sensory events in he appropriate modalities that* **trigger load** *conditions of stress responses. Also check the appropriate items to identify the specific type(s) of stress response(s) (e.g., the doctor's cold stethoscope produces high intensity crying that is difficult to soothe within 20 minutes; therapist jots event in tactile modality and checks the third stress response—flooded).*
Hypoalert (e.g., shuts down, avoids) Hyperalert (e.g., anxious, vigilant) Flooded (e.g., cries, tantrums)	Hypoalert (e.g., shuts down, avoids) Hyperalert (e.g., anxious, vigilant) Flooded (e.g., cries, tantrums)

(Continued)

Worksheet 7.3. Continued

Resources and Strengths Toward Allodynamic Coordination	Risk Factors for Conditions of Allodynamic Load

Sight
Event:_____
    Hypoalert   Hyperalert   Flooded
	Sight
	Event:_____
	    Hypoalert Hyperalert Flooded

Hearing
Event:_____
    Hypoalert   Hyperalert   Flooded
	Hearing
	Event:_____
	    Hypoalert Hyperalert Flooded

Touch
Event:_____
    Hypoalert   Hyperalert   Flooded
	Touch
	Event:_____
	    Hypoalert Hyperalert Flooded

Smell
Event:_____
    Hypoalert   Hyperalert   Flooded
	Smell
	Event:_____
	    Hypoalert Hyperalert Flooded

Taste
Event:_____
    Hypoalert   Hyperalert   Flooded
	Taste
	Event:_____
	    Hypoalert Hyperalert Flooded

Proprioception
Event:_____
    Hypoalert   Hyperalert   Flooded
	Proprioception
	Event:_____
	    Hypoalert Hyperalert Flooded

Vestibular
Event:_____
    Hypoalert   Hyperalert   Flooded
	Vestibular
	Event:_____
	    Hypoalert Hyperalert Flooded

8

Functions and Behaviors of the Relevance System

The relevance system reveals what is salient to us through the three large domains of emotion, memory, and meaning-making. In the relevance system, we think of *energy* as the degree of emotional reactivity and *information* as the content of memories and meanings. When working with the relevance system, we facilitate the child's ability to express and inhibit both positive and negative emotions, as well as blends of emotions, in a way that is appropriate to age and context.

Early experiences provide the context for learning. Learning determines the shape of memories in the present and influences memories that will be formed in the future. The combination of these factors is intrinsic to the process of meaning-making regarding the self, others, and the world. The foundation for relational and emotional health starts with reliable and loving long-term relationships. Having at least one such adult present in a child's life is pivotal for children to develop emotional balance and to learn to thrive within primary relationships.

When early beginnings do not have the necessary ingredients for a healthy relevance system, long-term effects and struggles emerge, as can be seen in the following case example of Anna.

Anna's parents contacted one of the authors (JT) seeking guidance to help their 5-year-old daughter. On the phone, Anna's parents, Paul and Nicole, told me the following story. Anna was adopted from a Romanian orphanage when she was 3 years old. From birth to age 1, she had lived with her mother and grandmother. She was taken to the hospital for a cluster of medical conditions, including a respiratory infection and acute diarrhea that required 4 months of treatment. When her caretakers did not return, she was sent to the orphanage. At the time of

the adoption, Anna had no speech and moved around by "scooting." Within an hour of taking her from the orphanage, disturbing behaviors emerged. When Nicole took her to the restroom for the first time, Anna was "completely terrified." For months, the parents could not take her to the bathroom. Once at home, they found that Anna had two distinct modes: (1) very restless with fleeting attention, or (2) "poker-faced, without emotion" and "checked out, staring into space."

Within a few months, Anna began to speak in single words and went from scooting to walking in her third year. Although she was showing progress, she was still very delayed in all milestones, and her disruptive behaviors were not improving. About 1 year after her adoption, her school conducted speech and language testing, and Anna began receiving 60 minutes per week of speech and language therapy. During the next year, her vocabulary increased, and she began speaking in phrases. One year later, at age 4, the school tested her motor skills, and occupational therapy services were added.

Overall, Anna's behavior at school was exemplary. From the time she began preschool, she was described as fidgety, inattentive, and distractible, but not at all disruptive. In fact, Anna was considered one of the happiest children the educational staff had ever seen. Meanwhile, at home, the parents faced increasingly defiant and oppositional behavior, which had begun 6 months after the adoption. When they tried to explain to the school what was happening at home, the response was, "She's fine at school!" This response led the parents to feel embarrassed that they were having so much trouble at home. As the parents recounted the details of their long journey to me, they were tearful, confused, and ashamed. Questions were flying. How could they make sense out of such divergent positive and negative behaviors? Why were they, as parents, getting all the disruptions at home and no one else was?

THE FUNCTION OF THE RELEVANCE SYSTEM

The relevance system links three crucial components of healthy functioning: the ability to experience emotions, to remember, and to learn in ways that create meaning. Each of these abilities involves complex capacities that interconnect.

Relevance Capacities

As noted, this chapter explores the capacities related to three large domains—emotion, memory, and meaning—in relation to the following three capacities:

- the capacity to flexibly experience, express, and modulate a full range of emotions in ways that are appropriate to context;

- the capacity to learn from experience by scanning and accessing a full range of memories that are appropriate to the context;
- the capacity to create meanings that accurately reflect self and others.

Emotion

There is no generally agreed-on theory of emotion. Endless debates surround questions related to what emotions are; where emotions begin; why emotions exist; how emotions develop; how emotions influence behavior, health, and relationships; and how to respond best when emotions go awry. When we consider the multiple perspectives and approaches represented in emotion research—emotions as appraisal of events, as subjective experiences, as continuums of valence, as a means of regulation, as degrees of reactivity (Friedman & Chase-Lansdale, 2002), facial and motor expressions; as somatovisceral contributions (Berntson, Sarter, & Cacioppo, 2003a, 2003b; Damasio, 1996, 1999), action tendencies, expressions of intent, and physiological changes, such as varying arousal patterns and electrical and/or chemical brain activities (Cacioppo, Berntson, Larsen, Poehlmann, & Ito, 2000; Moscolo, Harkins, & Harakal, 2000; Panksepp, 2000; Roesch, Fontaine, Scherer, Ellsworth, & Shen, 2007)—it is apparent that emotions are "complex and multiply determined" (Cacioppo & Gardner, 1999, p. 193).

Professionals who work with children, even in limited ways, can readily observe the rich complexity of influences on their emotional tendencies and expressions. We see that there are often emotional patterns and consistencies that are unique to each child, and we also recognize how much the emotional picture can change in response to changes in the environment, the interpersonal interaction, or the learning challenge. With more clinical experience, we see the limits of diagnostic categories and the dangers of simple answers for emotional problems. Many come to realize that assessment and treatment of emotional problems are best thought of as a work in progress—new pieces of the puzzle may emerge, and the way the pieces fit together may change.

For this reason, the neurorelational framework not only holds an awareness of the complexities of emotion with respect to the multiple biological, cognitive, and social factors that influence a child's emotional development but also acknowledges the dynamic opportunities for change. From this perspective, emotional development is shaped by both intrinsic and bottom-up factors (e.g., physiological patterns, malnutrition) as well as extrinsic and top-down factors (e.g., the environment, appraisals) (Lewis & Granic, 2000). Behaviorally, the neurorelational framework presents a

developmental progression of emotional development, whereby, starting in infancy, emotions are described according to a broad valence ("positive" and "negative") and marked by behavioral parameters that either possess or lack coordination (e.g., regular rhythms, modulated shifts in valence). With age, emotions take shape in more discrete and dimensional forms as well as in more rhythmic patterns, and they become increasingly integrated within relational exchanges.

Two selective dimensions that are considered primary contributors to emotion are arousal and valence (Berntson, Bechara, Damasio, Tranel, & Cacioppo, 2007). The *arousal* component of emotion refers to the degree of activation or inhibition, and the *valence* component refers to the degree of positive or negative salience.[1] Moods differ from emotions in terms of their duration (Lewis, 2000). *Emotions* are fleeting, lasting from seconds to minutes, whereas *moods* are emotion states, lasting for hours, days, or longer. The duration element of mood is why certain negative or high positive moods are a risk factor for a load condition.[2] Positively valenced emotions, such as love, laughter, happiness, and satisfaction, usually reflect contextual safety and tend to promote social affiliation. When a child "feels positive," he or she is more likely to absorb, engage, and explore. A predominance of neutral or positive valence is associated with the alert processing state, which means that in the context of optimal regulation, a neutral or positive affect or mood will dominate. Negatively valenced emotions, such as hate, anger, sadness, and disappointment usually reflect some degree of contextual challenge or threat and promote social isolation. When a child "feels negative," he or she is more likely to be defensive, aggressive, or withdrawn. A predominance of negative valence is associated with the stress response states, which means that in the context of load conditions, a negative affect or mood will usually prevail.

Studies indicate that adults have a tendency to show characteristic positive and negative response patterns (Cacioppo, Larsen, Smith, & Berntson, 2004; Ito & Cacioppo, 2005). The majority of us tend to have a neutral or positive baseline in the absence of negative triggers. In other words, we are just fine when not provoked. This is referred to as the *positivity offset* (Cacioppo & Gardner, 1999; Cacioppo, Gardner, & Berntson, 1999). However, once the negative alarm signals danger, we tend to react quickly and experience strong negative feelings that are easily fixed in memory. This is referred to as the *negativity bias* (Baumeister, Bratslavsky, Finkenauer, & Vohs, 2001; Cacioppo & Gardner, 1999; Cacioppo, Gardner, & Berntson, 1999; Ito, Larsen, Smith, & Cacioppo, 1998). One explanation for this common response pattern comes from an evolutionary perspective. An animal is more likely to survive and adapt to its environment if it continues to approach and explore when all appears benign or appealing (positivity offset); conversely, when an event signals the potential for

devastating effects, it is best to have a swift reaction and remember the dangerous cues to better guide behavior in the future (negativity bias). This evaluation between positive and negative is a dominant and immediate factor in human judgment (Crawford & Cacioppo, 2002). Indeed, the distinction between positive and negative evaluation "occurs at the earliest processing stages, within 140 ms of encountering a new stimulus (Cacioppo, Larsen, Smith, & Berntson, 2004; Morris, Ohman, & Dolan, 1999)" (Crawford & Cacioppo, 2002, p. 453).

There are individual differences in positive and negative reactivity; that is, some people interpret neutral information as positive and some will interpret it as negative (Ito & Cacioppo, 2005). Leanings in either direction carry advantages and disadvantages. A stronger negativity bias may save one from danger, embarrassment, or disappointment but may also support impressions that are false, hurtful, or unjust (e.g., when one quickly or harshly judges others or exaggerates information that fuels discrimination). A stronger positivity offset may promote social contact and feelings of well-being but may also support positive assumptions that are equally false, hurtful, and unjust (e.g., when one fails to see inequality or to consider the possibility of abuse due to "Pollyanna-ish" views). It may seem counterintuitive that there could ever be too much positive, but when it leads to denial of a potential reality that perpetuates harm, it is much more apparent how this tendency can be maladaptive. A common example of this tendency would be a refusal to believe the possibility of bad behavior from someone in an authority role or respected position. In another variant, a person might be repeatedly surprised because he or she cannot accept the reality in life that some people are simply not trustworthy, and thus, the person never learns when *not* to trust. In addition, an elevated positive emotion can be a risk factor for mania (Gruber, Johnson, Oveis, & Keltner, 2008).

Traditionally, the positive and negative valences of emotion are thought of as opposing one another, or on a bipolar continuum; in other words, as one type of valence emerges, the contrasting valence must recede. For example, one is either happy and not sad, or sad and not happy. Recall that a similar bipolar conceptualization used to surround the understanding of the two branches of the autonomic nervous system in that one was either being activated or inhibited in the reciprocal mode of control (see Chapter 4). A bivariate model of valence (Cacioppo, Gardner, & Berntson, 1997; Larsen, McGraw, & Cacioppo, 2001) allows for greater variation in potential combinations of positive and negative valence (e.g., being happy and sad at the same time, shifting from happy to sad). Interestingly, these emotional variations of positive and negative valence are similar to the expansion of the activating and inhibiting features of arousal (uncoupled or coupled modes of control) in the regulation system, as discussed in Chapter 4.

In applying the foregoing theories within the neurorelational framework, *a child's ability to tolerate and work through a full range of positive emotions, negative emotions, synchronous positive and negative valences, and blends of emotions, modulating at varying degrees of intensity, is a core developmental process.* We refer to this process as developing the emotional self or the emotional muscle. The nature of a person's response to life events, especially stressful events, plays a crucial role in developing the strength and flexibility of the emotional muscle. A study of coping from the bivariate model perspective (Larsen, Hemenover, Norris, & Cacioppo, 2003) posits an optimal emotional response pattern that varies according to the degree of stress involved. Low-stress events, or events that produce low levels of activation, evoke either generally positive or neutral emotions. For example, situations such as running late or discovering that one is out milk are a part of life's little mishaps that are best brushed off with a neutral or positive response. Moderate stress events warrant both positive and negative activation. A moderate stressor (e.g., a friend who is moving away) typically involves what one deems important in life, and the resulting negative feelings are a natural part of disappointment and loss. Consistently avoiding the negative denies authentic expression of loss or disappointment. At the same time, one's ability to inhibit the *degree* of negative and activate the positive is important to stress recovery. Although it is healthy to acknowledge the negative, it is best not to drown in your sorrows or hold on to your anger in a way that exacerbates the stress response. Severe stress events (e.g., death of a loved one), however, warrant a strong negative response with a weaving in of the positive that grows in strength over time. Expending the cognitive effort to find positive in the negative gradually creates meaning for the experience and thereby assists the stress recovery process. When a person creates some degree of positive meaning in response to a severely stressful event, he or she "turns adversity into advantage" (Larsen et al., 2003, p. 211).

In summary, the degree of stress reactivity in relation to the type of stressor is an important variable. High reactors to mild and moderate stressors may be at greater risk for disease susceptibility, whereas low reactors may have more resilience. "High reactors may therefore show selected signs of diminished immunosurveillance because of the long-term suppressive effects of sympathetic activation and stress hormones [HPA] on the immune response to viral and infectious agents" (Cacioppo et al., 1998, p. 672; see also Cacioppo, 1998).

Memory

Emotions influence learning and memory. Exactly how this influence occurs and under what specific conditions remain unclear, but research into

the bidirectional influence of emotions and memory reveals some general patterns. One well-known concept is that of *state-dependent retrieval* (Bower, 1981), which refers to the tendency for individuals to show better retrieval for memories that are similar to their current emotional state. In other words, when a person is sad, he or she can more easily recall events that were experienced when he or she was sad (Bower, 1981; Harkness & Tucker, 2000). A second, related pattern is that of *state-congruent process- ing*, which means that a person's current mood will bias him or her to take in information that is in keeping with that mood. Thus, a current depressed emotional state may bias one to attend to negative and sad in- formation (Dalgleish et al., 2003; Schacter, 1996). In this way, a pre- dominance of certain emotions (or life experiences that generate certain emotions) during the course of development can come to shape the va- lence of meanings and thus expectations. In other words, because our memories are a reflection of prior learning and experience, those memo- ries come to guide our expectations about relationships and the world.

To understand more fully how emotions and memories interact to shape meaning for the individual child, it is important to have a basic un- derstanding of learning and memory processes. Whatever the professional field, from medicine to psychotherapy to motor rehabilitation, learning and memory processes are at work and are central to the process of change—a goal that is common to all interventions. We begin with a few global prin- ciples of memory to set the stage and then briefly discuss the temporal processes of memory—encoding, storage, and retrieval—and two types of memory—implicit (unconscious) and explicit (conscious) (we discuss working memory in the next chapter).

First, *memories are not exact recordings of events.* What is relevant to us influences what we attend to, and what we attend to influences what we remember. Thus, it should not be surprising that people remember events differently depending on, for example, what was important enough to them to harness their attention at the time of the event. The nature of the situation itself may also influence memory. For example, emotionally arous- ing events (as opposed to neutral ones) lead to a narrowing of focus, such that information in the periphery is less likely to be attended to and there- fore less likely to be remembered later (Reisberg & Heuer, 2004). This phe- nomenon accounts for what has been called "weapon focus," whereby victims of crime may recall highly specific details about the weapon but much less about everything else (Loftus, Loftus, & Messo, 1987). One's in- ternal situation may also influence memory. For example, with depression, memory is thought to be impaired due to difficulties with elaborating the details of the experience during the encoding stage, such that the experi- ence is never really stored in memory in the first place (Elliott, 1998).

Second, *our memories are the product of distortion and bias.* Memories are reconstructions, and we fill in the gaps without realizing it. Thus, memories may lose time distinctions, become intermingled with other events, or be altered by new information or others' comments. People may even recall an event as having happened to them when it actually happened to someone else (Anderson, Cohen, & Taylor, 2000; Loftus 1994, 1997; Schachter & Dodson, 2002).

Third, *forgetting is typical.* We all forget. Take a moment and try to reconstruct your entire day yesterday, every single experience from waking to going to bed. Even if you isolate your recall to your behavior alone, exempting your thoughts and feelings, it may be surprising how little you actually remember. Fortunately, what you forgot is not likely to matter much—which is probably why you forgot it.

Children learn about the world and relationships by establishing associations among repeating events, referred to as *associative learning* (e.g., in essence, "When I shake the rattle, it makes a certain noise," "When I hear the *m* sound, I see that Mom's lips are in a certain position," and so on). The sensory and motor features of these events must be processed (encoded) in the brain to be stored in memory and thereby available for later retrieval. Thus, it stands to reason that if some features of these events were not encoded accurately (e.g., the baby hears the rattle but cannot see its features very well; the toddler sees the *m* shape of Mom's lips but cannot discriminate the *m* sound), the later storage and retrieval of the memory would contain the same inaccuracies or incomplete representations. As well, disruption in the processing or integration of sensory and/or motor signals may impede encoding and storage, which could account for some of the memory problems observed in children with learning disabilities.

One does not need to consciously remember a past event, or even be consciously aware of encoding it, for the event to exert an influence on behavior. A classic example of this phenomenon is demonstrated in the behavior of an amnesic patient with her physician, Édouard Claparède (1903). Because the patient's memory disorder did not allow her to form new memories, she greeted Dr. Claparède as a stranger at each visit. During one such visit, Claparède positioned a needle in his hand so that it poked her when they shook hands. On subsequent visits, she continued to greet him as a stranger but declined to shake his hand again. This behavior was guided by her *implicit memory*, the type of memory that we rely on to go about the procedures that we do every day (for example, prepare a meal or drive a car) without consciously thinking about the task. Procedural forms of implicit memory are most often involved in routines, habits, and acquired skills, but these three arenas may also include simple forms of associative learning (establishing associations among

events) and nonassociative learning (the processes of habituation and sensitization discussed in the last chapter). As such, implicit memories usually (but not always) require a period of time to form by means of repetition but are then resistant to forgetting (Charness, Milberg & Alexander, 1988; Cohen & Squire, 1980; Graf & Schacter, 1985). For example, memory disorders are characterized by loss of conscious memories but retention of routine habits and skills.

At some point around 2 years of age, children are thought to recognize the self as separate from others (Courage & Howe, 2002). The emergence of autobiographical memory, or the ability to recall past events from one's own experience, coincides with this stage of development (Howe, Courage, & Edison, 2003). Autobiographical memory represents a type of *explicit memory* comprised of those memories that are available to conscious access. There are other types of explicit memory, such as memory for acquired knowledge and facts (semantic memory) and preverbal memory for information or events that can be elicited through recognition and imitation. Explicit memories usually require less time to form than implicit memories, but they are also more vulnerable to rapid forgetting (Tulving, 1985).

Not all events that are encoded will be stored in memory; in fact, most will not be. A multitude of factors can facilitate storage either with or without conscious effort. The negativity bias discussed earlier ensures that an event with a strong negative valence, especially when it carries the potential for harm, is much more likely to be stored in memory than a neutral event (Baumeister et al., 2001). This storage occurs automatically, without effort on our part. Often, it is the gist or the implications of an event that are stored, not exhaustive details—which makes sense because the gist holds the information that is relevant for future behavior (Brainerd & Reyna, 1990). For example, people tend to remember the gist of what others have said, not necessarily what was said verbatim (Poppenk, Walia, Joanisse, Danckert, & Köhler, 2006). We are also more likely to store (1) information that is familiar and that easily links up with prior knowledge (Bjorklund, 1985, 1987; Chi, 1978; Ornstein & Haden, 2001); (2) information that is organized in a way that makes it more accessible and meaningful (Flavell, Miller, & Miller, 1993; Greene, 1999); (3) information that is self-generated (Slamecka & Graf, 1978); and (4) information that we share with others (Ybarra et al., 2008). It is well known that storage is also facilitated by activities that require cognitive effort, for example, repetition, practice, elaboration, and critical thinking (Craik & Lockhart, 1972; Hasher & Zacks, 1979). These more effortful activities are thought to underlie the dramatic improvements in memory that are seen as children mature (Howe & O'Sullivan, 1990; Schneider & Pressley, 1997).

The term *retrieval* typically refers to an active, conscious process and thus is associated with explicit forms of memory. Just as with encoding and storage, a multitude of factors affect retrieval. One already discussed is that of state-congruent retrieval, the tendency to recall events characterized by a valence in line with current mood. The context effect, or the tendency to recall information better when you are situated in the same context, is also known to facilitate retrieval (Parker, Gellatly, & Waterman, 1999; Schacter, 1996). Walking the halls of your high school and being flooded with memories of that time and place would be an example of the context effect.

Learning and memory problems of various types are implicated in numerous developmental disorders (attention disorders, learning disabilities) and insults such as very low birth weight, epilepsy, and traumatic brain injury (Anderson & Catroppa, 2007; Gozal & Molfese, 2005; Nolan et al., 2004; Swanson, 1993; Taylor, Klein, Minich, & Hack, 2000). Thus, understanding the general processes and types of memory opens up endless avenues for assessment and intervention. For example, simply observing a child's gaze and reactions or asking a child to repeat back what he or she just saw or heard can provide a great deal of information about encoding. Experimenting with different ways to present information may assist storage, and using various cues or contexts may facilitate retrieval.

A metalevel view of learning and memory for a child, a dyad, or a family begins with the question of what type of learning system is operating and, especially, whether there is an *open learning system*. The neurorelational framework defines open learning as the ability to (1) encode events with a range of qualities (positive/negative, gist/verbatim), (2) retrieve events with appropriate accuracy, (3) guide behavior based on those experiences, and (4) be open to new information that has the potential to reshape or update meanings. In an open learning system, the individual, dyad, and family are flexible enough to take in new or unexpected changes in information, tolerate negative feedback that may promote self-correction, and take in positive feedback that may promote self-esteem. Conditions of safety provide the backdrop for an open learning system.

However, some children, dyads, or families function within other types of learning systems that usually lead to less coordinated states. A *closed learning system* is both narrow and rigid. Closed learning systems are reflected by engrained patterns that block the influence of certain types of information or valence, usually those that threaten cohesion. In a closed learning system, the individual, dyad, or family absorbs only information that fits with existing knowledge or, when pressed, may distort information to make it fit (e.g., reinterpreting, assigning too much private meaning). There is often a quick rejection of the novel or unfamiliar and a very limited ability to adjust or adapt to changing contexts.

A *chaotic learning system* is one that is too open—too broad and too flexible. Here, there is a lack of stable knowledge and memories such that the relevant nuggets for storage that come from ongoing experiences cannot anchor into a solid network. In other words, without a stable structure, memory traces are too numerous or too weak to establish cohesion. In a chaotic learning system, new information continually distorts or replaces old information and fuels ambiguity and inconsistency. In short, without building on the relative stability of one's knowledge of feelings and concepts, not enough is learned. In intervention, the goals are to increase stability in the chaotic system and to increase flexibility in the closed system.

Meaning

What the child brings into the world, in conjunction with his or her relationships and environment, provides the raw data for emotions and memories. The integration of emotions and memories in real time shapes the ongoing and dynamic process of meaning-making. Meaning emerges through positive and negative emotions and through implicit and explicit memories. Sharing these meanings facilitates social bonding, such as the bonds that emerge from common knowledge or expertise, from a mutual interest or hobby, from shared values or cultural background, and so forth. Shared meanings connect us.

Both private and shared meanings shape what becomes relevant for the individual child. When trying to understand a child, one can begin by trying to understand the various contexts that provide the backdrop for emotions and memories that ultimately shape meaning. First, the child's internal context—what he or she brings to the world—will shape meaning. Any type of disruption to the typical developmental trajectory, regardless of etiology, will become integrated into what is meaningful for that child. For example, a physical disability will influence how the child views his or her abilities and expectations, how others respond to him or her, and what aspects of the environment are viewed as opportunities or constraints. All of these components become woven into the fabric of the child's private and shared meanings. Second, the child's environment shapes meaning. A community culture that provides support, interesting stimulation, and positive relationships will shape very different meanings than a community that breeds fear, withdrawal, and isolation. Multiple aspects of family culture also influence meaning; for example, rigid versus flexible parent roles, demanding versus permissive parenting styles, parental expectations of values such as family loyalty and education, or sibling profiles (e.g., one of whom is a high achiever and one of whom is severely delayed).

The parent–child relationship is a primary source of emotions and memories and is integral to meaning-making. In addition, the relationship with a parent is the fundamental context for the child's developing awareness of self and other, as well as a child's expectations in relationships. The meaning-making influence of this primary relationship is bidirectional and a co-created process; that is, a parent can influence the meanings that a child holds, and a child can influence the meanings that a parent holds (Tronick, 2007).

Meaning-making takes shape in the context of three common modes of dyadic interaction that can be characterized in terms of their degrees of responsiveness and directiveness ("response and demand"; Baumrind, 1971, 1991; Maccoby & Martin, 1983) as well as reflectiveness. These three modes parallel the triad of characteristics introduced in Chapter 2 of heart (response), hand (directive), and head (reflection). Although we focus mainly on the respond–direct–reflect patterns within the parent–child dyad, these modes apply to all relational dyads (spouses, therapist–client, etc.). Each of these modes requires a particular set of abilities, and most people show stronger tendencies toward one or two of these modes. Ideally, one should be able to express a comfortable blend of all three; such a balance reflects an open learning system that facilitates coordination across all brain systems. When parents have the ability to flexibly blend these modes in interactions with their children, there is a greater likelihood that their children will learn to express these modes flexibly in relationships. Rigid adherence to one specific mode or erratic expression of any given mode reflects a closed or chaotic learning system that fosters load conditions. Table 8.1 details parental versions of each style of interaction in both coordination and load conditions.

Physiological Underpinnings of the Relevance System

Emotions and the formation of memories, or learning, are affiliated with a large inner and older region of the brain known as the limbic system. Building on the information presented in Chapter 2, we now delve deeper into the brain regions associated with emotions and memory: (1) the limbic connections to lower and higher brain structures, or the bottom-up and top-down emotion pathways mediated by the amygdala; (2) the limbic connections with multisensory regions in the formation of memories, mediated by the hippocampus; (3) the role of mirror neurons in imitative learning and social connectedness; and (4) the neurochemicals that underlie stress and stress recovery.

Table 8.1. Examples of Coordination and Load Versions of the Three Interpersonal Modes: Parent

Respond	Overaccommodate	Direct	Demand	Reflect	Detach
Coordination	Risk Factors for Load Conditions	Coordination	Risk Factors for Load Conditions	Coordination	Risk Factors for Load Conditions
• Follows the child's lead • Seeks nurturing interactions • "Feels" the child's emotional experience • Tolerates tender and positive feelings within self and child ("softer" side of emotions) • Emotional tone is warm, nurturing, and tender toward child (or spouse/partner) • Experiences closeness and connection between self and child • Mirrors the child's experience (empathy) • Greater focus on shared meanings	• Overly permissive and ingratiating • Child is too often "rescued" or the behavior denied • Negative aspects of child are not mirrored, so child is rarely forced to contend with relational stress or challenge • Falsely positive affect dominates • High compliance toward the child or partner • Overly relies on child or others to function • At the extreme, leads to enmeshment	• Takes the lead with child • Holds expectations of child's (or spouse/partner) behavior • Can express own needs clearly and assertively • Willing to risk conflict and rupture • Tolerates tougher and negative feelings within self and toward child ("tougher" side of emotions) • Emotional tone is firm, stern, and assertive with child	• Overly controlling and aggressive • Child is too often challenged or suspect • Negative aspects of the child are emphasized, so child is too often confronted with mistakes and failures • Negative affects dominate • High defiance against child • At the extreme, leads to abuse • Emotional tension or discomfort that leads to attacking and blaming the child • Entrenched meanings lack those of child's perspective	• Observes interactions before taking action • Considers the truth/facts about self and child • Can problem-solve with self and with child (or spouse/partner) • Willing to make conscious choices about changing behavior • Can detach from emotions and consider them on a meta-level	• Overly detached and unresponsive • Child is left to function or cope on own • Child not given adequate feedback through either nurturing or guidance • Lack of positive or negative affect; neutrality dominates • High avoidance, turning away from child • At the extreme, leads to neglect • Emotional tension or discomfort leads to detaching from or stonewalling child • Escape to one's private meanings predominates • Under stress, may favor the hypoalert state

(Continued)

Table 8.1. Continued

Respond	Overaccommodate	Direct	Demand	Reflect	Detach
Coordination	Risk Factors for Load Conditions	Coordination	Risk Factors for Load Conditions	Coordination	Risk Factors for Load Conditions
	• Accommodates others' meanings at the expense of private meanings • Under stress, may favor the hyper-alert state	• Experiences boundaries between self and child • Supports self-modulation and limit-setting abilities • Greater focus on personal meanings	• Under stress, may favor the flooded state	• Can simultaneously hold tenderness and firmness in emotional tone • Experience of autonomy and separateness • Acknowledges both private and shared meanings	

The Amygdala and Emotion

The amygdala processes a wide range of negative and positive emotions. Although the role of the amygdala was once primarily associated with the experience of fear, it is now viewed more broadly as a "relevance detector" (Sander & Scherer, 2005, p. 217) that evaluates the emotional significance of an event. The research from Damasio's lab (e.g., Bechara & Damasio, 2005; Bechara, Damasio, Tranel, & Damasio, 2005; Damasio, 1994, 1996, 1999, 2003), among others (e.g., Joseph LeDoux and fear conditioning, see LeDoux, 1996, 2002), illuminates the complexity of the brain structures and the bottom-up and top-down processes that form the emotional experience, but there is general agreement that the amygdala takes a leading role. The amygdala has reciprocal connections with structures that are affiliated with each of the brain systems in the neurorelational framework (Iversen, Kupfermann, & Kandel, 2000); thus, these pathways support the integration of emotion with physiological (regulation system), sensory (sensory system), and motor (executive system) processes. For example, amygdalar connections to the hypothalamus influence autonomic experiences associated with emotions such as "a broken heart" or "a knot in the stomach" (Lieberman & Eisenberg, 2005); connections to lower (brainstem) motor regions mediate rapid motor responses when necessary (LeDoux, 2000); connections to multisensory regions (insula) and memory regions (hippocampus) facilitate encoding and storage for emotional events (Kilpatrick & Cahill, 2003). Furthermore, the degree of activation in the amygdala has been shown to correlate with the degree of recall for emotionally intense events (Canli, Zhao, Brewer, Gabrieli, & Cahill, 2000; Changjun & Michael, 1999; Mesulam, 2000b).

The Hippocampus and Memory

The Hebbian rule—neurons that fire together wire together (Hebb, 1949)—still holds as the neural foundation for learning. Memories are created through the strengthening of connections between neurons to form a memory trace. Memory traces are viewed as collections of basic elements (sensory pieces) that link current information with knowledge already stored in memory. Damasio (1994) contends that memories represent the binding of "sensory fragments to one another and to preexisting knowledge, thereby constituting complex records of past encodings" (in Schacter, 1996, p. 66).

The hippocampus plays a primary role in the binding process as new memories are being formed (Mesulam, 2000b). The hippocampus is connected to several brain regions that have major pathways linking up with

areas involved in the integration of sensory and motor signals (Suzuki & Amaral, 1994). As stated in Chapter 2, memories are not stored in the hippocampus but are distributed throughout the cortex. Like the amygdala, the multiple interconnections among regions within the other brain systems indicate that memory is mediated by a highly complex and distributed network (Markowitsch, 2000).

Mirror Neurons

Imitation and empathy are thought to be supported by the mirror neuron system. In macaques, the same mirror neurons fire both when the monkey is doing something and when it is watching someone do the same thing (Rizzolatti & Craighero, 2004). In other words, these neurons mirror the behavior of another. There is evidence that the same types of neurons exist in motor, medial frontal, and parietal regions in humans (Fadiga, Craighero, & Olivier, 2005; Fadiga, Fogassi, Pavesi, & Rizzolatti, 1995; Gazzola, Rizzolatti, Wicker, & Keysers, 2007; Mukamel, Ekstrom, Kaplan, Iacoboni, & Fried 2007). The human mirror neuron system is thought to guide imitation learning and support functions such as understanding others' intentions (Fogassi et al., 2005), empathy (Wicker et al., 2003), and perspective taking (Gallese & Goldman, 1998). As such, mirror neurons would then support the response mode that plays such a crucial role in the early stages of parenting (and in any therapeutic relationship). An impaired mirror neuron system has been hypothesized to underlie the functional deficits in autism, and there is some research support for this idea (Dapretto, 2006).

Neurochemical Effects

A variety of neurotransmitters and hormones involves the emotional experiences of contentment as well as excitement and joy. Oxytocin facilitates bonding (e.g., as in maternal behaviors) and social recognition as well as calming behaviors, such as the down-regulation of the stress response (it mediates the potential negative effects of cortisol) (de Oliveira, Camboim, Diehl, Consiglio, & Quillfeldt, 2007) and the feeling of warmth in the tummy when happy (Sunderland, 2006)—all experiences that fall with the relevance system. Oxytocin, along with dopamine and opioids, supports high-intensity emotions, such as excitement and joy. The brain is also showered with norepinephrine during high-intensity relational events, which enhances memory (Sunderland, 2006).

As noted in Chapter 2, dopamine is central to the brain's reward mechanisms, which help us improve detection of reward cues and our prediction

as to the likelihood of reward, both crucial aspects of learning (Montague & Quartz, 1999; Schultz, 2000).[3] Opioids are best known as pain relief chemicals (by producing natural versions of morphine), but they also give us a general sense of well-being (Sunderland, 2006). These examples merely scratch the surface of how the brain's various chemical messengers contribute to the emotions and memories that shape meaning.

Several studies have suggested that the chemicals underlying the experience of emotional stress can damage the hippocampus and thereby negatively impact the formation of memories. For example, sustained stress has been shown to damage cells in the hippocampus when cortisol remains in the brain too long (Sapolsky, 1994). As introduced in Chapter 2, research with at-risk infants and young children within the foster care system or adopted from international agencies has further suggested that chronic stress leads to alterations in the hypothalamus-pituitary-adrenal (HPA) axis in humans, which may then interfere with subsequent brain development and emotion regulation (Fisher, Gunnar, Dozier, Bruce, & Pears, 2006; Gunnar, 2000; Hart, Gunnar, & Cicchetti, 1996; Kaufman et al., 1997; Rogeness & McClure, 1996).

Activation and Inhibition

The various states of arousal reflect varying degrees of physiological activation and inhibition that are expressed through behavioral cues. (The arousal-related contributions to emotions, memories, and meanings are summarized later, in Table 8.4.) The stress response states (hypoalert, hyperalert, flooded) are accompanied by characteristic emotional expressions. The hypoalert state is often the backdrop for depression; the hyperalert state, the backdrop for anxiety; the flooded state, the backdrop for fear and anger. These are, of course, very general rubrics, and emotional expressions can also involve much more variation in arousal.

Consider the emotion of happiness. One may experience it as comfort when drowsy, as quiet contentment in the hypoalert state, as modulated happiness (talking, hugging, laughter) in the alert processing state, as excited in a hyperalert state, and as overjoyed or ecstatic in a flooded state. The same variation exists for negative emotions, such as sadness. One may be quiet and withdrawn (hypoalert), sharing the sad event with a friend (alert processing), ruminative and blaming (hyperalert), or sobbing and tantruming (flooded). These are typical variations in emotional expression, and just like with optimal regulation, they shift into a load condition only when there is a predominance or absence (too much or too little) of emotions at the extremes without adequate recovery.

As noted earlier in this chapter, we contend that people can experience more than one emotion at a time and at varying degrees of activation. For example, a woman may feel both happy and anxious at the thought of her approaching wedding day. Furthermore, the degrees may shift, at one point happier than anxious and at another point more anxious than happy. An example that reflects greater tension may be feeling happy and excited at being accepted into a competitive school but equally sad and upset that a best friend was rejected. More chronic emotional blends are reflected in an anxious or hostile depression.

The relationship between emotional arousal and memory is not straightforward. We noted earlier in this chapter that people are more likely to remember emotionally charged events over neutral ones and that this effect holds whether the valence is positive or negative. For example, when you tried the exercise of reconstructing your day yesterday, a memory of laughing with a friend or a disturbing news event might have sprung to mind before you recalled what you wore or what you ate for breakfast.

It stands to reason that a predominance of stress states (load conditions) would have consequences for memory; as noted, animal studies have shown that severe stress can damage the hippocampus and cause memory impairment (McEwen, 2002; Sapolsky, 1994). However, studies in humans have shown mixed results, indicating that stress can either enhance or impair memory. One recent study (Buchanan, Tranel, & Adolphs, 2006) suggests that the differential effect may be due to individual differences in cortisol reactivity. The participants in this study who showed a cortisol response to a cold pressor test (stress test) recalled significantly fewer neutral and emotional words than did controls and fewer than those participants subjected to the same test who did not show a cortisol response.

Research indicates that learning and memory processes may be disrupted in various emotional disorders. The findings with posttraumatic stress disorder (PTSD) are mixed; however, there is evidence that memory effects are related to the co-occurrence of depression with PTSD. The research findings indicate that depression impacts the attentional processes necessary for encoding (Elliott, 1998; Mesulam, 2000a). Studies investigating brain activation have found amygdalar hyperresponsiveness to negative stimuli in PTSD (Hendler et al., 2003; Protopopescu et al., 2005) and in borderline personality disorder, and the latter was also associated with cognitive dysfunction (Hurlemann, Hawellek, Maier, & Dolan, 2007).

Another way to view the effect of arousal on memory is by considering the degree of cognitive effort required for learning to occur. We have stated that more arousing events (positive or negative) are more easily remembered. Kensinger and Corkin (2004) found that the encoding

arousing events was automatic; that is, it did not require top-down effort. These data imply a linear relationship between arousal and memory—the higher the arousal, the stronger the memory. However, this relationship stands in contrast with studies of learning that show that high levels of stress often impair both attention and memory. Here, the relationship is curvilinear and in keeping with the Yerkes–Dodson law—the higher the arousal, the weaker the memory. According to Diamond, Park, Campbell, and Woodson, (2005), the distinguishing factor for these seemingly discrepant findings is the degree of cognitive challenge involved in the learning process.

Self- and Interactive Regulation

A child's ability to self-regulate is supported when a parent can adopt a predominantly responsive mode of interaction early on. Responsive parenting means that the parent can take the child's perspective, mirror the child's experience, and "feel" the child's emotions. Parental mirroring involves focusing on the child's emotions, positive or negative, and acknowledging his or her cues with facial expressions, tone, words, and touch. Infants and young children will often mirror others' emotional tone in a more primitive imitative fashion. The bidirectional process of mirroring supports the child's access to a full range of emotions. If the mirroring process breaks down on either end (e.g., a mother with depression, a child with autism), then there will be a constricted range of emotions in the dyadic interaction. Empathy involves taking the other's perspective and allowing oneself to feel the other's emotional condition. Infants older than 6 months have been shown to exhibit a distressed look at the discomfort of others; toddlers will try to comfort the other, even bringing over their own mother to help (Hoffman, 1978).

These two processes—mirroring and empathy—are powerful promoters of relational bonds because they facilitate and expand shared meanings. Experiences of mirroring and empathy are also essential for the development of a self. Mirroring helps the child see his or her image through the eyes of another, and empathy helps the child tune into the other's perspective. They also set the stage for the predominance of positive emotions that support the child's alert processing state and ability to recover from stress.

In infancy, a baby's arousal states, emotions, and behavior often change rapidly, making it difficult for even the most responsive parent to keep up. During this period of learning how to respond to the infant's nonverbal directives, experiences of mismatch, or rupture, dominate the

dyad's interaction. Tronick (2007) found that episodes of mismatch (3-month, 6-month, and 9-month-old infants) can make up more than 70% of the interaction during this period. As a parent learns to meet the infant's nonverbal directives and the frequency of mismatches diminishes, a foundation of procedural (implicit) memories forms, involving a rich blend of experienced safety, met needs, positive emotions, and shared meanings—which increase the efficiency of both self- and interactive regulation. This developmental shift is noticeable at about the age of 10 months, when emotional distress decreases and pleasure increases (de Weerth & van Geert, 2000).

As a child's motor abilities develop and allow for increased exploration, the parent must simultaneously increase limit setting and corrective feedback. Safety concerns increase along with use of the word *no*. As the directive elements of parenting increase, the dyad is again more often out of sync. The child experiences distress as he or she bumps into the boundaries set by the parent. At this stage, parental responsiveness is vital to repair these more intentional ruptures initiated by the parent's limit-setting. A "dance" now emerges between directive behaviors, which are needed to assert the self and guide the other, and response behaviors, which are needed to connect and reconcile with the other. The give-and-take of responsive and directive behaviors leads to secure relationships that can negotiate a full range of emotions within the self and with the other. As children grow older, the cycles of directing–rupture and responding–repair grow increasingly nuanced and elaborate. With age, the directive element begins to function more in a supportive role, helping the child internalize self-modulatory and self-limiting skills. Increasing maturity means that the parent must constantly update expectations, degrees of challenge, and respect for the child's growing autonomy in relation to deepening connections.

The Emotional Self

During development, children learn about their own and others' emotions. Infants do not need to be taught about things such as discomfort; they express it quite naturally with tears and other signals of distress. Babies *are* taught, however, about the meaning of emotions. A parent who consistently reacts to a baby's distress with agitation creates a very different emotional meaning than the parent who consistently reacts with tenderness. In the context of adequate mirroring and empathy, the child learns to read the signals coming from his or her own body, from others, and in the world—others' gazes, movements, tones, and so forth, become associated

with various events and feelings. Babies also learn about emotions and further develop their emotional self by imitating others. Through imitation, they learn to "catch the feelings of another, particularly if strongly expressed" (Goleman, 2006a). By the age of 4 months, babies exhibit some ability to read emotions, evidenced by their different reactions to different facial expressions (Flom & Bahrick, 2007; Montague & Walker-Andrews, 2001, 2002). The babies stared at and showed interest in an adult's smiling face; they looked away and would not look back in response to a sad face; and they stared with vigilance in response to an angry face. It appears that infants' ability to observe and follow the gaze of those around them (beginning at 10–12 months) is an important early step of the journey toward beginning to infer and to understand other's minds (beginning by 14–18 months) (Brooks & Meltzoff, 2002, 2005; Meltzoff, 2007; Meltzoff & Brooks, 2007). Thus, the relevance in what an infant does with his or her eyes has important developmental consequences.

The child's experience of positive and negative emotions fluctuates within the context of responsive and directive interactions. Response-based interactions in the dyad provide the foundation for the accomplishment of "merger" experiences, whereas directive-based interactions are the foundation of experiences of separateness (Stern, 1985).[4] In the neurorelational framework, these two modes occur in a fluctuating manner across the life span, with the goal being to flexibly modulate, shift, and integrate needs of self and other according to the context (more to come in the executive system). With early mismatch experiences, babies learn to tolerate a range of emotions, such as frustration and anger, within the context of safety. Mismatches also provide opportunities for implicit learning about the "other." When a parent's timing is off or when he or she misreads cues, there is an implicit meaning that the parent actually cannot "read the child's mind." If repair follows this rupture consistently enough, then procedural memories form that allow the child to hold the tension of shifting back and forth from "self" to "other," alongside the expansion and contraction of positive and negative emotions.

The child's emotional muscle is strengthened by stimulation of the negative range of emotions that are typically elicited by the directive aspects of parenting. Directives come in the form of "no" expressions, restricting behavior, correcting behavior, directing and guiding, insisting on social values, engaging in conflicts, expressing differing emotions (i.e., *not* mirroring), and expressing different intentions and goals. A child who must contend with these bumpy types of challenges within a loving relationship learns the emotional flexibility that is a defining characteristic of an open learning system. This process also builds resilience (Tronick, 2007). In contrast, when parents do not challenge children in this way, the

emotional muscle is not exercised within a negative range. As a result, the child may not learn emotional tolerance and flexibility, may not learn about appropriate expectations for others in relationships, and may not learn to self-soothe in the face of relational disappointments. This scenario predisposes one toward a closed or chaotic learning system.

Helping the child develop an emotional self presents a challenge for the parent. The parent must have a healthy emotional muscle at the outset to withstand the tension and "messiness" (Tronick, 2007) of this process. This process varies depending on the child's and the parent's tendencies to respond, direct, or reflect. Initially, there are not many pat responses or preset answers for parents who are trying to titrate directives appropriately and with the right dose of emotional responsiveness. For the most part, the nuances get worked out in real time, and consequently, mistakes will be made. Although this may seem like common sense, the ability to tolerate and negotiate the messiness of mistakes is where many parents may easily become stuck. It is uncomfortable!

For some parents, the discomfort comes with standing firm while inhibiting the impulse to let responsiveness take over, for example, holding firm to require a child who is uncomfortable expressing a desire to do so before getting what he or she wants, or following through on a consequence despite the child's tears. For other parents, the challenge comes from a need to offer mirroring and empathy for the imposed distress of directives; for example, acknowledging how difficult it was to express a desire and offering praise for doing so, or showing empathy for the child's sadness about a consequence, even though the child was warned about what would happen. A parent who experiences discomfort when using either a responding or a directing style may be signaling that it is time for reflecting to take center stage. Reflection is the tool with which parents can help themselves to further develop their *own* emotional self, so that they can feel comfortable being both firm and empathetic. The child's reflective capacities also mature through observing the parent's reflective behaviors and through practicing problem-solving behaviors with the parent. It is vital that parents (and spouses, as well as therapists and teachers) have the ability to step back and reflect on not only the child's emotional range but also their own respond–direct process. Note that reflective capacities involve primarily executive components from the executive system, which will be discussed in Chapters 10 and 11.

As the telling of Anna's history ended, I (JT) asked about the current state of affairs at home and at school. Paul and Nicole knew that Anna was significantly delayed in her functional abilities but felt that this delay was minor compared to her disruptive and atypical behaviors at home. First, Anna was still not bonding

with her parents. She made eye contact, could be soothed at times, and would "tolerate" affection, but she did not seek comfort and affection from them; she lacked the responsive behaviors we want to see exchanged between parents and child. Second, Anna had frequent tantrums. Any type of directive situation, no matter how benign, set her off. For example, she refused to leave the house. Every day, the parents went through severe tantrums that often ended with them physically carrying her to the car as she kicked and screamed. Third, Anna was fixated on controlling events, and if anything occurred outside of her expectation, she insisted that it be redone or fixed somehow. The parents' requests were always met with an automatic "No!" Fourth, although she was 5 years old, Anna was not yet toilet trained. She wore disposable pants to school, and children were beginning to tease her. Her father stated, "I know that something happened in that orphanage around going to the bathroom." The parents had literally organized their schedules around cleaning up after her, timing things so that she would not be publicly embarrassed, avoiding many situations that carried too much risk, and so on. They also lost sleep on a regular basis; both were chronically sleep deprived. Finally, the parents had tried giving Anna medication (a stimulant) to treat her behaviors, but this "made her worse," and they were not interested in pursuing the pharmacological avenue any further.

Anna participated in 3 half-days of testing with me. Consistent with her behavior at school, she was a pleasure. Granted, her attention was fleeting and she was very distractible, but she could be redirected easily, and she sustained a pleasant and cooperative attitude. However, knowing that it was important to see the other side of Anna, I began to slowly push the envelope with her. I started to redirect her more quickly when she was off task, I refused breaks more often, and I pushed her a bit harder to attempt responses on challenging items. It did not take long for this new, firmer, and structured behavior from me to elicit a tantrum. In line with the parents' report, she did not respond to soothing, distraction, negotiation, or bribes. She could only be monitored for safety as she worked it through.

During the feedback session with the parents, I first organized the sheer volume of concerns by using a bottom-up sequence of the brain systems within the neurorelational framework. In the *regulation system*, Anna's difficulties involved early illness and malnutrition, significant physiological stress due to illness and separation–abandonment, poor bladder and bowel control, and ongoing sleep problems. I suspected that her failure to toilet train was related to a poor connection to the visceral self. Anna spent most of her time in hypoalert and hyperalert states, with daily swings into a flooded state.

In the *sensory system*, I explained that Anna had multiple delays in visual processing, receptive and expressive language processing, and phonological processing. In some areas (more so in comprehension) her language was much better developed than her visual abilities. After observing Anna recoil and tense up when touched, I also suggested that tactile issues may trigger some of her fears and tantrums.

In the *relevance system*, Anna was clearly struggling to cope with a history of trauma, and her sense of meaning was shaped by experiences of loss, neglect,

unresolved grief, fear, and probably terror. Her emotional range (expression) involved a predominance of superficial happiness on the "outside" and protest and rage on the "inside"—at home. I framed her behaviors as attempts to cope with implicit or explicit memories of trauma and explained how, through her eyes, they could be quite adaptive. Her development of an emotional self was rudimentary. Given Anna's history, it is likely that the availability of mirroring, empathy, and repair of her emotional states went from minimal to almost nothing as she was shuffled from her mother's home to a hospital, and then into an orphanage, with not only low ratios between caregivers and children but also serious lapses in emotional care. This underpinning of relational neglect was the likely cause of Anna's emotional constrictions and distinct positive and negative polarities. Although her verbal and visual memory showed areas of relative strength, her poorly developed sensory system offered little compensation that could bolster her resilience.

In the *executive system*, Anna also exhibited numerous difficulties. Her large motor skills were much improved on testing, but this improvement did not come through in her functional behaviors. Her fine motor skills were weak when precision was involved. Her abilities to sustain attention, inhibit her impulses, and shift her attention were extremely poor, more akin to a 2- or 3-year-old level. As a result, she was not yet developing higher abilities within the executive system, for example, working memory, problem solving, and ability to generate alternatives when blocked.

As the first step of an ongoing process of assessment and intervention, I shared that the sleep disruptions for Anna and her parents (regulation) and the trauma and attachment issues (relevance) needed to take priority in treatment. Second, I concluded that Anna's therapies to bolster her sensory system delays were inadequate. She was not receiving remediation according to a developmental hierarchy, and she was not acquiring new skills to automaticity. Although not meeting formal diagnostic criteria for a learning disability, she was clearly struggling to learn in all academic domains. The parents were referred to a counselor (CL) to begin dyadic sessions in which the sensory system was used to address both the regulation and the relevance priorities. The executive system would be addressed not only through increased occupational therapy to work on coordination in the motor system but also through dyadic therapy with efforts to expand attention, switch attention, and strengthen inhibition. It was too soon to address academic issues and higher levels of the executive system as a priority. We agreed to touch base again in 3 months to review how things were going, and the parents gave me permission to share all the findings with CL.

CLINICALLY RELEVANT BEHAVIORS OF THE RELEVANCE SYSTEM

In this section, we present information about the behaviors and developmental markers of emotions, memories, and meanings. We culminate by

presenting the relationships among these components with the states of arousal.

Emotions and Development

One definition of emotion emphasizes the movement aspect, e-*motion*, and views emotions as the behaviors that signal intent to others (Freeman, 2000). Researchers such as Izard, Ackerman, Schoff, and Fine (2000) (for infants) and Ekman (2003) (for adults) focus on the muscular movements of facial expressions that comprise discrete emotions that are hypothesized to be genetically (innately) hard-wired (Izard et al., 2000). The research study by Bennett, Benderksy, and Lewis (2005), which includes a review of debates and other studies, suggests that at birth, infants display disgust; by the age of 4 months they show joy, interest, anger, and sadness; by the age of 6 months they show surprise; and fear emerges between the ages of 4 and 12 months (Bennett et al., 2005). In general, there seems to be research support that the organization of facial expressivity matures into emotional specificity over time during infancy. "Over time, the emergence of increasing specificity toward a particular facial expression in response to a given situation is likely to occur, for example, anger in response to arm restraint or disgust in response to a sour-tasting substance. Expressions are expected to show an increasing degree of situational specificity during infancy" (Bennett et al., 2005, p. 168).

However, not all researchers agree that a facial expression represents a discrete emotion. For example, Camras posits that the same facial expressions may "serve many masters, both affective and nonaffective" (Camras, 2000, pp. 120–121) in nature. Furthermore, these expressions are hypothesized to reflect a "softly assembled" (Camras, 2000, p. 120) dynamic system that responds "in the moment" (i.e., not innate) to novelty and complexity in the environment.

In the neurorelational framework, we take a broad view of emotional development by discussing the emotional range that is present within the child, parent, and dyad over time. Optimally, a child shows both positive and negative emotions, with a predominance of positive, and the range expands over time. The behavioral markers that we present (adapted from Greenspan, 1996) have the following developmental progression:

- showing a positive (3 months) and negative (5 months) emotional range through nonverbal cues of face, sounds, body movements;
- negotiating these emotional expressions through vocalizations (3 months), movements, and gestures (13 months) that mature from

basic forms in infancy to activities such as reaching up (9 months), declarative pointing (12 months; also referred to as joint attention, pointing with motivation to influence the intentions of others; Tomasello, Carpenter, & Liszkowksi, 2007), and walking (13 months), all of which provide the "vocabulary" of approach and avoid behaviors;

- talking about emotions with expanding language skills (24 months);
- engaging in symbolic and pretend play that reflects an emotional range (24 months).

We aim to grasp the larger gestalt of emotional expression by using the phrase "emotional themes" (introduced in Chapter 3). Emotional themes do not depend on discrete facial expressions or any single behavioral marker; rather, they embody movements, gestures, sounds, words, and symbolic play that capture the overall gist of positive and negative ranges. For example, consider the baby who, though working hard to suckle while breastfeeding, is making gurgling sounds, placing a hand on Mom's breast, molding to her body with closed eyes, and ultimately reflecting a picture of closeness, dependency, nurturance, and pleasure.

Table 8.2 summarizes the developmental behavioral markers in the context of emotional themes. These markers reflect aspects of the socioemotional milestones. Note that the first priority is to establish positive expressions that continue and expand in their range as the developmental markers unfold (i.e., the ability to show, negotiate, tell, and play). Similarly, once the negative range begins, it continues to expand. Although Table 8.2 provides a developmental timeline for these emotional themes, it can also be adapted as an assessment tool of an adult's emotional range.

Younger children, of course, have less ability to modulate emotion and will more often show extremes of emotion—very angry, very happy. Adults typically delight in the "unbridled" emotional expressiveness of children—when it is positive. However, such high-intensity, fast-rhythm emotions may be difficult for young children to modulate downward on their own. Some children may shift rapidly across emotions with parallel intensity (e.g., from shrieks of joyful laughter to screaming tears) and have trouble shifting back to an alert processing state, even with positive emotions. These children require emotional scaffolding and coaching from adults, who help them slow down the rhythm and decrease the intensity. Working the child's emotional muscle in this way helps him or her develop the capacity for a range of emotions that can speed up or slow down and increase or decrease in intensity while staying within the alert processing state.

Table 8.2. Developmental Progression (Shows, Negotiates, Tells, Plays) of the Expression of Emotional Themes

| Approximate Typical Age | Shows Emotional Theme | | Negotiates Approach/Avoid | Tells | Plays |
	Positive	Negative			
3 months	Interest Curiosity Pleasure		Vocalizations and movements to expressing positive (coo/cuddling) and negative (cry/arching)		
5 months	Comfort Excitement	Sadness Anger	Vocalizations and movements showing more variations of positive/negative		
9 months	Closeness Pleasure/excitement Assertive exploration	Protest Anger Fear	All the above plus gestures and sounds to initiate emotional themes thus far	Beginning basic word-like sounds in connection with themes (babbling, "Ma, Da, Ba")	
13 months	All of the above	All of the above, plus caution	Gestures, vocal, and advanced motor activity to initiate and respond to themes thus far (walking toward/away)	Jabbering, basic words in connection with themes (ba-ba for bottle, sounds for sources of comfort)	
18 months	Closeness/dependency Pleasure/excitement Assertiveness/exploration	All of the above, plus caution or fearfulness Anger ~ 19–22 months,	All the above plus gestural, vocal, and motor activity responses to outside limit setting	Simple words to express emotional themes	

(Continued)

Table 8.2. Continued

Approximate Typical Age	Shows Emotional Theme			Negotiates Approach/Avoid	Tells	Plays
	Positive	Negative				
		embarrassment (Aksan, Van Voorhis, Weber, & Georgeson-Dunn, 1999)				
24 months	All of the above	All of the above, plus recovery from and dealing with distress Shame (Mills, 2005)		Gestural, vocal, and motor activity dominates during stress	Two-word sentences to recover from distress or express at least one theme ("Me scared," "Want Mommy")	Pretend and early symbolic play that expresses at least one theme
30 months	All of the above	All of the above, plus recovery from and dealing with distress		Gestural, vocal, and motor activity dominates during stress	Words used to recover from stress and express at least two themes	Pretend and symbolic play that expresses at least two themes
36 months	All of the above	All of the above, plus recovery from anger		Gestural, vocal, and motor activity is linked more strongly to words and play	Words used to link up two or more logically connected themes	Play that links up two or more logically connected themes
42–48 months	All of the above Love/empathy	All of the above, plus loss/separation		Gestural, vocal, and motor activity supports the use of words and play	Words used to link up three or more logically connected themes that show cause/effect, awareness of time and space	Play that links up three or more logically connected themes that show cause/ effect, awareness of time and space

Note. From material in "Assessing the Emotional and Social Functioning of Infants and Young Children," by S. I. Greenspan, 1996, in *New Visions for the Developmental Assessment of Infants and Young Children*, by S. J. Meisels and E. Fenichel (Eds.), Washington, DC: ZERO TO THREE. Adapted with permission of ZERO TO THREE.

A poorly developed emotional muscle may be expressed through (1) the absence of the behaviors in Table 8.2 that indicate an inability to show, tell, or demonstrate by means of age-appropriate emotionally based play themes; (2) the presence of constricted themes (all negative or all positive); and (3) extreme expressions of negative play themes that include repeated aggression, destructiveness towards self or others, victimization, or paranoia, as summarized in Table 8.3.

When I (CL) met Anna's parents, they were visibly exhausted and seemed apprehensive. I spent time with them alone initially to carefully assess Anna's history from a socioemotional milestone perspective, talk about JT's assessment results, and introduce them to my dyadic play approach. I started our first session by following Anna's lead. She settled into playing with a little dog puppet, and within a few minutes, her puppet was attacking my cat puppet. My first response was to talk for my puppet, saying, "Wow, you seem really mad at me! I wonder why?" Immediately, Anna dampened down into a mute response with gaze aversion. Suspecting that I was running into her developmental and socioemotional delays, I shifted to a vocal but nonverbal means of interacting with her puppet by having my puppet begin to meow. Anna brightened and reengaged by having her dog puppet bark at my cat puppet. I slipped the mother a puppet, and soon we were an animal family having a lively "conversation" with each other. Eventually, Anna began to express clear pleasure with smiling and giggling.

Anna's quick shift to shut-down during the play was a clear message, and I needed to accurately decipher the meaning. Given her testing and functional socioemotional delays, I suspected that I had overshot her abilities on several counts.

Table 8.3. Load Condition Expressions of Emotional Themes

Constricted Themes	Extreme Expressions
Child shows, tells, or demonstrates through play:	Child shows, tells, or demonstrates through play:
1. No affect	1. Repeated aggression
2. Only brief and intermittent positive affect	2. Self-destructive behaviors (e.g., head banging, self-biting)
3. Predominance of negative range, with no positive affect	3. Destructive actions to vulnerable objects (e.g., younger siblings, pets, baby puppets [symbolically])
4. Predominance of positive range, with no negative affect	4. Repeated victimization scenarios (e.g., beaten up on playground, teased and tormented by others)
	5. Repeated themes of suspicion and fear regarding the motivations and intents of others (e.g., adults/authority figures/peers are always "out to get" the child)

With the language I used in my comment that her puppet must be "angry" and in asking her a why question, I was possibly hitting on several delays all at once: (1) delays in her receptive processing skills (my saying too much, too fast), (2) delays in her expressive language processing skills (her not being able to organize a verbal answer), (3) her emotional delays in accurately labeling facial and motor movements with words, and (4) her inability to verbally and emotionally link up emotional events (being angry) with emotional reasoning (i.e., "I'm angry because you hurt my feelings"; the sixth emotional milestone that requires cause-and-effect thinking). I also wondered whether I had induced an embarrassment. To test these hypotheses, I shifted my means of communication downward to a developmentally younger behavior, which was successful in reengaging the emotional "juice" between us.

What occurred in this slice of time demonstrates how crucial it is to be tuned in to shifts in arousal and then to immediately alter the intervention to get to the meaning of the shift. In this case, timing was everything. Had I not suspected that I was "shooting too high" for her cognitive abilities to handle (by asking an age-appropriate question), then we surely would have entered into a frustrating sequence of interactions that would have reinforced her mute withdrawal. The information I learned became highly valuable in future sessions. Furthermore, this seemingly small insight had the potential to promote more positive exchanges across settings, especially at home. I encouraged the parents to visualize Anna as a much younger child when talking to her and, when listening to her, to give her plenty of unpressured time to respond and scaffold her responses instead of speaking for her or making assumptions.

Although the parents' urgent need was to address the toilet training issue because it was a major contribution to load conditions for them, I had to hold that need in tension with following Anna's lead during the sessions. I knew that if I focused on the pressure to get her potty trained, she would probably feel that pressure, and we could easily move into a collapse. As I held in mind the need to explore Anna's connection to her body (her visceral self), I saw that she was showing excitement in our play, with glimpses of shared joy with her mother that had occurred in the first session. Because Anna's emotional expressions to her parents were stark and lacking vitality (apart from protest and rage), I felt compelled to follow this spark toward fostering genuine joy between mother and daughter.

Quickly I noticed that Anna enjoyed swinging. In our first session, she became calm and almost docile in the swing and kept asking to return to it. I used this sensory preference to create a bridge, a shared meaning between mother and daughter by saying, "You both like the swing! Some people don't like the swing. You like it, and Mommy likes it!" Within a few sessions, at Anna's insistence and initiative, both she and Nicole were in the swing together. Specifically, Anna wanted to be held by Mom while they both swung quietly together. The silence was important; words would have ruined the experience. These were powerful preverbal conditions where Anna's sensory preference could facilitate a mutual alert processing state, and genuine, quiet feelings of comfort, safety, and pleasure could be co-created. These conditions, of course, simulated early developmental experiences that had been so lacking.

During one particular session, after swinging together, Nicole went to sit on the couch, and Anna climbed up and curled onto her lap, molded into her body, and settled into her mommy's bosom. They cuddled in stillness for a long time while Nicole stroked Anna's hair—another new experience for them. These sensitive, loving moments turned into spontaneous "I love you" and kissing moments at home with both Nicole and Paul, for the first time.

In terms of developmental priorities, we can see here that in following Anna's natural inclinations along with my clinical judgment, I used a bottom-up approach (whereby one begins at the earliest point in the delay to focus on the relational (socioemotional) milestones of (1) regulation and (2) shared emotional engagement. These milestones were facilitated by using Anna's sensory preference. Though remediation in any brain system may be an early priority in the treatment setting, if that remediation is not done in tandem with fostering the relational milestones, we believe the gains may not be as great. By facilitating the attachment relationship, Nicole and Paul had renewed energy. For now, the toilet training priority was still on hold.

Memories and Development

Babies are able to exhibit simple forms of nonassociative learning in the womb, for example, habituation to a sound that at first caused a startle response (Hepper, 1997a, 1997b; Rizzo, 2001). Late in gestation, human and chimpanzee fetuses show the ability for simple forms of associative learning, such as classical conditioning (Hepper, 1997a, 1997b; Kawai, Morokuma, Tomonaga, Horimoto, & Taanaka, 2004). At the age of 6 weeks, babies can retain and reproduce facial expressions and head movements that were modeled by an adult 24 hours earlier (Courage & Howe, 2002, p. 258). By the age of 3 months, babies exhibit simple forms of explicit memory (referred to by some as "pre-explicit"; Nelson 1995, 1997); one of these forms is recognition memory (Diamond, Werker, & Lalonde, 1994), but a more conservative estimate would be that they exhibit an explicit form of memory the end of first year (Rovee-Collier, Hayne, & Colombo, 2001). At the age of 9 months, babies demonstrate brief memory storage for objects and events and they can repeat an imitated behavior sequence up to 24 hours later (Courage & Howe, 2002; Meltzoff, 1988a, 1988b, 1988c). The delay period expands between 2–4 months in 14- to 16 month-olds and up to 4 months in 24-month-olds (Meltzoff, 1995). Autobiographical memory and the more apparent forms of explicit memory (memory for events, facts) emerge by age 2 years.

Implicit forms of memory are predominant in infants and young children. The early forms of explicit memory already noted are demonstrated through behavioral means (e.g., looking time) prior to the emergence of language. Explicit memories in the traditional sense (e.g., verbal

recall) are not as recognizable until a child has language. Implicit and explicit forms of memory are separable in terms of general content but act together in the real world. In fact, they "behave" identically after retrieval (Rovee-Collier et al., 2001, p. 250). The underlying brain mechanisms involved are also separable, although the precise mechanisms for this implicit–explicit distinction are still not well understood and are the subject of ongoing research (e.g., is there a unitary process that governs both, or what is the nature of their overlap? Rovee-Collier et al., 2001).

For younger children, we can assume that most memories are not going to be organized with clarity and that a child may not be able to demonstrate or verbalize all aspects of a memory explicitly. Even when a child can use language to share a memory, it does not mean that he or she will state (or show) the aspects that are most disturbing or have the greatest influence on behavior. Aside from the influence of language on memory, a very important developmental marker for memory is that of autobiographical memory. A child cannot relate memories about the self until the onset of "the cognitive sense of self" (Howe & Courage, 1993, 1997a, 1997b), or the awareness of self as separate. Once this takes place, the ability to observe and absorb information from this new vantage point opens the door for a "meta"-level of encoding, storage, and retrieval (Howe & Courage, 1993, 1997a, 1997b; Howe et al., 2003).

Table 8.4 summarizes the progression of memory development in infants and toddlers.

The fundamental processes that govern learning and memory do not appear to change during the course of development. In fact, many of the

Table 8.4. Age and Types of Memory Development

Approximate Normative Age	Type of Memory Development
In utero	Habituation to sounds (nonassociative learning)
Birth	Imitation (e.g., tongue protrusion) and simple forms of associative learning
6 weeks	Retain and produce facial expressions and head movements modeled 24 hours earlier
3 months (more conservative estimates: by the end of the first year)	Simple forms of explicit memory
9 months	Memory storage for objects and events; can imitate a behavior sequence 24 hours later
14–16 months	Imitation ability sustained for 4 months
2 years	Autobiographical memory; more apparent forms of explicit memory

same principles that operate in the encoding, storage, and retrieval of memories are present even in very young, preverbal children (e.g., arousal, attention, emotional valence; Courage & Howe, 2004). The learning and memory improvements seen with development are due to factors such as efficiency, emergence of the "self," and top-down strategies. The following processes show progressive improvement with age:

- *Encoding*—Children encode things faster with age (Rose, Feldman, & Jankowski, 2002), their ability to encode the context in which information was acquired improves (Drummey & Newcombe, 2002), and the use of effective encoding strategies increases (Schneider & Pressley, 1997).
- *Storage*—Children are better able to maintain information in storage (i.e., forgetting due to storage failure decreases), the amount of information they can hold is greater, and they can hold it for longer periods of time with age (for review see Howe & O'Sullivan, 1990, 1997).
- *Retrieval*—Children acquire a broader range of effective retrieval cues and strategies with age, and reminders are more likely to retrieve a forgotten memory with age (Schneider & Pressley, 1997).

Memories and Load Conditions

Memory is greatly affected by emotions and the states of arousal embedded within them. Too frequent or prolonged experiences within a hypoalert, hyperalert, or flooded state will prime one toward anticipating arousal states and the emotional fluctuations within them, creating a sensitized memory system (Harkness & Tucker, 2000) and shaping meaning, from a bottom-up perspective. In turn, negatively valenced meanings tend to trigger these stress arousal states from a top-down perspective.

Hypoalert: Depression. Depressed individuals recall more negative memories than positive or neutral memories and selectively recall material previously learned in a depressed mood (Bower, 1981; Dalgleish & Watts, 1990; Dalgleish et al., 2003). When depressed, individuals will magnify negative events and minimize positive events (Harkness & Tucker, 2000). In recalling autobiographical events, those in a depressed mood tend not to focus on sources of challenge or threat but to ruminate on negative outcomes such as personal losses and defeats (Levine & Pizarro, 2004).

Hyperalert: Fearful vigilance or fearful withdrawal. Recall that the hyperalert state reflects gradations of activation and inhibition that result in responses along a continuum from escalating vigilance that can include

forms of withdrawal (inhibition) or combinations with the hypoalert state. "Fearful [vigilant] individuals display enhanced memory for threat-related information and poorer memory for threat-irrelevant details" because the person focuses all of his or her attention on the threatening object (Levine & Pizarro, 2004, p. 544). The memory-enhancing effects of heightened emotional activation may be partly attributed to adrenaline and other stress hormones (Berntson, Sarter, & Cacioppo, 2003a). In PTSD, for example, intrusive memories related to past threats temporarily overwhelm the individual (Levine & Pizarro, 2004).

On the other hand, fearful individuals prone toward vigilant withdrawal may "turn their attention away from threatening stimuli and later show poorer recall or recognition of it" (Levine & Pizarro, 2004, p. 545). Extreme inhibition in young children has been studied by some researchers, documenting that very shy children tend to have high and stable heart rates, suggesting a long-term increase in SNS activity (Kagan, Reznick, & Snidman, 1999), with a risk for developing affective (especially anxiety) disorders (Rosenbaum et al., 1988). The expectation has been that cortisol levels of highly inhibited children should be elevated as well. Although one of the wear-and-tear effects of the overactivation of cortisol appears to be related to poorer memory of daily events, information such as people's names, places and things, and the context of events (McEwen, 2002), the exact nature of how cortisol evolves during typical and atypical childhood contexts is still being discovered. Increased inhibition in young children is associated with unusual fears and phobias (Bierdman et al., 1991; Kagan, Reznick, & Snidman, 1987, 1999), with some cortisol studies showing elevations and others not (Gunnar, Bruce, & Donzella, 2001). Cortisol has both activating and inhibiting features, as well as fast and slow effects. For example, fast-acting cortisol can be arousing and improve concentration, whereas slower versions of cortisol production can slow down the stimulating effects of activation (Gunnar et al., 2001). Due to the complexities involved, how, when, and whether a highly inhibited child will have an overactivation of cortisol and suffer the consequences of memory loss are yet to be determined (Gunnar et al., 2001).

Flooded: Hostility. Adults deemed high in hostility in Mollet and Harrison's (2007) research could effectively recall negative emotional words but did not effectively remember positive words. On a similar line of research, children from high-conflict homes perceived more anger and more fear during simulated disputes; that is, they drew on negative memories more than positive ones (Friedman & Chase-Lansdale, 2002). Friedman and Chase-Lansdale (2002) in discussing the work of Dodge, Pettit, and Bates (1997), note that "hypervigilance to hostile cues would lead children to assume hostile intent in others and because of this misattribution

and highly accessible aggressive responses in memory, they would be more likely to behave aggressively" (Friedman & Chase-Lansdale, 2002, p. 269) (see also Crick & Dodge, 1994, 1996; Dodge & Somberg, 1987).

Emotion, Memory, and Meanings

A child is more likely to experience the world as a safe place when he or she has procedural memories of predictable routines, pleasurable sensory exchanges, modulated arousal, and an overall positive (or neutral) valence. In this context, a child may develop the expectation that future events will be safe rather than dangerous and positive rather than negative. This child can come to anticipate that similarly safe and positive experiences also may evolve within other relationships and in the world. Conversely, a child with procedural memories of unpleasant sensory exchanges, unmodulated arousal, and predominantly negative valence is more likely to experience the world as a dangerous and threatening place. A child with relatively few sensory exchanges, long periods of isolation, and an absence of interactive regulation is more likely to experience the world as a potentially dangerous and lonely place. When these components are mixed and there is a lack of predictability, the child is more likely to experience the world as dangerous and chaotic. In general, emotions and memories create meanings that become biased toward predictable or unpredictable, positive or negative, safe or dangerous, and connected or alone. What a child comes to expect from relationships and the world emerges from this blend of meanings.

Table 8.5 presents a snapshot of the potential interactions among emotions, memories, and meanings and their underlying states of arousal in both coordination and load expressions. Two caveats should be held in mind in using this table. First, it is intended as a starting point for thinking about the complex relationships that may exist among arousal, emotions, memories, and meaning. It is not exhaustive, and it is not a summary of research findings. Second, the way that emotions are organized according to arousal states in this table is intended as a rule-of-thumb rubric that is based on both clinical experience and some research support. For example, studies have associated low arousal (the hypoalert state in the neurorelational framework) with sadness (Harkness & Tucker, 2000; Mauss, Levenson, McCarter, Wilhelm, & Gross, 2005); a sympathetically dominant uncoupled pattern of both autonomic branches (the hyperalert state in the neurorelational framework) with fear responses (Berntson, Cacioppo, & Quigley, 1991); and high sympathetic arousal (the flooded state in the neurorelational framework) with anger (Schore, 1994). A guiding

Table 8.5.   Emotions, Memories, Meanings, and Their Underlying States of Arousal

Alert Processing State	Hypoalert State	Hyperalert State	Flooded State
Emotions			
Interest, joy, curiosity, pride	*Adaptive:* Sadness Shame	*Adaptive:* Anxiety Embarrassment Guilt Jealousy	*Adaptive:* Disgust Anger Fear Panic
Moods			
Pleasure Contentment	*Load Condition:* Depression Apathy Dissociation	*Load Condition:* Vigilance Paranoia Passive–aggression Dissociative hypervigilance	*Load Condition:* Mania, grandiosity Rage Panic attack
State-Dependent Memories			
Adaptive: Biases memories toward comfort and retrievability Balance of safety, challenge, and threat Cohesive network of stable memories that supports new memories (learning and skills)	*Adaptive:* Remembering a event that stimulated sadness, causing one to avoid a similar situation	*Adaptive:* Remembering an event that stimulated anxiety, causing one to better prepare for future event to avoid embarrassment or rejection	*Adaptive:* Remembering an event that stimulated anger, and preparing an assertive response
	Load Condition: Biases encoding, storage, and retrieval toward negative Imbalance toward threat Prone toward prolonged rumination on negative events (Levine & Pizarro, 2004)	*Load Condition:* Biases encoding, storage, and retrieval toward negative Imbalance toward threat Prone toward frequent memory intrusions (vigilance) or may turn attention away from negative events (withdrawal) (Levine & Pizarro, 2004)	*Load Condition:* Biases encoding, storage, and retrieval toward negative Imbalance toward threat Prone toward heightened memory of hostile events; may misattribute hostile intent towards others and increase aggressive behavior (Friedman & Chase-Lansdale, 2002)

(Continued)

Table 8.5.   Continued

Alert Processing State	Hypoalert State	Hyperalert State	Flooded State
Meanings			
I feel good	*Adaptive:*	*Adaptive:*	*Adaptive:*
I am not afraid	I don't want	I'm scared	This is too much for me
I am loved	anymore	I need help	I'm too uncomfortable
I love you	This isn't	This isn't safe	I'm too frustrated
I can do it	interesting	I need to negotiate	Stop!
I can survive negative	I'm not getting		I'm upset about this; I
experiences	enough out of		need to make other
Things will turn out	this; I need to		plans
okay	consider		I need to be assertive/
I can be flexible but	walking away		protest
not give up my			
needs			
	Load Condition:	*Load Condition:*	*Load Condition:*
	Nobody loves me	I'm never safe	I'm frantic
	I will always be	I'll never do this	Where are you?!
	lonely	I always fail	I hate you
	I will never make	I'm too scared to try	I hate myself
	it	You'll be sorry; I'm	You'll never get me to
	I wish I were dead	going to get you	do this
		back	I can do whatever I
		He's out to get me	want

motif is that *the organization of state governs the quality of inner experience* (Sander, 1988); thus, we view awake states of arousal as background containers that can hold the multiple dimensions of emotions, memories, and meanings. However, keep in mind that emotions are not exclusive to only one arousal state. Both positive and negative emotions can span the full range of awake states of arousal; these specific emotional expressions are not a one-to-one correlation with the more generalized state of arousal.

As the love relationship was being ignited, there was a sense of freedom that emerged in our dyadic play sessions. Anna began creating simple emotional stories. One time, Nicole's purse was stolen and while Mom was calling out for help, Anna, being Superwoman (while wearing a cape), swooped down to retrieve her purse. Anna loved being the hero for Nicole. During these times of imaginative play, the simple emotional themes of good guys and bad guys were establishing basic positive and negative valences. Anna was beginning to make correct associations about what was good and what was bad, and she was beginning to feel a sense of control over the outcome of good and bad. Thus, a progression began to emerge. First, Anna had the experience of safety, which led to her experiences and expressions of attachment and loving connections. In that context, she began

to play with a range of positive and negative emotional experiences through good guys and bad guys. Subsequently, she brought to us her own lived experiences of trauma, which she could only then begin to slowly master and alter.

Anna was using my costume box on a regular basis. She found a ghost's mask that was frightening to look at. This mask completely covered one's head and was reminiscent of the image portrayed in the movie *Scream*; features of this face were deep set, with wide-open eyes and a very elongated mouth wide open in horror. Spontaneously, during one play session, Anna took this face mask in hand, turned out all the lights in our play room, and forcefully closed the door behind her. When she came back into the play room, she was wearing the ghost mask. She pointed her index finger at us, and roared "Freeze!" Needless to say, both Nicole and I were surprised, and we did as we were told. We froze, literally in the middle of whatever we were saying, with our bodily gestures in mid-air. The tone in the room was somber, riddled with fear, shock, and terror. Anna was vigilantly watching us and any time we went to slightly move or relax a muscle, she would roar "Freeze!" or "Don't move!" Our bodies were stiff, tight, and frozen in the dark.

Once these enactments began, Anna periodically cycled back into them on a spontaneous basis over the next year. Although she was grave during these sequences, the next time she orchestrated the same event, she clearly enjoyed hearing our screams on her return into the room (she briefly cracked a smile). My comment to Nicole after the first time this happened to us was that although I had no idea exactly what this meant, I thought that she was enacting implicit (procedural) memory traces of some lived events that she now had the freedom to show us—just as with Laura in the last chapter, we saw as important what was being enacted through her terrorizing and biting the babies, even though we did not have the exact history. In addition to tapping into implicit memories, this was the first time that Anna began to command genuine negative emotions from us while she was in charge of creating them. As her positive palate had begun with genuine moments of quiet pleasure, her negative range began with authentic immobilized states of fear and hypervigilance that she could begin to master by creating them in our bodies. These episodes lasted for 10–20 minutes at a time; an oscillation of conditions of threat and safety occurred during these episodes. While she was in the dark room with us, her commands would alternate between "Freeze!" and "Unfreeze!" The "unfreeze" times allowed for short periods of bodily relaxation before the next command. An element of unpredictability ensued and we didn't know when the next command would take place or when she would leave, during which time we could temporarily relax until the next surprise. On more than one occasion, in addition to commanding us to not move a muscle, she also commanded, "Don't move your eyes" and "Don't blink."

When asked what this play enactment meant to her, Anna associated this freeze play with the intermittent nightmares that she still had; they were frightening dreams that woke her up but that she could not remember. In the dyadic therapy, Anna was making new associations regarding safety and threat: first, associating safety with her mother and, then going deeper into attachment, bringing to us her terror and accurately associating that trauma with her nightmares. She

made these connections within an environment that she accurately determined was safe enough for her to do the work she needed to do.

Inadvertently, about 7 months into these enactments, Nicole and Paul stumbled on actual video footage of the day they came to pick up Anna from the Romanian orphanage. Nicole decided to bring the videotape to our next session so that I could see what Anna looked like at that transition time. As we all gathered around the camera, we unmistakenly saw the state of arousal Anna was in during the entire visit and exchange. As Nicole held her in her arms, Anna maintained a frozen posture, with her arms suspended at mid-air, barely breathing, not blinking. Even though women she knew were talking to her, repeatedly calling her name out, and trying to engage her with a toy, she remained utterly detached and unavailable.

Following this tape and noticing the similarities of how she was on tape and what she had created with us, a slight shift began to occur during the next 6 months that led to progressive alterations of these states of terror into playful interactions. Anna first became a little less vigilant with us during the "freeze" episodes. Nicole and I could blink and breathe and even adjust our bodies a little. We became more playful with our screams and began to complain about the ghost who was scaring us. We actually had little conversations with the ghost, who was less commanding and, though still directive, more flexible in her allowances.

The final "working through" of these enactments turned another corner when Anna began to alter the ritual. In the new version, she spontaneously put on the ghost mask, came up to us, and said, "Boo!" When Nicole and I playfully acted scared, she would take off the mask and we would laugh together. The last few times she did this, she picked a smaller and less frightening ghost mask. As she lightheartedly scared us, while taking the mask off, she laughingly claimed, "It's just me!" Eventually, Anna would sometimes hide behind the door and "scare" me as I walked into the play room. Over time, we participated in helping Anna thaw from frozen hypervigilance into playful conditions where momentary emotional blends of fear and laughter, surprise and humor could coexist.

In the next chapter we consider how behaviors associated with emotions, memories, and meaning-making are organized into relevance system capacities that either support coordination or lead to load conditions.

NOTES

1. Pfaff's research reminds us, however, that the influences on arousal extend far beyond emotion. Arousal is also influenced by the sensory system, or the degree of sensory alertness, as well as the executive system, or the degree of motor activity (see Chapter 2, p. 51).

2. Our use of the term *mood* reflects the entire spectrum of affect. It is not specific to disorders involving depression or bipolarity, as in the *Diagnostic and Statistical Manual of Mental Disorders, Fourth Edition* (*DSM-IV*) (American Psychiatric Association, 1994).

3. Interestingly, "dopamine and opioids in combination have to be activated at optimum levels in the brain if we are to feel joy" (Sunderland, 2006, p. 92). Dopamine, referred to as part of the reward system, is also stimulated by food (sugar), drugs, and video games, all of which carry potential for addiction (Bozarth, 1994). The parallel makes one consider how relational joy during development might serve as a natural antidote for later potential harmful addictions, and how the context of positive therapeutic relationships can serve as an important component of healing during the addict's recovery process (Walant, 1995). One program which emphasizes positive affect as part of the therapeutic model is Developmental Skills Training (DST), used for treating adult and childhood obesity whose goal is to teach self- and interactive regulation skills to parents (www.solutionmethod.org) and children (www.shapedown.com). In shifting from high stress to joy, high-level well-being is promoted, which naturally becomes a preventive measure for allostatic load, thereby decreasing the risk of using artificial rewards and addictions as a way to manage stress (Mellin, 2004, 2009).

4. This idea of fluctuations between merger- and separation-based interactions stands in contrast to Mahler's (Mahler, 1967; Mahler, Pine, & Bergman, 1975) linear developmental theory that contends that infants are initially "merged" with others and progressively establish separateness. In her theory, "autonomy" is the goal of this progression and ideally is achieved at a fixed point in the developmental continuum.

9

Assessment and Intervention Principles, Priorities, and Strategies for the Relevance System

In the relevance system, we focus heavily on parenting skills in assessment and intervention priorities. We do this not only because parents are so obviously important to emotions, learning, and meaning-making for children but also because the principles underlying these parenting skills apply equally well to the professional role (e.g., the therapeutic relationship, the teaching relationship, the physician–patient relationship).

ASSESSMENT AND INTERVENTION PRINCIPLES AND PRIORITIES FOR THE RELEVANCE SYSTEM

In discussing the emotional range, we expand on the concepts of the positivity offset and negativity bias to demonstrate how an underdeveloped emotional muscle can influence stress responses in a way that negatively impacts a child's development and relationships. In discussing learning and memory, we highlight the important interplay among emotions and learning that influences development of the emotional self as well as the child as a learner. We present a four-phase model (Kort, Reilly, & Picard, 2001) that highlights the dynamic process of learning and helps us understand where and how both emotional disruptions and developmental delays can cause learning to break down. In discussing meaning-making, we consider the triad of interpersonal modes—respond, direct, reflect—for both adults and children. Finally, we discuss what these modes look like when out of balance. Whereas the focus is weighted toward the parenting role, we try to continually acknowledge the two-way street aspect of dynamic relationships by reminding the reader that children, too, bring

their own tendencies into the interaction. In the parent–child dyad, meaning is co-created.

Capacity 1: Building a Full Emotional Range

Building a full emotional range starts at a preverbal level and involves the implicit procedural learning that takes place through various forms of emotional experience, including the infant's observation and imitation of others' emotions. Research by Davidson and Fox (1982) showed that by 10 months of age, infants could experience positive and negative emotional reactions that registered neurophysiologically (although they were not outwardly manifested) while simply observing high-intensity positive and negative emotions in others. This finding may suggest that observation of emotion has similar underlying mechanisms as observation in imitation; that is, the emotional effect on the observer parallels what is observed in the other. Consequently, what the child observes or imitates in parents who have mood disorders (i.e., depression, anxiety, bipolar) may lead to a constricted range of emotions.

Coordination

The developmental process of building the emotional muscle involves parent and child equally. The parent needs to be able to experience (and tolerate in the child) a full emotional range, including simultaneous expressions of positive and negative valences (Cacioppo, Gardner, & Berntson, 1997; Larsen, McGraw, Mellers, & Cacioppo, 2004) and emotional blends of positive and negative valences (Larsen et al., 2004), and exhibit coordinated expressions of responsive, directive, and reflective modes. The child must be directive enough to communicate needs as well as responsive to interactive regulation to recover back to a positive baseline. The developmental sequence presented in Table 9.1 can be used to assess the strength of the emotional muscle within a dyad.

Risk Factors for Load Conditions

The etiology for emotional problems in children is certainly complex, but we feel we can state at least one point definitively: a child's emotional problems are *never* the result of a single causal factor and should never be addressed with a single treatment approach. We should be wary of defaulting to the explanation that "it's all about sensitive parenting" and equally wary of the explanation that "it's all in the genes or temperament." Indeed,

Table 9.1.   Emotional Muscle Markers for the First 4 Years

Time Period	Emotional Muscle Markers	Exercising the Emotional Muscle
Early in the first year	As an infant, the child responds to appropriate caretaking with pleasure, expresses needs with distress, and is soothed by a responsive parent.	Over time, the child learns how to move out of a stress response into a positive affective core (Emde & Harmon, 1984).
Later in the first year	By the age of 5 months, the dyad exchanges loving smiles, cooing, and playfulness, and shared joy (Greenspan, 1996).	Younger children often shift rapidly from one emotion to another. The experience of shared joy becomes a valuable tool for interactive regulation of these extremes.
Second year	The dyad's experience of a full range of negative emotions and modulations back to baseline are increasingly efficient. The child's expansion into the negative range in response to an unpleasant event is not only inevitable but desirable, and the recovery back to baseline is the important focus initially.	Over time, with the increasing procedural memories of emotional upset *and* recovery, the child learns that he or she can indeed "survive" intense unpleasant emotions. This is an important process that builds resilience for coping with life's inevitable upsets that bring disappointment, shame, embarrassment, jealousy, envy, defeat, loss, hurt, fear, and anger.
Third year	The dyad learns to negotiate ongoing emotional shifts and to stabilize into a predominantly positive baseline.	Over time, the energy expenditures that come with extreme emotional shifts should lessen and also be more and more adaptive when they do occur. In other words, there is less repetition of "wasted energy," or expenditures that have no learning value.
Fourth year	The dyad is able to experience the blends of positive and negative emotion that come with increasingly complex challenges in life (e.g., feeling happy to win a game but sad for the parent who lost).	Over time, the negotiation of life events that hold both positive and negative elements at the same time helps the child learn how to modulate the emotional range in relation to varying degrees of stress. This is an important developmental stage for teaching children how to maintain an optimal response pattern to mild, moderate, and severe stressors (i.e., positivity offset, negativity bias).

the dynamic interactions of genes and environment have resulted in new interdisciplinary efforts between ecological genetics, developmental biology, and evolutionary theory into such explorations as "phenotypic plasticity," which studies the property of a given genotype to produce varying phenotypes in response to environmental differences (Pigliucci, 2001). Dynamic questions are aimed at ascertaining the balance between constraints and opportunities and how organisms respond to stressful environments. We believe these provide important analogies to clinical situations that emphasize the interactive role between parental and child predispositions that may be more "set" (constrained) in their ways in the context of stress, with a lack of stress recovery expressed through individual and interpersonal dynamics. Our focus here is to point out how different types of parent pathology (constraints) and different ways of handling stress under conditions of imbalance have potentially detrimental effects on children.

Clinical convention has informed us that punitive, harsh, overly controlling, or overly permissive parenting can contribute to a wide array of childhood emotional problems and psychopathologies. Psychopathology is a more severe expression of emotional imbalance and has been defined as "'diminished flexibility and constrictions of . . . adaptational patterns' (Overton & Horowitz, 1991, p. 3) . . . overlearned and automatized . . . patterns that are insensitive to environmental change" (Hollenstein, Granic, Stoolmiller, & Snyder, 2004, p. 596; see also Cicchetti & Cohen, 1995; Mahoney, 1991). These patterns will be discussed as automatic default modes in the executive system chapter. We want to point out that this definition emphasizes the inflexible and entrenched nature of maladaptive patterns, paralleling one of the load condition characteristics (rigidity) of the neurorelational framework presented in this chapter. In addition to closed learning systems with constrictions in emotional range, the neurorelational framework recognizes the patterns of chaotic learning systems with an unmodulated emotional range (that may include a "full" range).

The potentially detrimental effect on children of parent depression, anxiety, and hostility is explored in a large body of research. In a review of the literature, Harkness and Tucker (2000) reported that infants of depressed mothers are less active, show poorer skills at orienting to sound and moving stimuli, have more frequent negative facial expressions, show less exploration of the inanimate environment, and have greater sleep problems (see also Beebe & Lachmann, 2002; Tronick, 2007). In using the Brazelton Neonatal Behavioral Assessment Scale, infants of depressed mothers showed more arousal and less attention to their mothers' faces and voices (Hernandez-Reif, Field, Diego, & Ruddock, 2006). McClure, Brennan, Hammen, and LeBrocque (2001) reported that mothers with anxiety disorders predict the presence of anxiety disorders in their children. In a 6-year longitudinal comparison study between anxious and

nonanxious parents, anxious parenting was significantly related to higher anxiety symptoms in their children (Ginsburg, Grover, & Ialongo, 2005). Interestingly, anxiety seems to be expressed physiologically through decreased heart rate variability, with the loss of the flexibility involved in healthy autonomic functioning (Berntson & Cacioppo, 2004), providing a metaphor for the constrictions and diminished flexibility that anxiety can bring about emotionally as well. Granic (2000) reported that once hostile interactions become an entrenched dyadic pattern, it takes only a slight sensory trigger, such as rolling of the eyes, to set off a full-blown aggressive interaction (see Dodge & Somberg, 1987). Hirshfeld-Becker et al. (2006) reported that there were significantly higher rates of behavioral disinhibition in the children of parents with bipolar disorder.

Previously (in the discussion of emotion in Chapter 8), we considered the adaptive response patterns to mild, moderate, and severe stressors in the context of the positivity offset and negativity bias. In the context of building the emotional muscle, this information guides our thinking about how much positive versus negative are appropriate to the context. With little or mild stress, we want to see a predominance of the positive emotional themes noted in Table 8.2. As the stress level increases, negative emotions should also increase, and weaving in the positive requires increasing effort.

Coordination for this capacity requires accessing a range of positive and negative emotions, as well as blends of the two, in ways that help create meaning. As stated in Larsen et al. (2003, p. 221), "coping depends not only on grappling with the stressor, but also on coming to grips with and gaining insight into it." Extremes in the behavioral dimensions of either positive or negative emotions that are not appropriate to the stress context contribute to load conditions for both the individual and the dyad. If a person has trouble accessing, negotiating, and blending positive and negative emotions that vary according to degrees of stress, then the meaning-making process is similarly limited. In this situation, chronic or severe stress in life brings increased risk for load conditions, which in turn begins to interfere with health and functioning. Here we consider two potential versions of load conditions in terms of response to stress: too much negative and too much positive.

Too much negative. A person experiencing too much negative (our shorthand) has difficulty maintaining a neutral or positive baseline state and often has trouble accessing the positive. He or she is not able to access and shift to a positive emotion in the midst of experiencing a negative emotion and has difficulty holding on to positive emotions alongside negative ones over time. In essence, the negativity bias is far too strong, and the positivity offset is far too weak. This load version is more characteristic of a demanding parenting style.

In response to mild stressors, this person is rarely able to brush it off, shifts quickly into negative emotional themes, and often lacks the resources to recover quickly. In response to moderate stressors, this person has an appropriately negative feeling but then escalates the negative into more severe forms or has limited ability to weave the positive into the experience. In response to severe stressors, the negative predominates without movement toward meaning-making. The negative response to the severe stressor may become all-consuming, affecting mood and potentially restricting functioning and daily activities. The event is never worked through such that some degree of resolution or acceptance is achieved; it often remains an "open wound" even after a long period of time. Thus, it is important to track the nature and amount of reactivity (intensity) one has to acute stressors, which have important implications for health. "Autonomic and neuroendocrine activation in response to stressors is beneficial up to a point, but excessive activation may also have long term costs . . . strong autonomic and neuroendocrine activation to psychological stressors . . . may diminish" the natural process in the aging of cells and health across time (Cacioppo, 2000, p. 19).

Too much positive. A person experiencing too much positive easily maintains a positive baseline but is overly resistant to shifting into a negative emotion—often having difficulty tolerating (in self and others) shifts into negative emotion, even in the face of a highly provocative stressor. These responses can appear to be adaptive and coordinated, but in fact, they serve as defensive maneuvers and can be quite deceptive to unsuspecting professionals. In this pattern, also known as naive optimism (Larsen et al., 2003), the positivity offset is far too strong and the negativity bias far too weak. This load version is more characteristic of an extreme accommodating or permissive parenting style.

In response to mild stressors, this person has no trouble maintaining a positive baseline and may be admired for being unfailingly optimistic. If life brought only mild stressors, this response style would pose little threat to coordination. The problem comes with the ways this style supports emotional rigidity and a closed learning system. In response to moderate stressors, this person exploits the positive spectrum of emotions to actually deny or defend against the negative impact of the stressor. The belief (albeit unconscious) is that a negative emotion has destructive power. It is important to note that this style entails its own version of energy expenditure that is not adaptive—it takes effort to suppress an appropriate and authentic negative emotional response. With close observation, there are often behavioral indicators of tension and incongruence—apparent distractibility out of sync with a cavalier demeanor, a smile on the mouth with worried eyes, or a sweet tone of voice that sounds a little pressured. In response to severe stressors, this person may go to extremes to avoid a negative range. There may be an innocent or "clueless" Pollyanna affect or

an outward expression that is strongly positive while thinly hiding a bubbling rage. Many children and adults with this style resist talking about a painful event and work hard to keep the negative "hidden" (both from others and themselves). If they share, then there is a quick and cheerful jump to a positive spin (e.g., "It doesn't really matter, I didn't want to go to that school anyway"—after being expelled or rejected from a school of choice).

Capacity 2: Achieving an Open Learning System with Full Access to Memories

We learn through interacting with the world, engaging in relationships, and having an experience of the self. Early on, most learning is implicit. It involves establishing links and associations, observation and imitation, and playing with cause-and-effect relationships. As motor skills increase from eye and head movements to independent locomotion, learning parallels the action-oriented doing. By the second year, explicit forms of learning are also functional. Explicit learning involves learning words and concepts and the process of reflecting on past events. As children mature and enter school, the demand for more focused and directed learning increases.

Coordination

The process of learning is dynamic. Just as emotions cycle from positive to negative to dimensional blends and are increasingly elaborated with age, the phases of the learning cycle, from novice to expert to various degrees in between, are increasingly elaborated with age. Although we rarely think of it this way, the process of learning is also emotional, and to promote optimal learning, one needs to consider the child's emotional state. In keeping with the curvilinear relationship of learning and arousal (Yerkes & Dodson, 1908), it stands to reason that any intense emotion will disrupt the concentration necessary for learning.

The effect of positive and negative emotions on learning is also influenced by whether the source of the emotion is internal or external to the learner (Ochs & Frasson, 2004). For the positive spectrum of emotions, there is a robust positive effect on learning if the emotion is internally generated (e.g., interest, awe), whereas positive emotion coming from outside the self (e.g., encouragement) is less motivating. For the negative spectrum, certain internally generated negative emotions can be motivating and aid performance (e.g., frustration), but emotions such as anger are not conducive to learning. With negative emotion coming from the outside, the learner switches focus to external matters and thereby reduces concentration and cannot fulfill or complete learning tasks.

Building on a model presented by Kort et al. (2001), we present a four-phase learning process that applies not only to educational but also other learning situations (see Figure 9.1). Phase I, the initial phase of a new learning situation, is characterized by positive emotions, such as curiosity, awe, interest, and excitement that can motivate the learner. In Phase II, more negative emotions, such as puzzlement and confusion, emerge; these can also motivate the learner to press on, gather more information, or ask for help to understand. Phase III occurs when one moves through Phase II but fails to understand, and puzzlement gives way to annoyance and frustration. Here, the learner may give up, push harder, or decide to shift to an entirely new strategy. This phase may also include an awareness that one needs to "unlearn" (or at least suspend) some aspect of acquired knowledge to absorb the new learning. Phase IV brings a positive emotional range back into the picture. Achieving new

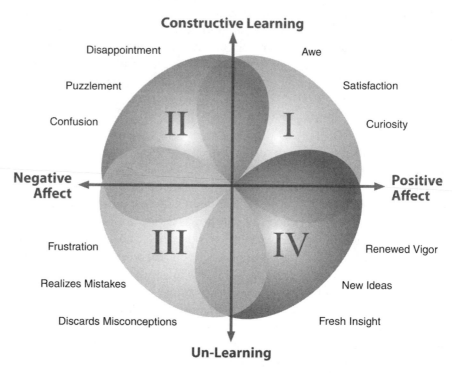

Figure 9.1. Four-phase learning process. (From *An Affective Model of Interplay Between Emotions and Learning: Reengineering Educational Pedagogy—Building a Learning Companion*, by B. Kort, R. Reilly, and R. W. Picard, 2001, paper presented at the International Conference on Advanced Learning Technologies, University of Madison, Wisconsin and retrieved September 10, 2007, from affect.media.mit.edu/projectpages/lc/icalt.pdf. Adapted with permission of Brian Kort.)

knowledge, a new perspective, or a new understanding inspires a surge of interest, curiosity, and a desire to learn more. In addition, learning from mistakes, false assumptions, or poor strategies may inspire an additional feeling of accomplishment, a new round of ideas, or help us consolidate previous work—all which brings us back into a positive range of pride, hope, and renewed vigor and keeps us moving forward.

The ability to cycle through each of these phases is necessary for an open learning system and equally important to the learning that occurs during the process of assessment and intervention. For example, professionals of all disciplines need to embrace the idea that course corrections and unlearning are an intrinsic part of the work. In doing so, professionals can also model an open learning system for parents and children, especially when negative feedback promotes learning together. By recognizing and accepting when a course correction is needed, we communicate the attitude that we are not afraid of mistakes and failures. For many parents, the implicit procedural experience of an open learning system will help them feel more at ease when receiving negative reactions from their children or negative feedback from their therapist.

Risk Factors for Load Conditions

Both emotional problems and developmental delays can negatively affect learning, especially when appropriate supports are not available. With too much negative, as in trauma situations, the child's memories can be sensitized to attend to anything that is negative in his or her world, thereby tipping the learning process in a negative direction. For children with developmental delays, the learning process itself can be traumatizing, again tipping the emotional range toward the negative. A blend of positive and negative emotions is integral to the learning process, just as it is integral to an open learning system. Thus, any conditions that cause the child to get stuck in an emotional state or a learning phase may predispose him or her to a closed learning system.

Trauma and memories. Memory for traumatic events is often more durable than nontraumatic memories. However, whether or not trauma has a negative impact on subsequent memory processes has been a matter of considerable debate. Recent reviews of the literature by Howe, Ciccheti, and Toth (2006) on this question conclude that memory performance per se is not impaired by trauma. These researchers found that regardless of whether they looked at the encoding, storage, retention, or retrieval processes of memory in groups of maltreated and nonmaltreated children, the maltreated children performed much like their nonmaltreated counterparts. In addition, other factors (such as dissociation, psychopathology,

intelligence, or PTSD) did not discriminate the memory performance of those maltreated and nonmaltreated children. Research in this area continues, and it is important that therapists, lawyers, and judges not view the memory of maltreated children as somehow distorted by trauma. Instead, they should expect that these children's memories are likely to be as accurate as other children of the same age.

With trauma situations of abuse, neglect, or both, or in the presence of a thought disorder, reversals can occur between perceptions of safety and threat. In other words, neutrality and calm are considered dangerous; vigilance or rage is considered safe. When reversals occur, it is thought to be a reflection of what the child has learned is typical and thus familiar. The emotional expressions of such children can be disturbing: laughter accompanies what is sad, and pleasure is expressed in victimizing through play, with animals, or with other children or adults.

Learning problems. Children with developmental delays of all types may have learning and memory problems. At times, the disruptions are related to direct hits to learning and memory structures, such as might be seen in epilepsy or brain tumors. Other times, learning and memory disruptions are commonly seen with particular risk factors or genetic and medical conditions such as very low birth weight, neurofibromatosis, or alcohol exposure. Typically, in these scenarios, learning and memory processes are affected more broadly and implicate a disruption to a basic memory process, such as storage or retrieval. In most of the developmental disorders, learning and memory are disrupted along more specific pathways (e.g., verbal memory in a specific language disorder, phonological memory in a reading disorder). The types of learning and memory problems probably most common across all disorders are those related to strategy and efficiency. For example, in academic learning disabilities, there is often an ability to acquire skills within the affected domain, but the learning may happen by means of alternate routes, and the skills are learned much more slowly. With ADHD, learning may be disrupted due to poor attention such that the encoded material is full of gaps. With brain injury, the executive processes involved in memory (e.g., organization, working memory) or those that govern strategies are often disrupted.

The potential for problems with learning and memory should be closely monitored when any developmental delay is present. Children may have trouble learning due to a disruption at some point along the sensory processing pathway (e.g., poor phonological discrimination leads to poor learning and memory for sounds and words); they may have problems with a particular memory stage (e.g., encoding may be scrambled in ADHD, retrieval is blocked in a mood disorder); or they may be unable to

develop, use, or expand memory strategies (e.g., singular reliance on a linear or serial encoding strategy in a nonverbal learning disorder).

When a child has difficulty learning, regardless of the etiology, he or she is at risk for getting caught in a negative cycle whenever his or her limitations are challenged. Applying the four-phase learning model already presented, a child with a learning problem may repeatedly drop out of the active learning process once the negative phase is reached. Initially, he or she may not lose motivation until reaching Phase III, where the going gets very tough; however, when a certain number of learning failures go unresolved (i.e., movement through the cycle is never completed), the child may lose motivation at the first hint of challenge in Phase II. Learning challenges can stimulate negative emotions whereby the negative comes to dominate the experience. With enough repetition, these procedural and explicit memories set up negative moods and meanings (anticipations). Some children begin to resist even entering Phase I of the learning challenge. The avoidance of learning and the ripple effect this avoidance has on parents and teachers stimulate a host of additional negative experiences. For some children, the learning problem itself becomes a source of chronic stress that further complicates learning. The cumulative experience of "repeated hits" (i.e., negative emotion) will eventually tip into load conditions, at which point the impact of the learning disability may disrupt emotional well-being and even lead to emotional disorders. Memory and emotional disruptions may exacerbate each other.

The importance of circumventing this negative cycle is one reason that early intervention is so crucial. Even in the situation where an emotional disorder or a developmental delay cannot be remediated by the time the child enters school, we can at least anticipate and prevent this negative cycle from starting. When a child is left to struggle and fail repeatedly without appropriate assessment or intervention, there are consequences for the emotional and motivational components of the learning process. These children do not know why they cannot learn or perform like other children; they only know that they are not meeting expectations and that this difference is bad. It was well stated in Briggs that "children rarely question our expectations; instead, they question their personal adequacy" (1975, p. 49).

Capacity 3: Creating Meanings That Reflect Self and Others

Self and other co-create meaning in relationships. Through the triad of responsiveness, directiveness, and reflectiveness, the flexible parent adjusts to the context and the developmental needs of the child. It is parents' capacity for reflection that supports these ongoing adjustments, which are

especially important to the rupture–repair cycle. Reflection enables parents to make the necessary corrections to their default mode of reacting (more about default modes in the executive system chapters 10 and 11). Reflection allows the parent to guide meaning-making.

Parents may have strong leanings toward specific tendencies to respond, direct, or reflect. The reflective abilities noted here are focused on the adult in the parent–child relationship, and they apply to both persons and in all relationships: therapist–parent, therapist–child, spouse–spouse, sibling–sibling, peer–peer, and so on. The larger coordination and load patterns that involve responding, directing, and reflecting pull together the ingredients we highlight for meaning-making.

Coordination

The parent's ability to hold the tension between responding and directing, between the needs of self and those of other, and between connection and separateness is contingent on the ability for reflection. Reflection is usually required to problem solve and negotiate when tension or discomfort is felt in a relationship. Reflection is not easy; it requires mental effort and sometimes courage. It means having the emotional muscle to tolerate uncomfortable feelings and thoughts that may carry negative meanings or may feel threatening (e.g., "I made a mistake" or "My child might have a problem" or "I don't like being around my child").

Reflection occurs on both macro and micro levels. On a macro level, parents reflect effectively by learning to become aware of the thematic nature and long-term patterns of their child's respond–direct cycles (e.g., "Whenever it's time to leave the house for school, my child always falls apart and I always get angry"; "Whenever my child rolls her eyes, I almost always feel a strong surge of anger"). During the macro process, a parent (1) honestly assesses behaviors, emotional reactions, and salient events for child and self; (2) identifies patterns and potential biases; (3) considers why a behavior occurred by using an observing ego (i.e., stands back and evaluates the event with less affect), and links history with the present, which highlights the parent's need to consider the meaning, intent, or motives that he or she attributes to the child's behaviors; and (4) thinks about problem-solving alternatives.

On a micro level, reflections are brief and frequent and often triggered by a sense of discomfort or tension. They occur in the moment when a parent observes the self and makes a quick adjustment based on that mini-reflection. In a child's early years, when a parent's task is to be more responsive, reflection involves focusing on reading the child's cues and making adjustments that promote self-regulatory capacities. As the

child matures and parents need to do more directing, reflection involves an honest assessment of the child's true capacities so that the directives actually fit what the child can handle. The micro process involves (1) being sensitive to those thoughts and feelings in the moment that trigger the need for reflection; (2) shifting mentally and emotionally away from the strong emotion to a more neutral inner position while holding the goal in mind and resisting the pull to jump to negative meanings; (3) making adjustments when appropriate; and (4) resisting emotional inertia and, instead, taking an uncomfortable step that will either prevent rupture or foster empathy or repair, when appropriate.

Optimally, a parent learns to hold not only emotional blends but also parenting style blends—for example, to follow through with the directive while continuing to be responsive (e.g., "No, you cannot have that piece of candy. . . . I see you are really disappointed and you are mad at me"). When a parent models blends, he or she can direct without being threatening and can nurture without being overly responsive. The combination of nurturance and limit setting, responding and directing, helps the child internalize the emotional warmth *and* the capacity for inhibition.

Risk Factors for Load Conditions

A number of factors can disrupt the respond–direct–reflect triad that shapes meaning-making in the family and, consequently, can impact the child's sense of self and relationship to others. The stress patterns we discuss here fall along a continuum from occasional to chronic experiences. A family stressor, such as an illness or death, can shift a family into a temporary load condition pattern. This pattern is in contrast to the type of chronic load condition in which one parent or the other has severe psychopathology and the effects may be dramatic. At times, a load condition pattern may result from relational dynamics. It is not uncommon for parents to polarize when one feels critical of the other's parenting style. For example, a father who believes that the mother is far too lenient with their child may try to compensate by being stricter. In these situations, parenting styles that may have been quite typical can shift into imbalance. Sometimes marital dyads co-create patterns that become entrenched. What the child brings into the world may also cause an imbalance. The three imbalances described next may occur as blends and are not always a pure mode of behavior.

Overaccommodation: Responsive patterns at risk for load conditions. An overly responsive parent is too permissive and ingratiating; thus, the child receives mirroring and empathy in situations where instruction and limit setting would be more appropriate. Consequently, the child is rarely

forced to contend with the stress of challenge or recognize the impact of self on the other. This child may even come to expect that others can magically know his or her needs and are obligated to meet them, dramatically increasing the potential that a mild social stressor may lead to an extreme stress response. Social difficulties emerge when the behavior the child has learned to rely on at home is rarely re-created in the real world. The world is expecting the child to exhibit self-regulation, but the child remains dependent on interactive regulation. For the overaccommodating parent, there is often a lack of clarity in the boundaries between self and other in the dyad. The parent may deny when his or her child has a delay, reasoning that it is most important to accept the child as he or she is, not make the child feel different, or not label the child.

An overaccommodating parent's behaviors may stem from anxiety and a desire to avoid negative affects (hyperalert), both of which may add overcontrolling behaviors to the accommodating parent's profile. In the context of relationships, perpetual overaccommodating behaviors can leave one feeling defeated, sad, or depressed. Likewise, an overaccommodating child tends to show *high compliance* in relation to others at the expense of developing his or her own self and personal meanings. If there is underlying anxiety, this type of child may also exhibit *overcontrolling* behavior. In either case, positive affects may dominate the relationship but, ironically, produce very negative effects.

Demanding: Directive patterns at risk for load conditions. A demanding parent is too rigid or aggressive; thus, the child receives instruction and limits in situations where positive mirroring and empathy would be more appropriate. Age-appropriate mistakes are consistently mirrored to the child as shameful neglect or willful disrespect of others, whereas behaviors that show achievement, compliance, empathy, or competence in some area are unrecognized, minimized, or devalued. Behaviors that accurately signal a problem in some domain are overamplified, such that the child becomes defined by the problem. This type of parent is prone to escalating into either an anxious (hyperalert) or a hostile (flooded) condition, which at an extreme could lead to abuse of the child. A propensity toward tough emotions and challenging others can lean one toward a combative, hostile, and arrogant edge. This type of parent consistently shows too much negative in response to any degree of stress. Negative affects dominate relationships.

In this rigid and critical world, the child does not learn enough about warm connections and consistent, nurturing intimacy. Receiving too much scorn and not enough tenderness and empathy, the child is constantly forced to contend with the negative impact of self on the other. A chronic lack of empathy disrupts the developing emotional self. In this context, a child who is overaccommodating may respond to a demanding

parent by being willing to be compliant and obedient, probably not developing a strong sense of self; anxiety may predominate. In contrast, a demanding child will continually "bump into" the parent, escalating high arousal, anger, and fighting. This child is also likely to show *high defiance* toward others and may develop an overly narcissistic set of meanings, expecting the world to adjust to him or her without being able to adjust to others.

Detaching: Reflective patterns at risk for load conditions. A detached parent is unresponsive and preoccupied in a world of private meanings. Even when a child is hurt or in need of response, this parent tends to stand back and weigh the options, staying perpetually neutral. The child receives reserve and caution where empathy (response) and guidance (directive) would be more appropriate. This type of parent is considered emotionally cold and distant and may be in a chronically hypoalert state that may reflect a variety of possibilities: chronic depression, frequent dissociative episodes from a trauma history, a schizoid personality type, or a person with a nonverbal learning disorder or autism spectrum disorder. In terms of affective range, there is not enough positive or negative; it is the *lack* of affect that dominates the relationship. An extreme of this behavior could lead to severe neglect of the child.

This child is often left to function on his or her own in a disengaged relationship, lacking connection and structure, and potentially feeling perpetually lost. The gap between self and other is so wide that there is neither enough connection nor enough bumping into another to enable the child to fully develop accurate meanings of self and other. A child in this environment may at first protest (show anger), which later gives way to depression and not caring (detachment, apathy) (Bowlby, 1969, 1973, 1978), or may turn into a chronically anxious and hypervigilant state when left alone for too long a time. A child with a tendency toward detachment is likely to show high avoidance of emotions and to disconnect whenever high-intensity emotions are expressed by others. A lack of purposeful connection to others may predominate, along with an undeveloped sense of self. A detached child may cut off affects as a way of coping. He or she may develop an overly private set of meanings, preoccupied with his or her internal world at the expense of shared meanings and is also likely to show *high indifference* toward others.

To complement Table 8.1 in the preceding chapter, Table 9.2 organizes coordination and load behaviors in relation to the child's modes of interaction.

Points to consider. It is important to note that particular parent–child combinations may actually be adaptive, or a good match, even when there are tendencies toward extremes. For example, a high-direct parent of a child with ADHD may provide useful structure for the child; a high-respond

Table 9.2. Examples of Coordination and Load Versions of the Three Interpersonal Modes: Child

Respond		Direct		Reflect	
Coordination	Overaccommodate — Risk Factor for Load Condition	Coordination	Demand — Risk Factor for Load Condition	Coordination	Detach — Risk Factor for Load Condition
• Follows the adult's lead • Seeks nurturing interactions from parents • "Feels" the parent's emotional experience • Tolerates tender and positive feelings within self and others ("softer" side of emotions) • Emotional tone is warm, nurturing, and tender • Experiences closeness and connection between self and others • Mirrors the other's experience (empathy) • Greater focus on shared meanings	• The "parentified" child who too often rescues a parent • Denies a parent's inappropriate behavior (e.g., alcoholism, sexualizing, stealing) • Falsely positive affect dominates • Overly compliant toward the parent • Overly clingy behavior toward the parent, even in familiar contexts • Overly reliant on parent, requiring constant reassurance • Unable to express own meanings • Under stress, may favor the hyperalert state	• Is able to take the lead when appropriate • Can express (includes nonverbal behavior) own needs clearly and assertively • Willing to risk conflict and rupture • Tolerates negative feelings within self and toward other ("tougher" side of emotions) • Is comfortable with separateness between self and others • Focuses more on own needs and wants being met	• Overly controlling and aggressive • Emotional tone is demanding and insistent • During emotional tension or conflict, child tends to challenge, verbally attack, and blame the other • Negative affects dominate • High defiance against the other • At the extreme, leads to oppositional or antisocial behaviors • Under stress, may favor the flooded state	• Observes interactions before taking action • Is able to solve problems with parent • Willing to change behavior on parent's request • Is not prone toward emotional outbursts, remaining steady and composed • Comfortable with separateness • Is willing to listen to the parent's viewpoints (meanings)	• Overly detached and unresponsive • Child tends to stonewall the parent during emotional tension or conflict • Lack of positive or negative affect; neutrality dominates • High avoidance, turning away from others • At the extreme, lacks the need for others • Escapes into private meanings most of the time • Under stress, may favor the hypoalert state

parent of a child with a nonverbal learning disorder may provide the extra help this child needs. These possibilities are not to imply that the other modes are not still needed or not important. The point is intended to highlight those situations where parents find themselves shifting toward an extreme style to adapt to their child's needs and are often criticized for it by outsiders who are not tuned into the child's needs.

Another important point is that of cultural biases. Most Western perspectives tend to view these three styles of behavior, when extreme, as less than optimal. However, many cultural groups (even within the "Western" purview) may consider some of these behaviors that we present as healthy as atypical and others we present as extreme as typical. For example, in some cultural groups it is typical for the parents to avoid high-intensity social interactions (Tronick, 2007), spank their children (MacArthur, 1998), have hostile interchanges on a daily basis (e.g., "road rage"), or for young children to be working (Associated Press, 2008). Our rule of thumb is that what is deemed *typical* is a dynamic construct that has to be reconsidered for each family within its cultural context.

ASSESSMENT AND INTERVENTION STRATEGIES

All intervention is a form of learning. The neurorelational framework emphasizes that it is important for professionals across disciplines to think about, on a meta-level, the approach used to promote learning in intervention and compare it to how the child and family learn best. In other words, is the learning environment a good match for the potential learner? The modes of *respond, direct,* and *reflect,* described throughout this chapter, are embedded in clinical approaches. Many mental health disciplines lean toward responding approaches (respond—emotions, implicit learning). Behaviorists, the medical professions, and rehabilitation disciplines that work with speech or motor delays lean toward directing approaches (direct—doing; guided extrinsic approaches that foster implicit learning). Rehabilitation disciplines that work with cognitive delays, cognitive therapies, educational approaches, and reflective practice within infant mental health lean toward the reflective approaches (reflect—thinking; making implicit meanings explicit). A relationship-based approach, as advocated by the neurorelational framework, requires an integration of respond, direct, and reflect orientations that are capable of adapting to the needs of a given family system. For more on how these heuristics apply to clinical theories within infant mental health and early intervention circles, please see CD-ROM Section 9.1, which links the respond–direct–reflect heuristic with clinical and parent education approaches.

The quality of the relationship among the professional, child, and parent significantly affects the emotion, memory, and meaning components for all participants. To assess the issue of fit for children and parents, it is important for professionals to consider their own style and approach both in terms of a personal comfort zone as well as their training history. Table 9.3 can serve as a useful aid in gaining awareness of your strengths and possible weaknesses regarding these modes of interaction. The neurorelational framework encourages professionals from all disciplines to expand into domains that are less familiar because all elements of responding, directing, and reflecting are necessary for healthy learning and relational development.

Table 9.3.   Clinical Modes of Interaction That Support Coordination or Trigger Load Conditions

Responding	Directing	Reflecting
Coordination		
Follows the child/ parent's lead	Therapist provides the lead	Therapist stands back
Allows the process to unfold; therapist may be hands-off in terms of providing directives	The process is guided by some type of structure from the therapist; therapist is hands-on	The process is co-defined by therapist and client and structured as it unfolds
Contains and mirrors feelings	Sets boundaries and limits	Stays even-handed, impartial while collecting information
Provides empathy, tracks emotional patterns	Provides direction, goals, guidance, skill building	Provides validation of experience and analysis of behavior patterns
Handles tender feelings; warm and engaging behaviors; tolerates closeness	Handles tough feelings; tolerates conflict	Handles staying neutral; tolerates reserve
Can repair a rupture	Can tolerate a rupture	Can problem-solve a rupture
Risk Factors for Load Conditions		
Overly permissive	Controlling	Emotionally detached
Process lacks a coherent focus, chaotic	Process is so predetermined that relevant information is missed, rigid	Process stays at a meta-level, lacks real-world relevance, detached
Indulgent	Authoritarian	Overly intellectual
Highly accommodating	Highly confrontational	Highly impersonal

The emergence of an open learning system in a child is crucially dependent on the quality of relationship the child experiences. Intervening by focusing on the quality of the relationship (parent–child, parent–therapist, child–therapist) is essential for ameliorating problems related to the capacities in this system. In an open learning system, emotional expression is flexible, wide-ranging, and modulated; memories are accessible and fluid; and meanings, derived from a complex blend of both emotions and memories, accurately reflect the context and support cohesion of the self.

Assessment and Intervention Steps

Because the full range of modulated emotions is so central to the co-creation of healthy memories and meaning-making as well as an open learning system, we emphasize building a healthy emotional muscle in which all practitioners and parents alike can participate. Rather than seeing emotional development as relegated to a "mental health" domain, we view it as *essential development* that interfaces with medical and physiological health (Cacioppo, Berntson, Larsen, Poehlmann, & Ito, 2000), the learning process and executive skills, developmental maturation, and relational health. Applying the titration principle to building an emotional muscle requires pacing the child's ability to tolerate emotional material, scaffolding the experience to just the right challenge, and then gradually expanding that window of tolerance. Further details are described in the following discussion. Because emotional reactions are such a part of everyday life—at home, in the classroom, or in a practitioner's office—there are multiple opportunities that often occur serendipitously that one needs to be equipped to manage on a regular basis.

Step 1: Review Developmental and Socioemotional Milestones and Consider the Potential Contributions of the Relevance System to the Presenting Problem(s)

Assessment within the relevance system means thinking about the emotions, memories, and meanings that may be having a disruptive effect on the emerging developmental and socioemotional milestones for any child of any age. An important question for the professional to ask is, "Which of this child's problems or delays may be due to the influence of relevance system components?" For example, a limited emotional range, poor modulation of emotional reactions, a closed learning system, and skewed meanings about the self might all be part of the clinical picture for a child who presents with learning and social–emotional delays.

Step 2: Assess Risk Factors, Strengths, and Resources of Child and Parent

Risk factors affecting the relevance system can be particularly disruptive to a child's overall development. These factors include:

1. *Relational disruptions,* as in marital distress (especially domestic violence), the absence of at least one adult who is lovingly and strongly committed to the child on an ongoing basis, such as occurs in foster care or orphanage placements (Lindhiem & Dozier, 2007), or a sibling with significant pathology;
2. *Familial psychopathology or addiction* (e.g., intergenerational predispositions toward anxiety-related, depressive, or bipolar mood disorders; the presence of a substance use/abuse disorder; parental history of abuse or neglect; parental history of having children removed from his or her care);
3. *Learning disruptions,* such as narrow, overly focused learning proclivities in either child or parent (closed learning system);
4. Lack of empathy or inappropriate eye contact in either parent or child; and
5. *Male gender* in preterm infants (Stanford Report, 2004) and male gender in contexts where there is parental psychopathology and early maltreatment (Howe, Toth, & Cicchetti, 2006; Stevenson et al., 2000; Tronick, 2007).

Recall that "as the cumulative number of risks increases, the developmental status of the child decreases" (Friedman & Chase-Lansdale, 2002, p. 264; see also Rutter, 1985; Sameroff, Seifer, Baldwin, & Baldwin, 1993; Sameroff, Seifer, Barocas, Zax, & Greenspan, 1987).

Intrinsic resiliency factors from the relevance system can have a robust impact and serve as the key to successful intervention. For example, a child with a vigorous capacity for joy provides the professional with almost infinite routes for establishing a sense of safety and repairing ruptures; a child who can tolerate all three approach styles—respond, direct, and reflect—provides the professional with multiple strategic routes. Other resiliency factors include "(1) dispositional attributes (e.g., temperament, cognitive abilities, self-beliefs); (2) family characteristics (e.g., warmth, closeness, cohesion); [and] (3) the availability and use of external support systems by family members" (Friedman & Chase-Lansdale, 2000, p. 264). To Friedman and Chase-Lansdale's third category, we add extended family, faith communities, and treatment teams. In addition, we contend that the practitioner/treatment team can make an important contribution in the second category. One can always use Worksheet 9.1

Worksheet 9.1.   History Worksheet for the Relevance System

Parental Risk Factors That Can Compromise a Parent's Ability to Provide Interactive Regulation	Global Questions That Assess the Overall Functioning of the Relevance System	Child Risk Factors That Can Decrease Self-Regulation and Increase the Need for Interactive Regulation
☐ A domestic violence participant ☐ Personal history of abuse and/or neglect ☐ History of children removed from home; abuse/neglect of other children ☐ Multiple children to care for ☐ Weak commitment to child ☐ Family history of mental illness ☐ Chronically depressed or anxious ☐ Rapid swings into high-intensity emotions; low frustration tolerance ☐ Lack of empathy for self and others ☐ Difficulty making eye contact and lacking warmth ☐ Negative appraisal of child as willfully disobeying or as not loving parent ☐ Parent unable to set boundaries and overaccommodates child ☐ Discrepancies exist among words, actions, or nonverbal communication ☐ Learning disruptions ☐ Inability to ask for help when necessary	• Is the individual able to express a range of positive and negative emotions flexibly? • How do experiences influence memories and appraisals? • Are emotionally loving, significant, and long-term relationships present? • Does the individual tend to attribute positive or negative meanings to experiences?	☐ Male preterm infant ☐ Exposure to domestic violence ☐ Abuse and/or neglect ☐ Traumatic memories ☐ Lack of emotional care due to foster care or orphanage placement ☐ Chronically depressed or anxious ☐ Rapid swings into high-intensity emotions; low frustration tolerance ☐ Lack of empathy for self and others ☐ Lack of eye contact, absence of interest in others, and/or lack of social referencing (overly detached) ☐ Highly demanding of others ☐ Overaccommodating to others ☐ Lacks one person in the family who is strongly committed to child and who provides loving care ☐ Discrepancies exist among words, actions, or nonverbal communication ☐ Learning disruptions ☐ Inability to ask for help when necessary

(a complete History Worksheet for all four brain systems is available for your use on the CD-ROM, Section 12.2) as an aid when evaluating the balance or imbalance of difficulties a child or parent is bringing to their dynamic interactions.

Step 3: Develop the Capacity to Flexibly Experience, Express, and Modulate a Full Range of Emotions in Ways That Are Appropriate to Context

Note that these recommendations apply to both child and parent. Assess the strength of the emotional muscle by evaluating the *range* and the *modulation* of emotional expression in child and parent. Be aware that emotions can span the range of awake states of arousal.

Next, assess whether the expression of emotion is appropriate for the child's age in terms of nonverbal ("shows"), verbal ("tells"), and symbolic ("plays") levels. For parents, assess their ability to demonstrate nonverbal and verbal expressions of emotion as well as their ability to use emotional themes during symbolic play with their children. Table 8.2 listed the typical progression of emotional themes and Table 8.3 provided an overview of typical load versions. (See Chapter 3 for more information on symbolic play themes.)

Last in this category, assess the capacity to experience positive and negative dimensions of emotions. For example, the child can protest the stopping of a game he or she is playing, yet be pleased and willing to transition to the next activity of going outside to play.

When assessing the child's emotional muscle, there are two ways to consider whether the emotional expressions are appropriate. First, think about the events that are known to trigger emotional responses that are too frequent, too intense, or too slow to recover (i.e., emotional load condition). For example, every night, the bedtime routine triggers a tantrum that lasts more than an hour. Next, assess for any specific emotions or themes that trigger emotional load conditions. For example, a child has a meltdown every time she feels embarrassed.

It is also important to look for those events and emotions that promote optimal or stable functioning of the emotional muscle. For example, the child transitions very well during the morning routine; the child has a wonderful sense of humor and handles mild stressors very well. Table 9.4 provides examples of load behaviors in relation to a limited range of emotions in terms of behavioral dimensions. The table focuses on the converse patterns from those noted in the optimal guidelines for mild, moderate, to severe stressors noted elsewhere in this chapter.

Four intervention goals shape the work in the emotional range capacity: (1) strengthen the ability to modulate emotion while within the alert processing state; (2) expand the emotional range in child and parent; (3) help the dyad begin to down-regulate intense emotional responses; and (4) develop an optimal midrange of emotional flexibility in the dyad.

Regulation strategies. The visceral self in the regulation system contains the precursors to emotional self-connectedness. Sensing bowel and bladder pressure, hunger and fullness, thirst and fatigue sets the stage for

Table 9.4. Examples of Load Behaviors Related to Limited Range of Emotions in Terms of Behavioral Dimensions

Duration	Intensity	Rhythm
Individual: There are predominant behavioral indicators of fearfulness, anxiety, defiance, sadness, withdrawal, or incongruent happiness that continue in the infant, child, or adult over time, even with mild stressors.	*Individual:* The infant, child, or adult is unable to modulate his or her own emotions by taking quick breaks and down- and up-regulating the intensity either within the alert processing state or in recovering from a stressor.	*Individual:* The infant, child, or adult makes jerky, abrupt, or chaotic shifts from one emotion to another and into stress responses, even with mild stressors.
Dyad: Has limited ability to engage in experiences of shared joy throughout the day, even without stressors, or does not use positive emotions to assist with stress recovery.	*Dyad:* Both infant/child and adult are unable to recover from high- or low-intensity emotions even with help from an emotionally safe person.	*Dyad:* Mild stressors produce rapid, negative emotional co-escalations between parent–child or parent–parent.
Dyad: Both infant/child and adult are unavailable for social interaction on a regular basis.		

discerning one's own fluctuating emotions. When the range of emotion is constricted, you can use a bottom-up approach by deepening children's connection to their visceral self and the parents' connection to their children's visceral cues (e.g., shaking their leg, touching themselves, mood shifts from hunger or fatigue, rubbing eyes). Promote an alert processing state and then guide the child's focus through his or her visceral connections. (Refer to Chapter 5 for intervention suggestions.) On occasion, use narrative of bodily cues (somatic markers) that are linked with bodily needs. The importance here is to make an explicit link between somatic markers and physiological need. One can use both descriptive language and queries to direct the child's focus to the physiological need. For example: "I see you are headed for the refrigerator. Are you hungry?"; "When you jiggle your leg, it usually means you have to go to the bathroom. Do you have to go to the bathroom?"; "When you lick your lips because they are dry it means you need to drink. Can you tell that you are thirsty?" This kind of linking extends the child's unconscious (implicit) procedural knowledge (learning) of visceral sensations into conscious (explicit), semantic knowledge (explicit actions—the child goes to the bathroom). Using visuals can help some children increase awareness and identification of their

somatic markers, thereby establishing somatic cause–effect connections (see CD-ROM Section 9.2 for an example of a tool that can be used). Linking physiological somatic markers with bodily needs provides the foundation for then making links between emotions and needs ("I feel sad—I need to cry; I feel happy—I want a hug; I feel angry—I need to take a break," etc.).

Some children may need medication to regulate their emotional state. The decision to use medication as a treatment with children should always involve caution and thoughtful consideration. We lean more toward medication when genetic risk factors are present, when the emergence of mood symptoms implicates a nature over nurture etiology, and when emotional dysregulation is causing significant disruption to ongoing development (further compromising meanings).

Parents who themselves cannot regulate emotions may need increased support (e.g., respite care, medication), an increased ratio of individual treatment sessions in relation to dyadic work, referral for individual mental health treatment with another therapist who can work on a treatment team, or some combination thereof.

Sensory strategies. We now shift to the sensory aspects of emotions (e.g., butterflies in tummy), whereas in the preceding section focused on sensory aspects of regulatory functions (e.g., hunger). We emphasize the sensory–motor transformation aspect of emotions because it provides a neutral framework within which to address sensitive emotional issues with parents. By describing emotions in sensory terms (e.g., intensity of sound, facial movements of furrowed brow, quickly shifting gestures), the match or mismatch between parent and child can be presented in ways that minimize defensiveness. In addition, increasing the child's awareness of and sensitivity to the use of sensory cues (e.g., lump in throat, hot tears, tense muscles) to identify a range of positive and negative emotions can help the child develop an emotional literacy. This focus is a high priority for children who do not feel or recognize any of their emotions. The following three-stage approach is one way to help children develop skills in this area:

1. *Use visual aids to increase awareness and identification of feelings and accompanying needs.* Here, one can make use of a visual medium for awareness and identification. Visual Talk Blocks (Brubakken & Lui, 2005) provide color-coded facial pictures and words for both "I Feel" and "I Need" categories that can be combined in various ways. The child is able to link combinations of feelings and needs, either to reflect an experience in the moment or to recall a previous experience. Having a child hold a "feeling" block in one hand and a "need" block in the other hand also expands the intervention to another sensory domain, by directly involving a kinesthetic and motor experience. In addition, the use of manipulatives

facilitates circles of communication that can go down a number of different paths depending on what thoughts and feelings are stimulated in the moment. In a more advanced version of this approach a child chooses several blocks that may be converging at the same time (i.e., calm, safe, happy; angry, sad, frustrated). If the appropriate feelings and needs are not found on the available manipulatives, then the child can be helped to articulate what is accurate for him or her. These attempts at self-expression that emerge in a more spontaneous way, can then be celebrated and the child can gain a sense of pride at being able to articulate something authentic about himself or herself without external referencing.

2. *Use an explicit/reflective intervention to recall an emotion*: As the child develops his or her basic emotional vocabulary, he or she can be led to begin practicing and exercising the use of these words in context. One might first want to lead the child into a relaxed state, using deep breathing. Once the child is adequately relaxed, ask him or her, "Do you remember a 'big' feeling you had in the past week?" Talk about the feeling with the child and take him or her through the somatic markers (Damasio, 1996) so that he or she can start to associate, even in a recall mode, bodily sensations with specific emotional responses.

3. *Use an action/procedural intervention to deal with a real-time emotion*: In the throes of a heightened emotional reaction during the session, use a "freeze-frame" approach to slow down and frame the child's reaction. For example, you might say, "Right now you're really sad. I want you to try to notice what you feel in your body. Do you feel tightness in your chest, a lump in your throat, tears in your eyes?" This type of exercise lays the foundation and connections for bodily signals that can enhance a self-modulation ability.

As Anna's emotional themes were unfolding, the toileting issue continued. Nicole was more used to it and less bothered by it; Paul was exhausted. Several months into our work together, now that there was much more emotional connection between Anna and her parents as well as myself, the timing seemed right to begin to include her body in our play therapy. As suspected, she initially had weak connections to her visceral and sensory selves. Since her adoption, her parents had noted that she had poor signals as to when she was hungry, full, feeling bowel or bladder pressure, or feeling pain.

Learned helplessness in the context of abuse and neglect often creates an accommodation to threat and an avoidance of or aversion to conditions of safety. Anna was originally forced to say "yes" to what was uncomfortable against her skin—wetness and feces. Under such conditions of threat (abuse and neglect) it is common for reversals between sensory conditions of safety and threat to occur. Signals that are meant to connote safety have to be ignored—hence rejected—and

signals that are meant to identify threat have to become familiar. During gentle exploration, it became clear that Anna actually disliked the sensation of wetness against her skin. After asking Anna to recall the sensations she did not like and the reasons she stayed in her diapers, she announced, "I'm used to waiting to be changed." The combination of poor visceral and sensory connections and learned helplessness was central to her ongoing inability to take control of what she did not like. Not long after this particular conversation, Anna began to exercise bowel and bladder control. Within a few weeks, she was diaper-free. In reflection, I realized that much of how I addressed the toileting issue was indirect: (1) The characters in our stories described sensory events; (2) in real time I was verbally narrating connections between her body and her behavior and making links; and (3) we talked openly about the discomfort she felt from wetness, even as she continued to accommodate it. Neither her parents nor I were certain how these interventions came together to facilitate the shift to this desired behavior. Seeing this reversal between safety and threat led me to further understand the inaccurate and inauthentic ways that Anna had accommodated unthinkingly to saying "yes" at school and "no" at home. Transitions from home continued to be increasingly uncomfortable. She refused to go anywhere, even if she loved where she was going. Smoothing these transitions was the next challenge.

Relevance strategies. The first focus here is to develop and strengthen the emotional self by applying the titration principle, an intervention principle (mostly based in procedural learning, although other forms are involved) that guides the child or parent in flexing and strengthening the emotional muscle. Strengthening a weak emotional muscle through the use of the titration principle requires a blend of responding and directing qualities from both parent and therapist. The titration principle can be applied whether one is expanding an emotional range to include new feelings that are uncomfortable or down-regulating high-intensity emotions to gain better modulation.

Experiences in which the child moves from a positive emotion to a negative one (e.g., when playing a game in which a child may shift rapidly from a winning streak to a losing streak) are excellent opportunities for the practitioner to begin to teach the child to tolerate heightened and shifting states of emotion. The following titration guidelines may be helpful (in addition, see the Flow Chart for Titrating on the CD-ROM, Section 9.3). Note that these guidelines include regulation and executive-based elements.

1. Prepare the child for the possibility of an uncomfortable feeling by developing the ability to anticipate (e.g., "Oh, wow, it looks like I might be able to capture you. What do you think you'll feel if I do that? Is this going to be a little bit of disappointment, a medium amount, or a lot?").

2. A simple 1–5 or 1–10 rating scale can help the child mark and learn to rate his or her intensity level. A child who is old enough to draw his or her own thermometer can make up a personal scale that describes the intensity levels along with the emotional words and phrases that accompany the escalation. Additional game-like tools are available to assist the children at different ages in learning to recognize, integrate, and modulate their degree of reactivity (e.g., Berg, 2004; Buron, 2008; Jaffe & Gardner, 2008; Weiss, Singer, & Feigenbaum, 2006).

3. Structure the activity (provide scaffolding) so that the child has control over the degree of intensity and always has an open door for escape. If the therapist feels that the challenge (losing the game or getting captured in the moment) will result in a flooded reaction that he or she will not be able to help the child modulate, then the therapist should give the child an escape hatch (e.g., "It looks like this is going to be too hard for you to be captured, so I'm going to make a different move, but next time maybe you'll be able to handle how it feels to be captured").

4. Allow an emotionally provocative event to unfold if the child has indicated a low to moderate degree of disappointment (e.g., the child starts to lose the game and may begin to cry and protest that it is not fair).

5. Narrate for the child the uncomfortable or threatening emotions by providing mirroring, validation, and empathy (e.g., "Oh, I know it's hard to be losing, I can see that you're really mad and sad. I can understand why losing would make you mad. Those emotions are like a wave that will go up higher and higher, and soon the wave will come down").

6. For children who have the ability, focus on meaning-making (e.g., "You are getting better and better at being able to stand the bad feelings and still have fun with the game"). In other words, begin to teach the child how to weave in the positive, or how to "do" meaning-making, through reflection. While reflecting on the experience afterward, listen to the child's narrative and pay close attention to his or her nonverbal cues; then plan ahead for next time (e.g., "Boy, this was a really hard turn for you and it made you really mad and sad; maybe next time when that feeling starts to come, you can take a really deep breath. How can I help you more next time? I wonder if it would help you if I . . .").

7. In future turns, the therapist can model not only a light-hearted way to lose ("Oh, phooey! Man, you got me! Doggone it! Too bad for

me!") but also a more affect-driven response (e.g., "Hey, this doesn't feel good; I've lost two times in a row. I'm disappointed").

When working with these guidelines, it is crucial to track the degree of congruency between the child's verbal and nonverbal communication; when nonverbal body language does not match the verbal statements, the nonverbal signals are more likely to accurately reflect the emotional tone. Children whose nonverbal and verbal emotional expressions are consistently incongruent may need to return to earlier developmental levels in order to more robustly develop somatic markers that are reliable. These children may also be unable to tolerate more vulnerable emotions (i.e., sadness, embarrassment, shame); in fact, such emotions may be driving the incongruities. Children whose parents also have discrepancies between their nonverbal and verbal expressions may need to work individually with the therapist to determine their level of disconnect or process their degree of discomfort among their visceral, sensory, and emotional selves.

The second focus here is to expand the range of emotional themes within a child through play activities. Some children with a constricted emotional range, which may include a background of traumatic experiences, present with a rigid identification with the bully in their play. Regardless of the diagnostic category (e.g., this type of play could characterize PTSD, Asperger or autism disorders, attachment disorders, bipolar disorders, and/or thought disorders), the goal is to expand the emotional themes into a richer, broader range. A child who focuses on aggressive play can be exposed to the role of the one hurt (victim) and the role of the protector who stops the bully, helps the victim, and scaffolds the bully and the victim into modulated assertiveness. First, modeling these other two roles of victim and protector, as described in Table 9.5, can be a way to expand the play (recall this is what occurred during Laura's play; see the case study in the sensory brain system chapters, 6 and 7). Later, fostering flexibility in the child is facilitated by role switching so that everyone gets a chance to be the bully while others are being hurt, others are helping the victim, and others are stopping the bully. Children learn from observation (watching others) as well as by acting out the new emotional role. Table 9.5 presents themes for each role (bully, victim, protector) that progress from most difficult/challenging/negative to healthiest behaviors. Using this table, practitioners locate the child's position in regard to each of these roles and then move downward to consider possible character roles that can be enacted to expressively shift the child out of a rigid identification with one or more of these roles.

As mentioned, an authentic emotional range was emerging in Anna, but it was still very early in its development. The most basic positive and negative valences can be associated with yes (approach) behaviors and no (avoidance) behaviors. It was clear that Anna felt safe at home, yet she also associated any change as a

Table 9.5. Increasing Flexibility in Character Roles Across Emotional Themes

Aggressor (Bully)	Victim	Protector
Has intent to commit or take pleasure in aggressive/ destructive actions, such as:	*Carries out nondominant role in such ways as:*	*Implements defensive safeguarding in such ways as:*
Hateful killing/destructive feelings	Feeling powerless	Stopping abuse
Intent or pleasure in destroying property	Showing pain	Mirroring the victim's pain
Intent or pleasure in hurting other's feelings	Accepting what can't be changed	Providing empathy/support for victim
Intent or pleasure in winning at all cost	Bearing difficulty/grief	
	Showing righteous anger	
Transition from taking pleasure in destructive acts to straightforward anger expressed in progressive developmental levels, such as:	*Transitions to more dominant expressions, such as:*	*Transitions to empowering others in such ways as:*
Using sounds to express anger (e.g., screams, yells, roars)	Making self-protective choices	Helping victim consider options, such as words/ actions for self-care (e.g., saying "Stop!", "I don't like this," or walking away)
Using body to act out anger (e.g., hitting, biting, kicking)	Expressing distress, shows pain	Mirroring the distress in the victim; mirrors the shift from destructiveness to angry feelings in the bully
Using words to communicate needs, wants, hurt	Wanting payback	Providing empathy for the victim's hurt; provides support for the bully to shift to the use of words instead of actions
Feeling own anger and at the same time, notice others' distress	Developing assertiveness and problem-solves what can be changed	Supporting the bully's use of words for self-expression
Wanting to repair	Rejecting repair effort	Considering problem-solving options for present problems between the victim and the bully
	Accepting repair effort	Anticipating, choosing, and planning for the future respectful problem-solving options

Note: This table was created in collaboration with Debra Kessler.

threat, and she associated avoidance of change as safety. Her rigid application of these automatic responses was crippling.

We began by intensifying expressions of *yes* and *no*. *Yes* was associated with any genuine positive experience we encountered during our play, and *no* was associated with negative and disappointing feeling we encountered. As we moved to playing board games, Nicole and I began to exaggerate the body language and vocalizations expressive of both joyful and disappointing moments. If I was losing, I would exaggerate my facial expressions and gestures and verbalize my disappointment. Snapping my fingers while I exclaimed an "Oh, phooey!" made Anna laugh. Here, she got to see that I was disappointed, and at the same time I was modulating the intensity of it. She began to mimic my disappointment when she was losing and my joy when she was winning. I very carefully titrated how much disappointment she could bear while playing a game. By using a scale of 1–10, she learned to cue me if she was going to be too upset or if she could handle whatever setback was about to ensue. Now she was using language to begin verbalizing the intensity of her distress. As time went on, she could handle more losses and more setbacks, with the appropriate facial and verbal expressions accompanying them. Over time, her negative repertoire of emotions expanded to include context-appropriate expressions of sadness, anger, jealously, hurt, nervousness, and upset.

Executive strategies. Children need to learn how to handle events and situations that they cannot control (excluding those involving danger, abuse, or neglect). Use the anticipation function of the parent's executive system to increase predictability for the child and thereby reduce the element of emotional surprise that can often trigger a stress response. In addition, develop a back-up plan for likely scenarios, for example, "I know you are really excited about going to the birthday party and you're especially looking forward to playing with Johnny. But if Johnny doesn't come or wants to play with someone else, what can you do to help yourself have a good time?" Wait a moment for the child to respond; if nothing is forthcoming, you could provide a few prompts (i.e., scaffold the strategy formation process) by saying, for example, "You could ask Johnny when he could play with you," "You could go play on the swing," "I wonder if there might be someone else there who you would enjoy playing with too?"

At first, the practitioner serves as an external executive system by noticing patterns, scaffolding executive skills, and teaching adaptable behavior. For example, the professional helps children and parents to do the following:

- Notice the pattern of events (and emotions and memories) that create disruptions (e.g., a sudden change in plans, not being told the plans for the day, feeling defeated or rejected, a spelling test, tired, hasn't eaten, a sibling is getting more attention) as well as patterns of events that go well.

- Learn from both positive and negative events or outcomes by modeling how the learning process can be useful. For example, "Now we know what *not* to do." By modeling for parents that the learning process can be facilitated whether things go well or not (e.g., "Mistakes are our friends, not our enemies") parents not only learn to accept their own mistakes more readily but pass on a valuable lesson to their children.

Over time, as they grow to trust what is safe and predictable, children take over more of their own anticipation and problem-solving functions. See Step 5 in the executive strategies in this chapter for more discussion of problem-solving skills.

Step 4: Develop the Capacity to Learn from Experience by Scanning and Accessing a Full Range of Memories That Are Appropriate to the Context

It is important for professionals from all disciplines to realize that memories may contribute to emotional regulation or dysregulation. In addition, *memories are evidence of prior learning.* For this reason, we recommend the following five-step assessment process for both child and parent:

1. Assess for memory-based triggers of negative emotion by noticing clues that either implicitly (e.g., play enactments) or explicitly (e.g., verbal communication) convey themes of distress or trauma being aware of particular implicit and explicit clues.
2. Assess for memories that reverse safe and threatening situations or stimuli (weighted toward psychotherapy) and for those that reverse learning strengths and weaknesses (weighted toward education).
3. Assess capacity to modulate positive and negative memories:

    - Does the individual get stuck in recalling *only* positive or *only* negative memories? The splitting off of one or the other is detrimental to emotional blending and maturity.
    - Is there open learning? For example, can the child take in new information as the parents try to shift their behavior in treatment?
    - In the learning phase model, can the child tolerate the negative phase, or have past memories of failed learning led to retreat?

4. Assess for possible learning problems:

    - Once a child enters school, learning problems usually (but not always) become more apparent. Sometimes difficulties can only

be inferred. It is important to consider not just whether a child is doing poorly in school but also whether the child appears to enjoy and find pleasure in the learning process. If the child seems to retreat from things that involve learning (e.g., going to a museum, watching an educational TV show) and never seems to get excited about learning something new, this could signal that there is some type of struggle or obstacle that is causing the child to anticipate failure.

- When there are more apparent learning issues occurring, it is very important to explore the context: How do these problems manifest in the classroom? Do the other children notice? Is the child ever teased? Does the teacher understand how to prevent exposing the child's difficulties? It is also important to explore the child's memories of hurtful or embarrassing events around learning, as these can fuel a negative cycle and keep it going. During testing, to get a feel for children's reflection capacity, I (JT) like to ask them how they would like me to help them. In response, a girl once said to me, "I would love to not always be the only one who doesn't get it." With comments like that, it is not hard to see how learning becomes synonymous with emotional pain.

- For younger children, emerging learning problems can be suspected with some of the same clues: Does the child retreat from learning games? Does the child's mood change more than seems reasonable every time the family plays a game that he or she is not good at? Basically, watch for signs that the child may be avoiding learning challenges rather than enjoying them.

5. Consider how the child's emotions, moods, and states of arousal are impacting learning and memory:

- Emotions that frequently shift a child into a hypoalert state will affect learning due to low activation (i.e., the child is not aroused enough to engage in learning tasks).
- Some children with learning delays will shift into a dampened-down, withdrawn state while at school or in the classroom, but may seem fine otherwise.
- Emotions that correspond to a flooded state will severely disrupt learning. Even after the flooded state has resolved (physiologically), the event can continue to drain cognitive resources (through rumination, denial) and disrupt learning.
- Learning can be enhanced or disrupted by the hyperalert state depending on the meaning of the trigger and the degree of activation. A trigger of worry over getting teased at recess, for which activation is high, is likely to interrupt attention and drain

resources. A trigger of worry over finishing a project by the deadline, for which activation is moderately high, is more likely to enhance learning.

- What is optimal in terms of degree of arousal and ratio of positive to negative emotion will obviously vary by child.
- Children whose default mode often goes into a negative range of emotion may (a) get "stuck" in a negative affect stage of learning (e.g., not experiencing enough progress to feel hopeful, not learning enough to feel satisfaction and curiosity) or (b) drop out during a negative phase of learning (Phases II and III of the learning process) to avoid the unpleasant experience.

Table 9.6 provides an overview of problems that typify constrictions in range of memories.

No matter the age of the child, intervention often involves taking the

Table 9.6. Examples of Limited Range of Memories and Learning in Terms of Behavioral Dimensions

Duration	Intensity	Rhythm
Individual: There is a predominance of negative memories (fearful, anxious, angry, sad) at the expense of building a full range.	*Individual:* Vague, limited recall of salient life events (e.g., births, weddings, funerals, accidents; involves episodic memory).	*Individual:* Unpredictable intrusions of nightmares and daytime flashbacks in the infant, child, or adult.
Individual: There is a predominance of positive memories (happy, naive optimism) at the expense of building a full range.	*Individual:* High-intensity recall or rumination of salient life events (e.g., births, weddings, funerals, accidents).	*Individual:* A predictable memory intrusion linked to a specific sensory cue of some kind (e.g., smell, setting, person).
Dyad: Parent has selective recall for focusing on what the child does well, what strengths the child has, or what the child does poorly or has problems doing.	*Individual:* Poor recall for repeated information or academic learning (semantic memory)	*Individual:* Frequent enactments or verbalization of negatively valenced events.
Individual: Child cannot learn new things without excessive repetition.	*Individual:* Poor recall for routines (procedural memory).	*Individual:* Frequent retrieval of prior learning that is accurate per se but out of sync with the current context (e.g., children who blurt out comments in class that are related to the topic but "miss the point" in the moment).

(Continued)

Table 9.6.   Continued

Duration	Intensity	Rhythm
Individual: Child can learn but is very slow to retrieve and demonstrate what was learned. Often the "moment is lost," and others remain unaware of what the child knows or can show if given more time.	*Individual:* Child requires multimodal approaches to learn	

child through a process of making something implicit into something explicit. The neurorelational framework differs from some approaches in that we oppose turning implicit knowledge into explicit knowledge too quickly. There may often be an urgency on the part of the practitioner to get a narrative out of the child. Especially when working with children who have experienced trauma, we advocate following the child's procedural memory system as it enacts old memories and then helping the child create new procedural memories as the precursor to narrative discourse.

It is always ideal, of course, to have a comprehensive history. Lacking that, the child's behavioral reenactments of implicit memories can provide substantial clinical information and guidance to the perceptive professional. Recall in the sensory system Laura's enactment of biting behaviors. Here in the relevance system, Anna reenacted her freeze condition. Remember that infants and young children will communicate through their behavior implicit meanings and memories that convey the gist rather than the verbatim aspects of an event. Our role as professionals is often to help the child gain control and mastery over fears, anxieties, and at times unpredictable events that he or she was not able to control. Procedural reenactments can be a way the child comes to terms with his or her implicit knowledge about a particular relationship. Such enactments can be healthy if the family and professional allow for the child's pacing and rhythm while also creating new rhythms and relational procedures based on loving, warm, connections.

Regardless of etiology for a learning or memory problem, the professional will not have much success if the child is not in a well-regulated state. Educational therapists and teachers may go too quickly into a teaching and instructing mode without first attending to the child's state of arousal. An alert processing state is best to help a child encode new memories related to academic subjects. In addition, new positive memories of the process of learning (Phases I through IV) need to be repeated to build a positivity offset toward learning in the child.

Regulation strategies. For children dealing with reversals of safety and threat due to traumatic experiences, the long-term goal is to shift the reversals so that stimuli such as memories that evoke a calm, alert state become safe experiences. One of the authors (CL) frequently uses a sensory–motor means of teaching relaxation that helps the child begin to identify somatic markers (Damasio, 1996; for more on somatic resources for creating safety, see Ogden, Minton, & Pain, 2006) of the heretofore averted state of calmness. For example, a child who likes swinging (a sensory preference) can be placed in a swing with his or her choice of a favorite object (e.g., a blanket). As the child relaxes in response to the gentle swinging motion, I might narrate and gently query, "Notice if your body feels more relaxed. Let's check your muscles . . . Oh, can you feel how your muscles are loose?" "Does your tummy feel tight and hard or soft and warm?" "I see your face is relaxing; notice that your eyelids feel heavy." Contrasting terms such as hard and soft, tight and loose, warm and cool can be used to help a child notice these distinctions. I also use a tension–release progressive relaxation exercise to help children with dissociative backgrounds feel more connected to their bodies and to help children with anxiety disorders learn how to reduce their arousal. (See, for example, Levine, 1997; Ogden et al., 2006; Rothschild, 2000 for body-based approaches to dissociative states.)

Sensory strategies. First, use multisensory approaches to access and elaborate (rehearse) memories that create safety. Sensory information is built into memory traces, and the goal here is to access those memory traces of safe experiences or events and elaborate all sensory components of the event (episodic memory). Specific techniques include the following:

- While in a relaxed state, have the child recall and describe specific memories that represent a safe place, relationship, or experience. For example, a child's safest haven might be his bed, or resting in Daddy's arms, or singing a favorite song with Mommy.
- Elaborate on the sensory preferences involved in that experience. For example, the child who loves his bed may also describe his beloved teddy bear, which he holds in a variety of contexts. The point here is for the child and the parents to become conscious of and be able to make use of this resource of safety in the form of memories. Parents who are so inclined can play an active role in rehearsing these memories of safe places with their children; such rehearsal reinforces associative learning.
- Teach the child to use the memory of the safe experience, event, or place as a refuge to "go to" when distressed (Levine, 1997).

- Use sensory–motor rhythms (e.g., music, drumming, creative movement) to enhance a feeling of safety (for more on this example, see Perry & Szalavitz, 2006).
- Drawing, for older children who love to draw, can offer a medium through which they can depict a continuum of experiences associated with safety or threat.
- Use routines and structure to enhance a feeling of safety and predictability (e.g., identify a "diet" of sensory preferences that can be incorporated into different aspects of the daily routine—morning, afternoon, evening). For example, include the beloved teddy bear in all transitions, use a swing (vestibular) or sources of proprioceptive input to help with modulation, or use a nightly routine of reading to or rocking the child.
- For children with learning difficulties, using sensory preferences is a great way to weave in positive emotion during challenging tasks. For example, set up the homework area with little things that are pleasurable to the child (but not too calming), such as a favorite snack, or pillow to sit on, or a stuffed animal on the desk. Little surprises are great for positive stimulation, for example, short visits from the dog every 15 or 20 minutes or a silly "thumbs-up" picture of Dad tucked in a binder. A child's intermittent amusement/smiles help support movement through the learning phases.
- For the child who has great difficulty tolerating the experience of challenge, increase the frequency of the sensory preferences and weave in tasks that leave the child feeling successful. A meaningful and effective way to do this is to create a family culture that values the child's strengths. For example, if the child loves Legos, then the parents (1) should become Lego fans, (2) be sure to praise the child's constructions, (3) join in on the projects regularly (even if just for a few minutes), (4) talk about how good the child is at it to others, and so on. Any strength can be used to build self-esteem, and the positive energy eventually feeds into the learning.

Next, use multisensory approaches (alternate pathways) to encode new memories (learning). Specific techniques include the following:

- Use alternate modalities to enhance learning. One pathway might be more accessible than another for encoding memories; for example, have the child write letters or numbers in sand or on your back, feel wooden blocks, make letters with body.
- Combine sensory modalities. For example, have the child say a letter while watching him- or herself in the mirror. Experiment with

differing combinations of two or more sensory modalities and evaluate which ones enhance encoding.

Relevance strategies. First, help the child master fears (negative emotions) through active, implicit procedural learning (doing):

- Use stimuli to which the child is drawn in the present that can trigger both positive and negative memories (and emotions) at the same time. For example, one child with whom I (CL) worked was drawn to the music (a sensory preference) of the jack-in-the-box but was terrified by the pop-up moment.
- Titrate the symbolic play to the right dose of anxiety, oscillating between safety and threat (Levine, 1997). For example, the little boy just mentioned wanted me to play the jack-in-the-box, but only from across the room. I gradually decreased the distance as he became able to tolerate being closer to the jack-in-the-box. Finally, he was able to hold the box himself and tolerate his startle response when the jack popped up. This symbolic play was a piece of the therapeutic work that helped him work through a single-incident trauma.
- When the child is in a relaxed state, practice placing a positive memory side by side with a negative memory as a way to facilitate modulation of emotion-infused memories and to expose the child to the experience of an emotional blend in a safe environment.
- Next, help the child master learning weaknesses by using strengths and working on weaknesses in relation to the four-phase learning process outlined earlier. Phase I (curiosity, interest): look for the child's strengths to engage his or her interests. Phase II (puzzlement, confusion) is likely skipped as the child drops immediately into Phase III (failures and frustrations) and falls apart. Now use the titration principle of building up the emotional muscle to handle the negative affect necessary to move through these learning phases.
- Break learning tasks down into very small increments, titrating the dose of challenge so the child feels success and pride. The child learns to trust that he or she can handle small doses of challenge, which creates a readiness for and a capacity to handle larger doses of challenge.
- Build a repertoire of positive memories regarding learning that include relational and individual accomplishments (e.g., go to the library and pick out books for child to read to parent, even if below developmental level, to enhance a shared experience of learning pleasure).

- Build a repertoire of Phase II experiences. For example, ask a question to which the child does not know the answer and use the child's mild frustration to give him or her an experience of working through the frustration to achieve learning. Celebrate the success. Such experiences prepare the child for successful learning in Phase IV (renewed energy).
- Scaffold an experience in which you help a child remember a positive memory of success (Phase IV) side by side with a mildly or severely frustrating memory (Phase II or III), depending on the child's capacity to tolerate a blend. Such experiences increase the child's familiarity with the different levels of learning and give him or her the perspective to anticipate success even in the midst of difficulty.

When working with children who have learning disabilities, professionals who are aware of the patterns of strengths and weaknesses within memory systems are well equipped to tailor intervention for optimal benefit. For example, a professional who knows that a child has poor memory for verbal information but a strong memory for visual information will know what strength can be accessed and used and when repetition and rehearsal would help.

Internal motivation for learning is optimal but may not be present. In this situation, consider the types of external rewards available to the child and whether those rewards are ones that (1) help promote and sustain the alert processing state and (2) engage positive affects. To turn external rewards into internal ones during an intervention, align rewards with the child's positive meanings. For example, for a child whose parents have their diplomas displayed at home, an official-looking certificate may bring immense satisfaction and pride; for a child who loves recognition, display his or her accomplishment; for a child who loves positive engagement, a joyful exclamation with applause and a hug would be most reinforcing; for a child who loves numbers, expressing gains made through charts with percentages or bar graphs might be very satisfying. Inducing a sense of pride is *always* good. No matter how small the achievement, most children will beam with pride if the goal is clear and approached with a titration of ease and effort.

A year and a half into treatment, Anna began to use her emotional language more accurately. She started to let us know that she was quite distressed about feeling that she was further behind in school. She felt embarrassed and could now talk about feeling "stupid" when others were ahead of her. She began protesting going to school, and with her words, she was able to describe her anxiety, what it felt like in her body, and she could tell Nicole that it was too hard to face.

We met with the school team and were able to discuss her distress as well as the positive and negative split that had existed between home and school. The school educators were open to hearing about the complexity of her situation and a little surprised to learn that her positive emotions were actually a detriment to her ongoing progress at this point, due to their superficiality. In describing the need for Anna to have access to a range of both positive and negative emotions at home and now at school, the school team realized that they had never seen her sad or mad in their setting. Strategies were set up for further learning support; an educational therapist for after-school hours was included so that Anna could get the extra support for homework that she needed in addition to the speech and language therapy, occupational therapy, reading and math support she was receiving during school hours. The challenge became to see whether Anna could allow herself to express her distress and her lack of knowing. The educational therapist established with her privately that it was safe to say "I don't know" in response to a question. All the staff could now see more clearly how her anxiety was underneath her bright smile and her quick responses to questions. As the rhythm for learning was slowed down and Anna said her first "I don't know" to the educational therapist and "I need help" to her teacher, she was on her way to establishing an open learning system both at home and at school.

Executive strategies. First, use the child's executive skills during treatment time.

- Use the child's memory of things done during the last session and his or her executive system to plan, sequence, and evaluate the processes involved in the current session. The sequence of events during a session can be determined by the therapist or the child, or it can be negotiated between the two of them. The process of the sequencing of the events can involve the child in a self-reflective activity, wherein he or she determines or selects his or her own preferences amid a plethora of choices. This lays the groundwork for later elaboration of more advanced self-reflection (developing the meta-level perspective that allows the person to see the whole even in the midst of an experience).
- For children who have learning difficulties, a therapist or parent can teach them a variety of memory strategies, which are a great tools for enhancing confidence as well as learning. Use trial and error to discover which strategies are most effective for each child, as this will vary greatly depending on the child's strengths and weaknesses. In the process of experimenting in this way, help the child self-reflect on each strategy and learn about what is most effective for him or her. For example, a child with a reading disability may find a mnemonic strategy to be just as hard as reading but

loves using a visualizing strategy. This type of intervention is also very effective for building good anticipatory skills. As the child becomes more acquainted with the nuances of his or her struggle and what helps most, he or she can much better anticipate and prepare. The Center for Development and Learning Web site (www.cdl.org) provides research-based information on memory and learning strategies for children: (go to the Library, browse by subject, choose Memory).

- Educate the child about the learning process, his or her own profile of strengths and weaknesses, and how to anticipate and plan for learning challenges.
- Teach the child about the effects of emotion on learning and narrate the process so that he or she can link his or her own process to the learning model.
- Teach the child how to titrate levels of difficulty to help maintain his or her motivation and cognitive resources for the duration of the task.

Next, to cultivate the reflective mode of parenting, use the parent's executive skills during his or her own treatment time to help the parent reflect on his or her memories and what those memories trigger, especially in reaction to his or her child.

The neurorelational framework does not emphasize a preordained point of clinical entry; the age of the child coupled with the child and parent's affective and cognitive functioning determine the initial intervention agenda. Although we often discuss using a bottom-up approach, the nonlinear nature of the neurorelational framework allows for flexibility as to the point of clinical entry. For example, for an older child (or parent) who enters treatment very detached from his or her feelings, the emphasis may be on making connections to visceral and emotional cues, whereas a child who is overwhelmed with emotions may need to develop more language skills to modulate and think about the meaning of his or her outbursts. With that information, a practitioner can apply the neurorelational approach in a more targeted manner, from either a bottom-up or a top-down starting point.

The practitioner's self-reflective processes are equally important in understanding emotion-based memory triggers that infants, children, and parents evoke (often referred to as countertransference reactions). Ideally, the professional uses his or her executive abilities (discussed further in the executive system chapters) to determine, "Should I contain this reaction or share it in an appropriate way with the client?" The practitioner who "speaks the countertransference" (Bollas, 1983, 1987) would first need to

work with a mentor, facilitator, or consultant to hone the reflective skills needed to discern when and how to share his or her visceral or emotional responses in an effective way that furthers the client's understanding of how he or she impacts others. Sharing the countertransference potentially expands the client's capacity to accurately understand him- or herself in relation to another.

Step 5: Develop the Capacity to Construct Meanings That (Accurately) Reflect Self and Others

A child's capacity to accurately construct meanings is greatly shaped by the parent's abilities (or lack thereof) to engage in responding, directing, and reflecting modes of behavior, each with the appropriate emotional valence. With infants and very young children, accessing reflection can help parents navigate the rapid fluctuations in the child and in the parenting mode required from moment to moment. As the child gets older, the reflective mode is especially useful for helping the child develop a language to verbalize feelings and sensations and, over time, cause-and-effect relationships in the self and others.

In an open learning system, the particular interpersonal mode expressed will fluctuate according to context and the needs and capacities of the individual child, and there will be more flexible movement across these mode boundaries. In a closed system, in contrast, the parent's emotional mode is expressed irrespective of context, and the parent is either stuck in one mode with little variation (rigid) or switches among modes in a way that is unpredictable (chaotic).

The following sequence can be used to evaluate the respond–direct–reflect triad as it affects meaning-making in the child, parent, and relationship:

1. *Assess responsiveness.* Is there too much accommodation toward others—that is, an undernourished sense of self? Is there too much emphasis on shared meaning at the expense of private meanings—that is, an enmeshed sense of self? Is there too much emphasis on positive feelings?

2. *Assess directiveness.* Is there too much reliance on demands for getting needs met, enforcing structure in the family, or both—that is, an exaggerated sense of self? Is there too much emphasis on negative feelings?

3. *Assess relationship between responding and directing modes.* Is the child or parent exhibiting emotional flexibility and resilience? Is the child or parent showing the capacity to shift his or her attention

from self to other or vice versa? The answers to these questions can help the professional guide the parents' ability to blend responding and directing modes.

4. *Assess reflectiveness.* Is there too much self-preoccupation with a private world at the expense of shared meanings within the child or parent? Is there too much detachment from feelings, in general, in the child or parent? Is the parent unable to gain self-reflective control while in the midst of a conflict situation with a child? Is the parent unable to recognize or admit problematic patterns involving overaccommodation, demandingness, and detachment between him or her and the child? With older children, are the child and parent unable to reflect together following a conflicted event?

5. *Assess for cultural propensities toward responding, directing, or reflecting parenting approaches.* As noted previously, cultural sensitivities often determine the degree of openness toward the positive and negative emotional spectrum. Do the parents believe that children should be primarily nurtured, disciplined, or taught to be stoic? Do the parents believe that some emotions are unacceptable or shameful? Do the parents strongly favor sharing over privacy or vice versa? Do the parents believe that children should not feel negative emotions or should not ever challenge parents? Do parents believe that emotions should be suppressed and that logic and rational thinking should prevail?

Table 9.7 provides an overview of problems that typify narrow or distorted meanings of self and others.

Use regulation strategies. The foundation of accurate meaning-making rests on an early experience of being "seen"—that is, an experience in which the parent accurately and consistently reads the infant's viscerally based cues. Parents can easily misinterpret the meaning of their baby's cues if he or she has a vulnerable nervous system (regulatory disorder). In such a case, it is essential to refer the parents to an infant mental health or early intervention specialist (occupational therapist) for targeted treatment of a regulatory disorder. To experiment with the matching and countering of sensory dimensions for arousal regulation, refer back to Table 5.3.

Regulatory difficulties can be seen as underlying many forms of child and adult psychopathology, especially mood and anxiety irregularities. Although medications at times can serve as an underlying physiological stabilizer that aids other intervention, especially in adults with chronic mood and anxiety disorders, using medication with children remains a controversial topic, and the general rule of thumb is to exhaust all other options first.

Table 9.7. Examples of Narrow or Distorted Meanings of Self and Others in Terms of Behavioral Dimensions

Duration	Intensity	Rhythm
Individual: Based on the infant's enactments or the child or adult's narratives, there is a predominance of narrow or distorted meanings of self and other (e.g., "I should always do it right the first time and so should everybody else"; "When I don't get what I want, it's because others are being mean").	*Individual:* Hyperintense preoccupation with one's internal world (private meanings).	*Individual:* The infant, child or adult rapidly shifts into negative interpretations or assumptions of ill will from others.
	Individual: Hyperintense preoccupations with cues, opinions, or concerns of others.	*Individual:* The infant, child, or adult is slow to understand and interpret the context and emotional meanings of events.
	Dyad: Sharing of distorted meanings (e.g., the folie à deux).	
	Dyad: Parent continually triggers a child's experience of shame, which, over time, may lead to paranoia in the child.	

Use sensory strategies. Parents need to be taught the subtle cues of reading (decoding) the cluster of nonverbal cues (eye contact, facial muscles, tone of voice, gestures and movements) that organize states of arousal. Table 9.8 is an excellent "cheat sheet" that is also available on the CD-ROM, Section 9.4. A parent's simple narration of what he or she observes in the child's body cues can help the child with receptive language skills learn to identify when he or she feels relaxed versus stressed ("Oh, you look so upset. I see that you're frowning and your jaw is tight when I rock you in this way"). This type of narration usually needs to be delivered in a slow vocal rhythm and low-intensity tone of voice; furthermore, it should be short enough in duration to engage but not long enough to lose the child's attention. This type of mirroring allows the child to accurately link up sensory signals with subjective arousal experiences, thereby laying the groundwork for an accurate sense of self.

Similar narrative processes can be used for tracking the sensory aspects of both positive and negative emotional valences. Of course, the

Table 9.8. Possible Regulation and Stress Response Correlates of Interpersonal Modes Across the Life Cycle

Arousal State and Interpersonal Mode	Just Right/Alert Processing	Too Fast/Flooded	Too Slow/Hypoalert	Too Vigilant/Hyperalert
	Stability with Flexibility	High Demand	High Detach	High Compliance or Control
Eye contact	• Bright, shiny eyes looking directly at other/object—gleam! • Gaze aversions for modulation of intensity • Appears to actively process information	• Eyes may be open, squinted, closed • May have direct, in-tense eye contact • May have avoidance of eye contact • Eye rolling upward • Scanning room very quickly, rapidly	• Glazed eyes, looking through rather than at the other/object • Prolonged gaze aversion • Appears drowsy • Eyes turned down • Eyes do not scan the room, looking for objects of desire • When interested, prefers looking at objects rather than people	• Eyes are wide open • Appears vigilant, in a state of panic or fear • Intensely focusing on something • Unable to break the gaze/fixation to the stimulus
Facial expression	• Joy, particularly smiles • Neutral • Can express a full range of emotions • Modulation with all emotions	• Wide open mouth • Anger, disgust • Distress • Grimace • Frowning • Clenched jaw or teeth • Forced smile (only mouth is upturned, corners of eyes are not)	• Flat • Turned down mouth, sad • Expressionless • No smiles or hints of smiles • Limited range of emotions	• Raised eyebrows, especially with inside corners turned up • Trembling lips or mouth • Facial expressions of pain, grimace • Mouth wide open (startle)

Tone of voice	• Melody and prosody • Modulation of tone • Fluctuations of tone • Laughing	• High-pitched cry • Loud • Hostile • Gruff • Yelling or screaming • Sarcastic, sneering • Hysterical laughter	• Flat • Lacks musical quality • Few or no vocalizations • Too quiet • Cold • Soft • Sad	• High-pitched nasal, "sing-song" voice • Moaning or groaning to indicate pain • Elevated tone • Quavers or fluctuates rapidly • Whimpering
Body posture, movement, and gestures	• Relaxed with good muscle tone • Stability • Balance • Moves arms and legs into midline • Coordinated movements • Varies according to rhythmic ups and downs • Body molds into other's	• Finger splays • Arching • Increased muscle tension in posture and in face • Constant motion • Demands space by pushing, shoving, intruding on others • Biting, hitting, kicking, jumping • Poor balance; falls, trips a lot • Bumps into things • Forceful or threatening gestures (shaking finger, shaking fist) • Throwing • Kicking	• Slumped • Low muscle tone • Decreased exploration • Lacks initiative in exploration • Will not protect his or her "space" • Avoids playground equipment • Lacks purposeful intent with movement • Wanders • Frozen or slow moving	• Tense or rigid body postures • Cowering • Rapid, repetitive body movements (wringing hands, jiggling foot) • Trembling hands • Clinging • Flailing • Grabbing
Rhythm and rate	• Fluctuating up and down • Midrange tempo	• Fast • Impulsive	• Slow • Delayed	• Fast • Jerky

Note: This worksheet was created in created in collaboration with Trevor Dobbs.

parent needs to be reading the sensory cues accurately, otherwise the meaning can become a projected meaning from the parent's private world. When meanings are misappraised by parents, the verbal child can provide a correction. However, when parents are unable to tolerate feedback from their children, the dyadic system will move toward a closed level of functioning. In this type of relationship, children will likely either accommodate to parents' "reality" or protest it. If protest is squelched by the parents' rigid directiveness, the child may slip into despair or depression after a period of time (Bowlby, 1969, 1973).

   Use relevance strategies. Practical implementation of the respond, direct, and reflect modes of parenting can be introduced to parents as a 1, 2, 3 system that they can put into practice in their daily home life with their children. (We note that this system involves a blend of relevance and executive capacities.) The gradations from 1 to 3 represent the shifts in progressing from firm parental limits to more engagement and involvement through parent–child negotiation to the child's freedom of choice. Here, directing is emphasized because a top priority in early childhood, for safety purposes, is to teach children to respond immediately to a "no." Children get the significance of the #1 item. In this system, then, the order is as follows:

- 1s: *Nonnegotiable rules*, limits, safety measures, and so on (comparable to implementing the directing mode).
- 2s: *Negotiable items* where needs and wants can be evaluated in relation to options and compromise (comparable to implementing the reflecting mode).
- 3s: *Child's choice*, wherein the child's feelings, wishes, and desires are honored (comparable to implementing the responding mode, especially the mirroring component).

   First, the practitioner helps the family identify which interpersonal mode(s) are most frequently used and to what degree that particular emphasis is useful or problematic. Highly directive parents may need to begin learning responsive or reflective skills (depending on their personal strengths or inclinations); similarly, overly responsive parents may need to learn and hold to directives or reflective skills; overly reflective (detached) parents need to learn to move into responding and directing expressions of emotional warmth and firmness, respectively. The goal is flexibility—that is, parents who are able to move comfortably among these three interpersonal modes in any particular context.

   Many parents disagree on what the 1s, 2s, 3s should be within their family system. When this is the case, parents often need to work with a professional in private discussions, further clarifying their differences and

finding ways to collaborate and compromise. Introducing the 1, 2, 3 system to parents can often naturally segue into an explanation of the three modes of responding, directing, and reflecting. When parents are polarized in this area, it often means that they are protecting (so to speak) one particular mode of parenting. Because all modes are essential, parents can be told that they are both right, and the strengths and weaknesses of each parent can be used more effectively. A parent who is not open to respecting one or more of these modes of parenting should be worked with individually to process his or her cultural differences, discomfort, and resistance to these ways of relating. Optimally, a united parental unit in which both parents agree on the 1, 2, 3 items and can enforce them with their individual and joint behavioral skills provides the best support for a child to develop an integrated sense of self and other. Table 9.9 shows helpful step-by-step sequences for developing respond–direct–reflect skills. The steps in this table can be used in a linear or a nonlinear fashion to assist parents in learning new interpersonal skills that underlie an interpersonal mode that needs to be strengthened.

Use executive strategies. The healthy clashing of demands between parent and child and the beneficial resolution of conflict are necessary precursors for the development of accurate meanings of self and other. The rupture aspect to relationships may need more than responsive skills to repair. Once a pattern of conflict emerges, problem solving may be necessary for repair efforts to change an established pattern. The neurorelational framework promotes problem-solving skills that emphasize the importance of the parent and child identifying their particular unmet needs (which usually underlie the conflict). Acknowledging that each person has a need promotes mutual respect and empathy toward self and other. The reflection sequence presented in Table 9.9 "holds the tension" between what the child wants and what the parent wants and promotes mutual respect and empathy. A co-created process is encouraged throughout each step. These skills can also be used for the negotiable 2s in the 1, 2, 3 system.

SUMMARY POINTS FOR PRACTITIONERS: RELEVANCE

Professionals can review their cases and consider whether any of the behaviors they observe might have contributions from the relevance system using the following points:

- There are historical implicit or explicit memory contributions to this pattern (e.g., child was in and out of the hospital for the first 2 years of life).

Table 9.9. Step-by-Sequences for Developing Responsive, Directive, and Reflective Skills

Type of Skill	Step-by-Step Sequence
Responding skills Comprise the mirroring and empathy skills involved in the "heart" components of responsive listening, which carefully track the range of a child's feelings, wishes, needs, and wants (skills often used for exploring 2s and 3s).	In this simple six-step model, parents are taught to do the following: 1. Listen with full attention. 2. Acknowledge feelings, wants, desires, etc., with a word or phrase ("Oh, uh-huh, I see"). 3. Give feelings, wants, and desires a name ("Sounds like you feel/want/like . . ."). 4. Narrate for the child ("I see that something made you mad. . . I wonder if [this or that] happened . . .") 5. Grant children their wishes in fantasy, for example, "I wish I had the magic power to make this go away (or to make this appear)!" 6. Be aware that although all feelings, wants, desires, and so on, are accepted, some actions may be prohibited.
Directing Skills Constructive directive language requires the parent to carefully modulate his or her nonverbal behaviors so that he or she does not give inconsistent cues to the child. For example, when setting a limit of not running out the front door, the parent would use a stern and firm voice; when setting up a transition for bedtime routines, the parent can use a calm and firm voice. These variations support the "hand" aspects of parenting, where parents take the lead in giving directives and requirements to their children.	The following suggestions require age-appropriate considerations (usually 2-year-olds or older): 1. Ahead of time, parents establish a clear structure and ground rules with their children, deciding what they agree are 1s, 2s, and 3s for their family. Agreement is critical. 2. Ahead of time, parents anticipate behaviors that are problematic and give instructions for expectations and consequences (should be executed when the parent is in a calm and friendly state of mind). 3. The parent begins the directive by stating expectations with a calm but firm tone of voice ("I expect you to brush your teeth in the next 5 minutes"). 4. The parent tells the child whether this directive is a 1, 2, or 3 category. If this is an area of conflict, give the child a choice between two 1s ("Do you want to brush your teeth now or in 5 minutes?" The focus remains on getting the teeth brushed as a nonnegotiable). For younger children (if a time limit is involved), use sensory signals such as a timer that mark the time with visual and auditory cues to signal the transition or directed behavior to occur. 5. Identify the consequences of not abiding by the request ("If you don't get dressed in time for school, you'll miss the bus"). The consequence needs to be logical (supporting cause-and-effect thinking) and as close to the actual time of occurrence as possible; consequences are seen as a natural result of the child's behavior, not as "punishment" per se (Faber & Mazlish, 2002). The consequence has to be something a parent can enforce, and it must match the child's behavior.

6. The parent can offer meaning and mirroring alongside the consequence, as long as they are congruent with his or her affect (e.g., in a calm voice, the parent states, "I love you even though it might not feel that way to you right now. I know you don't want to do this, but this is a No. 1 in our home. Enforcing this consequence doesn't mean that I don't love you").

Reflecting Skills

Once a pattern of conflict emerges, problem-solving may be necessary for repair efforts to change an established pattern. A co-created process is encouraged throughout each step (which can be used in a simplified way with as young as 3-year-olds). These skills can also be used for the "negotiable" 2s in the 1, 2, 3 system. These skills correlate with the "head" aspect of parenting, where flexible problem-solving dynamics in a two-way flow are co-created.

1. Talk about the child's feelings based on what he or she needs. Allow and, if necessary, assist the child to fully describe the need or desire underlying the problematic behavior (e.g., Child: "I don't want to go to the dentist; I'm afraid I'll find out I have cavities"). This step requires active listening–response skills (e.g., Parent: "Hmm, I hear how much you don't want to go to the dentist and you're afraid to find out if you have cavities").

2. Talk about your feelings as a parent based on what you need (e.g., "I need you to go to the dentist because it's important to me that you learn how to take care of your teeth").

3. Mutually brainstorm about how both needs can be met. If possible, let the child take the lead. The parent should model respect for the child's suggestions, no matter how unacceptable they may be to the parent (e.g., Child: "Mommy, I promise to brush my teeth every morning and every night without being told if I don't have to go." Parent: "That's a good idea! My suggestion is that we go to the dentist and find out how well you've been brushing your teeth. Maybe we can do something fun afterward together for your being so brave").

4. Together, identify which ideas each of you is uncomfortable with and which you like (e.g., child agrees to go to the dentist with something to look forward to afterward; child crosses off a suggestion of getting a sticker from the dentist as the "reward"; Mom crosses off having ice cream afterward; both agree to go to the park and play after the appointment).

5. Together, choose the top one or two solutions and set up a plan to follow through (for older children).

6. Check in and repeat process if necessary.

Note. The data in column 2 for responding and reflective skills are adapted from *How To Talk So Kids Will Listen and Listen So Kids Will Talk*, by A. Faber and E. Mazlish, 2002, New York: HarperCollins. Copyright 2002 by Adele Faber and Elaine Mazlish. Adapted with permission from both authors.

- There is a predominance of issues stemming from conditions of threat (e.g., child/parent exposed to domestic violence, child/parent history of abuse or neglect, child/parent history of being in foster care).
- There are issues stemming from a reversal of safety and threat (e.g., a child avoids calm situations and seeks out erratic, chaotic ones).
- There is pervasive anxiety, fear, sadness, or anger present in child or parent (e.g., possible mood disorder).
- The child or parent cannot express and modulate a wide range of emotions.
- The child cannot express a wide range of emotions through symbolic play.
- The parent does not know how to engage in symbolic play with his or her child.
- The child or parent does not have access to both positive and negative memories.
- The child or parent cannot link emotions with causes when asked (e.g., "Why do you look sad today?).
- The child or parent cannot learn from mistakes.
- The child or parent appraises self or others with an imbalance of strengths or limitations.
- Parent rigidly or chaotically uses accommodating, demanding, and detached interpersonal styles with his or her child.

In addition, professionals can make note of the disciplines weighted in this brain system and begin to create professional networks that can be used for referrals, when necessary. Disciplines weighted in the sensory system include the following:

- infant and child mental health professionals;
- adult mental health professionals;
- psychiatrists;
- educational therapists;
- child development specialists.

In terms of intervention, parents can play an important role. In particular, involving them in the following strategies can be beneficial:

- Balance positive and negative choices or consequences (for every *no* there is a *yes*).
- Develop empathic listening skills.

- Assist in modulation of emotions by helping one quantify the intensity level (on a scale of 1 to 10 how strong is this feeling?).
- Scaffolding the building of an emotional muscle across the full range of emotions.
- Help anticipate emotional responses that are difficult with a plan of action and support.
- Build positive emotional experiences as baseline for dealing with traumatic memories.
- Enhance joy within primary relationships, using sensory preferences to support connection.

In addition, all practitioners can consider the following possible strategies for assessment and intervention:

- Support building an emotional muscle.
- Support modulating emotional energy.
- Support building emotional joy in relationships.
- Support an open learning system.

Worksheet 9.2 summarizes the relevance concepts and can be used to assess the relevance system in infants, children, and parents. (This worksheet is also available on the CD-ROM, Section 9.5.)

Next we turn to understanding how the executive system communicates with regulation, sensory, and relevance networks as well as its own contributions to the underlying meaning of behavior.

Worksheet 9.2. Assessment of the Relevance System in the Infant, Child, and Parent

Resources and Strengths Toward Allodynamic Coordination	Risk Factors for Conditions of Allodynamic Load
Check whatever applies to the child and circle what applies to the parent (including those that apply to the parent's developmental history).	*Check whatever applies to the child and circle what applies to the parent (including those that apply to the parent's developmental history).*
☐ Primarily interprets sensory information as safe and pleasurable	☐ Has difficulty finding meaning in relationships
☐ Expresses joy in each significant relationship	☐ Has (or had) multiple caretakers or institutional care
☐ Looks back to see if parent is tracking with his/her eyes when pointing to an object of interest (by 12 months)	☐ Has (or had) experiences involving acute or chronic trauma

(Continued)

Worksheet 9.2. Continued

Resources and Strengths Toward Allodynamic Coordination

- ☐ Able to locate and track visceral and bodily experiences of emotions (butterflies, tight throat)
- ☐ Able to accurately read nonverbal signals in others (notices sad, angry, anxious, happy faces)
- ☐ Able to accurately appraise the intention of others (can tell the difference between an accidental affront and someone angry for a reason)

Range of emotional expressions: how often does the individual show the following emotions and in response to what?

	Not Present	Frequent
Joy	☐	☐
Safety/pleasure	☐	☐
Interest/curiosity	☐	☐
Assertiveness or protectiveness	☐	☐
Protest or aggression	☐	☐
Caution/fear	☐	☐
Sadness or disappointment	☐	☐
Shame or embarrassment	☐	☐
Empathy/love	☐	☐
Limit setting	☐	☐

- ☐ Rewards can be experienced through relationships
- ☐ Rewards can be experienced through inanimate objects such as stickers or toys
- ☐ Modulates the intensity, duration, and rhythm of emotions
- ☐ Shows a capacity to express range of emotions through pretend play and a variety of media such as toys, costumes, and puppets
- ☐ Shows a capacity to find meaning in emotional events and their consequences
- ☐ Can handle making mistakes and learning from them

Risk Factors for Conditions of Allodynamic Load

- ☐ Has (or had) experiences involving acute or chronic neglect
- ☐ Unable to locate or track visceral and bodily experiences of emotions
- ☐ Interprets typical levels of sensory information as a challenge or threat coming from within own body or from others (comments):
  ____
- ☐ Poor reading of others' nonverbal emotional expressions (comments):
  ____
- ☐ Holds negative or fearful appraisals of others (comments):
  ____
- ☐ Behaviors suggest implicit memories of sensory information as a threat (e.g., traumatic events or sudden loss) (comments):
  ____
- ☐ Conveys explicit memories of sensory information as threat (e.g., traumatic events or sudden loss) (comments):
  ____
- ☐ Shows little or no joy in relationships (comments):
  ____
- ☐ Shows a constricted range of nonverbal emotional expression (comments):
  ____
- ☐ Shows a constricted range of verbal emotional expression (comments):
  ____
- ☐ Poorly modulates the intensity, duration, and/or rhythm of emotions (comments):
  ____
- ☐ Unable to or refuses to access safety-based memories or threat-based memories (comments):
  ____
- ☐ Behaviors indicate themes of taking pleasure in violence, destructive acts, or being victimized (comments):
  ____

(*Continued*)

Worksheet 9.2.   Continued

Resources and Strengths Toward Allodynamic Coordination	Risk Factors for Conditions of Allodynamic Load
☐ Parent flexibly uses a range of respond–direct–reflect interpersonal styles that are developmentally appropriate ☐ Older child's or parent's appraisals of self and other show a balanced recognition of strengths and limitations ☐ Can recognize the need for help and can ask for help when needed ☐ Other:_____	☐ Tends to rely on scripted play instead of spontaneous verbal discourse (comments): _____ ☐ Cannot handle mistakes or learn from them ☐ Parent rigidly or chaotically uses accommodating, demanding, or detached interpersonal skills ☐ Older child's or parent's appraisals of self or other show an unbalanced focus on strenghts and limitations ☐ Cannot recognize the need for help and cannot ask for it ☐ Other: _____

10

Functions and Behaviors
of the Executive System

As noted in Chapter 2, *thinking* beings are first and foremost *acting* beings. Similarly, executive functions should be thought of as demonstrated in the context of adaptive and flexible action; they reflect the capacities that emerge in the context of engaging and guiding behavior in the world, or in the context of *doing*. Whereas rational thought and acquired knowledge may be involved in doing, executive functions are not confined to the quality of rational thought, nor are they measured by acquired knowledge and skills. Rather, the quality of executive functions is determined by the optimal fit of behavior to *context* and to *goals*. Good executive functioning is reflected in behaviors that adapt to the demands and opportunities of the context in light of one's goals, and are also flexible enough to shift as circumstances change. Executive functions are adaptive in that they access the past and the future to inform the present, without losing sight of broader implications and goals. They are flexible in that they are responsive to internal needs, emotions, and goals and, at the same time, responsive to external limitations and opportunities posed by others and the environment.

The executive system organizes what to do, how to do it, and when to do it in accordance with the context and goals. For example, when socializing at a party, one is hopefully feeling enjoyment and being spontaneous and not having to work too hard to inhibit inappropriate behavior. When working to meet a deadline, one is hopefully focused and steady rather than constantly wrestling with distractions. When engaged in a collaborative project, one is hopefully strategic and assertive yet able to modulate the intensity and enjoy an occasional laugh or distraction without losing sight of the goal.

Many people are familiar with the phrase "executive functioning" only as it relates to high-level thinking abilities, such as planning, reasoning, and problem solving. Although executive functioning certainly involves these things, it need not always be so challenging or deliberate. For example, searching for pen and paper to jot down a good idea, deciding to take a break to watch a favorite TV show, or taking a friend's call even though you are busy are all somewhat effortless adaptive, flexible, and goal-directed behaviors. As noted, executive functioning is not defined by rote skills and acquired knowledge. In fact, tests of intelligence and academic achievement have low correlations with tests of executive functioning (Delis, Kaplan, & Kramer, 2001; Lezak, 1995). Persons who have suffered a frontal brain injury may have severe deficits in executive functioning, while their intelligence and academic skills remain intact (Lezak, 1995). Similarly, a child may have a high IQ but weak executive abilities, or the reverse. These discrepancies raise serious issues when considering the important decisions that often rest on intelligence and academic test scores in our society.

Because executive functions are ultimately concerned with real-time, real-world behavior, they are intimately connected with motor abilities. Our brains are geared toward interaction with the environment, especially social interaction, and all inter*action* involves movement. Babies' brains develop within a context of engaging their immediate world, and this involves movement (e.g., shifting the eyes to meet gaze, playing in the crib, turning away from the dog's wet tongue). Thus, the very early seeds of executive abilities, such as initiating goal-directed movements and shifting attention, emerge within the context of movement. As motor abilities expand, the child extends his or her "reach" into the world with actions that develop alongside increasingly sophisticated executive abilities (e.g., learning how to negotiate new environments, learning about give-and-take in friendship).

The developmental ingredients that make up the executive system emerge very early and continue to emerge and expand throughout childhood. There is a general hierarchy in terms of developmental processes (e.g., attention span increases with age, complex reasoning emerges later), but so far there is no established sequence of milestones for executive development. Research in developmental neuropsychology and neuroscience provides clues as to which executive abilities emerge early and which emerge later. For example, studies indicate that cortical control over eye movement emerges at around 2 months of age (i.e., smooth pursuit; Aslin, 1981), and by 3.5 months an infant can predict visual events when exposed to visual patterns (i.e., an infant can look ahead to the right location before the stimulus actually appears there; Canfield & Haith, 1991; Haith, Hazen & Goodman, 1988), which implies selective attention or the ability to shift attention. The A-not-B task is the classic test for the emergence

of motor inhibition at around 7 months of age (Diamond, 1985). Simple working memory (i.e., holding information in mind over a brief delay period) emerges at around 5 months of age in the form of recall for one of two locations where an object was hidden (Pelphrey & Reznick, 2002). Joint attention (e.g., when infants follow adults' gaze, use adults' emotional expression to guide action, and use signals to direct adult attention) emerges at around 9 months and is considered a prerequisite for theory of mind (e.g., Carpenter, Nagell, & Tomasello, 1998; Meltzoff, 2002; Moore, 1996; Sodian, 2005).

In addition, test development informs us about the emergence and variability of executive abilities. For example, out of a total of seven subtests that assess components of the attention/executive domain, the NEPSY-II provides normative data for only one test at age 3 (motor inhibition), four tests at age 5, and all seven by age 7 (Korkman, Kirk, & Kemp, 2007). There are probably fewer tests available for attention and executive abilities at younger ages than for any other cognitive domain tested, which is primarily related to two issues. First, there is less clarity in terms of agreed-on rubrics and methods for objectively defining and eliciting separate aspects of executive functions than for other cognitive domains (validity). Second, it is more difficult to achieve the reliability standards for a good test with young children in this arena. Most attribute these challenges to the developmental variability within and across children for any specific executive function. The challenge is also likely related to the fact that tests of executive function must necessarily overlap with abilities in other domains (e.g., motor skills, receptive language, visual scanning), which introduces another source of variance in performance.[1] Thus, in early childhood, the research provides guidelines as to what to expect at what age in terms of the basic developmental ingredients of higher-order executive functions. Tests that directly assess aspects of executive function begin at age 3 and approximate the options for adult assessment by about age 8.

Two cognitive abilities, *working memory* and *processing speed*, are important to note here because they support not just executive development but arguably all cognitive development. At a basic level, working memory refers to the ability to hold information in mind; at a more complex level, it involves both holding in mind and manipulating information while working toward a goal. Working memory has been described as the foundation for control of behavior because it allows children to bring to mind and consider things/events that are not present in the here and now (e.g., Barkley 1997; Davidson, Amso, Anderson, & Diamond, 2006; Mesulam, 2002). Mesulam refers to working memory as "one of the most distinctive specializations of prefrontal cortex" (2002, p. 15) and points out that it

supports a broad range of activities "from keeping a telephone number in mind to considering alternative facets of a moral dilemma" (2002, p. 16). Processing speed refers to the amount of time it takes to adequately absorb or demonstrate a skill or behavior (i.e., efficiency). Speed of processing is important to consider in the context of working memory because slow speed (i.e., when more time is needed to absorb, learn, or demonstrate an ability adequately) places additional demand on working memory and limits other potential processes. For example, when reading, by the time a child reaches the end of a sentence what was read at the beginning is lost. In addition, the longer it takes for a child to complete a mental or physical task, the less available he or she will be to self-monitor, take in feedback, or adjust an approach.

The significant advantage to understanding the multiple facets of the executive system is that they inform nearly all developmental tasks and presenting problems and are relevant to all disciplines. If a delay or a presenting problem involves top-down control, or can be aided by using top-down control, then having a better understanding of executive processes becomes immediately valuable.

When Susan first contacted me (JT) by phone about her son, Mark, she had a very difficult time relating their story. She was anxious, flustered, spoke rapidly, and jumped from one topic to another. She seemed relieved when I interrupted her to take charge of the conversation by asking questions. Mark was just beginning the second grade at a local public school. His current teacher suggested to Susan that it would have been better to hold Mark back and have him repeat the first grade—and that this might still be an option. Susan and her husband, Jerry, were alarmed. They had no idea his delays were this serious. The school district had tested him halfway through the first grade and decided to provide resource support in math for 45 minutes a day. The parents were told that Mark's other academic skills, although not strong, were within the expected range. Susan and Jerry, though alarmed at this report, were also relieved because they felt that Mark's reading and writing skills were way behind what other children his age seemed to be doing.

Susan went on to report that toward the end of the first grade, Mark became increasingly obstinate about doing his homework. He seemed unable to read the books he was assigned and became frustrated quickly with any homework that involved using a pencil, whether it was math or writing. Susan's good intentions to help him always ended up in disaster with Mark screaming and crying, stubbornly refusing to finish, and with Susan imposing consequences and often losing her temper, as well. Jerry was a stay-at-home dad who ran a computer consulting business from his home office. He seemed to have more success in the helping role with Mark, but homework still took far longer than it should and Mark still often broke down in tears. This year, things were already beginning to escalate and Susan feared the same scenario was about to unfold.

Susan felt much more uncomfortable talking about Mark's behavioral issues. She responded honestly to direct questions but had to be asked to elaborate. Her anxiety clearly mounted as the details of Mark's rages slowly emerged. The first serious incident occurred in kindergarten. Some of the kids were bullying Mark, calling him names, and goading him to do things that would get him into trouble. Susan stated that Mark was very innocent and socially naive, so he was slow to catch on that he was a target for teasing and that these boys were not really his friends. One boy in particular frequently coerced Mark to throw balls at other children, initially promising to be his friend if he did, and then later threatening to beat him up if he didn't. At some point, Mark finally caught on and told his parents and teacher what was happening. His teacher took the bullying seriously, talked to the other boy and his parents, and offered support and empathy to Mark. Unfortunately, soon after, this boy managed to corner Mark on the playground and taunted him, repeatedly calling him a tattle-tale. Mark "apparently just lost it." The other children were screaming wildly as the teacher arrived on the scene to find Mark sitting atop this boy, choking him.

Even before this, Mark did not have many friends. Susan found herself initiating all of the play dates but had chalked this up to other parents' busy schedules. When he had play dates, it was not uncommon for them to end badly because of some disagreement, and with Mark pronouncing, "I hate him and never want to see him again!" However, Mark would soon forget his upset and want another play date, so Susan surmised this as "typical boy" behavior. It was only after she began to have trouble arranging play dates that she started to suspect that these little squabbles might not be so typical.

Another alarming outburst occurred toward the end of last year. Mark raised his hand to give an answer and when the teacher did not call on him, he abruptly jumped up, screamed in protest, forcefully turned over his desk, and ran from the classroom. The intensity of this incident was deeply upsetting for the teacher and the other students, and especially for Mark. Although he never stated it openly, Susan knew he was devastated and humiliated. Soon after, he began complaining that his teacher was "mean" and that other children were mean to him. Between this disturbing episode and the difficulties the parents were having around homework, school was clearly becoming more than just challenging and stressful for Mark—it was severely threatening. Mark had become so dark and unhappy, Susan and Jerry hoped that the summer would bring calm and happiness back into his life. They initially tried to incorporate some learning games into the summer routine, but Mark protested so severely that they decided it wasn't worth it and let it go.

But here it was, only 3 weeks into a new school year, and Susan had already received two calls from the school. The teacher was concerned about his behavior in the classroom and on the playground. She stated that he was daydreaming, not paying attention in class, and not responding to her prompts. She also stated that Mark seemed sullen and touchy and was not engaging with the other children. The teacher's calls were motivated by Mark's sudden explosions into angry outbursts toward her or one of the children. The outbursts were triggered by

something that seemed to the teacher to be benign or clearly accidental, but Mark would insist that it was done on purpose. Susan admitted that this type of behavior was not a surprise to her. Mark had exhibited this same behavior at home—the insistence that something was done on purpose or that it was directed specifically toward him when it was not. However, she had always assumed that he was "just trying to push our buttons" and "trying to manipulate us." She had not seriously considered until very recently that he actually believed that his parents were purposefully trying to hurt him. Mark was also beginning to protest going to school. At this point, Susan was extremely worried and confused and she pressed for immediate answers. Despite being told that it was far too soon for conclusions and that I would not speculate, she could not take this in and asked repeatedly what the problem might be and what the treatment might be.

After this initial phone contact, Mark's refusals to go to school escalated. At first, he claimed to be sick with a headache, stomachache, or cold, but when that ran its course, he began declaring, "I'm not going to school and no one can make me!" Mark refused to get out of bed or to get dressed and was not swayed by any reward or negative consequence. At my first meeting with both parents, Mark had refused school for the prior 3 days. The parents had notified the school about what was happening and arranged a meeting to brainstorm what to do. During this meeting, I learned more about Mark's history. He was described as a very rambunctious child who was easily excited. As soon as he could crawl, there were frequent accidents where he clumsily slammed into things, tripped, or fell down. He often misgauged his proximity and force with people and objects. He was described as "always happy" and "never went through the terrible twos." However, at age 3, his moods became "dark" at times, which the parents described as "turning into Chucky." When disappointed or upset from natural consequences that had nothing to do with the parents, he would scream and accuse them of causing the unwanted occurrence on purpose. He had occasionally, but not often, thrown things when upset. When Jerry saw it coming, he was able to playfully distract Mark or come up with other creative ways to help him stay out of this angry place. Susan took a more authoritarian approach that inevitably escalated Mark's reactions. When Jerry was home, she backed off and let him handle everything. The different parenting styles created obvious tension, yet there was still a clear sense of mutual respect between them. Despite knowing that Jerry's approach was best, Susan resented how Mark controlled things with his temper and felt he got away with far too much. She also admitted feeling afraid that Mark might become violent toward her.

By the time our first scheduled testing date arrived, Mark had been out of school for three weeks. The school district provided a home tutor, but this plan failed within two weeks. The tutor saw Mark as very capable and prompted him to continue when he complained that he was tired or that the work was too hard. As soon as the tutor left, Mark would explode, stating angrily how "awful" and "mean" the tutor was to him. Just before the tutor arrived, Mark began to complain of illness; he would hide under the bed and refuse to come out. Two days in a row, just prior to the tutor's arrival, Mark had bolted from the house and ran

without stopping. Because these incidents were not only alarming but also dangerous, Susan and Jerry discontinued the tutoring.

Given this history, it was clear that testing with Mark would need to proceed cautiously and I was quite certain that a standardized administration would not be possible. I could easily trigger the same pattern—that I was trying to hurt him "on purpose"—and he might shut down and refuse to participate, or bolt from my office. The parents warned me that Mark was not easy to read, that he may present as okay but then fall apart later. I decided to do whatever possible to create an experience of safety for him during the initial session. The parents and I brainstormed the potential triggers and preferences and planned carefully. We decided that success would be most likely if Jerry, the parent with whom Mark seemed the most comfortable, remained in the room during our sessions. Jerry suggested that he bring along a game that he and Mark enjoyed playing together at home, letting Mark know that they could play the game during breaks. We decided to keep the first session fairly brief, to 90 minutes. I told Jerry that I would take a slow approach, always let Mark know what was coming next, and give him plenty of opportunity to ask questions. I also told Jerry that I would look to him to alert me to Mark's signals of distress, in case I missed them and, if needed, I would find a reason to excuse myself and give Jerry a chance to calm him before things escalated. The parents decided to refer to the testing sessions as "special time with Dad" but also to be very clear about what was expected of him.

As expected, Mark presented as apprehensive and sullen. At the same time, he clearly trusted his dad and wanted to please him. My challenge was to achieve a relational blend that was weighted toward responsiveness but with enough of a directive style to give him structure and clarity as to what was expected of him. Our planning paid off. The first session went as well as we could have hoped. Most of our time together was spent in play and light-hearted conversation with his dad providing a lot of prompts to help him along. With the little testing that was done, Mark was given a lot of control. He was allowed to opt out of a task if it looked too hard, and allowed to quit a task whenever he chose. I encouraged Mark to let me know by either choosing a feelings sticker (stickers with various facial expressions) that best matched his feelings, or pointing to a place on a thermometer to show me how difficult a task was. We agreed together that if he pointed to the "hysterical" face or the "10" on the thermometer, we would stop. His dad assured him that it was "completely fine" and "no big deal" for him to opt out, and Mark was clearly comforted by his reassurance. He was anxious and opted out almost immediately with the first two tasks, and then found a task he could tolerate. I titrated the degree of challenge by using tests I thought he could handle and that could be broken down into small chunks. I monitored for signals of distress, such as his tone of voice, slouching posture, rubbing his eyes, and sighs. We got through the session with only one near escalation, which Jerry handled well. Surprisingly, when we were done for the day, he asked if he could try one of the tasks he had earlier declined. The approach, along with ample praise and being told that he was exceeding expectation, was actually quite effective, and we were able to complete most tasks that we started.

During a phone conversation with the parents after the initial session, I learned that Mark had a meltdown after he left. However, they said that it felt like more of an "anxious release" than a "real tantrum." Even though he called me "mean," he did not resist when he was reminded later that he would return. Given the degree of Mark's anxiety, we decided to allow him to bring his dog to his testing sessions. The dog was old and slow and had a calming effect on him.

THE FUNCTION OF THE EXECUTIVE SYSTEM

In many respects, the executive system reflects a convergence of the other brain systems. We are now concerned with how the regulatory, sensory, and relevance capacities are organized and expressed in behavior relative to changing contexts across time. What is the nature of the thought patterns, emotional patterns, and action patterns that have formed? How do these patterns influence the pursuit of goals? How do these patterns influence perceptions of self and its continued development? How do these patterns feed into the co-created patterns within the dyad? Thus, although the executive system has a unique set of abilities that must be considered in assessment and treatment, these abilities converge with those presented in other brain systems. In this section, we provide descriptions of the many facets of the executive system. We address an array of executive abilities and their potential implications for enhancing coordination or contributing to load across tasks and settings.

Executive Capacities

This chapter explores three large domains within the executive system in relation to the following three capacities:

- the capacity to express spontaneous, automatic, and consciously controlled behaviors in a flexible and purposeful manner;
- the capacity to integrate the bottom-up influences of emotions with the top-down contribution of thoughts;
- the capacity to assess, integrate, and prioritize internal (self) needs in relation to external (context/other) needs.

Capacity 1: The Capacity to Express Spontaneous, Automatic, and Consciously Controlled Behaviors

The functioning of the executive system, conceptualized broadly, can be thought of in terms of three fundamental behavioral formats: spontaneous,

automatic, and consciously controlled behaviors. Assessing a child's behavior according to these formats, although broad, provides numerous
insights into the potential breakdowns that may occur at a more fundamental level of the executive system, insights that may also help define
problems within the other two capacities. For example, a child with an
overreliance on the automatic format (and thus less reliance on spontaneous and conscious control) may potentially have a fundamental weakness
in his or her ability to shift attention and behavior, thereby remaining
stuck in a narrow range of preferences and activities and leading to what
appears to others as rigidity and self-absorption.

The *spontaneous format* is reflected in a free flow of activity, thought,
and emotion. In this mode, one is more likely to be creative, energetic,
novelty-seeking, and impulsive. The mention of impulsivity in this context suggests resilience. According to Eisenberg et al. (2004), resilience involves some impulsivity, including the tendency to approach people and
situations, which is reflected in spontaneity. One is also more likely to
absorb external information and be open to experiencing a variety of
emotions and considering a variety of options. The spontaneous mode
does not lack structure entirely, but the structure is flexible and loose. The
spontaneous mode captures distinctive features (e.g., playfulness, curiosity) of the executive system that are often neglected, yet key to positive
affect. This format is likened to one of Mesulam's core functions of the
prefrontal cortex: "the active pursuit of choice and novelty" (2000a,
2000b), and also similar to Polak-Toste and Gunnar's (2006) construct of
exuberance. The spontaneous format supports positive emotions, such as
amusement, playfulness, and surprise, and lends to enhanced flexibility.

The *automatic format* is reflected in overlearned activities, routine
thoughts, and modulated emotions. It occurs when one is familiar enough
with a routine or process that it can be carried out without exerting a lot of
mental effort but, at the same time, still requires some effort to sustain focus
and to inhibit distraction. In this format, one is more likely to be steady, predictable, and productive and engage in routines, carry out decisions, and
complete tasks. One is less likely to absorb external information or to be
open to novelty and options. The concept of automaticity, discussed in the
sensory system, is a corollary because once an efficient routine is established,
fewer problem-solving resources are required. Thus, the automatic format
supports efficiency and expertise as well as positive emotions, such as
confidence, pride, and the comfort that comes from known pleasures.

The *conscious control format* is reflected in an effortful focus of activity, thought, and emotion. It involves accessing spontaneous and automatic formats as needed (i.e., a mix of structured, goal-focused activity
alongside an openness to novel solutions and risks) without giving in to the

extremes of distraction or perseveration. In the context of resiliency, Block and Kremen noted that "the human goal is to be as undercontrolled as possible and as overcontrolled as necessary. When one is more undercontrolled than is adaptively effective or more overcontrolled than is adaptively required, one is not resilient" (1996, p. 351). In this mode, one is more likely to draw on a broad range of information, memories, and emotions; use a broad range of executive abilities to consider cause and effect; and take a part-whole perspective. This format includes the ability to access thought processes and emotions but without becoming immersed in them; conversely, conscious control should be able to "take over" abruptly. For example, socializing at a party, someone makes a political statement that you find repugnant. In a flash, conscious control takes the helm. Not only do you resist the impulse to blurt out a retort, you manage to maintain a pleasant expression. Such impressive restraint requires effort, and studies indicate that it also comes at a cost. In a review of the relevant research, Muraven and Baumeister (2000) concluded that the resources required for such efforts at self-control are actually limited and subject to depletion. The authors liken self-control to a muscle and assert that things like coping with stress, regulating negative affect, and resisting temptations all weaken the muscle and make subsequent attempts at self-control during that immediate time period more likely to fail (Muraven & Baumeister, 2000).

To maintain adaptive and flexible behavior, conscious control requires monitoring the outcome of actions as well. When all goes well, conscious control is not needed. However, despite our best efforts, outcomes do not always go as predicted, and to do better in the future, it is important to detect errors (i.e., mismatches between the expected goal and the actual outcome have to be registered). Humans are quite naturally adept at error detection. Prediction of outcome and monitoring expectancies are wired in to the brain's processing from the simplest motor acts up through the highest levels of reasoning (Rotman, Troje, Johansson, & Flanagan, 2006; Schubotz, 2007; Wolpert & Flanagan, 2001). Those occurrences that do not match what we predicted, expected, or "thought" we knew grab our attention, a function referred to as conflict monitoring (Botvinick, Braver, Barch, Carter, & Cohen, 2001; Carter et al., 1998).

In a study that investigated the impact of unexpected similarities and differences (i.e., learning two things presumed similar were actually different, and vice versa), participants indicated greater surprise when the unexpected revealed a difference versus a similarity, and differences also had greater emotional impact than similarities (Olson & Janes, 2002). In a study of the effect of feedback on learning, it was found that the participants

best recalled information that contradicted what they thought they knew. In other words, when students were asked to rate how confident they were that individual test questions were answered correctly, those rated with highest confidence, yet incorrect, were more likely to be recalled correctly on subsequent testing (Butterfield & Metcalfe, 2001). Thus, conscious control is activated by detection of a mismatch, which suggests that conscious control, at least in some respects, depends on how well one is able to detect conflict between expectation and actual outcome. This raises the possibility that some children who seem to lack conscious control may simply be unaware of the mismatch.

Capacity 2: The Capacity to Integrate the Bottom-Up Influences of Emotions with the Top-Down Control of Thoughts

Executive abilities are needed to achieve a balanced flow of thought and emotion. This capacity spots the emotional muscle with top-down strategies to predict, modulate, and respond to emotions. Using this capacity, children begin to learn what facilitates positive emotions and what triggers negative ones. They learn ways to modulate emotions in the moment, such as by inhibiting the impulse to hit when angry or by shifting attention when something funny tempts them to joke around during class. They learn to better predict emotional outcomes, plan ahead, and view an emotional incident as a problem to solve. Zelazo and Müller (2002) postulated two routes to decision making, called "cool EF" (EF stands for executive functioning) and "hot EF." The cool component represents the more rational path to decision making, whereas the hot component, as you may have guessed, represents the more emotional/visceral path to decisions. An example of the latter might be taking the call of a friend in distress when it is not convenient even though you could stand on solid ground, logically speaking, by deciding to finish what you are doing and call him or her back later. In the Cartesian tradition, the hot route has been relegated a lowly status, whereas the cool route has been exalted. But for several years, this tide has been shifting (e.g., see Damasio, 1994) as studies nudge us toward a paradigm shift where emotions hold great value in our thinking about thinking. Ultimately, this capacity lays the groundwork for fulfilling relationships, ethical judgments, and altruistic values in adulthood.

We specify two executive abilities that are needed to achieve a balanced flow of thought and emotion: cause–effect associations and temporal integration. *Cause–effect associations* provide the reasons for events. Some cause–effect associations are universal to all (e.g., I bumped the glass off the table and gravity took over; the cookies are gone because I ate them), and some are specific to an individual's context (e.g., the joke I made hurt

my husband's feelings). In this context, the latter category of cause–effect associations is crucial to one's ability to predict both personal and social outcomes and more fully realize both personal and social potentials. *Temporal integration*, a term borrowed from Joaquin Fuster (2002), involves a process of "mediation of cross-temporal contingencies between the action plan, the goal, and the acts leading to the goal" (p. 96). We use the term to convey a process of "mental time travel" that allows us to consider selective features of past, present, and future as a loose collective with interchangeable parts. Through *hindsight*, one can review the past cause–effect scenarios that are important to the current situation or goal. *Insight* involves knowing oneself—being aware of one's actions, thoughts, and feelings in the moment and being able to self-correct or modify behavior in the moment. *Foresight* involves using hindsight and insight to anticipate needs, resources, and likely outcomes as well as to rehearse alternatives. Having a flexible ability to shift between these various temporal perspectives allows one to better blend information from emotional and thinking levels and sharpen preparatory sets. As noted in the introduction to this chapter, these executive abilities may be constrained or facilitated by the limits of working memory. At about age 3, young children are able to passively hold two items of information (Hulme, Thomson, Muir & Lawrence, 1984) but are not able to actively manipulate those two items until around 4–5 years of age (Carlson, 2005).

Capacity 3: The Capacity to Assess, Integrate, and Prioritize Internal (Self) Needs in Relation to External (Context/Other) Needs

This third capacity supports a balanced accommodation of self needs in relation to others and the context. Using this capacity, a child or adult can pursue personal interests and enjoy relationships and at the same time meet personal obligations and respect the needs of others. To reach personal goals, one must be able to sequence a plan of how to get there, monitor progress against predictions, and come up with a new strategy when something is not working (i.e., problem-solve). One is usually better off if he or she knows how to make use of strengths, avoid or compensate for weaknesses, and accurately gauge available resources and limitations. To establish healthy relationships, one must be able to respect the desires and goals of both the self and the other, without allowing the self or other to dominate consistently. This means one must be aware of the social rules and expectations in a particular context, recognize the impact of one's behavior on others, take another's perspective, and consider others' feelings.

We specify two executive abilities that are needed to achieve a balanced accommodation of self and other/contextual needs: theory of mind and part–whole reasoning. In keeping with Goleman's idea of "catching" the feelings of another to describe empathy (Goleman, 2006a), *theory of mind* reflects the ability to "catch" the perspective of another, as well as consider the implications of that perspective. As originally defined (Premack & Woodruff, 1978), theory of mind enables one to understand that others have mental states and intentions that are different from one's own and to understand that these states and intentions can be the cause of behavior. Thus, theory of mind helps us understand and predict others' behavior. With this ability, children are better equipped to read social cues, develop social connections, and consider social values. When children show concern for others, they are likely to have more positive interactions, receive more positive attention from others, and have more positive feelings about themselves. They are also more likely to handle negative feelings in more socially appropriate ways, learn more about the needs of others, rely more on others, and have more social resources.

Part–whole reasoning expands the shift of perspective between self and other to include shifts of perspective among the features of the context. This ability may include focusing on the sequence of details or stepping back to see the big picture; attending to the verbatim communication or absorbing the gist; and focusing on the present content or seeing the present as one small part of an ongoing process.

When negotiating the appropriate balance of self and other/context, the components of temporal integration also come into play. For example, pursuing an interest or goal is more effective if the child knows his or her strengths and weaknesses (insight—"I'm good at playing one-on-one basketball but not good at hitting a baseball"), attending to the relevant aspects of past events (hindsight—"Last time when we played basketball and I won, I felt good, but my friend was sad"), and predicting the implications of potential actions and plans (foresight—"Maybe my friend and I should play baseball first today"). This example also involves holding in mind multiple pieces of information (e.g., one's strengths and limitations, a friend's strengths) in relation to the larger context (e.g., the historical context). In this way, part–whole reasoning is critical to making good decisions about what to prioritize between oneself and others or oneself and goals.

Physiological Underpinnings of the Executive System

The brain is often organized functionally into right and left divisions (right hemisphere = visual–spatial; left hemisphere = language), lower and higher

divisions (subcortical = primitive functions; cortical = advanced functions), and back and front divisions. In this last organization, the back/posterior regions mediate "incoming" information (sensory), and the front/anterior regions mediate "outgoing" information (actions, intentions). Motor is thus integrated within the executive system because flexible, adaptive, goal-oriented behavior is integrated within this outgoing movement.

Executive functions are associated with the frontal regions of the brain, or frontal lobes. The posterior frontal regions contain motor structures: the primary motor area controls large motor, the "hand area" coordinates fine motor, the frontal eye fields direct ocular motor, and Broca's area controls oral–motor (speech). "Lower" motor regions, such as the cerebellum and the basal ganglia, which are densely connected to higher motor regions, mediate the learning of rules, patterns, and motor programs. The anterior frontal regions, or prefrontal cortex (PFC), receive integrated sensory information from both internal and external sensory sources with reciprocal feedback connections. The dorsal-lateral (top-side) regions are associated with reasoned thought/action and the external world (e.g., the rational cool EF, the environmental or social context), and the ventral-medial (bottom-middle) regions are associated with emotional thinking/action and the internal world (e.g., the emotional hot EF, personal context) (Happaney, Zelazo, & Stuss, 2004; Rolls, 2002; Tranel, 2002). The prefrontal regions are associated with higher-level executive functions such as planning and creativity (Delis et al., 2007; Lezak, 1995), as well as adaptive behavior in real time (Clark, 1997).

The brain's decline in energy use as motor learning progresses provides a good example of the adaptive advantage of the automatic format of behavior. When an action sequence is novel, the period of active learning recruits multiple brain regions, including prefrontal areas. As the action sequence approximates a rote skill, brain activity becomes more streamlined along specific pathways. We have discussed this same principle with respect to automaticity in the sensory system; when a new skill is overlearned, less brain energy is consumed when performing that skill. This helps us understand why a child with a reading disorder may have trouble sustaining the effort required to finish a reading assignment. This child's brain is expending a lot more effort, and as we saw in the review of social inhibition studies, brain effort often comes at a cost.

More broadly, conscious control formats selectively activate a large number of brain regions and pathways to support behaviors that are ultimately most adaptive and efficient for the long term. Once decisions are made or plans are in place, less brain activation is typically needed to reach the goal, which is why the process of developing a good plan often

feels more taxing and mentally fatiguing than actually carrying it out. We think of this capacity as "expanding" into wisdom. Similar to the efficiency that comes with automaticity, wisdom is supported by the brain's capacity to selectively learn and preserve in memory those components involved in not only success but also failure. Wisdom informs when the energy demands of conscious control are truly needed.

All behaviors are supported and mediated by attention. Attention plays a role in the "selective and orderly activation" (Fuster, 2002, p. 100) of cortical networks. Three different aspects of attention recruit different prefrontal regions: (1) motivational drive recruits the anterior cingulate regions; (2) inhibition and the screening out of distraction recruit orbital regions; and (3) attentional focus (orienting, selecting) recruits lateral regions (Fuster, 2002). The cingulate region is also associated with error monitoring or conflict monitoring, which was mentioned as the ability to detect a mismatch between expected and actual outcome. In two similar studies (Carter & van Veen, 2007; van Veen & Carter, 2002), the authors concluded that "the anterior cingulate cortex (ACC) contributes to cognition by detecting the presence of conflict during information processing, and to alert systems involved in top-down control to resolve this conflict" (van Veen & Carter, 2002, p. 477). These researchers also discuss how certain mental disorders (e.g., obsessive-compulsive disorder) may be related to these performance monitoring functions of the ACC. In another study, it was found that the conflict-related activity of the ACC predicted both greater prefrontal cortex activity and subsequent adjustments in behavior (Kerns et al., 2004), which supports the important role of error detection in the engagement of cognitive control. Posner and Rothbart (2002) found that activation in ACC regions corresponded to both conscious control of mental events and automatic activation of those same events. Furthermore, they found that it was possible to separate brain activation related to conscious control from the brain activation related to automatic processes.

Activation and Inhibition

In the executive system, a broad and flexible range of activation–inhibition patterns are necessary to support adaptive behaviors in real time. Four core functions of the executive system—the ability to initiate, shift, sustain, and inhibit action—begin to organize the potential variations in autonomic patterns. The first two core functions, initiate and shift, are more associated with activation, whereas the latter functions, sustain and inhibit, are more associated with inhibition.

Initiation promotes the child's active engagement with others and with the environment. In addition, it supports activities crucial to development, from speech and walking to conversation and exploration. These examples are all observable, and initiation may also promote invisible mental or emotional activity. It is the foundation for pursuing interests, risk-taking, discovery, and creativity. *Shifting* reflects a change or an adjustment in attention, action, thought, or emotion that again may or may not be observable to others. Shifting often serves a modulatory role because it supports ongoing adjustments relative to error detection or changing circumstances. Shifting supports a child's ability to take another's perspective, take on a new challenge, go inside when recess is over, track the conversation in a group, and figure out how to solve a problem. These two executive functions involve activation and correspond with the spontaneous behavior format.

Sustaining is linked to vigilance, persistence, and the maintenance of adequate resources. To develop abilities and relationships, a child must be able to sustain purposeful action, thought, or emotion long enough to reach a goal, which sometimes can be for prolonged periods. The amount of activation needed to sustain depends on the degree of challenge involved in the activity relative to the resources of the child. For example, in the relevance system, we discussed how the ability to sustain focus when involved in a high-level learning challenge was dependent on the context. The child who believes that he or she is capable and anticipates a feeling of pride will have far greater resources to sustain him or her through to the end than the child with low self-esteem and anticipation of failure. *Inhibition* is crucial for a child's social and emotional development (discussed later). It reflects the ability to resist impulses and stop behavior at the appropriate time. Like shifting, inhibition also often serves a modulatory function, especially for prosocial behaviors. Inhibition is required to modulate intense emotions, resist provocative but unwise options, delay gratification, and resist responding in the same ineffective way. These two executive functions involve inhibition and correspond with the automatic behavioral format.

In the conscious mode, a dynamic mix of these core functions (i.e., initiate, shift, sustain, and inhibit), with their varying blends of activation and inhibition, is required, depending on the goal or challenge and what is most adaptive given the circumstances. For example, a study by von Hippel and Gonsalkorale (2005) administered a test of cognitive inhibition to participants and then offered a rather disgusting meal (a chicken foot) to some, under conditions of social pressure to pretend that the food was actually appealing. The researchers found that better performance on the inhibition task predicted the degree to which participants

were successful at restraining a negative response. Like the cocktail party scenario, this is an example of the rapid recruitment of conscious control. Much of the time, the need for conscious control is interlaced within each person's unique life circumstances, some brief and some enduring. For example, a child with a learning disability must continually adjust to the changing demands that arise with each new assignment and each grade level, but at the same time, the themes that define the enduring dynamics of the experience become more familiar, more practiced, and even mastered. For this child, the degree of prolonged conscious control has been streamlined to a set of efficient strategies, and the meanings that evolved gradually made room for a more adaptive sense of uniqueness and pride.

Table 10.1 provides examples of executive abilities associated with activation and inhibition.

Self- and Interactive Regulation

The top-down abilities that support the three executive capacities are all involved in self-regulation. Thus, self-regulation is supported by having insight into one's own triggers/preferences and personal weaknesses/strengths, the ability to use past experience to inform present activities

Table 10.1.   Examples of Executive Abilities Associated with Activation and Inhibition

	Spontaneous	Automatic	Conscious
Activation			
Initiate	Exploration, creativity	Selecting and engaging a routine	Goal setting, planning
Shift	Novelty-seeking novel associations	Sequencing; changing routine/strategy when necessary	Strategizing, problem solving
Inhibition			
Sustain	Stick with one creative endeavor	Sticking with a routine to completion; resisting distraction	Weighing the relevant factors; prioritizing self and other needs
Inhibit	Suppression of excess activation according to context	Delaying gratification; impulse control	Resisting impulse reactions when inappropriate to context; resisting impulse decisions

and predict future outcomes, and the ability to consider and respect one's own needs alongside those of the other. In the executive system, maintaining optimal regulation requires the ability to express the format of behavior that is most adaptive, given the context, and to flexibly shift as the context changes. Allowing each behavioral format to fluctuate between foreground and background, depending on the context, is a marker for healthy self-regulation from an executive system perspective.

A crucial developmental aspect of self-regulation in the executive system is the ability to shift from external control (i.e., interactive regulation from the parent) to internal control (i.e., self-regulation via, e.g., gaze aversion, turning of the head, walking away, and verbalizing distress) (Kopp, 1982; Rothbart, Ziale, & O'Boyle, 1992). Individual differences in these abilities, noticeable even in infancy, likely reflect the interactive effect of physiology and the child's primary relationships (Gralinski & Kopp, 1993; Holden & West, 1989; Manian, Strauman, & Denney, 1998). Beginning control over self-regulatory behaviors emerges by the end of the first year, with further development in the second and third years of life (Gralinski & Kopp, 1993; Kaler & Kopp, 1990). An older child is better able to maintain self-regulation when he or she is mindful of the social context and others' expectations, has personal goals and activities that are interesting, and has a sense of the amount of time and effort that will be required to achieve them. For example, if a child is aware that she has to clean up her toys before leaving for a family event, she can enjoy her spontaneous play, shift into clean-up mode (i.e., inhibit the desire to continue playing and initiate a different behavior) with her mother's reminder, begin to get excited as she thinks about seeing her cousin, and leave the house on time and happy.

The parent's executive system is necessary for interactive regulation. Parents rightly assume a lack of executive abilities in the infant, but more are expected as the child develops. For example, when a child is first potty trained, the parent anticipates the child's needs and gives a prompt such as, "You need to go potty now because we'll be in the car for a while." With time, the parent shifts to a reminder, "Do you need to use the bathroom before we go?" Eventually, there is a solid expectation that the child has the executive ability to anticipate this need independently. "You should have thought about that before we left!" might be the exasperated response of a parent whose old-enough child left the house without using the bathroom. In normative circumstances, parents can do a lot to encourage strong development of a child's executive capacities. For example, with the first capacity, a parent can encourage a healthy balance of spontaneous (e.g., "Let's go to the park"), automatic (e.g., "You need to finish now"), and conscious formats (e.g., "I'll try harder to listen. What will you try to do differently?").

When a child has a disorder, the challenge to the parent's executive system is far greater. In this situation, parents often need help in developing and strengthening their own executive skills above and beyond what is typically required for good parenting. These children will inevitably need help in maintaining an alert processing state, and the parent's temporal integration skills are crucial to this process. For professionals (and the parent), hindsight involves reviewing the child's history of stress responses and teasing out the cause–effect relationships; insight helps professionals identify how the parents' behaviors are disrupting or supporting regulation; and foresight allows parents to learn to anticipate the potential for a stress response and to plan and troubleshoot to prevent them.

Some parents tend to provide too much support, especially when their children have significant difficulties. The titration principle discussed in the sensory system applies here as well. It is important that parents find the right balance among pulling back, scaffolding, and stepping in. A parent who shifts into an automatic format and sequences through the daily routines while doing everything for the child is not allowing enough challenge to prod development of the child's top-down control. The optimal zone of titration is that of maximizing challenge (i.e., working the "executive muscle") without losing alert processing or resources for self-control. However, we do not intend to imply that pulling back completely is the ultimate goal. In fact, executive challenges that are undertaken collaboratively can work the executive muscle in ways that independent work cannot.

For example, in a recent study on problem solving, participants either worked alone, worked alone while being videotaped with the opportunity to observe themselves later, or worked with a partner (shifting every 20 seconds from observing the partner to being observed). The results showed that role exchange between *doing* and then *observing* a partner (i.e., the observational and collaborative approaches) had a facilitative effect on insight-based problem-solving (Kiyokawa, Izawa, & Ueda, 2007). This finding conveys an important message for parents and professionals in terms of the benefits of giving children the opportunity to both observe and share in problem-solving tasks. Whereas we fully acknowledge the value of observation and practice when it comes to teaching children things such as how to ride a bike or flip pancakes, we tend to ignore its value when it comes to higher-level abilities such as problem solving.

Executive Self

Conscious control supports the ability to direct and sustain behavior in the service of reaching short- and long-term goals, modulating emotional

responses, and negotiating the needs and interests of the self in relation to others and context. We already discussed several ways that automatic behavior facilitates efficiency and accomplishment; here we expand on the importance of spontaneous behaviors.

Recall the review of research on self-control already mentioned, which suggested that inhibitory efforts increased the likelihood of subsequent inhibitory failures. In other words, our resources for conscious control can be depleted. A recent follow-up study examined the possibility that positive affect could have a restorative, replenishing effect (Tice, Baumeister, Shmueli, & Muraven, 2007). Following an initial act of self-regulation, participants who watched a comedy video or received a surprise gift were able to self-regulate on various tasks as well as nondepleted participants. Furthermore, the positive-emotion group performed significantly better than participants who experienced a sad mood induction, a neutral mood stimulus, or a brief rest period. These results indicate that positive emotion can counteract depleted resources.

Positive emotions are also associated with creativity and flexibility. A study investigating sense of humor found that being prone to smiling or laughing correlated positively with creativity (Wycoff & Pryor, 2003). In a study that examined the link between positive emotions and cognitive flexibility, Hirt, Devers, and McCrea (2008) found that participants in a happy mood (as compared with a sad and a neutral mood) consistently exhibited greater cognitive flexibility. When faced with a mood-threatening task, the happy participants were able to creatively transform the task so as to maintain positive mood and interest.

This research makes the point abundantly clear that positive emotion is essential for a healthy executive self. It highlights the importance of fun, pleasure, laughter, joy, surprise, excitement, discovery, delight, eagerness, satisfaction, fulfillment, warmth, and any other positive emotion you can think of! We suggest that the experience of joy, which is so important to an infant's world, should expand to encompass a broad and increasingly varied range of positive emotions throughout childhood, adolescent, and adult years. These are the life experiences that inspire, replenish, and, when need be, keep us afloat in the midst of troubled times. The spontaneous format is just as important and requires just as much "flexing" and practice as the others . . . it is simply more fun to do so.

After our first meeting, I (JT) realized that the testing was going to proceed even more slowly than I had predicted, which was a concern because Mark was now at home without any educational support. Susan and Jerry had hired a nanny whose main task was to ensure their son's safety, but she was not capable of meeting his educational needs. In fact, Susan reported that his threats to run away from home

were increasing. He would make this threat when he was disappointed or especially when she said *no* to some activity or request. Because the situation was escalating, I decided to gather a team and initiate treatment prior to having test
results. Based on the history, clinical interviews, and the functional assessment
information I was able to obtain up to this point, I provided the team with the
following information.

In terms of the *regulation system*, Mark's arousal patterns had been out of
balance for several years. He slept well but spent little time in an alert processing
state during the day. Most of his time was spent in a hypoalert (shut down) or
hyperalert (vigilant, paranoid) state with frequent abrupt shifts into a flooded
(rage) state. Overall, there was a chaotic pattern with frequent rapid shifts
throughout each day.

In terms of the *sensory system*, I suspected processing disruptions in both
the auditory and visual domains. Given Mark's significant difficulty with math,
his poor spatial arrangement with drawing and writing, his immediate frustration with using a pencil, and his poor reading of social cues, I suspected that his
visual processing problems were the more severe of the two domains. Mark's auditory processing difficulties were evidenced by the nature of his reading delays.
He also had sensory sensitivities. He had been hypersensitive to sound since infancy and held his hands over his ears if sounds were high-pitched or loud or if
onset was abrupt. He was also extremely sensitive to tone of voice such that any
firmness in tone with an adult was heard as "mean."

Turning to the *relevance system*, Mark was warmly connected with his father.
Their relationship seemed to be his lifeline to a feeling of safety. His father's
strength was his engaging, warm style; his limitation was his own distractibility
that could get him off topic and tended to reinforce Mark's chaotic pattern. Susan
was overly anxious. In her eagerness for control of the situation, she conveyed
tension, irritability, and set a "pressured" tone in the home. Mark was triggered
by any escalation in her anxiety. Mark was unable to modulate negative emotion,
quickly shifting into flooded states of anger that took on paranoid meanings. He
had very few periods of sustained positive emotion. Mark seemed to have immediate access to negative memories of being hurt, victimized, and bullied by other
children at school and at Boy Scouts. In addition, he had been very upset by a
couple of teachers who were dismissive of the bullying and taunting, either viewing him as somehow bringing it on himself or as needing to toughen up. Susan's initial directive style of parenting, which had become more demanding,
triggered Mark's sense of being treated unfairly and ultimately his rage. Mark
seemed to believe that both adults and children were potentially dangerous and
not to be trusted, and also that negative emotions were destructive, not tolerable,
and not manageable. In other words, his meaning-making system was pervasively
negative.

In terms of the *executive system*, Mark's processing speed was very slow, but
at the same time, he rushed through things impulsively and made multiple errors
along the way. He did not detect the errors and did not self-correct. Mark had
both gross- and fine-motor difficulties. His movements were awkward and overly

rushed, his motor planning was poor, and his fine-motor skills were severely delayed. Mark was unable to inhibit impulses and shift attention in ways that were adaptive and appropriate to the context (conscious control); rather, he shifted chaotically from spontaneous behaviors (e.g., when he was drawn to novelty, he would become quite disorganized) to his default automatic modes (e.g., when he was certain others were hurting him on purpose and would fly into a rage or shut down, retreating to solitary safe activities) (Capacity 1). Mark could not integrate emotions with his thoughts in an adaptive way (Capacity 2). Most of the time, his distorted thoughts only fueled his emotional disruptions, and he clearly lacked sufficient positive emotion to support flexibility or enhance inhibitory abilities. Mark did not accurately assess others' cues or make accurate inferences about others' mental states. He experienced himself as under constant threat and therefore was absorbed in self-protective maneuvers that left little room for the needs of others (related to Capacity 3). When forced to contend with others, he retreated into his own world for safety. In addition to this functional profile, Mark's behavior provided starting points for several working diagnoses: ADHD (combined or inattentive type), a probable mood or anxiety disorder (likely mixed, with thought disorder features), a possible nonverbal verbal learning disorder, possible sensory processing delays, and sensory modulation difficulties in other areas.

My highest priority was getting Mark and his parents into treatment with CL to stabilize the negative emotional escalation and then to a psychiatrist for a medication consult. Although the neurorelational framework advocates trying other interventions prior to medication whenever appropriate, Mark's emotional disruptions were both severe and chronic and were escalating into situations that were dangerous, and I suspected that he would benefit most from immediate medical help. In addition, with such chaotic arousal patterns, there was a very small window within which learning could occur. This, combined with the chronic conditions of load Mark experienced, made it unlikely that therapy alone would be effective. In addition, I saw virtually no inhibition capacity and no top-down conscious control, indicating a closed/chaotic learning system. Thus, it seemed imperative to gain medical support to stabilize the situation quickly so that CL could begin her work and other team members could be added once there was enough of an alert processing window in which to work. Understandably, Susan and Jerry were not eager to approve the use of medication for their son, but they agreed that their situation was critical and needed rapid stabilization.

CLINICALLY RELEVANT BEHAVIORS OF THE EXECUTIVE SYSTEM

The executive system guides our bodies through complex motor sequences, focuses our thoughts, generates interesting ideas, and modulates our emotions in the service of goal-directed and prosocial behaviors. The executive

system also allows us to shift among all of these processes, quickly if necessary. For example, for those times when we feel frustrated by a perspective different from our own, our executive system supports a shift to consider another's mental state, to better understand another's values and desires, inhibit our impulse to protest, and maybe even change our minds. These types of flexible shifts reflect good use of our executive abilities to balance thought and emotion and to balance self and other.

Clearly, this complex set of behaviors would not be expected of a 6-year-old, yet all of the abilities that feed into this description are in full swing at this age. Children may not be able to negotiate all of these behaviors simultaneously or at the same pace as adults, but they are fully engaged in the component processes—for example, meeting responsibilities, thinking into the future, negotiating conflict in a friendship, inhibiting the urge to yell in protest. Many executive abilities begin to emerge in the first few years of life that support such developmental accomplishments.

Motor Abilities

Executive abilities are associated with social and goal-directed action in the world and thus are ultimately expressed by the motor system. In fact, most of what we know about the emergence of the executive milestones presented in this section comes from the motor and temporal parameters of behavior. Infants cannot follow verbal commands or talk about their experience, so researchers present carefully devised scenarios and take note of the infant's responses. For example, they observe how long an infant's eyes remain focused in a particular location (e.g., to inform recognition memory), the frequency of kicking when the movement causes a rewarding event to occur (e.g., to inform implicit memory), and looking/search behaviors (e.g., to inform response inhibition) (Diamond, Werker, & Lalonde, 1994; Johnson, 1995; Nelson & Collins, 1992; Posner, Rafal, Choate, & Vaughan, 1985; Rovee-Collier, 1993; Tipper, Bourque, Anderson, & Brehaut, 1989). Motor functions also reflect a culmination of abilities across the four brain systems. For example, the emergence of speech involves alert processing (regulation), looking at faces and hearing sounds (sensory), imitation and emotion expressions that stimulate back-and-forth communication (relevance), and the coordination of breathing with oral–motor sequences to vocalize, babble, and eventually articulate phonetic streams (executive).

Next, we review general principles of motor development and a developmental trajectory of the motor accomplishments that support learning about the other and the environment. As we noted previously, the presentation of behaviors as separable skills is somewhat artificial. Just as a

perception is multisensory, a child's actions involve a coordinated whole-body organization. In addition, we noted that sensory perception and action are coupled in a continuous coordinated process, such that movement itself is a form of sensory perception (e.g., walking is integrated with proprioceptive and vestibular information) and vice versa. Furthermore, we pointed out that sensory and motor processes are not always linked in a continuous chain of stimulus → response sequences. In other words, motor functions are not bound to the perception of sensory information to organize an adaptive response. They also precede the presentation of stimuli based on the ability to anticipate patterns, predict outcomes, adjust errors, and ultimately learn to rely on executive memory. Rather than present the sequence of development for specific motor skills, we focus on motor abilities as they develop within social and learning contexts—in other words, as the child actively engages with others (e.g., speech) and with the environment (e.g., exploration). In this context, Table 10.2 presents the development of motor abilities in both coordination and load forms. A discussion of domain-specific motor skills (i.e., gross and fine motor skills, muscle tone and strength, and motor sequencing and planning) can be found on the CD-ROM, Section 10.1.

Motor development follows a general head-to-toe, proximal-to-distal sequence. Head and trunk control emerge first to support turning, rolling, and sitting, followed by arm control for reaching and grasping, leg control for crawling and walking, and last, the fine-tuning of finger and oral motor muscles for object manipulation and the articulation of phonetic sequences for speech. Motor development is both an interactive and iterative process. Infants and children discover opportunities for exploration as they learn about the world and others, and each new skill that is acquired opens the door to new learning opportunities. Individual differences in children's body dimensions, muscle qualities, and inherent energy levels will affect the timing and quality of skill acquisition. In other words, "low energy children with large limbs may have to learn different adaptive strategies than small, wiry, highly energetic ones" (Thelen, 2000, p. 392).

Once a motor skill is learned, it supports additional adjustments and variations to the core skill. Thus, motor abilities that emerge for newborns or young children become core abilities that expand in complexity with maturation. Motor development is function-specific, not muscle-specific. A toddler who is able to walk has the muscle strength for climbing, but needs experience to learn how to climb. Conversely, once a toddler figures out how to navigate the steps at home or retrieve her pacifier, she can easily expand this procedural function to all types of climbing and retrieval tasks. With motor learning, an initial period of instability is

Table 10.2. Developmental Progression of Motor Abilities and Their Contribution to Functional Behaviors

Approximate Age	Observable Motor Ability	Function	Coordination	Load
Newborn	Reflex and orienting movements such as rooting, sucking, eye movements, crying Orients to stimuli in environment; with visual, salient features include motion and contour (Bertenthal, Bennett, Campos, & Haith, 1980); with auditory, can detect changes in frequency, loudness, and timbre of voice (Molfese & Molfese, 1985)	Supports survival behaviors; supports engagement with others; supports increasing familiarity with regularities in the environment; supports phonemic development for native language	Has good suck, swallow, breathe coordination; able to cry robustly Shows reflexive and orienting movements, turns head to sounds, voices, motion, objects, especially if novel	Has poor suck, swallow, breathe coordination (feeding difficulties; may be at risk for speech production problems; may signal poor vagal tone); does not cry (risk for delay in speech production) Under- or overresponsive in turning head and shifting attention to listen to sounds and look at mouths and objects
Newborn	Strong bias to orient toward faces and	Supports preferential learning of socially relevant information,	Sustains attention to eyes, faces; meets gaze	Does not attend to faces, does not meet gaze; over- or

	eyes, especially eyes that return their gaze (Farroni, Johnson, Brockbank, & Simion, 2000; Fogel & Melson, 1988)	interpersonal connection, bonding, gestural communication		underresponsive to other engagement
Newborn	In general, eyes move on to the new and novel rather than to the familiar	Supports initiation behaviors, agency, exploration of others and the environment and learning	Shows flexibility in ocular-motor skills; orientation to novelty indicates learning through habituation	Does not shift eyes to novelty, does not explore the surround with eye movements; stares "through" versus "at"; darting eyes that flit from location to location without seeming to register responses
Early infancy	Predominance of spontaneous/self-generated movements (i.e., movements that are not solely response-based)	Strengthens connectivity of central and peripheral nervous system pathways that support movements	Initiates self-exploration and meaningful movements toward others (hands reaching for face, breast, or bottle) and objects of desire	Is very still and motionless, lacks purposeful initiations, appears to show a restricted variety of movements
Infant 3–6 months	Visually orients to near and far space localizes and orients to voice and sound; grasps with hands	Supports understanding of temporal and causal dynamics in others and of object movement (establishing associations); supports study of object properties; supports localization of sounds, objects, events in space	Can orient to location of an expected object of desire (face, toy, dyadic game). Orients to voices, orients when presented with novelty (shifting attention) and appears attentive to a variety of sensory stimuli (sustaining attention)	Does not build on previous routines, does not show surprise or anticipation of established patterns of care and play. Shows vacant gaze with an inability to sustain eye contact. Does not reach and grasp

(Continued)

Table 10.2. Continued

Approximate Age	Observable Motor Ability	Function	Coordination	Load
Infant 3–6 months	Respiratory, facial, and oral–motor muscles coordinate to produce primitive sounds, emotional vocalizations, and facial expressions	Supports ability to initiate relational interactions and express emotion Supports speech production and playing with mouth movements and vocal variations, which are the building blocks for speech	Sustains attention according to relevant information for appropriate durations Responds to playful engagement attempts with cooing and babbling Facial expressions respond to emotional content (e.g., responds with smiles, frowns, grimaces, furrowed brows, downturned mouth) Coordinates oral–motor movements for eating and speech production (e.g., uses jaw, lips, and tongue well)	Is vocally nonresponsive to attempts at emotional engagement Facial expressions are over- or underresponsive in emotional range Sluggish use of oral–motor muscles for eating and speech production (e.g., excessive drooling, poor chewing, poor articulation of sounds)
Infant 6–9 months	Imitates other's facial movements and sounds; produces more organized speech-like babbling; initiates interaction	Supports reciprocal communication, learning about the other, and emotional expression Supports babbling as "conversation" with an emotional tone	Exercises oral and vocal muscles, produces babbling and early speech Communicates emotion and preferences/triggers with voice tone, volume, babbling, and facial expressions	Fails to imitate other's faces and sounds Fails to use vocal-motor muscles for babbling and speech Fails to communicate emotional tone with facial expressions

Infant 6–12 months	Sits, crawls, makes pincer (thumb–index) grasp	Supports development of visual–motor skills; supports expansion of movement, spatial, and object/other processing; supports vestibular and proprioceptive processing; allows for increased control over grasp	Explores! Initiates movements for volitional change in location; "plays" with balance abilities (leans, wiggles, etc.); initiates interaction with others; seeks out distant interests, toys; investigates the source of noise	Sluggish in initiating movement (still, slow) or is overly active; in either case, reduced or excessive movement leads to a lack of sustained, purposeful engagement with things or others
Infant 6–12 months	Reacts differently to variations in facial expression and acoustic parameters in vocalization; responds with increased clarity of emotional content (e.g., smiles, frowns, grimaces, furrows brow, raises brows)	Supports learning about the meanings conveyed through vocal tone and facial expression	Is able to initiate vocalizations with emotional tone/facial expression; is able to respond appropriately to another's emotional tone/facial expressions	Tone of vocalization does not match facial expression; vocalizations and facial expression seem to lack emotional tone or contain excessive negative emotional tone; appears unaware of emotional tone from others' vocalizations, facial expressions
Infant 9–12 months	Watches and listens intently when another person speaks to him or her directly; speaks first words alongside more consistent speech-like	Supports language development that is specific to the child's relational world and social learning; speech supports ability to communicate needs/wants with more ease and clarity; supports early language and conceptual	Shows greater attention to, awareness of, and participation in social communication; has back-and-forth "conversations"; says first words and uses them appropriately; initiates standing and shows appropriate mix of emotions at the challenge	Is not responsive to, or does not engage in, back-and-forth communication; is not using any words; first words are unusual or used inappropriately; makes no attempt at standing; is unresponsive to praise or becomes excessively upset if falls

(Continued)

Table 10.2. Continued

Approximate Age	Observable Motor Ability	Function	Coordination	Load
	utterances; is pulling up to standing position and attempted walking with support	development (e.g., categories, object/action words)	(laughs with praise, cries briefly or tries again when falls)	
1–2 years	Picks up small objects (e.g., beads); can make increasingly precise and subtle finger movements	Supports ability to manipulate surroundings; supports grasping and holding ability for visual and tactile exploration of small objects; supports learning of causal connections; supports ability to show and share objects; creates novel configurations	Coordinates fine motor alongside visual–motor movements (e.g., picking up finger food to place in mouth, dressing oneself, grasping a pencil, drawing, writing) with appropriate initiation and inhibition of these activities	Is clumsy, uncoordinated, or impulsive in use of fine-motor and visual–motor coordination to accomplish tasks, with too much or too little initiation and inhibition of motor activities
1–2 years	Crawling, walking	Supports more distant exploration; supports progressive development of motor coordination; supports ongoing development in spatial perception and movement perception	Coordinates smooth gross motor movements with appropriate initiation and inhibition of these activities	Is uncoordinated with gross motor movements, often clumsy, stiff, or awkward in use of body to accomplish tasks, with too much or too little initiation and inhibition of motor activities

2–3 years	Stands, bends, runs, climbs with balance; able to coordinate a sequence of movements	Supports increasing flexibility, range, and efficiency of movements; sequencing of movements supports perceptions and planning about motor planning (e.g., how to obtain something out of reach)	Modulates body movements according to the context (e.g., can sit still, can inhibit walking and running on command); can negotiate environment and, when appropriate, plan alternate ways to navigate a challenge (e.g., path obstruction, object out of reach)	Makes impulsive body movements; unable to inhibit body movements (e.g., runs into the street, constantly fidgeting with hands and feet); falls constantly; does not navigate well in the allotted space (e.g., bumps and knocks things over)

followed by stability with practice. With age, motor abilities show increased coordination (smoothness), accuracy, flexibility, and speed. Well-established motor memories (i.e., procedural memories) are not forgotten and are highly resistant to disruption (Carlson, 2001). (For an additional summary of coordination and load characteristics of this capacity, see Markers for Purposeful Motor Actions, Attentional Behaviors, and Speech, which can be found on the CD-ROM, Section 12.5, p. 94.)

When assessing the motor aspects of behavior, it is important to bear three points in mind: (1) some problems are more disruptive to ongoing development than others, (2) the principle of automaticity is essential, and (3) the functional goals of movement must be considered. First, significant balance (vestibular) issues, for example, can be expected to have a greater impact on a child's successive skill acquisition than difficulty with coordination. Second, when a skill is automatic, it is more efficient because it requires little or no conscious thought and, thus, fewer resources. For example, if a child dismounts from a chair slowly and clumsily, or correctly dons socks and shoes only with verbal prompts, these motor skills are not automatic. Third, it is important to be aware of the functional goal as well as the motor ability in question. Recall that motor development is function-specific but not muscle-specific. When you consider the child's goal state, you can assess how and whether the child compensates to attain the goal. This assessment focus can provide valuable information as to the degree of challenge experienced by the child as well as his or her cognitive executive abilities. For example, if a child bypasses the option of using a step stool to retrieve a toy from the counter, in favor of climbing up and down stairs to fetch the mother for help, you can infer that this motor task is a significant challenge for him or her. You can also deduce that this child is comfortable seeking help and possibly does so too often. In contrast, if the child picks up a plastic bat from the floor and uses it scoot the toy off the counter to the floor, you can be impressed by his or her planning and sequencing skills.

Cognitive Processes

Although the executive system has a unique set of abilities to be considered in assessment and treatment, these abilities also converge with the abilities presented in the other brain systems. For example, although theory of mind (executive) does not *depend* on language (sensory), there is a strong enough relationship between them that one should not be assessed without considering the other (Astington, 2000; Astington & Jenkins, 1999; Hasselhorn, Mähler, & Grube, 2005; Tager-Flusberg & Sullivan, 1994).

In addition, because the executive system integrates information from all other systems, it is largely dependent on the quality of information received. If the executive system receives information of poor quality from the other brain systems, that information will shape goal-directed behaviors. But that is not the end of the story. Because the executive system also has the role of a traffic controller (e.g., scans, selects, retrieves, emphasizes, and organizes available information), it can also serve a strong compensatory role, adjusting the skills relied on and making use of external resources to scaffold the process. Finally, if the information is good but the executive system has difficulty using and responding to it appropriately (e.g., cannot inhibit, cannot detect errors), then the true nature of the clinical problem changes. For the professional, the clinical challenge is to distinguish between these two potential etiologies (or identifying some combination of the two), which can be tricky when the behaviors look very similar on the surface. Nonetheless, this is clearly an important distinction to make, given that the sources a professional considers in assessment will ultimately guide the course of intervention.

To assist in making such distinctions, it is necessary to understand the components of the executive system, which are presented according to the three executive capacities in Table 10.3. In reviewing the table, it is important to bear in mind that research in this area is recent and dynamic. Thus, on one hand, there is still much to be learned and agreed on, such as how terms are best defined and how experiments are best designed to tease out the ability in question. For example, in this literature, it is not uncommon to have findings called into question because it was discovered that varying the nature of the task yielded different results, often indicating an earlier emergence of the ability in question. On the other hand, countless groups of researchers across different fields and philosophical perspectives are rigorously pursuing answers to fundamental developmental questions in a way that sometimes sparks controversy and always inspires thoughtful debate.

Table 10.3 focuses almost exclusively on the development of executive abilities from birth through 5 years for two reasons. The developmental information that is available for this age range is scattered broadly across professional domains and peer-reviewed journals, making access complicated. Furthermore, due to the instability of executive measurement early in development, valid and reliable neuropsychological tests are not available for this age range (but are available for older children, e.g., NEPSY-II, Korkman et al., 2007; the Delis-Kaplan Executive Function System, Delis et al., 2001); thus, a general guide as to what to expect at what ages is needed. Although the material in Table 10.3 represents merely the tip of the iceberg, it is intended to fill a need for clinical access to developmental information regarding early executive processes.

Table 10.3. Development of Executive Abilities from 0 to 5

Executive Task	Initial Age	Research Description	Functional Implications
Simple Working Memory			
Forward span tasks (auditory and visual)	3	Child repeats a series of words or a series of digits in the same order as presented: Age 3: 2 items Age 4: 2–3 items Adult: 6–7 items (Hulme, Thomson, Muir, & Lawrence, 1984; Isaacs & Vargha-Khadem, 1989)	Simple working memory tasks involve only immediate holding; no updating or additional processing is required. Span tasks are intended to indicate the "capacity" or the limits of what can be held in mind without rehearsal. Information held in working memory is highly vulnerable to interference and lost quickly if not rehearsed.
	4	Child watches examiner tap a series of blocks and then child repeats the same sequence: Age 4: 4.5 squares Age 10: 7.5 squares (Gathercole, 1998; Strobl, Strametz, & Schumann-Hengsteler, 2002)	Simple working memory reflects emergence of the ability to "hold in mind" something that is not immediately available to the senses. The object (or caregiver) is "known" to be in a particular location not because of a current sensory experience, but because of a prior sensory experience held actively in mind.
Complex Working Memory			
Backward span tasks (auditory and visual)	3	Backward digit span: Age 3: 1.58 Age 5: 2.88	Complex working memory tasks require additional updating or processing, not just "holding." Such tasks reflect an emerging ability of children to "perform operations" on information as it is held in mind.

5	Backward block span (Corsi block test):
	  Age 5: 2.5 blocks
	  Age 15: 6 blocks
		A recent model proposes that phonological working memory is a "major pacemaker" of cognitive development (Hasselhorn, Mähler, & Grube, 2005, p. 234). Working memory limitations can be bypassed with strategies (e.g., chunking; Cowan, 2001).

	As compared to retention tasks, the auditory modality is more difficult to reverse than the visual (Carlson, 2005; Davis & Pratt, 1996; Garon, Bryson, & Smith, 2008; Schumann-Hengsteler & Pohl, 1996).	Task performance may improve when working memory demands are minimized.

CAPACITY 1

Inhibition

Simple response inhibition	2	Snack delay: Child is asked to wait until the examiner rings a bell before eating a goldfish cracker, with four trials of 5-, 10-, 15-, and 20-second delays (Kochanska, Murray, & Harlan, 2000); 50% of the two year olds were able to wait 20 seconds (Carlson, 2005).	Simple inhibition tasks require either withholding or delaying a response tendency. These examples are both delay-of-gratification tasks.
	3	Child is told that he or she can have a smaller treat/prize now or wait for the larger treat/prize (i.e., smaller immediate reward vs. larger delayed reward) (Prencipe & Zelazo, 2005). Out of nine trials, 3-year-olds were able to delay gratification on just over 30% of the trials; 4- and 5-year-olds were not	The ability to withhold/delay a response paves the way for all sorts of mental processes. If one can withhold an impulse response, then one can respond based on information not immediately available; one has additional time to consider other options; and one can work out scenarios in the mind versus in the world.

(*Continued*)

Table 10.3. Continued

Executive Task	Initial Age	Research Description	Functional Implications
		significantly different and able to wait just under and over 70% of the time, respectively (Hongwanishkul, Happaney, Lee, & Zelazo, 2005).	
Complex response inhibition	3–4	Bear and Dragon: Child is told to do what the bear asks but not do what the dragon asks (Reed, Pien, & Rothbart, 1984); 51% of the younger 3-year-olds are able to inhibit, as compared to 88% of the younger 4-year-olds (Carlson, 2005).	Complex inhibition tasks require inhibiting a response tendency and responding instead according to a rule that is held in mind, which creates more of a conflict situation than a delay task. This ability is important to self-control and social behavior. In the study presented earlier, it allowed for the feigned positive response to the disgusting meal to be expressed, rather than the immediate, but inhibited, disgusted response.
Shifting			
Response shift	6 mos.	A-not-B task: The infant retrieves a hidden reward from location A several times, then has to successfully retrieve when object is switched to a new hiding place (location B). At 6 months, the infant no longer perseveres by returning to the old location (Diamond, 1985).	Shifting involves shifting of response, attention, tasks, or rules. Shifting taxes both working memory and inhibition and involves overcoming the inertial tendency to continue in the same mindset (Davidson, Amso, Anderson, & Diamond, 2006).
	2	A-not-B task variation: A reward is placed in one of three "A" locations. Once the child	Here, the child is able to hold the new location of the object in mind, update working memory during the delay period, and also

		retrieves it three times, the object is visibly switched to location B, and the child has to wait 10 seconds before retrieving it (Diamond & Taylor, 1996).	override a previously learned and rewarded response in favor of a new response.
Attention/rule shift	4	Card sorting: Children are given a deck of cards. An image on each card contains two features (e.g., color and shape). The child is asked to sort according to one dimension, and after a response set is established, the child is asked to sort according to the other dimension. Prior to age 4, children cannot shift even when prompted before each response, a "knowledge-action dissociation" (Schneider, Lockl, & Fernandez, 2005).	The ability to shift is one of the early supports for self-control. It aids in adapting to change by opening the door for alternative behaviors in the face of challenge or unexpected changes. Shifting is an early reflection of an open learning system because the child is no longer "bound" to a learned stimulus–response behavior but can allow behavior to be guided by new information.

CAPACITY 2

Cause-Effect Contingency

	2–3	Child has ability to follow a single "if–then" statement or rule.	An important aspect of development is the ability to manage increasing complexity. The cognitive complexity and control (CCC) theory is a theory of executive development. According to CCC theory, age-related changes in executive functioning are due to the complexity of rules that a child can use; each new rule system permits a new level of cognitive control, eventually allowing reflection and higher-order rule use (Frye, Zelazo, & Burack, 1998; Zelazo, Qu, & Müller, 2005).
	3	Child has ability to follow two different "if–then" statements or rules.	
	4–5	Child has ability to represent a higher-order rule: "if–then, if–then" (Frye, Zelazo, & Burack, 1998; Zelazo & Frye, 1998).	

(Continued)

Table 10.3. Continued

Executive Task	Initial Age	Research Description	Functional Implications
Mentalistic terms	2	Wish–emotion terms emerge and are used to refer to internal mental states.	Early use of mentalistic terms and epistemic terms reflects an emerging conceptual understanding about one's mental state. Making statements such as "I wish" and "I think" suggests a developing knowledge of the self. Such awareness is also important to be able to infer the mental state of another, or develop theory of mind.
Epistemic terms	3	Begin to use words such as "think" and "know" (Bartsch & Wellman, 1995).	
	4–5	Master the fundamental features of additional epistemic terms such as "guess" and "forget" (Johnson & Wellman, 1980).	
Causal reasoning	4	Child can correctly answer questions, "What will happen if . . ." After witnessing a few events in which there is a causal structure, children are able to make reasonable judgments about causal properties: that is, that one thing caused another to occur (Gopnik, Sobel, Schulz, & Glymour, 2001; Gopnik et al., 2004; Schulz & Gopnik, 2004; Sobel, Tenenbaum, & Gopnik, 2004).	As children come to understand causal relationships, they develop a greater appreciation for both antecedents and consequences. Much younger children can appreciate that behaviors cause things to happen, but at this age, they begin to understand causal relationships such that predictions and judgments can be made. They also develop awareness that *thoughts* and *feelings* can cause things to happen, as well. Such causal reasoning, as it relates to self, can also be transferred to the other.
Sensory knowledge source	4	Child responds correctly to "How do you know?" questions (e.g., "I saw it, I touched it . . .") (O'Neill, Astington, & Flavell, 1992).	Young children are not adept at identifying "how" they know what they know. One of the earlier expressions of this ability comes with associating sensory experience with a way of learning and "knowing" about the world. This is followed by whether knowledge was self-obtained or came from another. An interesting achievement occurs

	Age		
Self-other knowledge source	5	Child can distinguish how knowledge was acquired whether from others or self-generated (Gopnik & Graf, 1988).	when the child becomes aware that knowledge need not come from an external source but can be deduced or inferred based on indirect information. As a child comes to understand how his or her learning is acquired, he or she can begin to infer how others learn, as well.
Inference knowledge source	6	Children can take inference into account as a potential source of knowledge (Sodian & Wimmer, 1987).	
Temporal Integration			
Past-to-present connections	3–6	Child able to explain past-to-present connections in behavior. Able to explain that a person felt sad because that person was reminded of a past event (a cue in the present reminded the person of a sad event; Lagattuta, 2007).	Developments in causal reasoning include past-to-present connections about self and others; 3-year-olds do not make these connections consistently. This reflects a child's emerging awareness that past-to-present connections are person-specific and related to that person's history.
Temporal duration	4	Child judges the times of past events using distance-based processes; can distinguish times of events based on impressions of distances into the past (Friedman, 2007).	Use of frames of reference, particularly time, to represent past and future desires and motives, independent of current state (Bischof-Köhler, 2000); contributes to "ability to organize and control one's actions."
Past-to-future connections ("mental time travel")	4–6	Child is able to explain past–future connections in behavior, e.g., that a boy's worry about the future was caused by an event in the past (4-year-olds can demonstrate this ability 88% of the time, 5- and 6-year-olds almost always) (Lagattuta, 2007).	Awareness that another person's feelings and decisions may arise from what the person *anticipates* will happen in the future. The child has an awareness that past-to-future thinking is person-specific and dependent on history. The child can span the range of hindsight–insight–foresight.

(Continued)

Table 10.3. Continued

Executive Task	Initial Age	Research Description	Functional Implications
		CAPACITY 3	
Theory of Mind			
Self-recognition	18 mos	Placing a mark on an infant's forehead, the infant can look in a mirror and touch mark on own forehead (Brooks-Gunn, & Lewis, 1984).	Awareness that the person seen is a representation of self rather than another person. This is an early form of self-awareness; self-awareness in the form of beginning introspection does not emerge until age 8 (Sodian, 2005).
Reads others' preferences	18 mos	Experimenter gave toddlers two foods, then showed a food preference opposite the child's, then asked the child to pick a food for both of them. The child offered food in line with the other's personal preference versus offering own preference (at age 14 months, child still offers own preference) (Repacholi & Gopnik, 1997).	Early differentiation between own and others' mental states, but this need not imply an understanding of the mental state of the other; a recognition that other may be different from self.
Switch self/other perspective	3.5	False belief task: Present puppet show to child: Maxi puts a piece of chocolate in location A, then Maxi leaves. Mom puppet enters, moves the chocolate from location A to location B. Mom leaves. Maxi returns. Child is asked, "Where will Maxi look for the chocolate?" (Wimmer & Perner, 1983).	Understands that a situation can be viewed from two different perspectives; can switch from one perspective (self) to another perspective (other). Variations on this task can yield different ages of emergence; a meta-analysis found a consistent developmental increase starting at age 3.5 (Wellman, Cross, & Watson, 2001).

Strategic deception	4	Mean monkey test: Children were asked to choose one of two sets of stickers, but once the child chose, the "mean monkey" took the child's selection. To get the desired choice, the child had to learn to deceive mean monkey by inhibiting the dominant response and instead choosing the option he or she did *not* want (Peskin, 1992).	Implies that an inference is being made about how the other will behave. The fundamental ability may be the inhibition of the dominant response to take desired object.
Explicit theory of mind	5–7	Child is able to demonstrate an understanding of another's mental state and make inferences about another's behavior.	Child has an explicit understanding of the representational relation between mind and world. Theory of mind necessary for a number of social competencies (e.g., social communication, conflict management, imaginative ability; Astington, 2003). Language development is the best predictor of theory of mind development (Astington & Jenkins; 1999; Jenkins & Astington, 1996).

Working memory development is presented separately because it is generally accepted as a fundamental ability that is distributed across domains. Probably for this reason, there is no simple or singular definition for working memory; in fact, an understanding of the term seems only to evolve in complexity. Towse and Cowan (2005) provide an excellent discussion of the relevant issues and, in considering the idea that an assessment of working memory can be accomplished by determining the number of items that can be held in mind during processing, they sum up the issues to consider with the following analogy:

> The situation is akin to that of the juggler, whose reputation is built solely on the number of balls, or sticks, or knives, or other items that can be juggled simultaneously. In our fascination with the juggling, we seem to ignore whether there are other issues to be considered. Does our juggler have the ability to interact with an audience, to make them feel involved in what he or she is accomplishing, as they laugh or gasp or cheer at the performance? Does our juggler have the ability to develop a story as part of the juggling act, to change the tempo and potentially break up the monotony of just juggling? Indeed, does our juggler have any other tricks [up his or her sleeve or anywhere else]? As we begin to generate, or reflect on, these and other questions, it becomes apparent that judging the quality of a juggler is more complex than it initially seems—and so it would seem with working memory . . . there is more to working memory than just remembering in sequence a large set of unrelated words. (Towse & Cowan, 2005, p. 20)

For Capacity 1, Table 10.3 highlights two broad executive abilities: inhibition and shifting. A much more detailed synopsis of the relevant research is available in a recent review of executive functioning in preschoolers (Garon, Bryson, & Smith, 2008). For Capacity 2, we focus on a few of the cognitive developments that support temporal integration, such as causal reasoning, inferences about why events occur, and the ability to connect feelings as causes of behavior. In general, for a young child to establish a cause–effect association, the antecedent and event must occur close together in time; for example, pushing the button turns on the television. As children age, they can manage increased temporal distance between events, but the links are often prompted by adults. As children begin to understand causal relations, they can reflect on the possible reasons for an event; this awareness of causality is often emphasized in the context of social mistakes. Most of the time, reflections on these connections are not initiated by young children but are prompted by adults. At about age 5 or 6, children will more often reflect on their own behavior to try to determine the causes for events without adult prompting. With a foundation of cause–effect reasoning, a child can exercise his or her conscious mode of behavior by accessing past

and present events to learn about self, others, and the environment and guide behavior in the present in relation to past experience and what can be predicted in the future.

For Capacity 3, we focus on precursor skills for theory of mind. Although theory of mind is now considered one of the core deficits in autism, the concept predates its association with this condition (Premack & Woodruff, 1978). Theory of mind goes a step beyond perspective taking (the ability to "stand in another's shoes") to include inferences about the reasons for another's behavior, assumptions about another's mental state, and speculations about what another person might do in the future. Theory of mind emerges with increasing complexity and has been examined across the life span from infancy to old age. It can also be viewed along a continuum of competency with severe limitations in abilities at one end, such as in severe autism, and a highly sophisticated integration of abilities at the other, such as we might expect to see in a highly skilled and effective psychotherapist. Advanced theory of mind has been defined as "the understanding of the mind as an active interpreter of information" (Lalonde & Chandler, 2002, as cited in Sodian, 2005, p. 113). It emerges around age 4 or 5, and its development continues throughout adulthood. Abilities associated with advanced theory of mind (or later developmental stages of theory of mind) include understanding stereotypes and prejudice, the appropriateness of a white lie, and the potential relevance of the reason for the breech of a commitment (Mant & Perner, 1988). A child (or a parent) may fall at any point along this continuum; we should assess for areas of potential compromise and contribution.

As I (CL) began to get involved in the case, I felt that the number of issues to be addressed was overwhelming; what should be addressed first? Consulting with JT, we agreed that although Mark's ADHD symptoms were pronounced, his mood shifts were clearly the most disruptive issue at this point. It seemed most important to first address the rapid and repetitive emotional escalations that were becoming dangerous. Our suggestion to the psychiatrist was to first try to stabilize his moods and then assess where we stood. In addition, because ADHD medication could provoke further arousal or mood dysregulation, it seemed important to avoid that situation if at all possible. The process was very slow, but over time Mark's moods were eventually regulated by a mood stabilizer. Later, a low dose of stimulant medication was added to address his distractibility.

The early phase of treatment with Mark required a high degree of caution and patience as well as a meticulous process of tracking his cues, being on the alert for signs of agitation as well as signs of pleasure and joy. After being forewarned by JT and Mark's parents and then personally observing the vulnerability in Mark, I found myself hypervigilant. The analogy that came to mind was that Mark was like a skittish horse that had never worn a saddle, and the slightest

mismatch or misreading of cues could send him bolting. Given Mark's extensive history of failed connections with adults, I knew that I had to slowly forge trust over time so that he could begin to relax and develop a sense of safety and confidence in his relationship with me. I began the dyadic sessions with Jerry because that relationship was the most stable for Mark. Jerry was very good at coaching me as to when to back off (a glance of caution) and when I was "right on" (showing me a subtle thumbs-up). Although I felt as though I were walking on eggshells, I also wanted to make it clear to Mark that I knew I was going to make mistakes along the way in either what I said, how I said it, or my tone of voice, and we needed to prepare for that inevitability. I knew that if I did not establish a format between us wherein I could make a mistake, and wherein Mark could let me know and experience my immediate self-correction, then I was likely to lose him with my first mistake. I reiterated several times that as soon as I made a mistake, I really wanted him to tell me so that I could learn from him.

Soon after we had that discussion, Mark experienced a huge disappointment that gave me more information. The leader of his Boy Scout troop had promised that if the troop won a contest, then the boys would get to go up on stage and each receive a ribbon, followed by a photograph of the whole group. Mark's troop did win the contest, but just as the children were starting to run up on stage, the troop leader abruptly announced that they were *not* to get up on stage. Instead, the troop leader chose two children to represent the troop in receiving the award on stage. Mark was enraged at the abrupt change of plans; his anticipated glory of going up on stage, getting a ribbon, and having his picture taken with his troop was suddenly taken away from him. The troop leader saw his change in mood and said, "I'm sorry, Mark, did I hurt your feelings?" Mark replied with a cold "no" but inside he was seething. He immediately bolted from the auditorium with Jerry in fast pursuit. While he was running, Mark ripped off his decorations and badges and threw them to the ground. By the time Jerry reached him, Mark was yelling loudly, "I hate him! He doesn't deserve to be alive!"

I recognized several things in this scenario that needed to be addressed. There was a clear lack of flexibility or tolerance for any spontaneity or abrupt changes in plans. Mark's emotions completely overrode his ability to exercise impulse control or read the context. He quickly made an inference that he was being purposefully hurt by the change in plans, showing faulty cause–effect reasoning. He could not admit his disappointment to the troop leader and problem-solve but, rather, quickly denied that he was affected at all, possibly as a result of his own embarrassment. He then spiraled into an intensely negative reaction that was not buffered by any other possibilities. The frank denial of his obvious rage in real time reminded me of a similar scenario in which Mark had stated that he did not want to tell the teacher he was scared at school for not knowing an answer because he felt too embarrassed.

This scenario only confirmed that my making a mistake was unavoidable and that a parallel process would likely ensue. Indeed, it was more important for me to anticipate and prepare for it rather than try to avoid it. Within the second month of our treatment, I made my first mistake. I have a gumball machine in

my office that is governed by "Connie's rule": A child can have one gumball if he or she chooses to have it during a session or two gumballs if he or she waits until the end. The rule is intended to support impulse control; most children prefer to wait and get two. Mark knew the rule and had always waited until the end of the session to get his two gumballs. However, on this day, he went toward the machine in the middle of a session and, after getting one gumball, initiated the process of getting a second one. Things happened very quickly at this point. I abruptly jumped up, got between him and the gumball machine, and reminded him firmly that he could not have two gumballs, only one. The good news was that, while he complied with the rule, he immediately signaled that I had made a mistake *and* reminded me that I had asked him to do so. I instantly understood and narrated my mistake of moving toward him suddenly and speaking in a tone that, for him, sounded harsh. He confirmed and I agreed that my sudden movement and tone of voice were things that upset him and triggered his anger. This was our first important turning point. I had averted an escalation and, by mirroring his experience and honoring my promise to self-correct, I began to gain his trust to tell me how he experienced things. My goal was to model flexibility and foster an open learning system between us, versus a closed system where my way was the only way. A co-existing focus, as noted, was one of creating joyful interactions.

For adults who value being "in charge" at all times, this approach smacks of accommodating a demanding child in a situation where the child should be accommodating the adult's demands. As we shall see, this fear of accommodating was exactly his mother's viewpoint and was also shared by some of the adults at his school. Yet it was clear that a directive approach would only breed further defiance in this child. Further, should a directive approach escalate to a demanding one, with all of its sensory components (e.g., abrupt movements, harsh tone), this would make matters even worse. We could not afford further dangerous escalations. In actuality, the more appropriate initial goal in this situation is to create an open learning system in which the rigid child can learn to trust that an adult will be responsive and flexible. However, being responsive and flexible as the adult is not an end point. It is a necessary beginning that establishes a new baseline of trust and enables the rigid child to take risks and find the flexibility to learn to express feelings, rather than act out feelings with the wish to protect the self and control others.

In the next chapter, we consider assessment and intervention principles, priorities, and strategies for working with deficits in executive capacities.

NOTE

1. However, the Delis-Kaplan Executive Function System (D-KEFS), a test battery that measures components of executive functioning for children and adults, reflects an important advance—it is the first to incorporate methods of analysis (e.g., contrast scores, error scores, methods of interpretation) for parsing out cognitive contributions from various domains (Delis, Kaplan, & Kramer, 2001).

11

Assessment and Intervention
Principles, Priorities, and Strategies
for the Executive System

Regardless of one's age, executive abilities always have the potential for further growth. Given that they are expressed within the context of goal-directed behavior, it makes sense that they should evolve with increasing complexity and nuance as both the capacities of the other systems and age-appropriate goals evolve and mature. For the three capacities of the executive system, there is a general progression of complexity. The sequence relates first to the regulation of broad behavior patterns, then the regulation of the self with respect to thoughts and emotions, and then the regulation of the self in the context of both personal and social goals.

The overarching assessment questions for the executive system include the following:

- Over time, does the child or parent show a balance of automatic, spontaneous, and conscious control formats?
- How does the child or parent integrate and manage his or her thoughts and emotions? In the relevance chapter, we were concerned with the balance of positive and negative emotion, whereas here we focus on the relationship of thought and emotion.
- Does the child or parent manage personal goals in relation to others and the context?
- Does the child or parent make use of strengths and weaknesses to pursue interests and meet responsibilities?
- How well does the parent make use of his or her executive functions in parenting his or her child?

- Are the capacities of the other brain systems facilitating or imped-
  ing the three capacities of the executive system?
- Are the child's or parent's motor abilities age-appropriate and able
  to support the capacities of all brain systems?

ASSESSMENT AND INTERVENTION PRINCIPLES AND PRIORITIES FOR THE EXECUTIVE SYSTEM

Executive abilities can be used to compensate for delays as well as to build resiliency for both the child and the adult. There is a growing awareness among professionals who work with children that a child's executive abilities are central to the development of flexible and adaptive behavior in the world. Studies that focus on resiliency in children (and adults) have recently begun to take a closer look at the relationship of executive functions to resiliency and overall functioning. For example, Martel, Nigg, et al. (2007) looked at a number of executive abilities, such as response inhibition, interference control (i.e., resisting distraction), alertness, shifting, and working memory, to evaluate their impact on children's functioning. They found that executive abilities not only contributed to academic competence but also showed a consistent linear relationship with resiliency (i.e., greater executive skills were associated with greater resiliency). In addition, resiliency and interference control jointly predicted social competence, whereas poor inhibition contributed to both internalizing and externalizing behavior problems. The growing awareness of the importance of executive functioning has led to treatment programs that teach and reinforce executive functions as a means of promoting resilience for both typical and at-risk children (Greenberg, 2006). Some of the executive targets for development include attentional control, inhibitory control, emotional control, planning, and problem solving—all of which are aspects of our executive capacities.

Capacity 1: Purposeful Adaptive Behavior

A child's ability to engage in and vary spontaneous, automatic, and conscious control behaviors in a way that is adaptive in relation to the context defines coordination in this capacity. All formats are important to
development, and conscious control regulates the balance.

Several studies have clearly shown the benefits of strong executive abilities, especially the ability to regulate behavior by means of self-control. Children who demonstrate this ability in various contexts show better social

and emotional adjustment and are considered to be more adaptive (Eisenberg et al., 1997). Several longitudinal studies have shown positive effects of top-down regulatory control on social and behavioral adjustment in the early school years (e.g., Denham et al., 2003; Eisenberg et al., 2003). Children ages 4 and 5 who were able to delay gratification (an ability supported by top-down inhibition) showed more social competence, positive coping abilities, and academic success 10 years later (Mischel, Shoda, & Peake, 1988). More specifically, when the children grew to be adolescents, parents rated them as more verbally fluent, rational, attentive, planful, and able to deal well with frustration and stress. A more recent longitudinal study found that response inhibition, switching (i.e., shifting), and sustained attention were among the executive abilities that predicted later behavioral competence and academic success—an effect that went beyond the effects of background characteristics and IQ (Jacobson & Pianta, 2007). A study by Wills, Sandy, Yaeger, and Shinar (2001) found that both the ability to sustain focus (i.e., focusing and persisting on tasks until finished) and positive mood (general cheerful mood) were related to a higher degree of resilience for preadolescents at risk for substance abuse. These studies underscore the importance of supporting and enhancing the development of a child's executive abilities early on.

Coordination Factors

The spontaneous behavior format promotes openness and learning. Interest and curiosity, primary features of the spontaneous format, motivate children to try new things, think about things in new ways, and be open to new emotional experiences. Curiosity introduces the child to novelty, and novelty promotes further interest and curiosity—the relationship is reciprocal. As previously noted in the relevance system, interest and curiosity also support the level of activation needed for persisting with learning challenges. In addition, when the topic of interest is both complex and seems understandable, then interest is more likely to be sustained (Alexander, Jetton, & Kulikowich, 1995; Morgan, Harmon, & Maslin-Cole, 1990; Ross, 1983; Sansone & Smith, 2000; Silvia, 2006). In other words, interest is likely to fade if the novelty turns out to be too complicated to be understood. The spontaneous format is supported by the ability to initiate and shift, as well as a healthy dose of impulsivity. Impulsivity that is not excessive can stimulate playfulness, surprise, and creativity.

The automatic format, as noted previously, is reflected in overlearned activities and routines that contribute to efficiency and productivity. In addition, the automatic format is also reflected in the familiar routines that reliably bring pleasure and contentment to our lives, such as favorite

pastimes, foods, music, and hobbies. These activities involve preferences, the things that are known and loved, the tried and true. A child will tend to gravitate toward these things when not in the mood for something new, when he or she wants calm and comfort instead of stimulation, and when he or she wants something simple instead of complicated. With respect to learning, the automatic format reflects a child's base of knowledge, the areas in which he or she has established sufficient familiarity that new information that is related to what is known feels within reach or understandable. The automatic format is supported by the ability to sustain attention and inhibit distractions (i.e., interference).

The conscious control format is reflected in an effortful focus of activity, thought, and emotion in the service of personal and social goals. In this process, conscious control detects mismatches between the current state and the goal state so that a child can consider what is needed to shift strategies or adjust the balance. In a learning task, there are often many points at which a shift in approach or a new strategy is helpful. For example, if one is struggling to learn something new, it is helpful to stop and think about the nature and goal of the learning activity. Is it something that is interesting and familiar enough to be understandable, or is the struggle with lack of interest? Is it a core topic that needs to be known well, or will a superficial understanding suffice? The answers to these questions dictate different shifts in strategy. In a social context, the conscious control format helps a child gauge the appropriateness of behavior. A mismatch might be detected by picking up on a gesture that what was just said was offensive rather than funny. Better yet, the child will predict the mismatch and the thought will be inhibited rather than spoken. As the cited studies highlight, this ability to inhibit an impulse response is often crucial to social and personal successes. The conscious control format also helps adjust the balance across the three formats. For example, the automatic format becomes too dominant when a child consistently defaults to what is familiar and comfortable. To prevent becoming stuck in a rut, the child can be encouraged to consider a new experience, take a risk, or take on a learning challenge of greater complexity.

Risk Factors for Load Conditions

When a child presents with a problem, it is both important and informative to assess the nature of the imbalance among these three behavioral formats. Is there an overreliance on the spontaneous, the automatic, or the conscious control behavioral format? In addition, how do the abilities to initiate, shift, sustain, and inhibit behavior contribute to the imbalance? The answers to these questions promise to yield additional insights and multiple potential routes for intervention.

Overreliance on spontaneous behavior. When behavior is weighted toward an overreliance on the spontaneous format, in general, there is too much activation, too much shifting from one thing to another, too much novelty seeking, and too much risk taking. Excess shifting can encompass actions, thoughts, and emotions. For example, distractedly picking up one toy after another with no apparent goal and no follow-through would be the product of too much shifting of actions; changing one's mind every time a new piece of information comes along would reflect too much shifting with thoughts; and too much emotional shifting might result in being overly vulnerable to taking on others' emotional states.

Attention-deficit/hyperactivity disorder, or ADHD (all subtypes), is an example of an overreliance on the spontaneous format. A lack of inhibition, or impulsivity, is a hallmark feature of ADHD. Impulsivity is often thought of in terms of impulsive actions, but it can be just as problematic when thoughts and emotions are impulsive. In this case, the lack of inhibition may be seen in impulsive or default judgments (i.e., without taking time to consider the available information or the alternatives), a continual shifting from one topic to another, shifting attention with every distraction (internal or external), or shifting emotions when a trigger is activated. (Children who have trouble inhibiting their actions often come to the attention of professionals quickly because their behaviors are bothersome and demand attention from others.) In addition, many studies of ADHD have found impairment on tests of executive functioning. For example, a recent study of adolescents diagnosed with ADHD found impaired performance on executive tests of shifting and inhibition (Martel, Nikolas, & Nigg, 2007).

Inhibition problems span several diagnostic categories and behavior problems beyond ADHD. Impulsivity is also associated with conduct disorders, substance abuse, mania, externalizing behavior problems, and social problems (e.g., Caspi, Moffitt, Newman, & Silva, 1996; Martel, Nikolas, et al., 2007; Olson & Hoza, 1993; Tarter et al., 2003). The bothersome impact of impulsive behaviors on others may also lead to secondary emotional problems, such as anxiety and depression.

Overreliance on automatic behavior. An overreliance on the automatic format is seen when there is too much consistency and repetition of the familiar. In this situation, there is too much inhibition and stability, and routines are dominant to the point that new things are nudged out. This child experiences too much simplicity and comfort and not enough challenge. In addition, when the child repeatedly returns to the tried and true, others' preferences and ideas may also be gradually nudged out, eventually making the child more isolated in his or her own interests and less social overall. A similar dynamic can occur with learning and knowledge, whereby

the child immediately assumes that the familiar and the known is the correct course without considering alternatives. This child may also adhere to controlling, rigidly engrained patterns of behavior that are guided by rules and laws. Here, inhibition is used to avoid deviation from the pattern. This type of thinking compels the child to make overly simplistic judgments, overlook alternatives, and repetitively focus on one detail that defines the self or others, usually to his or her disadvantage or shame (e.g., "I'm always a failure"; "You're *bad!*"). This type of overreliance on negative thoughts can be an underpinning to depression.

Overreliance on conscious control. An overreliance on conscious control means that the child or adult places too much value on thinking through all matters and emotional detachment. There is often a need to feel in control of events and outcomes and to filter thoughts according to what is considered acceptable. Too much conscious control is similar to an overactive superego, whereby rigid standards dictate the actions, thoughts, and emotions that are "allowed"; for example, when things that are provocative within one's culture are considered wrong and a great deal of effort is expended to avoid these things. A person who overrelies on conscious control may deny emotional pain and become skilled (or conditioned) at masking negative emotional responses or feigning positive ones. There may also be such a strong preparatory set for avoiding the anticipated negative emotion that the child or adult becomes hypervigilant for associated cues. For example, a child may reject or disavow things he or she actually likes to avoid potential disappointment. The rigidity in this format is more about control of emotion than the rigidity of the automatic format, which is about sticking with the familiar.

Bear in mind that children and adults who evidence overcontrolled behaviors, such as rigidity and social withdrawal, may not be simply bearing down with voluntary control but, rather, may be reacting to inherent inhibitory tendencies that are more endemic to their constitutional physiology (often referred to in the literature as "reactive control"; Derryberry & Rothbart, 1997; Eisenberg et al. (2005). It is quite possible that voluntary, conscious control teams up with reactive control to create a strong propensity toward too much inhibition. Children who fit this description are often more naturally fear-based, shy, and prone to withdraw when activated (a range within the hyperalert state). An overreliance on conscious control may also be reflected in a hypersensitivity to mismatches, such that the slightest nuance in another's tone or gesture becomes cause for excessive worry or rumination (e.g., "Is she mad at me?" "Did I say something stupid?"), or the slightest indication of a cognitive challenge creates a surge in anxiety about one's ability to learn (e.g., "Oh no, this is too hard, I'm going to fail!" "I'll be up all night, I'll never get this!").

Assessment Questions

For this capacity, the assessment priorities and issues to consider include the following.

The spontaneous format:

- Does the child or parent demonstrate curiosity and interest in novelty and discovery?
- Does the child or parent exhibit an openness and willingness to learn about things that are unfamiliar?
- Does the child or parent have the ability to "go with the flow" without a specific plan or explicit rules?
- Can the child or parent adapt to relatively benign changing circumstances?
- Does the child or parent exhibit appropriate ability to initiate behavior and to shift behavior (i.e., action, thought, emotion)?
- Does the child or parent show enough stability such that everything is not experienced as novel?

The automatic format:

- Does the child or parent exhibit efficient/effective use of over-learned routines and procedures (e.g., getting ready for bed, getting ready in the morning, doing chores, doing homework)?
- Has the child or parent established an age-appropriate knowledge base, and is he or she able to expand that base with related learning?
- Does the child or parent demonstrate a set of acquired preferences and interests that reliably bring pleasure and comfort?
- Does the child or parent show an appreciation for familiarity and predictability?
- Is the child or parent able to sustain behavior and inhibit distractions?
- Does the child or parent show enough openness that routines and preferences do not become rigid?

The conscious control format:

- Does the child or parent appropriately detect mismatches between current state and personal or social goals (i.e., the child or parent is neither oblivious nor hypersensitive)?
- Can the child or parent respond to mismatches with appropriate adjustments to behavior (e.g., inhibit an impulse when socially appropriate to do so)?

- Is the child or parent able to experience emotions without denying or inhibiting them?
- Can the child or parent reflect on alternatives and ideas and problem-solve without shutting out information that comes from either general knowledge or academic or emotional domains?
- Can the child or parent use conscious control to rein in an overreliance on automatic or spontaneous formats?
- Can the child or parent use conscious control to bolster development of executive abilities?

Capacity 2: Integrating Thoughts and Emotions

In the relevance system, we discussed the precursors for and the patterns of positive and negative emotions; in the executive system, we turn our focus to the interactive patterns of emotion and thought. Optimally, our learning and behavior reflect a harmony of thinking and feeling that supports adaptive behavior. Whether emotions are implicit or rise to the level of awareness, they should promote growth (e.g., to work better, be a better parent, make better decisions, be happier). Conversely, it is equally important to make use of thinking to modulate our emotional world (e.g., to explore a negative emotion, consider our role in a success or a failure, hold back a hurtful remark). The emphasis here is on embracing the value of emotions to thought processes as well as the value of thought to emotional modulation. One of the primary benefits of the bidirectional influence of emotions and thoughts is the ability to learn from mistakes, an important component of an open learning system.

Coordination Factors

Coordination for this capacity is reflected in a harmony of thinking and feeling that supports adaptive behavior. Emotions promote better thinking and decisions, and thinking promotes both the healthy expression and inhibition of emotion. Thinking and feeling are dynamic processes within the context of hindsight, insight, and foresight, whereby emotions present almost limitless potential for self-reflection, and thinking provides meaning and structure to emotional experiences. Our contention is that in the executive system, this capacity for mental time travel is what allows us to engage in meaning-making and integrate emotional experiences into our conscious thought in constructive and growth-oriented ways. Supporting this viewpoint is a study that examined the relationship of temporal

perspectives to substance abuse and found that a predominantly present focus was associated with more substance abuse, whereas a future focus was associated with less substance abuse (Wills, Sandy, & Yaeger, 2001).

The value of emotions to thought. Emotions can be an excellent springboard to insight. When we experience an emotion that captures our attention, pondering it is bound to yield some type of insight about the self. For example, a parent's strong and unexpected surge of anger when his or her child begs for a toy in the toy store can prod the parent to consider the implicit meaning that this behavior holds for him or her, likely from his or her own childhood (Siegel & Hartzell, 2003). In this sense, emotions can "tell on us" and "teach us" by revealing things that we were unaware that we thought or felt. To gain insight from emotions, however, one must first be able to tolerate emotions—to feel the sensation in the muscles and the gut and feel the full course of them. One has to be able to first *accept* an emotional experience (as opposed to rejecting, denying, minimizing) before it can open the window to insight. In other words, the potential value of emotion to thinking cannot be fully realized in the context of disavowal. Once the emotion is acknowledged and accepted, one can begin to ponder its meaning—for example: Why did that upset me? What did that mean to me? What did that remind me of? The honest answers to such cause–effect questions may be painful or difficult to ponder, but are very likely to pay off with increased understanding or insight. Over time, engaging in this process has the potential to enhance emotional resilience and encourage more flexible thinking. If we come to view emotional discomforts as opportunities or as problems to solve, we may find that there is a universe of insights available at our fingertips.

We noted in the relevance system that this ability to tolerate a range of emotions takes time to develop; it is a process. The younger the child, the more likely he or she is to be overwhelmed by an emotion and, in this state, incapable of weaving thought into the picture. However, the structure of thought is what begins to provide containment for a child's emotional experiences. When parents place an emotional experience in a cause–effect context, they build on mirroring and empathy (foundations for insight) and expand the structure of meaning-making into a broader temporal realm (i.e., promote hindsight, insight, foresight). It is important to highlight the crucial role that this activity plays in promoting the development of executive abilities, especially temporal integration. It helps expand a child's focus of attention beyond the here and now and thus raises the possibility that the child's ability to apprehend and discern the motivations and causes for behavior can likewise extend beyond the present. Providing a cause–effect template for emotional experience encourages the child to consider the value of emotions to thinking.

The value of *positive* emotions to thinking is often overlooked. Positive emotions enhance executive functioning, replenish resources so that the executive system has the fuel it needs to function optimally, and promote goal-directed and prosocial behaviors. In the last chapter, we noted that positive emotions can replenish the mental resources needed to inhibit inappropriate social responses (Tice, Baumeister, Scmueli, & Muraven, 2007). We also pointed out that positive emotions enhance cognitive flexibility (Hirt, Devers, & McCrea, 2008). For example, when in a good mood, you may be more likely to view a novel activity as a fun adventure than a dreaded obligation, or an intimidating activity as a challenge rather than a threat. In the relevance chapter, we noted how positive emotions, such as curiosity and awe, promote the learning process, giving the learner more mental energy to persist when the going gets tough. Furthermore, recent research suggests that a baseline positive mood supports our routine daily goals (i.e., taking care of business) as well as our social behaviors. In other words, subtle positive emotions motivate us to continue pursuing a goal as well as to engage in prosocial behaviors (Custers & Aarts, 2005a; Custers & Aarts, 2005b). Positive emotions provide a baseline that might be compared to the idling of a car; as long as we do not inhibit movement with the brake, the idling itself will compel us forward. All of these noted processes—inhibition of inappropriate responses, cognitive flexibility, learning persistence, goal-directed behavior—represent various components of thought that are enhanced by positive emotions. Clinical experience provides numerous examples of the same. For example, during the testing process, it is quite clear that a child in a good mood will often show more persistence and resilience with cognitive challenge than a child in a bad mood, and that having fun for a while often brings a renewed energy and alertness to the next task.

The value of thought to emotions. Thoughts provide hindsight and foresight to structure emotional experiences. When emotions such as guilt or regret or sadness feel overwhelming, thoughts gradually emerge and cohere to organize and frame the experience, making it increasingly comprehensible. Thoughts access the past, prompting us to consider the possible antecedents and to begin to make cause–effect associations. These associations prompt us to think constructively about past situations and consider what we might have done differently (hindsight). Thoughts are also valuable to emotions by allowing one to predict emotional outcomes (foresight).

Studies by Baumeister, Bratslavsky, Finkenauer, and Vohs (2001) indicate that when we anticipate a future negative outcome, we tend to overestimate the impending magnitude and duration of the negative outcome, which can have a powerful influence on present thinking and decision making. The anticipation of potential criticism or conflict may compel us

to exert extra mental effort or action in the present, for example, taking an hour to carefully word a one-paragraph e-mail in a delicate professional situation. According to a review of the literature and work by Baumeister and colleagues (Baumeister, 2005; Baumeister, Vohs, & Tice, 2006), emotions may stimulate thinking more reliably than they stimulate behavior. Negative emotions may help stimulate counterfactual thinking (i.e., thinking outside the boundaries of what is known, or assumed to be known), challenging us to rethink past choices or reactions as well as contemplate new ones for the next time. In other words, positive emotions tend to be affirming, indicating that our actions were on target, we made the right choice. Negative emotions, however, signal that something was off and prompt us to consider that a different choice or a behavior might have yielded a better result. According to Baumeister, Vohs, DeWall, & Zhang, "The affective residue provides the push to support future behavior change" (2007, p. 173). Studies have also shown that it is more effective and adaptive to use reappraisal strategies (e.g., reframing emotional experiences) to cope with *anticipated* emotions than to use suppression strategies (e.g., inhibition) to cope with a *current* emotion (Gross, 1998). These types of studies highlight the importance of using executive abilities to promote emotional well-being and avoid the costs of unnecessary emotional disruptions.

The more familiar value of thought to emotion is the regulatory role that thoughts serve to keep emotions in check and keep us from running amok. In other words, allowing fleeting or strong emotions to continually dictate our actions is not an adaptive way to function in the world. Phrases such as "level-headed" and "cool under pressure" espouse the value as well as the difficulty of being able to think in the midst of intense emotion. The value of this type of top-down control is well established. For example, one study found that emotional competence (defined by patterns of emotional expressiveness, emotional regulation, and emotion knowledge) at 3 and 4 years of age contributed significantly to children's later likeability and social competence (Denham et al., 2003).

Risk Factors for Load Conditions

Load conditions are more likely when emotions and thinking are out of balance. An imbalance in either direction—too much thought or too much emotion—disrupts one's ability to make sound cause–effect connections, learn from mistakes, and use thoughts and emotions to inform hindsight, insight, and foresight. Consequently, negative patterns typically emerge. Imbalances between thought and emotion contribute to false/weak assumptions and conclusions, disorganized thoughts, and sometimes

distortions. For example, in the case example for this chapter, Mark's auditory sensitivities contributed to a keen awareness of and vulnerability to tone of voice. As a result, he was unable to clearly distinguish past events when an adult had used a harsh tone from current events when an adult's tone was firm and assertive but not harsh. To him, they were the same, which drove his very quick (albeit false) conclusion that all adults exercising authority were "mean."

Overreliance on emotion. A child who is too often overwhelmed with emotion will have difficulty making use of thought to structure the emotional experience. This child will be too busy coping with emotions in the present to have the resources to access the past, make cause–effect associations, or anticipate the future in an adaptive way. For some children, the means of coping itself can prevent thought from bringing coherence to emotional experiences. For example, a child who has experienced trauma may continually focus on the cause–effect connections that signal threat and thus be unable to use thought to see beyond the anticipated negative. This stance only serves to reinforce the same triggers and encourages reactions such as withdrawal and hypervigilance versus problem solving. Similarly, significant disruptions to mood (e.g., depression, bipolar disorder) have a narrowing impact on the thinking process, such that thought becomes bound to the task of coping with the present, or hindsight and foresight are skewed toward only the negative information.

Another type of overreliance on emotion comes from a lack of access to thinking, such as a distrust of potential sources of knowledge or a rejection or avoidance of effortful thinking. For example, one may have an overly strong preference to rely on hunches and gut feelings as sources of knowledge (e.g., clinical wisdom) and reject sources of information that have become associated with the potential for negative outcomes (e.g., clinical research). More commonly with children, the thought processes required to make cause–effect connections and see patterns in behavior are either perceived as too threatening or too cognitively challenging and may be due to limited working memory capacity or weak cause–effect reasoning abilities. These children tend to shift quickly into blame or into overly simplistic cause–effect connections.

Overreliance on thought. A very different style is shown by those who actively deny and disavow feelings and use thought to escape as well as distort emotions by transforming them into an intellectual experience. Denial and intellectualization are the primary tools of disavowal. Denial can occur along a continuum, from a conscious, effortful process of repression to an unconscious process in which emotions never make it to the level of awareness. A simple way to distinguish between these conscious and unconscious processes is to think of someone who *doesn't want*

to feel or remember versus someone who *can't* feel or remember. With intellectualization, the focus of attention is much more dedicated to thinking about feelings and trying to understand them from a logical perspective, perhaps incessantly. When overused, this process greatly reduces the potential for emotions to lead to insight and distorts their value in terms of informing hindsight and foresight. This type of overreliance on thinking restricts or even eliminates certain emotions from being incorporated into thought as acceptable experiences. In a potential variant of this process, an individual attempts to fit every experience into a rigid system of thought, such that certain emotions are never experienced (e.g., "I never cry, only losers cry" or "I'm never disappointed"). Children with these tendencies have trouble attending to a broad range of information, may draw conclusions or make judgments without considering alternatives or integrating feedback, and may become angry with others for not adopting their view. These children are also likely to exhibit a lack of empathy or sympathy for others—an emotional disposition that has been associated with an increase in aggression (Rothbart, 2007; Shechtman, 2002).

When an overreliance on thinking causes distortion in the interpretation of events, this inaccurate information influences present reactions as well as anticipations of the future. Some children and adults are constantly anxious about the future, and this hypervigilant state fuels expectations of dreaded outcomes, such as feelings of shame or criticism from others. A child or adult with such a stance is so busy projecting negative possibilities that he or she is unable to accurately associate outcomes with antecedent causes. Some children with executive weaknesses (e.g., in planning, cause–effect reasoning) may attempt to avoid negative outcomes with weak strategies, such as plans that are too difficult to be feasible or that do not take into account their own strengths and weaknesses. Some children may come up with only very general plans that are not likely to work without the details (e.g., "I'll study harder") or come up with fantasy plans to cope with unwanted emotions (e.g., "I'll tell the teacher to make him go to another school").

Perhaps the most serious variant of an overreliance on thinking comes from fundamental distortions in thought processes. Young children with thought disorders may be prone to projecting blame onto others or fearing that others are there to harm them, while not being able to understand their own effects on others (e.g., consequences of hitting others, breaking things). For such children, double binds in reasoning are common, whereby the child places demands on others that cannot realistically be met (e.g., demands that the parent come close and at the same time pushes him or her away, or demands that the parent "leave"). Indications of more severe thought disorders include paranoid, grandiose,

and nonsensical thinking. The causes of thought disorders appear to "lie in a complex interplay of genetic, prenatal, and developmental factors, as well as precipitating events in later life" (Role & Talmage, 2007, p. 263). (For a summary of coordination and load characteristics of this capacity, see Behaviors Indicating the Relationship Between Emotions and Thoughts on the CD-ROM, Section 12.5, p. 95.)

Assessment Questions

In assessing the child's or adult's balance and integration of thought and emotion, one must consider the quality of cause–effect reasoning as well as the ability to use temporal integration (hindsight, insight, foresight) to guide behavior.

In assessing the value of emotions to thought, consider the following:

- Previously, we discussed the importance of being able to connect with (visceral self) and tolerate (emotional self) emotional experiences. In the executive system, does the child or parent allow the visceral/emotional self to influence and become integrated with the thinking process (the executive self)?
- Do emotional experiences (positive and negative) promote insight? Do they prompt the child or parent to think about the feelings experienced in the moment (or on reflection) and then use the emotional experience to see patterns in his or her own behavior? Do emotional experiences help the child or parent gain understanding of triggers and preferences, of personal strengths and weaknesses?
- Does the child or parent use emotional experiences to reconsider past choices and behaviors? Do negative emotional experiences stimulate counterfactual thinking so that new choices and behaviors can be considered in the future?
- Does the child or parent demonstrate empathy or sympathy in his or her thinking about others' circumstances?
- Does the child or parent experience enough positive emotion to drive goals and enhance executive functioning?

In assessing the value of thought to emotions, consider these questions:

- Does the insight gained from emotional experience stimulate cause–effect associations with respect to antecedents (hindsight), and are those associations accurate?
- Once the child or parent is able to see his or her role in a negative emotion or outcome, can he or she engage in productive thinking

around the problem—for example, consider more details, consider another's perspective, generate alternative responses, or plan to try something new the next time?

• Can the child or parent use a past emotional experience to better anticipate a future event? In other words, can the child recall the lessons learned to accurately detect and respond to the antecedent signals and cues?

• Can the child or parent make use of anticipation to modulate negative emotion? Does the cognitive preparation enhance top-down control in the moment?

• Can the child or parent problem-solve and plan reasonable ways to avoid the negative emotions for others as well as self?

• Can the child or parent recognize and understand when it is socially desirable or appropriate to regulate his or her emotions?

Capacity 3: Shifting Between Self and Other/Context

For this capacity, optimal behavior is reflected by a harmony of internal self and external (other/environmental) contexts. It is concerned with the self in relation to both personal and social goals. This capacity requires well-honed feedback mechanisms to monitor approximation toward goals, detect potential mismatches, and determine the need for adjustments to bring present the state in line with a desired state. It also involves an evolving and maturing understanding of self in relation to context. For example, are the child's personal goals appropriate, and do they allow for the fulfillment of personal responsibilities? When is it appropriate to keep the inner world of thoughts and emotions private versus share it with others? What is the appropriate balance to achieve between self-interests and other interests? When is it appropriate to advocate for the self versus give to the other?

Theory of mind and part–whole reasoning contribute to coordination for this capacity. Part–whole reasoning allows one to assess self needs, interests, and goals relative to the larger context to weigh and gauge the appropriate approaches for pursuing different types of interests and goals. Theory of mind enables one to better read others' mental states and infer their intentions. With this awareness, personal interests can be integrated with one's need for social belonging, and one can defer to others' needs and interests as appropriate. An important focus for this capacity is the ability to *use executive abilities in real time*, meaning that one must be able to continually shift and update behavior according to the larger context. In addition to theory of mind and part–whole reasoning abilities, this capacity integrates aspects of former capacities as well.

Coordination Factors

In chapters on the relevance system, we referred to the development of an autobiographical self that emerges around 2 years of age, wherein the self is experienced as separate from others—the beginnings of self-awareness— and is able to recall memories from one's own experience. Here we present a heuristic regarding the internal development of this self-awareness in relation to others. This development involves the emergence of three types of self-awareness that complement the three interpersonal modes from the relevance system: the private self (reflect), the assertive self (direct), and the giving self (respond). The heuristic of the interpersonal modes is focused on external behavioral expressions, whereas this heuristic concerns the internal world of self-awareness, self-identity, and self-image. Kagan notes, "Although [the] term [self-awareness] has no standard definition, most psychologists use it to refer to those processes that permit recognition of one's ability to act, to feel, and to regard self as an entity different from others" (Kagan, 1981, pp. 1–2); his research supports the roots of self-awareness as emerging during the second half of the second year of life. The neurorelational framework's view of self-awareness is consistent with Cicchetti's (1991) position that the emergence of self evolves from the complex interplay of biological, caregiving, cognitive, and environmental factors. In discussing self-other awareness, Beeghly and Cicchetti (1996, p. 127) note, "The ability to talk about the internal states and feelings of self and other is an age-appropriate development of late toddlerhood hypothesized to reflect toddlers' emergent self-other understanding and to be fundamental to the regulation of social interaction." As self–other awareness matures in the developing child, the behaviors we observe could be conceptualized as the private self, the assertive self, and the giving self. The private self is the container of self- and other-awareness from which one draws information and through which one develops a sensibility of both asserting one's needs (assertive self) and giving to others (giving self).

The private self involves the accumulation of self-knowledge that is recognized as reality-based by the child or parent. This self-knowledge includes the person's awareness of his or her responses (e.g., feelings, reactions, meanings) to others. The private self draws on the capacities of all the brain systems in the sense that self-awareness includes knowledge about one's arousal in terms of what constitutes safe versus threatening conditions (e.g., "I always love being in my bedroom; I get anxious before a test"), knowledge of strengths and weaknesses (e.g., "I tend to be too hyper; I am a good reader, but I struggle with math"), knowledge about one's sensory preferences and triggers (e.g., "I love learning about music; I hate crowded noisy places"), knowledge about one's emotional tendencies

(e.g., "I am compassionate; I get mad easily"), and knowledge of one's top-down control abilities (e.g., "I am not so good at putting on the brakes in the moment, but later I can accept responsibility and problem solve"). The private self is also about maintaining a balance between personal/ private information and public/shared information. It reflects the growing maturity to keep quiet when it is not appropriate to blurt out something personal about self or others and also to begin to discern when it is safe and appropriate to trust another and self-disclose. The private self is closely associated with the reflective self (presented in the relevance system), in the sense that the private self is the storehouse of information and observations from which the reflective self draws. In psychodynamic terms, the private self represents the intrapsychic world. The reflective interpersonal mode is a *process* of reflection that makes use of the private knowledge about self and other. To acquire self-knowledge, the private self must be attuned to feedback from others and from one's own efforts.

The assertive self involves the tasks of self-responsibility and self-advocacy. It reflects the child's (or parent's) ability to use the knowledge gained from self-awareness to promote both personal and social self-interests. It is expressed in how well a child is able to use self-awareness to meet responsibilities, formulate goals that are in sync with strengths and interests, allocate time spent in various activities, know when to ask for help, and know when it is appropriate to assert one's needs, thoughts, or feelings. The assertive self is internally driven and motivated and less vulnerable to external distractions and diversions. It is supported by a strong sense of self needs and interests as well as a desire to explore and learn more about those things that are interesting and stimulating. Another aspect to the assertive self is knowing when one has encountered a challenge that taps into a weakness or an area of low interest so that one can then strategize about the best way to meet the responsibility.

The giving self involves maintaining a self-other balance. It reflects the child's (or parent's) ability to use the knowledge gained from both self-other awareness to make judgments about what to give, when to give, and how much to give. The giving self rests on age-appropriate development of theory of mind, the ability to weigh the relevant parts of a situation in relation to the whole, a solid private self, and a healthy assertive self. Theory of mind supports the ability to read and make inferences about others and thus be able to better anticipate others' expectations and respond when appropriate. When a child can read others well, he or she is able to get in sync with others and meet social responsibilities with less mental effort and thus greater efficiency. Theory of mind also supports a child's ability to see another's situation and be able to feel empathy, set aside one's own interests, and offer help and support when appropriate. The private self helps the

child discern when giving to another is not safe, is not appreciated, or is out of balance. Having an understanding of both self-interests and other-interests, a child is better prepared to gauge when it is appropriate to focus more on the self and when it is appropriate to focus more on others.

Risk Factors for Load Conditions

An overreliance on any aspect of the self will impact the others but an overreliance on the private self can be most problematic. The private self provides the foundation of knowledge and awareness from which assertive and giving behaviors originate; thus, distortions in the private self will distort the others as well.

The load patterns of this capacity place a child at increased risk for social rejection. This is an issue of crucial importance, given the serious negative consequences to actions, thinking, and emotions that result from social rejection. A series of studies indicate that social rejection causes decrements in self-regulation (Baumeister, DeWall, Ciarocco, & Twenge, 2005), increases the likelihood of aggressive behavior (Buckley, Winkel, & Leary, 2004; Twenge, Baumeister, Tice, & Stucke, 2001), is associated with thinking deficits such as impaired logical reasoning (Baumeister, Twenge, & Nuss, 2002), is associated with an emphasis on the present versus the future and an avoidance of self-awareness, and contributes to an increase in self-destructive behaviors (Twenge, Catanese, & Baumeister, 2003). Social exclusion has also been associated with emotional numbing, a reduced sensitivity to physical pain, increased emotional insensitivity, and decreases in empathy for another person's physical or psychological suffering (DeWall & Baumeister, 2006).

Imbalance of the private self. One type of imbalance within the private self is reflected in an excessive focus on the internal world that has little adaptive value for personal or social behaviors. There may be little translation or generalizability of self-knowledge to purposeful actions. An imbalance of the private self can be expressed in many other variations. There may be an obsessive rumination on specific features of self-knowledge while completely ignoring others—for example, a focus on past failures that becomes ruminative and all-encompassing to the point that a child develops an anxious hypervigilance for cues of potential failure scenarios and then withdraws at the first hint of challenge. To avoid potential mistakes, this child (or parent) sidesteps learning situations, neglects interests, and declines any type of risk taking. A very different type of rumination involves a child who obsesses on how others have hurt his or her feelings. This child holds an ever-evolving script of perceived injustices in active working memory and, as a result, is always primed to interpret others'

behavior as part of the same script. This child is so focused on the anticipated negative that he or she cannot see alternatives or access contrary past evidence and may respond to benign situations with hostility and even aggression.

Another variation of imbalance within the private self occurs when there is a distortion in self-awareness that promotes maladaptive goal-directed behaviors. For example, a child with little connection to the visceral self will not receive internal cues that are strong enough to clearly define pleasure/preferences or discomfort/triggers and, as a result, may pursue goals that are both beneficial and sabotaging at the same time. For example, with the goal of wanting to be a "good student" or "just like my sister," a child may study for hours every night for advanced placement classes that are not even in sync with the child's own strengths or interests. Whereas the child may attain the goal and make good grades, this may be at the cost of neglecting self-care (e.g., unaware of physiological stress cues), not having time left for social activities, and allowing strengths to lie dormant. A distortion in self-awareness is also likely to cause a child to misjudge strengths and limitations. This child does not detect the mismatch between perception of performance and actual performance. Last, any distortions in self- or other-awareness will impede the child's theory-of-mind abilities, leaving him or her at a disadvantage in the social arena.

Overreliance on being assertive. An overreliance on the assertive self reflects an imbalance in the "self" direction. It is exhibited in too great a focus on self-interests and a dominance of self-interests in goal-directed actions, thoughts, and emotions. This child (or parent) is too internally oriented and not sufficiently responsive to external cues. This child may become preoccupied with his or her own strengths/preferences, spend an excessive amount of time pursuing personal hobbies and goals, and focus excessively on his or her own opinions and emotions. The dominance of self-focus means that the needs and interests of others are easily overlooked and often neglected. This child may not notice enough about the other and the context to realize what is expected and, thus, may be often caught off-guard because he or she is poor at anticipating what is next. For example, a child may play with his or her video games and trains for hours each day and neglect to help with chores, fail to be ready to go on time, or fail to spend time with others. Even during a play date, this child may assume that his or her friend will be entertained by the same activities. Although an overreliance on either the assertive self or the private self can create a type of behavioral self-absorption, the imbalanced assertive self *intrudes* on others by imposing self-interests, whereas the imbalanced private self can be characterized by a withdrawal into oneself that *excludes* others.

Overreliance on giving. An overreliance on giving is an imbalance in the "other" direction, reflected in too great a focus on other-interests and

a dominance of other-interests in goal-directed actions, thoughts, and emotions. This child (or parent) is too externally oriented and not sufficiently responsive to internal cues. He or she is often not in touch with his or her own preferences/strengths or triggers/weaknesses due to a need to remain flexible so that others' interests can always be accommodated. (The causes for a disconnect from internal cues may be varied. One may be disconnected from visceral cues due to visceral disruptions very early in development and, thus, one uses external rather than internal cues to guide behavior. In another variation, one may have robust visceral connections but disavow these internal cues in order to escape abuse or avoid interpersonal conflicts. This variation may result in internal resentments and conflicts or a blunting of visceral cues over time.)

The ability to use part–whole reasoning is important for the balanced and smooth functioning of the private, assertive, and giving modes. This ability requires working memory skills to mentally hold and manipulate the various parts in relation to the whole. Part–whole reasoning can break down for many reasons. Deficits in perceiving the parts may result from (1) a tendency to ignore or deny aspects of the self (e.g., ignoring own bodily cues, denying feelings; poor connection to visceral self; an imbalance in integrating thoughts and feelings) or (2) failure to attend to the relevant features of others or the context (e.g., weak theory of mind, processing problems, cannot distinguish the important points in a story). Deficits in perception of the whole may result from (1) an inability to hold or consolidate the meaning or implications of the parts (e.g., a 7-year-old child at a birthday party who falls apart because he or she doesn't have any presents to open; possibly due to poor working memory, poor cause–effect reasoning, or weak theory of mind), (2) overfocusing on the parts, getting lost in the details (e.g., anxious child who often gets stuck on one detail out of numerous details that comprise an activity or task), and (3) overfocusing on the whole (e.g., the visionary who sees the big picture and the goal but cannot organize the details needed to make it happen). (For a summary of coordination and load characteristics of this capacity, see Behaviors Indicating the Relationship Between Self and Others on the CD-ROM, Section 12.5, p. 96.)

Assessment Questions

Assessment of the private self:

- Is the child or parent's self-knowledge accurate or distorted?
- Does the child or parent overemphasize aspects of the self while ignoring or denying others (e.g., ignoring feelings; poor connection to visceral self; poor awareness of weaknesses)?

- Does the child or parent translate self-knowledge into behavior (e.g., "I hate crowds, so I won't go to Disneyland!")?
- Is the child or parent able to discern what should be private and what should be shared?

Assessment of the assertive self:

- Does the child or parent use self-knowledge to formulate personal goals and strategies?
- Are the child or parent's self-interests and goals in sync with preferences, strengths, and interests?
- In the context of pursuing personal goals, does the child or parent remain aware of others' expectations and what is appropriate behavior in context?
- Does the child or parent advocate for self needs and interests when appropriate (e.g., ask for help, ask about expectations and rules)?

Assessment of the giving self:

- Does the child or parent exhibit age-appropriate theory-of-mind development? Does the older child or parent show the appropriate higher-level theory of mind abilities?
- Is the child or parent able to attend to the "parts" of self and others that are most relevant, given the context (e.g., is not distracted by background noise and can accurately track an interpersonal exchange)? Does the child or parent weigh self-interest relative to other-interests and balance the roles of giving versus receiving (e.g., child can let guests at his or her birthday party take a turn first)?
- Is the child or parent able to understand the relevant implications of the broader context or environment (e.g., being in church means being quiet)?
- Does the child or parent recognize and appreciate the meaning when there is a shift in the other or the context (e.g., child responds to Mom's serious tone of voice, knowing to get ready for bed)?
- Does the child or parent understand the roles and expectations of different relationships?

Table 11.1 presents a synthesis of executive capacities as organized by our three behavioral formats under conditions of coordination and load.

Table 11.1. Synthesis of Executive Capacities Organized by Foundational Behavioral Formats for Coordination or Load

Spontaneous		Automatic		Conscious Control	
Coordination	Risk Factor for Load Condition	Coordination	Risk Factor for Load Condition	Coordination	Risk Factor for Load Condition
• Able to flexibly use spontaneous and creative actions, emotions, and thoughts • Able to respond quickly to situations that warrant immediate action for self and others (e.g., danger; assisting a friend or relative in need) • Able to shift into exploring new ideas or activities/jobs • Shows curiosity and interest in new things	• Overrelies on spontaneous activity, emotions, and thoughts • Distracted attention and impulsivity dominate actions • May have difficulty staying on task when sequencing is required • Unihibited; socially inappropriate • So much in the present, shows little or no awareness of cause and effect or learning from the past • Offers impulse fantasy solutions during problem solving, leaps to quick-fix approaches	• Able to flexibly use automatic actions, emotions, and thoughts, avoids rigid adherence • Has efficient morning, afternoon, and evening routines that support health • Has a number of preferences and traditions that reliably bring pleasure • Able to stay calm, providing a soothing presence to others	• Overrelies on autopilot activities or default emotions and thoughts • Automatic habits are unhealthy or sabotaging (i.e, autopilots for poor nutrition, fast foods, poor sleep patterns) • Automatic habits involve an inefficient use of time during morning, afternoon, and evening transitions/routines • Engages in routines and preferences to the degree that the external world gets shut out • Usually shifts quickly into a stress response as a default mode, in response to slight provocation from	• Able to flexibly use conscious control of actions, emotions, and thoughts • Able to stay thoughtful and fair minded, providing integrated advice for self and others • Can integrate past, present, and anticipated judgments, viewpoints, and emotional responses from others into own perspective • Able to hold the past, present, and future reflections	• Overrelies on conscious control of activity, emotions, and thoughts • "Overthinks" things wherein thinking is not influenced by emotion; too "logical" • Overly cautious and slow to act, with too much inhibition • May either not anticipate an upcoming event or perseveres on upcoming plans • Perceptions of cause and effect may be inaccurate or distorted • Offers fantasy solutions based on magical, internal world solutions that are unrealistic • Highly self-absorbed

(Continued)

Table 11.1. Continued

Spontaneous		Automatic		Conscious Control	
Coordination	Risk Factor for Load Condition	Coordination	Risk Factor for Load Condition	Coordination	Risk Factor for Load Condition
• Willing to take on appropriate challenges and risks • Able to generate ideas and experience creative "bursts" without losing focus or drifting off task • Able to flexibly shift into a variety of interpersonal modes	that are unrealistic • Tendency to look for excitement and novelty in the environment, at the expense of ignoring or not seeing danger • Highlights aspects of novelty in the environment without keeping current task in mind • Lacks integration with healthy automatic and conscious control behaviors	• Default modes are oriented toward maintaining the alert state, or shifting into adaptive or mild stress responses with recovery • Default modes include giving to others, asserting own needs, and keeping things private	others • Relies on hypoalert, hyperalert, and flooded states with slow or no recovery • Interpersonal default modes resort to an over-indulged or undeveloped private world; making no demands or rigid demands of self and others, or giving too little or accommodating too much to others • When problems are mentioned, automatic defensive reactions may include denial, forgetting, procrastination, or blaming others • Lacks integration of healthy spontaneous and conscious control formats	of oneself and others • Able to hold and manipulate information during part-whole reasoning • Makes thoughtful decisions as to when to give to others, assert self-needs, negotiate self in relation to others, or when to keep things private	in own internal thoughts and fantasies • Cannot read, misreads, ignores, or is unaware of the nonverbal cues of others and often is oblivious to others' needs • May be oblivious to safety or danger in the environment due to preoccupation with internal world • May consciously choose to be reclusive, vindictive toward, or overinvolved with others • Lacks integration of healthy spontaneous and automatic formats

While waiting to see the effect of medication, I (CL) began working with Mark's parents. I wanted to explore how we could maximize the strengths in the parent–child relationships and simultaneously decrease the escalations. Jerry's style was warm, playful, and engaging, and he usually could prevent escalations with Mark. Susan's style was stern, a demanding style of interpersonal mode, which usually escalated Mark and left her feeling ineffective with her son. Interestingly, both Susan and Jerry had been raised by parents who were quite demanding, but Jerry was naturally responsive and had consciously rejected the parenting style that he'd experienced growing up. That's not to say he didn't have his moments, but overall he projected warmth and acceptance. Susan felt torn. On one hand, she clearly saw the painful reality that Jerry's style was effective in preventing an escalation, whereas hers was not, but on the other hand, the permissiveness of it just felt wrong to her, and she wondered if this approach was contributing to Mark "turning into a monster." Was Jerry actually "feeding and catering to the monster?"

Although Jerry was the more responsive parent, he sometimes triggered Mark by making an impulsive promise (e.g., to buy him a toy as a way to avert an escalation) that he realistically could not keep. Jerry's distractibility and impulsivity tended to encourage spontaneous "solutions"; thus, he needed help to slow down his thoughts, use more conscious control and hindsight (recalling past events where he had promised something he could not deliver), become more aware of current and future time constraints, and see the big picture before he offered quick resolves. It appeared that a polarizing pattern had developed between Jerry and Susan, a pattern in which each was adapting his or her behavior in an attempt to compensate for the other; therefore they were both moving to extremes: that is, Dad was overly accommodating and Mom was overly demanding. I felt that the polarizing pattern was escalating behaviors in a way that was dangerous, and the parents agreed. Because Jerry was able to modulate Mark's behavior, we agreed that Jerry would continue to be the primary parent to engage Mark. Susan did not know how to mirror and track Mark with empathy (skills that she would not be able to learn overnight), so we decided that initially she would practice being emotionally neutral with Mark to see if this would reduce the co-escalating pattern. When interacting with Mark, she would stop talking or walk away the second she detected that Mark was escalating. Despite her fears of feeding the monster, she understood that our first and highest priority was to decrease the escalations, and she accepted this strategy as our starting point. I reassured her that as we gained more stability, we would slowly introduce more directives, boundaries, and consequences and titrate them appropriately into Mark's relational repertoire.

At this point, however, it seemed that Susan and Mark's history together had created a large number of highly sensitized cues that easily triggered Mark's stress responses. Life at home had reached critical mass. Mark's sensitivity to sounds, there from infancy, now launched into an escalation every time Susan said *no* to him or gave him a directive. Susan also soon admitted that a pattern of co-escalation was common between her and Mark. She would give an order in a harsh tone of voice, Mark would react with a protest, and both of them would quickly escalate

into a rage. Susan admitted that she often said inappropriate things when she was in a rage, but she also justified her response by pointing out that this occurred primarily when she was provoked by Mark. For his part, Mark did an excellent job of provoking his mother; his rage toward her was often accompanied by obsessive pleas to Jerry to "leave Mom." Susan admitted that she had experienced impulses to hit or physically punish her son but had never done so. Nonetheless, the inclinations to abuse him were terribly disturbing to her.

The situation was clearly a dangerous one, so in addition to dyadic treatment with Mark and Jerry, I began individual sessions with Susan so that she could process her emotional distress and work on building her responsive and reflective skills. Furthermore, we set up intermittent conjoint parenting sessions in which we tracked the escalations and triggers with Mark and worked on how they could begin to manage them as a team.

ASSESSMENT AND INTERVENTION STRATEGIES

Executive abilities are involved in nearly all target behavior and all diagnostic categories. Executive problems are associated with disorders such as ADHD, autism, and learning disabilities as well as acquired syndromes resulting from early deprivation or insult. Any disorder that involves problems with attention will involve the executive system. The range of behaviors involved and the interventions that are possible relate to all disciplines, so no single discipline can cover this domain. In fact, all treating disciplines should have the executive system in mind.

Executive abilities are responsive to practice, and the benefit of intervention appears to generalize to other relevant cognitive and behavioral domains. Two separate studies examined the change in response inhibition and cognitive flexibility with training and feedback in typically developing preschoolers (Dowsett & Livesey, 2000; Kloo & Perner, 2003). Children who failed the initial executive task were then trained and did better on the retest than those children who were not trained, and their performance improved on other tasks, as well. Klingberg and his colleagues (2005) trained working memory in a group of normal participants for 25 minutes per day for over 20 days and found that working memory improved as well as performance on other tasks, indicating more widespread benefit. A follow-up study found that working memory training improved symptoms in a group of ADHD participants (Klingberg et al., 2005). Rueda, Rothbart, McCandliss, Saccomanno, and Posner (2005) improved performance in selective attention and rule use in 4-year-olds who underwent five training sessions.

In the process of assessment and intervention, several primary principles can be kept in mind: (1) the need to use one's own executive system

while teaching parents about and supporting their use of their own executive systems; (2) the need to scaffold and weight priorities across brain systems in relation to the big picture; (3) the importance of looking for recurring relational and behavioral patterns and themes; (4) the value of using formal assessments and formal/established programs of interventions; and (5) using movement and technology as assessment and intervention resources.

1. As a professional, one can think of one's own executive system as a support for the parent's and the child's executive systems. By using various methods (e.g., modeling, coaching, teaching), convey to parents the processes you want them to begin to learn and emulate; over time, you gradually transfer the processes to them. It is common for parents to assume that a child's behavior is intentional. A child's weak executive system can often be interpreted by the parents as "My child is lazy," "My child is forgetting on purpose so he [or she] doesn't have to do the work." Teaching parents about the executive system helps them (a) better understand their child, (b) better understand themselves, (c) use the principles to adjust their own behavior (e.g., to inhibit the automatic "He's just being lazy!" response), and (d) use executive skills such as planning and problem solving to provide more optimal interactive regulation (e.g., anticipate situations that will create problems or that can be exploited for teaching, to generate alternatives).

Educating parents about executive functions also helps them structure the priorities and goals of intervention as well as hold the temporal process of intervention over time. For example, with an understanding of the executive system, a parent is better equipped to appreciate that the current focus of intervention is to bolster the child's ability to reflect on past situations and consequences (hindsight) and that a focus on insight and foresight will come later. Knowing the long-term plan, the parent can hold the process and inhibit the temptation to try and force insight on the child before he or she is equipped to learn the lesson. Modeling an open learning system in discovering your own executive strengths and weakness and how you cope with those limitations may be useful to parents (e.g., "I use a daily planner to write down the details that I'd have trouble remembering"; "I have to organize our goals on paper"; "I remind myself of where we are in the sequence before each session").

2. As the professional begins to hold the big picture of all the brain systems in terms of the strengths and weaknesses for each individual, priorities for intervention need to be established. High-priority items become whatever is causing the greatest distress or disruption in the child's life. One begins to think about the interventions in terms of balancing the short-run items that will bring relief fast in relation to the long-run categories that

bring optimal change over time. For example, if a child cannot read and his or her self-esteem is plummeting, immediate help may mean having a parent decrease the stress by reading to him or her and advocating to the teacher to reduce the workload during and after school, and the long-term solution would be remedial intervention for the learning disability.

3. Identify the relational patterns and themes from both bottom-up and top-down perspectives. Because all brain systems influence each other in complex ways, certain behavioral patterns can be discerned for individuals, dyads, and the family system. A bottom-up pattern would involve automatic arousal tendencies that occur under nonstressful as well as stressful conditions. For example, a child may have a tendency to favor the hyperalert state of arousal for both adaptive and load conditions. Top-down patterns would involve the interpersonal modes of behavior from the relevance and executive systems that also occur under stress-free and stressful contexts. For example, the previous child mentioned, who tends to be hyperalert, may develop a responsive interpersonal mode that, under pressure, becomes too accommodating toward others. Of course, there are bidirectional influences between bottom-up and top-down contributions to the relational patterns that emerge. Table 11.2 considers how these various interpersonal modes and arousal patterns can intersect and influence each other. Intervention is needed whenever a child or parent shifts into an interpersonal stress mode with load conditions.

Table 11.2. Interpersonal Modes of Behavior from Executive and Relevance Systems Under Coordination and Load Conditions

	↓ Top-Down Influence ↓		
Executive	Private Mode	Giving Mode	Assertive Mode
Relevance	Reflect Mode	Respond Mode	Direct Mode
	Detach Mode	Overaccommo-date Mode	Demand Mode
Regulation	Hypoalert	Hyperalert	Flooded
	↑ Bottom-Up Influence ↑		
Coordination	Flexible use of all three interpersonal modes according to the context with an open learning system (use of alert processing state); shifts into detach, overaccommodate, and demand modes are temporary and contextually driven		
Load Conditions	Stress responses used too quickly, too frequently (chaotic system); stress responses used chronically, too rigidly (closed system)		

The behavioral dimensions of duration, rhythm, and intensity, introduced in Chapter 4 and used throughout the brain systems, can continue to assist a professional in assessing and intervening with a relational pattern. Each category can give useful information in targeting one or more ways that the patterns may need to be altered.

- *Duration.* Under conditions of coordination, a child, dyad, and family can play together for extended periods of time. The quality of play includes a blend of give and take, with both self and others' ideas, needs, and emotions taken into account. There is a strong predominance of positive emotions, such as joy, surprise, playful teasing, pleasantness, gratitude, and graciousness. There is flexibility, yet not too much catering to one person at the expense of another. Implicit in play that goes on for an uninterrupted period of time is a modulated degree of both rhythm and intensity. When the child is unable to play for any meaningful block of time (i.e., duration is short), look to the components of rhythm and intensity for possible problems.
- *Rhythm.* The rhythm within dyads or a family system may include a quick disruption, wherein play comes to a crashing halt, or slow pace, wherein the play ends on a sour note with a gradual deterioration over time.
- *Intensity.* While playing, one particular dyad among four or five family members may begin to escalate such that the event turns into a fight, with demands flung back and forth. In another scenario, a family member may get his or her feelings hurt, shut down, and abruptly detach and walk away. Another individual may be so anxious about everyone else's feelings (overaccommodating) that he or she is unable to engage in the playful yet competitive aspects of winning a game.

As these patterns are identified, they can begin to be altered, one aspect at a time. For one family, the main goal may be to slow down the quick eruptions into flooded states and demanding, high-intensity interpersonal modes. For another family, the first goal may be to reduce anxiety, keeping the rhythm flowing, so that there is more freedom to have spontaneous fun. For yet another family, the primary shift may be to stay engaged and not walk away with detachment even when disappointed.

4. It is often helpful to assess the executive system through testing. Formal testing of executive functioning requires a high level of training and knowledge of brain functions. The interpretations of these tests are complex

and open to multiple variations, with no pure, one-to-one correspondence between the child's score and his or her ability (for information on testing executive functions and general assessment and intervention guidelines, see material on the CD-ROM, Section 11.1).

Depending on the professional setting, it may be appropriate to consider the use of a formal program or curriculum designed to enhance or support various components of executive functioning. The PATHS Curriculum (Promoting Alternative Thinking Strategies) was designed to be implemented by teachers and rests on the theory that executive functions support and mediate social and emotional competence (Kusche & Greenberg, 1995). The primary components of the curriculum involve inhibition/self-control, the management and recognition of emotions, verbal self-talk and expression of emotions, and interpersonal problem solving. Several studies involving both regular education and special education elementary students (and more recently, preschool students) have demonstrated the program's effectiveness (Greenberg & Kusché, 1993, 1998; Greenberg, Kusché, Cook, & Quamma, 1995; Kam, Greenberg, & Kusché, 2004; Riggs, Greenberg, Kusché, & Pentz, 2006), including a large randomized prevention trial involving 48 U.S. schools (Conduct Problems Prevention Research Group, 1999). Carroll Izard and colleagues' Emotion-Based Prevention (EBP) program focuses on emotional knowledge and self-regulation, whereby teachers and parents coach and guide young children in the moment, during the emotional experience (Izard, Trentacosta, King, & Mostow, 2004). Studies of the program in urban and rural Head Start systems found that increased emotional knowledge and regulation resulted in decreased aggression, anxious/depressed behavior, negative peer and adult interactions, and negative emotional expressions (Izard et al., 2004, 2008).

In a preschool program known as Tools of the Mind (a Vygotskian approach developed by Elena Bodrova and Deborah Leong, 2001, 2007), the daily routine and activities are designed to build executive functions such as working memory, cognitive flexibility, and, primarily, self-regulation. The program rests on the idea that children do not engage in as much unstructured peer play as they did in the past and, as a result, do not have as much opportunity to practice skills, such as controlling emotions and resisting impulses, that are integrated within the self-generated, detailed rules of children's pretend play scenarios. Adele Diamond and colleagues (Diamond, Barnett, Thomas, & Munro, 2007) conducted a 2-year randomized study and found that the preschoolers in the Tools of the Mind program did significantly better across a series of tests of executive functioning than the children who were in the regular education program. Levels of

self-regulation among the Tools students were also correlated with performance on achievement and language tests (Diamond et al., 2007). Other studies have also demonstrated the program's effectiveness for self-regulation and learning (Barnett, Jung, Yaroz, Thomas, & Hornbeck, 2008; Bodrova & Leong, 2001).

These and many other programs with demonstrated effectiveness are geared toward the development of social competence, a construct with multiple parallels to the capacities of the executive system. Social competence has been defined as involving the ability to regulate and adapt behavior in dynamic interpersonal situations (Sroufe, 1996), and requires social information processing, emotional and behavioral regulation, and flexible responsiveness to social feedback (Bierman & Welsh, 2000: Fabes, Gaertner, & Popp, 2006; Sroufe, 1996). Overall, the effective programs focus on: (1) cooperative play skills, (2) language/communication skills, (3) emotional knowledge and regulation, and (4) social/interpersonal problem solving and control of aggression (Bierman & Erath, 2006). For a review of programs that are specific to the treatment and prevention of conduct problems in early childhood (ages 2–7), see Webster-Stratton and Reid (2006).

5. The executive system can be developed through movement. For example, walking through and "doing" a sequence of actions will enhance learning more than listening to someone describe the sequence. Assessment and intervention should always include components that are interactive and action-oriented. Furthermore, movement is good for the brain; exercise stimulates the growth of new neurons (Churchill et al., 2002; Cotman & Berchtold, 2002; Kemper, 2001; van Praag, Shubert, Zhao, & Gage, 2005); thus, the actual practice of new emotional and educational skills, not just talking about them, is paramount to lasting change.

Movement can be considered in terms of the duration, rhythm, and intensity of speech and gross motor: How fast or slowly does a child or adult talk and move? Is the individual constantly talking or in constant motion or often quiet and still? Are words and actions deliberate and thoughtful, or do they seem rote, scripted, or on auto-pilot? The duration–rhythm–intensity extremes provide a gauge of too much activation or inhibition, wherein the middle ground that conscious control or a well-modulated system can bring is lacking. Such a baseline assessment, easily made during a session, can give any professional a starting point to ascertain the strengths and weaknesses of the child's executive system.

An interdisciplinary tool that assesses motor movement and nonverbal communication is provided by Tortora's Movement Signature Impressions

Checklist (Tortora, 2006). Tortora notes that for very young children (birth to age 2), music and dance can enhance natural self-expression by encouraging simple movements such as "rocking, rolling, crawling, clapping, bouncing, swinging, stamping, and running" (Tortora, 2006, p. 443). For preschoolers, obstacle courses with elements of going "in, under, over, swing, crawl, squeeze through, jump, balance, and roll" (Tortora, 2006, p. 444) assist with the regulation and sequencing of movement as well as modulating attention. For older children, music or drumming can encourage the modulation of movements by interspersing free-style movements with having to randomly shift movements from quick to slow to stopping and freezing positions. Perry also notes that using music, dance, drumming, and other basic rhythms, wherein gestures and bodily expressions are the focus, may be the place to begin intervention with traumatized children whose arousal systems remain dysregulated (Perry, 2006; Perry & Szalavitz, 2006). Again, whatever modality is used to promote and enhance movement and gestural/nonverbal communication, the three arousal intervention benchmarks (supporting sleep, promoting and expanding alert processing, and enhancing efficient stress recovery) should guide the process of ascertaining which sensory–motor experiences will optimize the achievement of these goals for each child.

In the near future, virtual reality (VR) applications will provide a resource for the assessment and treatment of a child's motor, cognitive, and emotional difficulties within multisensory and interactive environments. For example, Rizzo et al. (2006) has developed a virtual classroom that has been used to assess attention in children with ADHD and pediatric brain injury (Parsons, Bowerly, Buckwalter, & Rizzo, 2007; Rizzo et al., 2006). Children don a VR headset and are whisked away into a simulation of a typical classroom wherein they follow the virtual teacher's instructions or turn to watch a car pass by the window or a paper airplane fly across the room. Using tools like this, wherein the stimuli of the virtual world can be selectively manipulated, clinicians will be able to better understand the sensory stimuli and the temporal parameters that enhance and diminish performance for the individual child—information that can then inform precise environmental adjustments and treatment goals in the real world. Researchers have developed virtual homes, public spaces, traffic-filled streets, and obstacle courses to teach children with autism or other developmental and motor disorders relevant functional behaviors such as social skills (Parsons et al., 2000), fire safety skills (Rizzo, Strickland, & Bouchard, 2004), safe street-crossing (Bart, Katz, Weiss, & Josman, 2006; Strickland et al., 1996), and earthquake safety (Raloff, 2006) and to evaluate the capacity to navigate safely using a motorized wheelchair (Inman, Loge, & Leavens, 1997).

A more recent development in this area is the intersection of VR with computer games (called the "games for health" movement; see www .gamesforhealth.com). The basic premise of these applications is that intervention efforts will be more effective and potentially more robust by using some form of embedded game play to enhance a child's arousal, motivation, and positive emotion (Grealy, Johnson, & Rushton, 1999). Recent research on the treatment of motor deficits associated with cerebral palsy, using game-based VR, was shown to promote better control and a greater range of ankle movements as well as greater interest in doing the exercise than did stand-alone exercise (Bryanton et al., 2006). A number of researchers have also begun work with game applications for children with autism that are designed to promote eye contact (Trepagnier et al., 2006), cooperative pretend play (Gal et al., 2006), turn taking, and social awareness (Tartaro & Cassell, in press). Games are also being used successfully to promote health behaviors in children undergoing chemotherapy (see HopeLab ReMission, www.hopelab.org) and for distracting attention away from common, yet anxiety-provoking medical procedures (IV insertions, spinal taps, etc.) to reduce pain perception and emotional dysregulation (Gold, Kim, Kant, & Rizzo, 2005).

Although research-validated VR applications like these will be more readily available in the future, most are still in development or in clinical trial phases. In the interim, there are several off-the-shelf games, some developed for entertainment and some for education, that can be used as fun supplements to other ongoing interventions (i.e., therapy aids). For example, many of the Wii platform games (us.wii.com) involve movement (e.g., boxing, dance), cooperation (e.g., tennis), and learning (e.g., sea exploration); Dance Dance Revolution (www.ddrgame.com) products provide practice for motor sequencing, coordination, planning, and timing; the Sim City games (simcity.ea.com) exercise abilities such as planning and problem solving, and the project can be selected according to a child's interests; and Tetris-like games (www.tetris.com) provide practice for visuospatial, processing speed, and attention abilities. Educational and brain training software programs have also burgeoned in the past few years. For example, the Learning Company (www.learningcompany.com) has developed several academic programs for all ages and subject areas, with some programs specifically targeting executive abilities such as critical thinking; the Brain Gym (www.braingym.org) engages motor and multiple cognitive areas, including executive abilities; and Posit Science (www.positscience .com) currently offers software programs that enhance auditory and visual processing skills and are in the process of developing programs to enhance executive functioning and motor control (these products were developed for adults but purport to be appropriate for all ages).

Assessment and Intervention Steps

For executive system interventions, we stress the importance of using consistent (daily) strategies to effect change, strategies that focus on the global dynamics within the executive system's purview. Interventions such as helping a child expand his or her ability to initiate and inhibit purposeful behaviors, build an ability to see the big picture, hold multiple parts (emotions, thoughts) while playing with and manipulating them, connect the memories of the past into the present with anticipation of the future, and make accurate cause–effect links bring the rich synthesis the executive system can provide. Development of executive skills in children often requires help from an adult to scaffold the learning process. When the executive abilities of the parent are weak, several different types of strategies can be provided, in individual to consultation with the parents, which we describe next.

Step 1: Review Developmental and Socioemotional Milestones and Consider the Potential Contributions of the Executive System to the Presenting Problem

Developmental markers for motor abilities are located in Table 10.2 and for executive abilities are covered in Table 10.3. In addition, the fifth and sixth socioemotional milestones require significant executive input; for example, creating emotional themes within a story that has a beginning, middle, and end, with accurate cause–effect linkages (see Chapter 3).

Step 2: Assess Risk, Strengths, and Resources of Child and Parent

Risk factors are those existing internal and external vulnerabilities for both the child and the adult. The family history, in utero history, and medical/developmental history all provide data about the severity and pervasiveness of presenting problems. One can always use Worksheet 11.1 (a complete History Worksheet for all four brain systems is available for your use on the CD-ROM, Section 12.2) as an aid to consider the balance or imbalance of difficulties a child or parent is bringing to their dynamic interactions. Diagnostic symptoms of executive disorders can be found at the following Web sites.

- ADD: Help for ADD (www.helpforadd.com); Emedicine, (www.emedicine.com)
- Autistic spectrum disorder: NIMH (www.nimh.nih.gov/health/publications/autism/complete-publication.shtml); UC Davis M.I.N.D.

Worksheet 11.1. History Worksheet for the Executive System

Parental Risk Factors That Can Compromise a Parent's Ability to Provide Interactive Support	Global Questions That Assess the Overall Functioning of the Executive System	Child Risk Factors That Can Decrease Self-Regulation and Increase the Need for Interactive Regulation
☐ Motorically clumsy, awkward, or lethargic ☐ High distractibility ☐ High impulsivity ☐ Unable to delay gratification ☐ Lacks stable routines ☐ Adheres to rigid routines and habits, avoiding novelty ☐ Difficulty anticipating the need to sequence and implement agreed-on clinical input ☐ Lacks a willingness to incorporate a new way to understand a child's behavior (e.g., mental rigidity) ☐ Is unaware of, or inaccurately judges, own strengths and weaknesses ☐ Difficulty using hindsight, insight, and foresight for self-reflection and problem sovling ☐ Lacks cause–effect reasoning ☐ Unable to hold self and others in mind at the same time ☐ Unable to consider the part in relation to the whole	• Does child/adult show purposeful movement that is both adaptive and flexible? • Can child/adult see the big picture? • Can the child/adult stay on track in expressing a thought, emotion, or narrative? • Can the child/adult complete tasks in a relatively smooth fashion?	☐ Motorically clumsy, awkward, or lethargic ☐ Lacks developmentally appropriate use of gestures to communicate needs and wants ☐ Lacks developmentally appropriate use of words to problem-solve ☐ High distractibility ☐ High impulsivity ☐ Unable to delay gratification ☐ Lacks developmentally appropriate abilities to sequence activities of daily living ☐ Adheres to rigid routines and habits, avoiding novelty ☐ Lacks a willingness to incorporate a new way to understand own or other's behavior (e.g., mental rigidity) ☐ Is unaware of, or inaccurately judges, own strengths and weaknesses ☐ Difficulty using hindsight, insight, and foresight for self-reflection and problem solving ☐ Lacks cause–effect reasoning ☐ Unable to hold self and others in mind at the same time ☐ Unable to consider the part in relation to the whole

Institute (www.ucdmc.ucdavis.edu/MINDInstitute), Autism Speaks (www.autismspeaks.org); The Help Group (www.thehelpgroup.org/index.php)

- Asperger syndrome: Asperger Syndrome OASIS (www.aspergersyn drome.org); Autism Speaks (www.autismspeaks.org); Autism Society of America (www.autism-society.org/site/PageServer?pagename =life_aspergers)
- Developmental coordination disorder: Hillier (2007) (see ijahsp .nova.edu/articles/vol5num3/hillier.htm); MentalHelp.net (www .mentalhelp.net/poc/view_doc.php?type=doc&id=14495&cn=37); National Institute of Neurological Disorders and Stroke (www .ninds.nih.gov/disorders/dyspraxia/dyspraxia.htm)
- Nonverbal learning disorder (NLD): NLD on the Web (www .nldontheweb.org/about_nld.htm); NLDline (www.nldline.com); Nonverbal Learning Disorders Association (www.nlda.org); LD online (www.ldonline.org/indepth/nonverbal)

As we were identifying the triggers at home and things were deescalating, and as Mark was gaining stabilization with the medication for the mood dysregulaton, JT and I began to contemplate putting together a team that could further stabilize Mark, provide necessary services for him, provide for his educational needs, and ultimately help him successfully reenter school in a setting that was more appropriate for his multiple needs. With so many issues co-occurring, what would be addressed first? While the testing process was still in progress (the testing was ultimately accomplished over a 100-day period), it seemed appropriate to at least begin bottom-up with an occupational therapist skilled with learning disorders who could initiate playful sensory experiences with Mark and at the same time begin addressing remediation on his educational needs that were making his daily experiences with school work so frustrating and painful (e.g., poor fine-motor skills, weak visual-motor skills, sensory modulation difficulties). At the same time, as JT and I continued to assess Mark, we collaborated on making two lists. The first included nonverbal and verbal triggers we had identified that could feed Mark's quick escalations and distractions. The second list included ways to deescalate and calm him so that the parents, JT, CL, and the occupational therapist could be using the same cues and methods, self-correcting as we went along. As we attempted to titrate all activities, we needed to read his cues—his tone of voice rising, his eyes rolling up in frustration, his tongue clicking against the roof of his mouth, his sighing, his legs kicking, and his comments ("I'm tired," "I'm bored," or "This is too hard")—red flags that an escalation was imminent if the situation was not adjusted. An adjustment could mean (1) taking a break and coming back to the activity; (2) changing tone of voice by lowering tone and slowing rhythm; (3) asking Mark to participate in problem solving ("What do you think we should do about having to get this done?"); (4) giving Mark a choice as to what was easy, fun, or a "just-right" challenge so he felt he was being included in the transition and not being told what to do; (5) giving him a reward

system for accomplishing an agreed-on not-overwhelming amount of home-work without a meltdown; or (6) giving him some sensory input that helped organize his attention for longer periods of time (the swing and trampoline became his favorites). Thus, titration principles took front and center stage for all team members.

Over time, the full team that worked with Mark and his family, in addition to JT and CL, included the psychiatrist, an occupational therapist, an educational therapist, and two tutors who were team-led by the educational therapist. Within 3 months, Mark was able to begin learning again in home schooling sessions for 3 hours a day, which was accomplished through the educational team, and to partici-pate in therapy twice a week with CL and the occupational therapist. This team functioned for the remainder of the school year and through the summer, helping prepare Mark for his transition into a private school that was a better match for his special needs. Table 11.3 shows the distinct areas each professional was in charge of and the overlapping areas they shared by using the neurorelational framework.

Step 3: Support the Capacity to Flexibly and Purposefully Express Spontaneous, Automatic, and Consciously Controlled Behavior According to the Context

As mentioned, the executive system's multiple processes are integrated and, along with the other systems' input, they form patterns and themes of individual and dyadic behavior. In previous chapters we organized the intervention section according to specific strategies for each brain system for each capacity. We deviate from that structure here because the execu-tive system is intended to represent a synthesis of multiple contributions to healthy behavior and, likewise, a synthesis of the multiple contribu-tions to a child's difficulties. Our goal for the process of assessment and intervention in the executive system is that the professional will begin to reconstruct the parts of the child and the dyad back into a cohesive whole. The executive system provides the platform for the bird's-eye view where the professional can see and monitor the global patterns that support co-ordination and contribute to load from across brain systems.

In the prior section, we addressed problems involving too much spon-taneous, automatic, or consciously controlled behavior. To address imbal-ances, interventions must be targeted toward developing the less dominant behavioral formats as well as encouraging the flexible use of each format relative to circumstances. Because we are looking for the smooth flow of movement across actions, emotions, and thoughts, noting imbalances or the inappropriate use across the three formats gives clues as to where to target executive interventions.

Overreliance on spontaneous format. If the child/adult overrelies on the spontaneous format, with too much initiation and shifting of behavior

Table 11.3. Individual and Collective Functions of the Professional Team in Mark's Case

Area	Primary Functions	Shared Functions
Psychiatry	Using psychopharmacology to physiologically regulate rapid mood shifts and ADHD	Using all the information from team members, funneled through Connie, to keep abreast of progress in reaching emotional stability, attentional stability, and thought processes.
Occupational therapy	Strengthening trunk support; visual–motor, graphomotor, and fine-motor skills	Finding ways to deescalate emotional disruptions and gain further attention (through vestibular, proprioception, and deep touch pressure) that all team members could incorporate as needed.
	Using the titration principle and automaticity in building up all skills related to visual–motor, writing, and fine-motor processes (shared with educational therapy)	Implementing synchronized strategies with OT and educational therapist: • Sharing the same writing program • Providing supports for sitting • Using similar angle to writing table and similar pencil grip • Using raised-line adaptive paper, giving Mark more feedback during his writing so he would know where the top and bottom of his letter should be • Reminding Mark of correct posture; feet flat on the floor, nonwriting hand to support the paper
	Using a variety of sensory strategies to help further hand–eye coordination, fine-motor strength in hands, and enhance gross motor coordination and motor planning	
Educational therapy	Creating an individualized curriculum for Mark based on playing and working with him	For all subjects, titrating the challenge to his individual cues for frustration and attention
	Setting up tutors, educating them as to his special needs, and holding educational team meetings	Using executive skills in educational therapy (shared with mental health and occupational therapy)
	Carrying his educational needs forward in reading, writing, math, and all subjects, highlighting his strengths (reading) and titrating subjects of challenge (writing, spelling, and visual-spatial concepts)	Using emotional muscle tools to verbalize his range of frustration and using his words to share how hard a subject is
		Narrating and mirroring for Mark when a team member sees how hard things are getting for him
		Encouraging Mark to ask for help and problem solve with team members rather than denying his own struggle or trying to be self-reliant, which only increases frustration later down the road

	Enhancing working memory through visual–motor tracking integration (shared with occupational therapy)	Asking Mark to participate in reading nonverbal facial cues between himself and team members as these relationships deepened
	Using automaticity principles for all subjects	
	Using executive skills for all subjects (sequencing skills, tracking the steps involved in a process, using a part–whole process to writing a paragraph, emphasizing cause–effect reasoning in reading comprehension, working memory games, using temporal integration of past successes and steps to apply to next process or skill)	
Mental health	Case coordinator	Sharing the information about Mark's hypersensitivity to sensory information from vocal tone, intensity, and rhythms
	Building his emotional muscle to tolerate disappointment in himself and others, tolerate feelings of embarrassment in himself, and increase emotional freedom for self and others to make mistakes	Encouraging an open learning system with all practitioners by titrating challenges so Mark can learn to tolerate the negative range of emotions necessary in learning
	Working through Mark's trauma history of being bullied by peers and unsupported by teachers	Supporting his growth in making use of others (all practitioners on the team), being able to ask and accept help from others
	Becoming more flexible in relationships and decreasing anxiety and rigidity to create a more open learning system	Encouraging Mark to think about his own needs in relation to others' needs, in terms of part–whole relationships and the big picture in educational therapy
	Taking on another's perspective and holding onto that in relation to his own needs	Using executive skills in psychotherapy

(Continued)

Table 11.3. Continued

Area	Primary Functions	Shared Functions
	Clearing up confusion about cause–effect in relation to his part and others' parts in the bullying events	
	Using executive skills in psychotherapy (cause–effect reasoning in creating emotional stories and processing real-life events, clarifying appraisals of "everyone is mean to me," learning from past events and applying that to present and future, using visuals on the white board to show part–whole relationships in how an emotional event was co-created, role-playing previous events and how to do them differently in anticipation of a "next time")	
Neuropsychology	Initial assessment	Setting up treatment team and initial treatment plan
	Documentation of neuropsychological strengths and weaknesses and educational needs	Interpretation of findings to treatment team. Providing an initial set of working hypotheses for problem behaviors (for example, the meaning of social distortions in the context of a nonverbal learning disability)
	Periodic follow-up testing of established neuropsychological deficits/delays	Initial weighting of priorities based on determination of primary and secondary issues (from a brain–behavior perspective)
		Ongoing consultation regarding treatment successes and failures viewed in the context of his neuropsychological profile
		Consultation about the potential executive contributions to learning issues and problem behaviors; brainstorming as to potential strategies for building executive abilities

(reflected through high activation behavior), the general rule of thumb is to increase the capacity for inhibition from multiple directions and brain systems. For children with ADHD, research indicates that a combination of medication with appropriate therapeutic intervention is the most effective approach (MTA Cooperative Group, US, 1999a, 1999b; Swanson et al., 2008a, 2008b; Wells et al., 2000). As adjuncts to treatment or alternatives to medication, calming interventions that utilize relaxation, meditation, and biofeedback have shown effects for ADHD (Weisz & Gray, 2008; Weisz, Hawley, & Doss, 2004). In emerging studies, neurofeedback resulted in improved self-regulation in children with attentional difficulties and were rated as "probably efficacious," according to guidelines established by the Association for Applied Psychophysiology and Biofeedback and the International Society for Neuronal Regulation (Monastra, 2005; Strehl et al., 2006).

From a sensory perspective, decreasing the degree of incoming stimulation to reduce the pull of novelty simplifies the environment (i.e., decreases the intensity), thereby modulating arousal. When working with a hyperactive child, a practitioner might first match the child's behavior by increasing the speed of turn taking, thereby extending the child's engagement with the board game. Over time, however, slowing down and elongating transitions (countering the speed of too many shifts by increasing the duration) by requiring the child to complete the current task, activity, or game before turning to the next desired activity may help increase inhibition. Longer durations slow down the rate in which shifts are made, so that slower rhythms become emphasized.

For those children with too many tendencies toward distraction, pairing learning tasks with what the child deems interesting (relevance) can help sustain attention and decrease impulsivity. For example, if a child loves writing on a white board or using colored chalk, then these may be ideal ways for him or her to practice writing letters, spelling words, and doing math problems. Using executive (cognitive) strategies, children can be taught to use self-talk to give themselves feedback to reduce their distractibility as well as to keep them going when making mistakes, so that they can stay on task and not become thwarted by their own distractions, even giving themselves positive praise and rewards when they do well (Camp, Blom, Hebert, & van Doornick, 1977; Weisz et al., 2004; Weisz & Gray, 2008). Checklists for sequencing and structuring work loads for homework, daily routines and activities, time management, and learning and problem-solving strategies can provide important feedback to help a child stay on task, as well as provide useful organizing strategies for parents.

Underreliance on spontaneous formats. For those children with too much inhibition, from either overreliance on automatic or conscious-control formats, using activities that encourage spontaneity may increase the activation side of arousal. Games with an element of surprise or that require participants to make shifts frequently (e.g., Sorry, Trouble) provide natural stimulation and opportunities for spontaneity in real time. Titrating these shifts to the child's arousal needs is important, although eliminating the stress of a challenge is not the goal. The goal is to support the child as he or she moves through the challenge (e.g., the distress of losing, upset from making a mistake, discouragement when a task feels too hard) in order to slowly build tolerance for emotional disruptions and promote the development of an open learning system (similar dynamics to the titration principle may be referred to in other treatments such as "reinforced exposure" used with anxiety disorders and related conditions; Weisz & Gray, 2008).

Overreliance on automatic format. If the child/adult frequently uses the automatic format, with too much sustaining and inhibition of behavior (often in a hypoalert state), the general rule of thumb is to increase the capacity for behaviors that involve initiating and shifting among activities. In this case, a practitioner might counter a child's slow pace by increasing his or her own rhythm and intensity as a way to inject more momentum into the interaction. For children with too many automatic tendencies, paring spontaneous activities with known routines may help expand flexibility (e.g., introducing a riskier game in between well-known and well-loved habits of swinging and coloring).

Underreliance on automatic formats. For those children who need an increase in healthy automatic routines (e.g., making their beds, cleaning their rooms, hygiene), breaking down the routine or task into small increments is advised. For example, take on one activity at a time, motor through a consistent sequence of the activity with the child for several days, and set up rewards until the process becomes rote. The first phase of developing useful automatic behaviors requires an emphasis on conscious control, which can be encouraged initially by narrating the sequence of actions as the child verbalizes the same in parallel. Conscious control can also be woven in by providing anticipatory reminders (e.g., stating at bedtime, "Let's think about the morning routine ... "), by prompting the child to anticipate distractions (e.g., the dog wants to play, a sibling turns on the television), and by problem solving as to when it might be okay to let the routine go (e.g., woke up late, so cut corners by not washing one's hair).

Overreliance on conscious control format. If the child or adult overrelies on the conscious control format (often in a hyperalert state), the general rule of thumb is to increase the capacity for initiating and shifting

into more spontaneous thoughts, emotions, and activities. For example, playful disagreements that challenge a rigid thought may be useful (e.g., playfully "arguing" about who is going to win or lose a game and subsequently modeling being a good sport while losing).

As noted, the maturation of executive skills builds resources and resiliency that help mitigate risk factors (e.g., substance abuse, dropping out of school). As the parent serves as the executive system for the child, the professional serves as the external executive system for the parent. Maturing the less developed formats builds resilience and restores balance to the executive system's foundational dynamics.

Underreliance on conscious-control formats. In general, developing conscious control means bringing behavior into attentional focus, or creating opportunities for the child to become increasingly self-aware of thoughts, emotions, and actions. Building a capacity for conscious control involves a slow, steady rhythm so that new variables can be held in mind and manipulated (working memory) as they are prioritized and integrated into a part–whole structure. In addition to slowing down the rhythm, giving only small amounts of verbal information at one time is useful while collecting the variables that a child or adult is trying to acquire. A child can be asked to repeat back what was stated as a way to help enhance the accuracy of information exchanged (especially for those with processing speed or information processing difficulties). Another helpful approach to support working memory is to speak in shorter sentences and give no more than three pieces of information at once. Having the child verbalize relevant aspects of a task, such as "state the rule" him- or herself rather than only listen to someone else state it, can enhance the child's performance (Kirkham, Cruess, & Diamond, 2003; Kray, Eber, & Karbach, 2008; Zelazo, 1999). In addition, have the child write down the sequential steps to a task or brainstorm a list and then numerically prioritize the items. As the child performs the steps, check off or line through each part (or allow the child to do this) so that the child can see his or her progress in relationship to the whole process.

As noted, conscious control is also aided by problem solving for anticipated events, especially those that are uncomfortable. As priority solutions rise to the top of the list, they can be practiced through enactments that take the child from the old way to the new desired way (e.g., role-playing; evidence-based research discusses the use of interpersonal therapy for adolescents; Weisz & Gray, 2008). Gaining facility with the conscious control format includes increasing top-down awareness of changes in facial expressions, vocal tones, gestures, and verbal expressions. Parents can take a lead role in modeling the conscious format for their children by thinking out loud, coaching them, talking them through situations and tasks, and so on.

Step 4: Support the Capacity to Integrate the Bottom-Up Influences of Emotions with the Top-Down Control of Thoughts

Interventions in this section are geared toward creating a dynamic flow of information through past, present, and future time frames to enhance the executive system's ability to modulate and integrate emotions and thoughts. In this step, we focus on the use of conscious control to assist in creatively changing default modes involving emotions and thoughts. Using the conscious control format to examine and learn from the problematic patterns is central to increasing the flexible integration of thought and emotion— the overall goal being movement toward an open learning system.

Treating imbalances in emotion. During the early phase of intervention, noticing the degree of balance between emotion and thought processes is important. When flooded emotions (too much arousal) shut down access to thoughts, the goal becomes building up an emotional muscle that better tolerates and modulates emotion, as described in the relevance system. Here, insight in the moment is virtually impossible because emotions are running too high. Thus, the ability to recall and learn from past events (hindsight), when arousal is more optimal, is pivotal in treating this imbalance. A top-down approach to overemotional expressions is to teach the child or adult to view the "big feeling" as a problem to solve. Although exploring affects is important for both children and adults, those who are easily flooded by bottom-up experiences may need more top-down help. Approaching overreactions as problems to solve shifts the focus to a thinking modality with support from top-down inhibition, rather than further fueling emotional connections that are already poorly managed.

For example, a child whose problem becomes how to manage embarrassment when being teased during recess, the brainstorming process might explore (1) what happened before he was teased (sets the stage for the larger picture); (2) if there is a pattern to the teasing (looks for recurring themes and patterns that might enable hindsight; e.g., a bully who teases everyone who wears glasses); (3) what has been tried already (enables insight by itemizing and prioritizing what has and has not worked); and (4) what new things could be tried next time (enables foresight by anticipating future occurrences, this time armed with new solutions to try). The new solutions can vary, for example, from walking away to hooking up with another peer for protection to getting adult help to practicing asserting oneself and standing up to the troublemaker. These problem-solving skills are often related to strategies employed in cognitive-behavioral therapy. In reviewing evidence-based research, problem-solving skills have been shown to be successful with conduct-related problems and disorders (Weisz et al., 2004; Weisz & Gray, 2008).

Treating imbalances in thinking. For a child whose thoughts dampen down access to emotions, the first step is to help him or her identify emotions that he or she ignores. Just the process of increasing self-awareness of an emotion is an insightful moment. The second step is to help the child become aware of underlying negative assumptions that exacerbate the shutting down of emotions or create rigid, default conclusions. The problem to be solved may be the assumptions, beliefs, and cause–effect reasoning that need to be altered. Here, the child may need help to deconstruct the assumption that, for example, he or she must get straight As so as to not fall apart, or that he or she can never be wrong about anything to avoid shame. Rigid thinking based on black-and-white assumptions usually undergirds faulty cause–effect reasoning and prevents one from reading the context and the inferences of others in real time. Increasing the child's capacity to understand that others may have opinions or varying assumptions that differ from his or hers helps the child become more curious about others' mental states, creating more flexible cause–effect associations by expanding theory of mind.

Treating simultaneous bottom-up and top-down imbalances. Many times, both exaggerated emotions and unhelpful thoughts converge to create difficulties in gaining hindsight about past errors, insight into current challenges, and foresight regarding possible future disappointments. For example, a child may fall apart, unable to bear losing a game (see the strategies in Chapter 9 for building the emotional muscle). Examining the thoughts accompanying this emotional display reveal beliefs, such as "If I don't win, it means I'm stupid" or "I have to be the best or I'm nothing" or "Nothing ever goes right for me—I must be bad." These beliefs create unrealistic internal demands on the child that are neither accurate nor attainable but that fuel the negative emotional tank. At times, these beliefs may come from a parent's demands of perfection. Other times, they are rudimentary deductions made by a child because the parent does not sufficiently mirror what the child does right. Still other times, the child brings this type of pressure into the relationship him- or herself, likely tied to heritable influences involving anxiety disorders, obsessive–compulsive disorders, bipolar disorders, and so on. Of course, all the foregoing situations can co-occur.

Modeling mistakes, loss, and imperfections within the therapist–child relationship is important for parents and their children to see. In "live modeling" (Weisz & Gray, 2008) the professional can model how to lose gracefully, with disappointment but not despair; to take a disappointing event (e.g., not getting what one wants during a turn) with a grain of salt, showing "flexible disappointment" ("Oh, well, maybe next time"). As emphasized several times, the ability to not only tolerate but also learn

from mistakes is essential for an open learning system to develop. Also salient here is helping the child accept these mistakes as a natural part of relationships. One can be aware that the child's likely focus on the other's mistakes mirrors the child's intolerance of his or her own mistakes. If the parent, teacher, or adult can show genuine concern about how these incidents disrupt the child's functioning, while at the same time staying steady in accepting that he or she made a mistake (blending responsive, directive, and reflective modes), the child can learn to begin to tolerate the normalcy of mistakes. This acceptance and tolerance of everyday mistakes and disappointments have to be mirrored and modeled—and celebrated—when the child shows flexibility in this direction in his or her learning through imitation. For example, the adult can praise a child who typically does not tolerate losing a game when the child succeeds by saying something like "Wow! Look at you! You just got captured and you handled that so well! What a big-boy thing to do!" Establishing a "proud bank," in which the child can collect and store experiences in which he or she felt pride about an achievement, can enhance the momentum towards further growth.

In the dyadic play sessions, we rotated between co-creating emotional stories and playing games that stimulated emotional upheavals from losing. At first, the emotional stories were all about random destructiveness. These stories reflected automatic default modes that permeated play at home and in my office. The "meaning" of these stories seemed to be in the re-creation of Mark's experience of being bullied and the volatile relationship between himself and his mother. In actuality, Mark was a very tender boy with a big heart underneath his rough exterior as the bully who laughed at his own destructiveness in the play. Eventually, he showed his responsive side to me (CL) and other team members, bringing in sweet surprises and gifts he had made for each of us. As I heard more of his history, I learned that he had always assumed that people were going to be kind to him. Because he was such a "happy boy," always laughing and smiling early on, easily engaging with everyone, he did not seem prepared for what hit him in preschool and beyond. In fact, at first (beginning as early as preschool), he always accommodated the bullies, trying hard to please them (e.g., allowing them to eat his lunch or throw it away; throwing the balls at others when told to), and was very confused as to why he was getting into trouble.

In parallel fashion, Susan was completely unprepared for Mark's onset of mood shifts. When Mark's moods did not dissipate, Susan began to feel oppressed by his bad temper. She relied on offering Mark what had been offered to her as a child: clear directives that involved being told what was right from wrong and how to obey. She felt that Mark needed limits, to be directed in what he was doing wrong. In addition, she expected Mark to comply, just as she had done as a child. Even though she cried as she recalled how she had been parented, she felt that the one way she knew how to parent was being taken away from her. Susan

felt perpetually attacked by Mark. Even though she recognized that he was only 7, she felt that he was abusing her. A vicious circle had developed wherein Mark's moodiness stimulated Susan's demandingness. She found herself oscillating between depression and rage. The more she demanded obedience, the more Mark attacked her and became violent. Both experienced the other as abusive, and they co-escalated in short order.

Amid the bullies at school and the escalating relationship with Susan at home, Mark's mantra of "everyone is mean to me" began during his kindergarten year. He emotionally shifted from naive optimism to a mild form of paranoia in his emotional journey, where distinctions in the range of good and bad behavior for self and others were lacking. It was necessary to take time to sort out what had happened, how it had hurt him, the effects of his being kind to bullies, and how he and his mother fueled each other's rage. While doing so, we inadvertently built up his private and assertive modes through implementing hindsight and reviewing the meaning of these events. Slowly, Mark became able to build into his stories realistic cause–effect relationships. In addition, he became more able to create temporal patterns that helped clarify how the past story related to the present circumstances and how it could be anticipated in the future. Finally, the ability to express empathetic and protective roles emerged (see material on the relevance system, specifically Tables 8.2 and 9.5).

As Susan's individual therapy with me progressed, she began to build hindsight and insight about her depression as a child as well as her urges to rage at her parents. However, she needed to do more to create a parenting shift in her daily life at home. Susan needed concrete, kind, yet firm directives from me to learn new ways of being with Mark. My first set of instructions included asking her to let go of the word *no*, which was to be replaced by a reflective remark in response to Mark ("It seems you really want this to happen; oh, wow, this seems really important to you"). Mark needed this type of reflection, and this instruction helped Susan think before saying *yes* or *no*. It also enabled her to get away from a yes/no orientation and focus more on understanding Mark's needs in relation to the context. In essence, Susan needed to become more curious about Mark's demands and their meanings. In addition, I suggested that she had to find a way to say yes to some aspect of Mark's request *before* she offered the no. This strategy, too, required her to shift out of her default automatic mode and use more conscious control as well as more spontaneous responses. These new responses began to alter the long-standing pattern of her demands for limits, which were predictably followed by Mark's attacks. To her surprise, as she began to "think on her feet" and offer other alternatives, Mark began to join her in spontaneous problem solving, and the two of them began to come up with creative solutions. This shift enabled Susan to slowly discover, through reflection, that her automatic no's had been provocative for Mark and that Mark had also felt abused and attacked by her. Over time, using conscious control, Susan began to catch herself offering a directive and was able to inhibit and shift to change this on-the-spot urge into creating a more productive comment (e.g., "Oh, I think you need a hug right now!").

In the couple's treatment, Jerry offered a great deal of support to Susan as she struggled to make these changes, and he expressed empathy for her sad history. His support inspired Susan to find the courage to make the changes. Susan, too, offered support to Jerry. She made a great watchdog, spotting Jerry's spontaneous gestures that would lead to Mark's rigidity, and she could begin to catch Jerry before he blithely promised to do something impractical or beyond their reach as a family.

Step 5: Support the Capacity to Assess, Integrate, and Prioritize One's Own Internal (Self) Needs in Relation to External (Context/Other) Needs

We have conceptualized the three modes of self-awareness—the private, assertive, and giving selves—as way to "operationalize" the complex movement involved in the multiple components of this capacity. Chronic imbalances in private, assertive, and giving modes are red flags signaling intervention needs in this capacity. These imbalances may be present for various reasons, including problematic (i.e., too slow or too fast) processing speeds and limitations or breakdowns in any or all executive capacities. Reestablishing balance between private, assertive, and giving modes requires the top-down help of conscious control.

Facilitating the maturation of the private mode. Someone who lacks access to a developed private mode may be prone toward spontaneous or automatic behaviors that never facilitate self-reflection. Always being on the go or externally focused does not allow for "being" time wherein one's own behaviors are noticed. Increasing the private mode for child and adult requires increasing conscious awareness of central aspects across all brain systems—their arousal, sensory, emotional, memory, and thought patterns. Can they notice a pattern (requiring hindsight or insight)? What meaning do they attribute to these patterns (requiring insight)? Are they making accurate cause–effect links between their part and how they impact others (also requires theory-of-mind abilities)? Do they hold all the parts of themselves or only certain aspects (requiring working memory)? Can they see the links between their contributions in relation to the group's/context's contribution (requiring part–whole relationships)?

Developing a private self requires this self-awareness, and it most often does not develop in a vacuum; on a most basic level, the private mode requires an ability to tolerate feedback from others while learning from mistakes. In addition, the private mode, to be healthy and accurate, must receive and process information from the visceral, sensory, emotional, and executive selves. For those with little connection to these selves, the practitioner may need to begin with a combination of bottom-up and top-down strategies

that help the child or adult learn how to identify and increase awareness of markers from the visceral, sensory, emotional, and thinking realms. A visual format that organizes the rich range of bodily markers from various sources can be a useful guide while building this fund of awareness. A sample of such a tool can be found on the CD-ROM, Section 9.2.

Children or adults who are overly engrossed in a private mode may appear detached, dissociative, or aloof due to their self-absorption. "Too much" of a private self often develops in the context of lacking feedback from others, such that a closed system with only internal, private thoughts, and often ruminations develops. The practitioner may need to help these individuals expand their ability to hold onto their reactions in relation to others. Tracking a sequential process, a previous troubling event can be broken down into components of "self" and "other" to help the child or adult gain a sense of his or her personal perspective in relation to the other. As the practitioner is tracking these two components, he or she needs to be sure to illicit the child's appraisal of him- or herself and others, including negative appraisals, misinterpretations of strengths or weaknesses, or denial of strengths or weaknesses.

Facilitating the maturation of the assertive mode. A child or adult who lacks an assertive mode may be (1) stuck in a reclusive inner world; (2) fearful of taking action due to current or prior abuse (see the material on the relevance system); (3) extremely shy (Kagan, 1987; Kagan, Reznick, & Snidman, 1999); (4) prone to shame (Covert, Tangney, Maddux, & Heleno, 2003; Keltner & Harker, 1998; Tangney, Wagner, Hill-Barlow, Marschall, & Gramzow, 1996); (5) overly accommodating and giving to others at the expense of self (Brandchaft, 1994; Connors, 2000); (6) unaware of, or not know how to compensate for, learning strengths and weaknesses; or (7) lacking in motor planning skills. Knowing these possible underlying dynamics is essential in facilitating a further maturation of an assertive mode. Because access to the private mode is essential for a healthy assertive mode, if the private mode is underdeveloped, that would need to be worked on in tandem.

Developing the assertive mode may be enhanced by movement (Tortora, 2006). Without movement through eyes, faces, vocal sounds, gestures, and actions (nonverbal cues), the private mode can remain locked up; needs, wants, desires, and responsibilities are not achieved and remain unknown to others. The same nonverbal cues we identified as essential communicators of states of arousal in the regulation system are key vehicles of communicating the shift from the private mode into the assertive mode of being known.

When working with children and adults struggling to cope with shyness or shame-based withdrawal, as well as traumatic histories, often the

most important factor is carefully modulating the dimensions of the interventions. Because these children and adults typically misappraise normal levels of sensory input as toxic, they respond best to slow rhythms, low intensity, and sensory input of short duration (e.g., when verbally communicating, use short sentences, only a few sentences at a time, and slowly and with a calm tone), whether verbal or movement-based. In every session, it is also critical to point out the positive attitudes, events, and skills a child has recently evidenced before launching into the problematic aspects of his or her behavior. Because a shame-based child will often consider any negative feedback an indictment against him or her, the overarching goal becomes helping the child build the emotional muscle to tolerate mistakes, errors, and unlearned skills.

The parent and the professional may need to scaffold the child's early attempts at self-assertion by tracking his or subtle cues and narrating the inferences drawn. For example, with a socially withdrawn child who glances wistfully at another child playing with a toy, the perceptive adult might query, "Oh, I wonder if you want to play with that toy? Shall we see if your classmate is willing to share this toy with you?" Being validated through mirroring can bolster a willingness to expose more of one's preferences and one's authentic self. If one actually knows one's preferences but is afraid to show them, role-plays can be used as a way to practice exposing and expressing one's needs in a safe environment. Ample practice with actions and words enables the child to develop more ease with initiating self-expressive behaviors, such that tremendous effort is no longer required in real time when on the spot.

For those whose weak assertive mode is due to giving too much, the challenge becomes helping the child or adult tolerate the anxiety that comes from saying *no* to others and *yes* to self. Again, this new behavior may best be facilitated in a safe relationship with a parent or professional who can support the child in practicing standing up for him- or herself through symbolic play, pretend play, and role-plays. Usually, children and adults who accommodate too much get angry later because they feel taken advantage of. This anger can be a useful motivator for them to brave the anxiety of setting clearer limits and boundaries. Mapping out what occurred when, for example, the child felt angry, and planning ahead for what to say the next time helps the child develop hindsight, insight, and foresight into events where assertion was lacking.

For some children, the assertive mode is weak due to learning or processing problems. Initially, these children need to be differentiated according to (1) those who are unaware of the mismatch between the task/activity and their ability to perform it and, thus, are caught off-guard when things do not go well; and (2) those who know that they are confronting a weakness but

lack the know-how to problem solve or compensate. For the first group of children, those seeming to lack awareness, the process of intervention should begin slowly and at a micro level by answering the following question: At what point along the sequence of confronting a weakness can the child's capacity for insight be stimulated? A simple reflection on a past experience of failure (hindsight) may be enough to stimulate a child's insight, whereupon the child might say, for example, "Yes, other kids seem to do better on tests than me," or "Yes, I do have a hard time listening to directions sometimes." More often, the insight will not come as easily, and the child will require a more gradual process of being exposed to the weakness, such as through (1) modeling (e.g., "Wow, this type of memory game is so hard for me!"), (2) breaking down the past in a "light" nonjudgmental way (e.g., "That test must have been really hard! Let's see if we can think of things that might have made it a little easier"), (3) reflecting on the process in real time ("You have that test tomorrow—do you think you're ready? What did you do to prepare?"), (4) checking insight in real time (e.g., "Let's play this game . . . do you think this will be hard? . . . Why/why not?"), or (5) structuring the child's anticipation (e.g., "How do you think you will do on the test tomorrow?").

For children aware of their weakness, the problem-solving process can begin immediately. The first step is structuring the cause-and-effect components: What particular aspects of tasks/activities cause the struggle, what makes them better/worse, what is the lowest/highest priority? Often, with the help of another person for tracking and monitoring, children are well able to answer these questions. The reason it takes time and mental effort initially may be simply that they have never attempted to structure it in a top-down way before, and sometimes just organizing the problem can go a long way toward helping children help themselves.

The second step is to ensure that there are opportunities and venues through which the child can pursue a strength/talent or an interest. A child's life should never be swallowed up by a focus on weaknesses, even if it means that additional remedial efforts must be postponed in lieu of an enjoyable or fulfilling activity. This does not mean that intensive interventions are off the table, only that they should be titrated appropriately and that something positive (i.e., replenishing) must always be woven into the child's daily life.

The next step is to problem solve the weaknesses: What skills could the child develop (e.g., better organization, study skills), what strategies are most effective (e.g., memory strategies, listening to books on tape, repetition), how much time does the child need (e.g., is the child allocating time poorly, not starting soon enough?), and what environmental factors can be manipulated (e.g., does the child need to stay after school to

finish things? Does the child need headphones to block out the noise?). It usually takes time and the regular assistance of a professional (e.g., tutor, educational therapist) to work through all of these components.

The last step is monitoring and enhancing: What is working and what is not, are the child's efforts sufficiently productive, what is giving the child the most bang for the buck, what strategies need further tweaking, and are the strategies enhancing self-esteem and resilience? As always, along the way, the child should receive positive rewards and feedback in a way that is meaningful to him or her. For example, some children will beam with pride at nothing more than a "good job!" whereas others may feel rewarded only if they receive something tangible. At the same time, rewards need to be titrated; they lose their impact when overdone.

Facilitating the maturation of the giving mode. Those who lack a giving mode often are (1) preoccupied with their inner worlds, (2) oblivious to social cues, (3) preoccupied with self-needs and self-aggrandizement, or (4) under tremendous pressures and responsibilities that consume them. Developing a giving self requires being given to by significant others in a responsive, nurturing manner—a heartfelt experience that one is valued. This sense of self-value lays a foundation for giving. Without this authentic security, giving too much becomes a compensatory behavior for warding off anxiety, rather than an act of caring about others as separate from oneself.

First, accurately reading others' nonverbal cues is just as important as being connected to one's own nonverbal cues, so checking out the connections on both levels is important. (For children who do not notice enough of their own cues, interventions would need to use previously mentioned strategies that link visceral and emotional cues.) Second, making distinctions between self and other is imperative for giving to match the need in others. A child or adult with an inability in this area is likely to give presents to another that he or she wants for him- or herself. For such children, using the white board can be useful to highlight the lines of demarcation between self and other. A previous event can be discussed in terms of four categories of information: what the child was feeling and meaning to communicate, what the child's nonverbal and verbal cues were, what the child saw in the other, and what the child's inference was about the other. By writing this information in four columns, the cause–effect relationships can be highlighted in the back-and-forth process. These four columns can be set up for each one of the following categories: (1) nonverbal and verbal cues from self, (2) private meanings about nonverbal and verbal cues from self, (3) nonverbal and verbal cues from others, and (4) inferences and private meanings about nonverbal and verbal cues from others. As the back-and-forth exchanges of relationships are deconstructed in this way, children

(and parents) gradually learn the degree to which they are aware of themselves and others. Skewed meanings, misread cues, and discrepancies between verbal and nonverbal messages are typically revealed. Using this four-column format, the therapist, parent, and child can review relational conflicts that the child has experienced. In addition, there are games available for older children that stimulate social conflicts and emotional dilemmas that require the player to, in essence, draw upon their private, assertive, and giving selves (Berg, 2004).

For some, the lack of giving is rooted in bitterness, anger, hatred, envy, or vindictiveness toward others (often from perceptions/experiences of unfairness). These strong emotional responses must be deconstructed in order for the giving mode to surface and blossom (Horney, 1945, 1950; Klein, 2001). Fear-based thoughts and assumptions that either the giving will not be noticed or will be denigrated, causing the giver embarrassment, may be prevalent and need to be deconstructed. Again, the importance of shame as a driver of negative thoughts and attacks towards self and others cannot be underestimated (Schore, 1994, 1998, 2003a, 2003b). As a nascent giving expression develops, a responsive other is often necessary to receive the gift and reinforce the giver. Tolerating the reality that not all gifts will be as appreciated as one might want is a hard lesson to learn, but a necessary one for healthy living.

As progress was being made on all fronts, the educational therapist and I (CL) made up a list of what kinds of things would be helpful for Mark to get ready for reentry into a school that could handle his needs. Things on this list included becoming more flexible and less rigid, thinking about others' feelings and needs in relation to his own feelings and needs, tolerating making mistakes and being disappointed in himself and others, noticing others' nonverbal cues and inferring their meanings, and being able to ask for help when needed. These abilities were shared with team members and were included in his educational goals.

It was a big step when the parents, Mark, and the team felt that Mark was ready to try out a new school that seemed to have the flexibility and emphasis on learning and emotional needs that Mark needed to succeed. JT's testing had confirmed that, indeed, his diagnostic categories had aligned with ADHD, inattentive type, NLD, and a mood disorder. I (CL) was especially intent on making sure that his new teaching team knew about his nonverbal and verbal signs of potential escalation. Whenever there was any type of emotional glitch that Mark would complain about in our sessions, I was on the phone the next day with the lead teacher to discuss the upset and help make decisions about how to proceed. We all wanted Mark to be successful and knew that a second school failure would not bode well for his future.

The new school was remarkable in its accommodations, which continued throughout the first year of attendance. First, Mark was allowed to come to school late, which he did almost every day. Mark struggled to get out of bed

every morning, and Jerry's main concern was to pace with him, not pressure him, and help him transition into the day. Second, 1 day a week, Jerry came to school and took Mark out to lunch so they could have some special time together. Though concerned about Mark's need to develop peer relationships during the lunch hour, they also adapted to accepting Mark's need for special contact with Jerry during the school week for Mark to continue to feel safe and supported during this stressful transition. Third, on more than one occasion, when the school mentioned that Mark was not working up to his potential, I reassured them that his school work was not as important as his ability to show up to school every day, even though he was late. I added that although we cared about his learning, it was enough that he was building his emotional muscle to endure the stress of being in a classroom each day and continue trying to learn despite his learning challenges. The school continued to titrate his workload so that it was just right for what he could tolerate. His new teaching staff took our feedback seriously, and we were able to create an open learning system between us as a team, similar to what had been accomplished through the tutoring educational team. Mark maintained his relationship with his educational therapist and continues to work with her on an after-school basis.

Susan progressed in her individual therapy to the point where she began to rotate into our dyadic sessions. Susan and Mark were able to learn to play together successfully, acknowledge their triggers with each other, and solve problems with each other. The early playfulness they once had shared during the first years of life returned. The next phase of treatment began with Mark learning to tolerate a boundary coming from Mom as well as Dad. Jerry slowly began to share his authority with Susan, and very slowly, Mark has begun to tolerate them parenting him as a couple. No longer are there cries from Mark pleading for a divorce, and he can now begin to tolerate that he both loves and sometimes hates his mother, mostly loving her.

Mark is in the early phases of taking responsibility for his own eruptions and occasional escalations. He admits how much he enjoys feeling powerful and in charge when he is angry, but he is also willing to admit that his rages negatively affect others. This two-pronged insight is motivating him to change. He is noticing the somatic markers in his body when he's on an upswing, developing his private mode with his internal cues. When problem solving, he is beginning to spontaneously come up with his own ideas for how to be assertive and starting to practice ways he can be assertive instead of aggressive. The monster is beginning to learn how to tame himself.

It is a pleasure to say that Mark has returned for a second year at his new school. Moreover, he has been able to get to school on time every day, he has participated in a school play, he is taking gymnastics classes after school, he is doing his homework on his own, he is able to ask for help when he needs it, he is on student council for his class, he was recently selected as student of the month, and he is now beginning to catch up academically. This child, who had been unable to recover and learn, is becoming successful, and we feel confident he will be able to reach his potential.

SUMMARY POINTS FOR PRACTITIONERS: EXECUTIVE SYSTEM

Clinicians can consider their cases and identify whether any of the behaviors they observe might have contributions from the executive system. These contributions may be identified from any of the following points:

- Does this child or parent have the ability to pay attention and to focus?
- Does this child or parent need help anticipating sudden or upsetting events?
- Can this child or parent handle transitions?
- Can this child or parent problem-solve with you and plan ahead for a different way to handle his or her upsetting reactions?

Furthermore, professionals can make note of the disciplines weighted in this brain system and begin to create professional networks that can be used for referrals when necessary. Disciplines weighted in the executive system include the following:

- neuropsychologists;
- psychologists;
- physical therapists (gross motor);
- occupational therapists (oral motor, fine motor, and motor planning);
- educational therapists;
- psychiatry (medical management for ADHD);
- behaviorists (sequencing and structuring in small increments).

In terms of intervention, parents can play an important role. In particular, involving them in the following strategies can be beneficial:

- Provide repetition to build automaticity.
- Teach a problem-solving sequence.
- Build impulse control through having to slow down and wait (e.g., take three more turns in the game before deciding to stop).
- Assist with sequencing through a story, task, daily activities, or problem (use pictures and narrative).
- Break things down into small steps.

In addition, all practitioners on the team can consider the following possible strategies for assessment and intervention:

- Scaffold emotional problem solving.
- Support building in impulse control.
- Support providing structures in session or classroom with planning, sequencing, and follow-through.
- Support the perception of cause–effect and part–whole relationships.

Worksheet 11.2 summarizes the executive concepts and can be used to assess the executive system in infants, children, and parents. (This worksheet is also available on the CD-ROM, Section 11.2.)

The final chapter weaves together the major components of the neurorelational framework, and walks readers through an application of its use.

Worksheet 11.2. Assessment of the Executive System in the Infant, Child, and Parent

Resources and Strengths Toward Allodynamic Coordination	Risk Factors for Conditions of Allodynamic Load
Check whatever applies to the child, and circle what applies to the parent (including the parent's developmental history).	*Check whatever applies to the child, and circle what applies to the parent (including the parent's developmental history).*
☐ Flexible attention between what is safe and dangerous in the environment and relationships	☐ Highly distractible ☐ Highly distractible with excessive body movements
☐ Modulates attention between familiar and novel sources of information	☐ Prolonged hypervigilance ☐ Easily tunes out
☐ Balance between flexing and extending arms and limbs; stays in midline position when safe	☐ Poor muscle tone (either too flexed/tight tone or too extended/low tone)
☐ Stability in motor system (postural stability of head and trunk; symmetry and alignment of body; able to right self and use protective reflexes if falling)	☐ Motor instability in crawling, walking, or sitting ☐ Lack of initiative to move ☐ Desire to move, but inability to mobilize motor system
☐ Mobility in motor system (rolling, crawling, creeping, walking, running)	☐ Does not use gestures (e.g., pointing) to communicate needs or wants
☐ Able to use gestures (e.g., pointing) to communicate needs and wants	☐ Tendency toward impulsive acts ☐ Excessive falling and tripping
☐ Bilateral coordination (symmetry in using both sides of body or back-and-forth use, such as in swimming)	☐ Poor fine motor coordination; difficulty holding and using a crayon or pencil (difficulty reaching, grasping, and manipulating objects)
☐ Able to use sensory and emotional information to create, sequence, and act on a plan	Comments:

(Continued)

Worksheet 11.2. Continued

Resources and Strengths Toward Allodynamic Coordination	Risk Factors for Conditions of Allodynamic Load
☐ Able to be spontaneous according to context ☐ Able to do things automatically ☐ Able to exercise conscious control ☐ Learns from past experience (hindsight) and incorporates into future plans and actions (foresight) ☐ Learns from current experiences (insight) and uses this information for future planning (foresight) ☐ Makes appropriate cause–effect links ☐ Appropriately reads the nuances and intentions of others' nonverbal and verbal communication ☐ Balances self–other awareness so there is the ability to shift between private, assertive, and giving modes ☐ Able to see the parts to the whole relationship ☐ Other: _____ _____	☐ Poor gross motor coordination: clumsy, awkward body movements (unable to co-ordinate acts with large movements like jumping, hopping, skipping, and throwing a ball) Comments: _____ _____ ☐ Favors one side of the body over another ☐ Left to right confusion ☐ Inappropriately spontaneous (impulsive) ☐ Difficulty performing rote/automatic tasks ☐ Unable to problem solve ☐ Poor working memory Comments: _____ _____ ☐ Slow processing speed ☐ Overly fast processing speed ☐ Inability to use sensory and emotional information to form, sequence, and act on a plan Comments: _____ _____ ☐ Lacks stable routines and interests, hobbies, preferences that reliably bring pleasure ☐ Avoids/resists appropriate challenges and risks ☐ Is easily overwhelmed by emotions or disavows emotions ☐ Does not seem to learn from past experiences ☐ Difficulty incorporating new information ☐ Difficulty using planning for the future ☐ Makes inappropriate cause–effect links ☐ Does not appropriately read the nuances and intentions of others' nonverbal and verbal communication ☐ Imbalances in self–other awareness so there is too much or too little expression of a private, assertive, or giving self

(Continued)

Worksheet 11.2. Continued

Resources and Strengths Toward Allodynamic Coordination	Risk Factors for Conditions of Allodynamic Load
	Comments: _____ _____
	☐ Gets lost in the parts/details without seeing the whole or sees the whole but cannot organize the details Comments: _____ _____
	☐ Other _____ _____

Bringing It All Together

12

From Parts to Whole

Here we review where we have been and draw the parts together into a comprehensive whole. Chapter 1 described four key problems we face in our various professions—disciplinary fragmentation, isolation, hierarchy, and specialization—that have evolved along with tremendous progress and gains in each profession. Two large bodies of clinical knowledge, *infant mental health* and *early intervention,* exemplify the divisions in our service delivery systems. The neurorelational framework is our attempt to provide a common language and a part-to-whole process that can bridge the boundaries across all related disciplines. Chapter 2 described the major concepts within the neurorelational framework, highlighting the neuroscience theories that support it and presenting an overview of the four brain systems. Chapter 3 emphasized the need for all professionals to have a working knowledge of dyadic socioemotional milestones and introduced an interpersonal triad of respond, direct, and reflect processes that relates to a wide span of clinical approaches, personality theory, and interpersonal dynamics. Next, we explored the parts of each brain system, wherein the function of each system, the behaviors to observe, and the assessment and intervention priorities and strategies were presented. Now, we return to the whole. This concluding chapter offers (1) a way to synthesize, at a meta-level, assessment and intervention information from each of the brain systems; (2) a step-by-step process by which to apply the information you have learned; (3) community applications of the neurorelational framework; and (4) visions for the future.

SYNTHESIZING THE NEURORELATIONAL FRAMEWORK

One of the major tenets of the neurorelational framework is that there are both discrete and shared (i.e., distributed) brain processes (Chapter 2). We believe that research, academic, and clinical professionals can (and should) function along both levels by expanding the discrete knowledge, competencies, and skills that characterize each profession as well as cultivating the shared knowledge and skills that all professionals can use working together. As mentioned in Chapter 1, interdisciplinary efforts require practitioners (or researchers, academic scholars, public policy experts, etc.) to branch out from one particular methodology and incorporate features from other disciplines and approaches into their work. This book is dedicated to expanding the clinical knowledge and skills needed to create shared knowledge across disciplinary boundaries; as such, we envision the creation of a new hybrid interdiscipline composed of professionals from all related fields who contribute to the care and treatment of infants, children, and their parents (Hongcai, 2007; Polikarov, 1995).

One way to create a shared knowledge base is to make use of global constructs, such as energy and information (Siegel, 1999; Tronick, 2007), activation and inhibition (Berntson, Cacioppo, & Quigley, 1991; Berntson, Sarter, & Cacioppo, 2003a, 2003b), and self and interactive regulation (Beebe & Lachmann, 2002; Tronick, 2007), which we have done throughout this book. Here we unfold an integrated "big picture" that includes both particular and global areas of knowledge. Self- and interactive regulation, the lynchpin of healthy functioning, hinges on the functioning across brain systems. In working with children and parents, it can be useful to gain a general sense of the quality of modulation and processing across brain systems and what emerges in the dyadic format. Table 12.1 provides a broad summary of how energy and information manifest in each brain system through the behaviors we observe. For example, by applying this table to a child who presents with symptoms assumed to be attention-deficit/hyperactivity disorder (ADHD), one can begin to see the potential distributed nature of the difficulties. He or she may have difficulties (1) making smooth transitions between states of arousal (regulation system); (2) tracking, processing, and modulating the flow of sensory information (sensory system); (3) modulating the negative range of emotions (relevance system); as well as (4) the standard difficulties associated with an ADHD diagnosis, such as executive problems in sustaining (focuses attention on tasks that are only of interest), shifting (cannot shift attention away from an interest to another priority), and modulating actions, thoughts, and emotions. This approach, then, widens the intervention lens to capture the big picture along points of strengths or limitations across domains. Rather than relying on a diagnosis that holds discrete

Table 12.1. Concepts Associated with Energy and Information in Each Brain System

Brain System	Energy	Information
Regulation	Physiological activation and inhibition/reactivity; states of arousal	Internal and external information organize into experiences/perceptions of safety, challenge, or threat
Sensory	Sensory reactivity: energy from the body and the world (e.g., thermal, chemical, mechanical, and electromagnetic forms of energy) is transduced via sensory receptors	Energies are integrated by means of sensory modalities, which organize into sensory information (e.g., sights, sounds, and pain) that reflects preferences and triggers
Relevance	Emotional reactivity: positive and negative valences	Energy and information organize to form emotions, memories, and meanings
Executive	Motor reactivity: initiate, sustain, shift, and inhibit behavior	Energy and information organize into purposeful actions, emotions, and thoughts

features only, a dimensional approach incorporates multiple variants at the same time.

As the large-scale networks of the brain (represented in the neurorelational framework's heuristic of four brain systems) continue to mature, there is an increase in complexity, coherence, and cohesiveness in the flow of energy and information. Thus, the distinctions between the flow of energy and information "within" each brain system become harder to parse, especially in moving up the brain hierarchy into the executive system. With maturation, there is greater integration, complexity, coherence, and cohesion emerging across all of the brain systems under conditions of coordination, increasing the development of a healthy, open self-organizing system (Siegel, 1999; Tronick, 2007). As is true in any theory that addresses the functioning of systems, the "whole" in this framework is greater than the sum of its parts (Gleick, 1987; Sameroff, 1989; Wachs, 2000).

The cumulative and gradated effect of activating and inhibiting levels of arousal, sensory perceptions, emotions, memories, meanings, thoughts, and actions, as noted in Table 12.1, does not happen in isolation; rather, these coalescing processes gain momentum toward coordination or create glitches for load conditions, often through the experience of self- and interactive regulation. This complex process is represented in Figure 12.1. The left side of the diagram depicts the development of self from each brain system, which is the culmination of self-regulation properties that

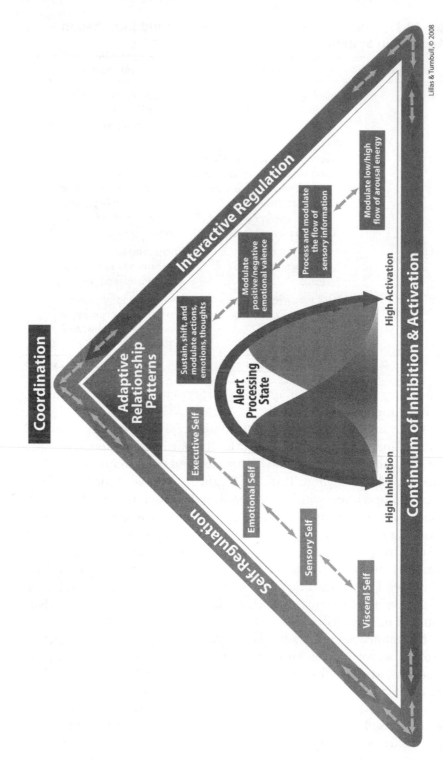

Figure 12.1. Self- and interactive regulation of the four brain systems, via inhibition and activation, resulting in coordination.

have been shaped by interactive regulation. The right side represents the modulatory aspects of interactive regulation with the features of behavior that each brain system manages, processes, and modulates. The center of the diagram represents the basic awake-arousal bell-shaped curve, which shows the gradation of arousal from high inhibition to high activation under stress and, at the center of the curve, the most optimal state of arousal for learning and relating—the alert processing state. At the top of the figure, self and interactive processes culminate in relationship patterns that are the product of bottom-up and top-down contributions.

The ultimate sign of coordination is the state of flexibility with stability, in which both the individual and the dyad have the adaptive ability to move into stress responses with adequate recovery. Depending on the actual stress responses involved, this coordination process will have different characteristics that nevertheless reflect the same basic level of responding—with hypoalert, hyperalert, flooded, or blended states, and then recovering back to baseline. Recovery may involve various forms of self- or interactive regulation. For example, self-regulation may require taking a long walk when angry, talking to someone when anxious, or listening to energizing music when in a slump. Interactive regulation might require a parent to actively help an upset child lessen his or her distress, or two partners might blow off steam together by "losing it" and then find humor in the outburst, repairing the conflict with a good outcome.

Any and all of the brain systems can contribute to self- and interactive regulation dysfunctions that perpetuate load conditions. At this juncture in our synthesis, it is important to consider the typical types of relationship *patterns* that emerge in all dyads, especially those that catalyze default-mode load conditions. Figure 12.2 shows the reverse of Figure 12.1—namely, the components that co-create load conditions and the maladaptive relationship patterns that are learned over time as a result of poorly functioning bottom-up and top-down processes. As the ability to sustain, shift, and modulate across brain systems becomes more dysregulated, activation and inhibition processes become increasingly imbalanced and disrupted. The dimensions of intensity, duration, and rhythm, used throughout this book, are important factors that ultimately differentiate adaptive stress responses from load conditions. Recall that load patterns occur under any one (or more) of the following conditions:

- too frequent stress responses to real or perceived stressors;
- inability to adjust (habituate) to challenges that, through repeated exposure, should no longer be threatening;
- prolonged stress response after the stressor is removed;
- inadequate stress recovery back to baseline.

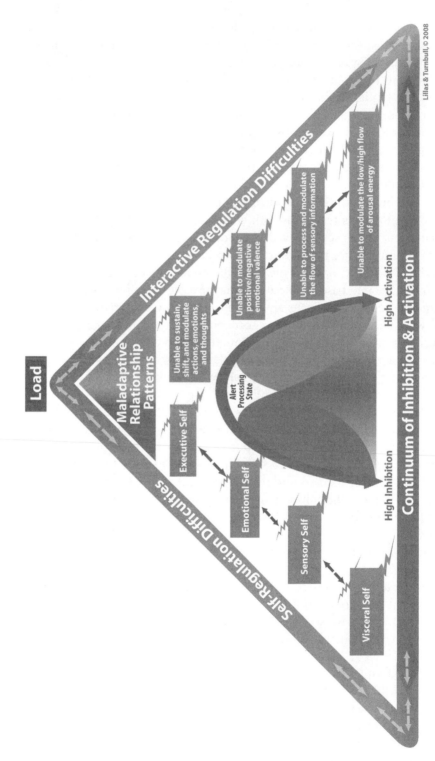

Figure 12.2. Self- and interactive regulation of the four brain systems, via inhibition and activation, resulting in load conditions.

Any stress response that occurs within one of these load conditions places the individual at risk for health problems—that is, health in the broadest sense (medically, mentally, developmentally, interpersonally, educationally; Cacioppo, 2000; Cacioppo & Berntson, 2007). Stress responses are varied, reflecting individual and dyadic differences; they can be rigid, such that the person always goes into one type of response, or they can be more chaotic, going "all over the map," or they may swing between two extreme responses.

The adaptive and maladaptive relationship patterns that are referred to in Figures 12.1 and 12.2 can be conceptualized as (1) co-occurring, (2) dissimilar, and (3) oscillating. In the *co-occurring pattern,* both partners rely on the same interpersonal mode. In the *dissimilar pattern,* partners rely on different modes. In the *oscillating pattern,* one or both partners shift from one interpersonal mode to another. Each pattern has both a coordination and load version. Under conditions of coordination, the co-occurring patterns create harmony, dissimilar patterns are complementary, and oscillating patterns reflect flexibility. In contrast, under conditions of load, co-occurring patterns become rigid, dissimilar patterns become polarizing (Dumas, LaFreniere, & Serketich, 1995; Granic, 2000), and oscillating patterns becomes chaotic. All three patterns in load conditions function in what we think of as in an automatic default mode.

As such stressful patterns become engrained over time, they are more quickly and easily triggered. In dynamic systems terminology, these patterns are known as strong attractors: "Over developmental time, dyadic attractors serve as cascading constraints; they are the product of past self-organization, and they increasingly narrow the possibilities for further development" Granic, 2000, p. 286). For example, troublesome behavior in children identified by preschool has been found to persist, especially with ongoing family stress (Campbell & Ewing, 1990) and negative, inconsistent parenting behavior within highly adversarial family relationships (Campbell, 1995).

Worksheet 12.1 contains the main concepts regarding three interpersonal modes from Chapters 8 to 11, with the addition of boxes to check. By checking the pertinent boxes in Worksheet 12.1, the practitioner can begin to identify the pattern(s) that characterize dyadic interactions (more on relationship patterns later in this chapter). (This worksheet is available on the CD-ROM, Section 12.1.) Keep in mind that this same form can be adapted to evaluate spousal relationships.

A STEP-BY-STEP APPLICATION PROCESS

Given this review of the big picture, we now guide you through a step-by-step process that integrates the information you have learned throughout

Worksheet 12.1. Interpersonal Modes That Support Coordination or Lead to Load Conditions in Parents and Child

	Interpersonal Modes That Support Coordination		
	Responsive Mode/Giving Self	Directive Mode/Assertive Self	Reflective Mode/Private Self
	☐ Parent follows the child's lead	☐ Parent takes the lead	☐ Parent takes observing stance
	☐ Parent can give to others and shift beyond own needs, modeling this shift when contextually appropriate	☐ Parent can stand up for own needs in relation to others' needs, modeling this stance when contextually appropriate	☐ Parent can self-reflect on personal meanings, using hindsight, insight, and foresight, modeling this reflective process when contextually appropriate
	☐ Parent provides warmth and engagement	☐ Child asserts needs, wishes, desires	☐ Child can wait and observe
	☐ Child follows the parent's lead	☐ Parent provides structure	☐ Parent can patiently gather information
	☐ Both parent and child listen while the other is talking	☐ Parent sets boundaries, limits, and logical consequences in a firm and clear way	☐ Parent can offer a neutral stance and can contain own reactions; is thoughtful of the big picture; makes appropriate cause–effect links; is fair and logical
	☐ Both parent and child can offer mirroring and empathy when appropriate	☐ Parent provides expectations	☐ Parent guides and models problem-solving skills
	☐ Mutual empathy is present	☐ Mutual respect for needs is present	☐ Mutual willingness to participate in problem solving

Interpersonal Modes That Can Contribute to Load Conditions

Overaccommodating or Anxiously Controlling	Demanding	Detaching
☐ Parent is consistently too permissive	☐ Parent is consistently harsh with discipline	☐ Parent is consistently avoidant
☐ Parent "caves" under pressure	☐ Parent becomes increasingly rigid under pressure	☐ Parent becomes increasingly unresponsive under pressure
☐ Chronically overanxious (either child or parent or both)	☐ Too demanding (either child or parent or both)	☐ Parent remains detached toward child even when need is pressing
☐ Parent is chronically overprotective of child	☐ Explosive reactions (either child or parent or both)	☐ Too cut off from emotions (either child or parent or both)
☐ Anxiously tries to please (either child or parent or both)	☐ Reactions frequently escalate (either child or parent or both)	☐ Too detached (either child or parent or both)
☐ Anxiously shadows adult figure; clingy	☐ Lacks empathy (either child or parent or both)	☐ Shows pervasive indifference toward any relationship (either child or parent or both)
☐ Co-dependent relationship	☐ Prone to abuse others (e.g., parent violates child's boundaries with harshness; child finds pleasure in harming others or pets)	☐ Lacks empathy and is disengaged (either child or parent or both)
☐ Prone toward poor boundaries (e.g., adult placates abusive spouse; child complies with bullies)		

this book. Having gathered detailed information about the functioning of each brain system, you can use this five-step process to pull all the information together in a meaningful way. We provide both the thinking process and worksheets that will aid your tracking of such large amounts of information into a cohesive whole. Keep in mind that you do not have to follow this sequence rigidly; as you gain more facility in using the neurorelational framework, the process can be adapted to individual circumstances. Professionals can benefit most by keeping in mind the awareness of where they are weighted in regard to the four brain systems and accompanying relational approaches (i.e., respond, direct, reflect). A practitioner's versatility in looking at a child's or adult's behaviors through the lens of regulation, sensory, relevance, and executive capacities may vary, as can his or her level of comfort with using the variety of response, directive, and reflective clinical approaches. Given these idiosyncrasies and the fact that learning is an ongoing process, we offer the following five steps for assessment and intervention:

1. Assess the self- and interactive regulation needs of the individual and dyad based on history.
2. Assess each brain system's current capacities and history of development.
3. Assess the interpersonal modes of interaction between child and parent.
4. Consider the ideal possibilities for parental and professional intervention strategies.
5. Determine intervention priorities in relation to real-world practicalities.

Table 12.2 summarizes the following material, including all the tools in tables, figures, and worksheets, and CD-ROM material that are used in these steps.

Step 1: Assess the Self- and Interactive Regulation Needs of the Individual and Dyad Based on History

Given the central role of self- and interactive regulation in the processing and modulating of different degrees of energy and types of information from each brain system, it is important to gain a gestalt of how much support an infant/child will need in relation to the available resources the parents have to give. We have stated that younger and more vulnerable children require more interactive regulation (as do more vulnerable adults).

Table 12.2. Summary of Assessment Steps and Relevant Tables, Figures, and Worksheets

Steps	Tables	Figures	Worksheets	Find on CD-ROM
Step 1: Assess self and interactive needs based upon history		See Figure 12.3 in text for Danny's filled-out History Worksheet for the four brain stems at 3 months of age		Blank History Worksheet for the four brain systems available in Section 12.2
Step 2: Assess each brain system's current capacities	See Table 12.2	See Figure 12.4 in text for Danny's filled-out Current Brain Capacities Worksheet at 3 months. See Figure 12.6 in text for Danny's filled-out Current Brain Capacities Worksheet at 3 years.		Blank Current Brain Capacities Worksheet available in Section 12.4
Step 3: Assess the interpersonal modes of interaction between child and parent			Worksheet 12.1	Potential Parenting and Professional Strategies Worksheet available in Section 12.6
Step 4: Consider ideal intervention strategies	Table 12.3	Figure 12.8		

Figure 12.3 consolidates the risk evaluations from the history worksheets used in prior chapters in relation to the case of Danny (a blank version of Figure 12.3 can be reproduced from Section 12.2 on the CD-ROM). The professional may use this worksheet to organize a big picture perspective of the factors that will increase the child's need for support, in relation to the obstacles that might prevent the parent from providing it. Historical factors that relate to the child's needs are listed in the column on the right; factors that influence the parent's available resources (or lack thereof) are listed in the column on the left. The subsections of each right- and left-hand column can be filled out by placing a checkmark in each box that applies. The middle column lists the brain systems and global questions relating to each system's capacities.

History Worksheet for the Four Brain Systems

Parental Risk Factors

That Can Comprise a Parent's Ability to Provide Interactive Regulation

- ☑ Significant prenatal stressors
- ☐ No or poor prenatal care
- ☐ History of, or current substance abuse, smoking
- ☐ Teenage pregnancy
- ☐ Poor nutrition
- ☐ Premature labor
- ☑ Multiple births
- ☐ Genetic disorder(s)
- ☐ Chronic medical condition(s)
- ☐ Chronic allergies
- ☑ Sleep difficulties
- ☐ Rigid or chaotic pattern of arousal energy that is entrenched (hypoalert, hyperalert, flooded)
- ☐ Low maternal education
- ☐ Few financial resources
- ☐ Inadequate food, shelter, or clothing
- ☐ Limited community resources

- ☐ Loss of hearing or vision
- ☐ Inaccurate processing of information
- ☐ Slow processing of information
- ☐ Speech abnormality
- ☐ Learning disorder(s)
- ☐ Overreactive, underreactive, or both to sensory information

Global Questions

That Assess the Overall Functioning of Each Brain System

REGULATION

- Are stress responses adaptive? That is, does a person show adequate recovery?
- Is the person's use of energy efficient and flexible or rigid or chaotic?
- How does the person conserve energy?

SENSORY

- How quickly and efficiently does the child/adult process sensory information?
- How reactive is the child/adult to sensory information from relationships?
- Is the child/adult leaning toward types of sensory information that are considered safe as opposed to those that are threatening?

Child Risk Factors

That Can Decrease Self-Regulation and Increase the Need for Interactive Regulation

- ☑ Prenatal maternal stress
- ☐ No or poor prenatal care
- ☑ Intrauterine growth retardation or fetal malnutrition
- ☐ Toxins in utero
- ☑ Premature birth
- ☐ Genetic disorder(s)
- ☑ Infant medical condition(s)
- ☐ Chronic allergies
- ☐ Feeding problems
- ☑ Poor suck, swallow, and breath coordination
- ☐ Poor nutrition
- ☐ Sleep difficulties
- ☑ Rigid or chaotic pattern of arousal energy that is entrenched (hypoalert, hyperalert, flooded)

- ☐ Loss of hearing or vision
- ☐ Inaccurate processing of information
- ☐ Slow processing of information
- ☐ Speech delay
- ☐ Learning disorder(s)
- ☑ Overreactive, underreactive, or both to sensory information
- ☐ Institutional care or neglect without adequate sensory information

☑ Male preterm infant
☐ Exposure to domestic violence
☐ Abuse and/or neglect
☑ Traumatic memories
☐ Lack of emotional care due to foster care or orphanage placement
☐ Chronically depressed or anxious
☑ Rapid swings into high-intensity emotions; low frustration tolerance
☐ Lack of empathy for self and others
☐ Lack of eye contact, absence of interest in others and/or lack of social referencing (overly detached)
☐ Highly demanding of others
☐ Over accommodating to others
☐ Lacks one person in the family who is strongly committed to child and who provides loving care
☐ Discrepancies exist among words, actions, or nonverbal communication
☐ Learning disruptions
☐ Inability to ask for help when necessary

RELEVANCE

- Is the individual able to express a range of positive and negative emotions flexibly?
- How do experiences influence memories and appraisals?
- Are emotionally loving, significant, and long-term relationships present?
- Does the individual tend to attribute positive or negative meanings to experiences?

☐ A domestic violence participant
☐ Personal history of abuse and/or neglect
☐ History of children removed from home; abuse/neglect of other children
☑ Multiple children to care for
☐ Weak commitment to child
☐ Familial history of mental illness
☐ Chronically depressed or anxious
☐ Rapid swings into high-intensity emotions; low frustration tolerance
☐ Lack of empathy for self and others
☐ Difficulty making eye contact and lacking warmth
☐ Negative appraisal of child as willfully disobeying or as not loving parent
☐ Parent unable to set boundaries and over-accommodates child
☐ Discrepancies exist among words, actions, or nonverbal communication
☐ Learning disruptions
☐ Inability to ask for help when necessary

(Continued)

Left box:

□ Motorically clumsy, awkward, or lethargic
□ High distractibility
□ High impulsivity
□ Unable to delay gratification
□ Lacks stable routines
□ Adheres to rigid routines and habits, avoiding novelty
□ Difficulty anticipating the need to sequence and implement agreed-on clinical input
□ Lacks a willingness to incorporate a new way to understand a child's behavior (e.g., mental rigidity)
□ Is unaware of, or inaccurately judges, own strengths and weaknesses
□ Difficulty using hindsight, insight, and foresight for self-reflection and problem solving
□ Lacks cause–effect reasoning
□ Unable to hold self and others in mind at the same time
□ Unable to consider the part in relation to the whole

Center circle:

EXECUTIVE

● Does child/adult show purposeful movement that is both adaptive and flexible?

● Can child/adult see the big picture?

● Can the child/adult stay on track in expressing a thought, emotion, or narrative?

● Can the child/adult complete tasks in a relatively smooth fashion?

Right box:

□ Motorically clumsy, awkward, or lethargic
□ Lacks developmentally appropriate use of gestures to communicate needs and wants
□ Lacks developmentally appropriate use of words to problem solve
□ High distractibility
□ High impulsivity
□ Unable to delay gratification
□ Lacks developmentally appropriate abilities to sequence activities of daily living
□ Adheres to rigid routines and habits, avoiding novelty
□ Lacks a willingness to incorporate a new way to understand own or other's behavior (e.g., mental rigidity)
□ Is unaware of, or inaccurately judges, own strengths and weaknesses
□ Difficulty using hindsight, insight, and foresight for self-reflection and problem solving
□ Lacks cause–effect reasoning
□ Unable to hold self and others in mind at the same time
□ Unable to consider the part in relation to the whole

Lillas & Turnbull, © 2008

Figure 12.3. Danny's History Worksheet, indicating the need for self- versus interactive regulation as determined by parent and child risk factors.

Once completed, practitioners can use this information in several ways. First, each column could simply be tallied. Are there more risk factors checked off on the child's side, on the parent's side, or are they roughly equal? As mentioned in Chapter 5, the ratio between the number of vulnerabilities/risk factors and strengths/protective factors provides a guide for understanding the degree of need and seriousness of conditions. If there are more factors listed on the child's side and fewer on the parent's side, one might conclude that the parents have resources and strengths that can be actively incorporated into the intervention process and the implementation of daily strategies at home. As a general clinical guideline, if both sides have four or more factors, one can assume that this family is very vulnerable; if the parents' vulnerabilities outweigh the child's, this family may be in crisis.

Second, practitioners can look for how the risk factors are distributed across the four brain systems. For the parents, the more risk factors there are in the regulation system, the more likely the parents will need extra support through case management assistance (e.g., financial assistance, transportation help, food supplies, medical care) to improve stability. Parents who have multiple medical, learning, emotional, and executive difficulties are more likely to need individual support from a professional who can provide interaction regulation, mobilize community support, and provide dyadic intervention. At times, a professional may need to work with the parent individually while teaming with another professional who works with the dyad.

To illustrate the process of applying the neurorelational framework using the worksheets in this chapter, we use the case of Danny (from the regulation system chapters). When this family sought professional help at the first sign of trouble, when Danny was 3 months old, a professional trained in the neurorelational framework might have created the completed history worksheet shown in Figure 12.3.

At a glance, the worksheet reveals that risk factors were weighted much more heavily toward Danny than toward his parents, the ratio being 12:4. The parents have a wide range of resources, from financial help that allows them to begin intervention services right away to emotional resources that allow them to extend themselves to Danny and Kenny. More important, they seem to have an open learning system that would allow them to engage in a collaborative relationship with practitioners and apply what they are learning in daily life. Danny's high number of risk factors suggests that even with their strengths, his parents need help in learning how to interactively regulate their son.

Figure 12.3 reveals that Danny's difficulties were heavily weighted toward the regulation system, with both sensory and relevance contributions. Given the nature of his risk factors, one could hypothesize that prematurity

and intrauterine growth retardation were the etiology for his feeding and sleeping problems as well as his difficulties in being soothed. Danny's choking episodes during feeding appeared to result from his inability to regulate the flow of the milk due to immature sucking, swallowing, and breathing abilities (an aspect of vagal functions). The repetitive choking experiences led to negative associations (implicit memories) such that he screamed in fear every time a bottle or breast nipple approached him. Danny was also beginning to show signs of gastroesophageal reflux (a medical condition wherein stomach contents flow up into the esophagus), so when he did eat, he had painful episodes afterward. Danny's nervous system was overreactive to sensory information, especially touch, sounds, and certain movements (e.g., he could not relax while being rocked in a rocking chair). This sensory overreactivity was another major contributing factor to his disrupted regulation and load behaviors, such as prolonged and inconsolable crying.

In Danny's case, we can see the cascade effect of an immature physiology and, specifically, the effect of a poorly functioning brake of the autonomic nervous system. Without adequate inhibitory capacity, functioning across brain systems was thrown off. In his immature and vulnerable state, Danny's nervous system was easily hijacked by internal (e.g., from choking, pain) and external (e.g., noise) stimuli. As a result, procedural memories were dominated by negative emotional experiences as well as their antecedents (e.g., nipple) and consequences (e.g., choking from the fast flow of fluid; pain from the reflux). In this context, arousal states could not organize into a stable pattern. Danny's awake arousal states were frequently flooded, and his baseline shifted between hypoalert (checking out, dissociated) and hyperalert (activated, hypervigilant). His sleep was poor. Shifts between states were abrupt and chaotic. This regulatory context did not support positive emotions and further primed the relevance system to shift into negative valences. As a result, negative procedural memories continued to accumulate, which then skewed his emerging appraisals of the world around him toward negative meanings. The information that he was able to integrate from relationships was likely to be similarly skewed in the negative direction. In summary, Danny's physiological problems drove his poor regulation and were further exacerbated by the cumulative traumatic memories (i.e., conditioned learning) that now served as triggers for dysregulation, in and of themselves.

Danny's history worksheet (Figure 12.3) provides a profile of an infant who needs a lot of interactive help. His parents, although sensitive and responsive, were not equipped to cope on their own with his feeding problems, sensory sensitivities, and arousal regulation difficulties. They would need the guidance of practitioners to help them begin to make gains in regulating Danny. Our hope is that Danny's case highlights the potential

error of defaulting too quickly to a simple answer (e.g., blaming the parent) or a predetermined one-size-fits-all approach (e.g., learned behavior to get attention) when faced with a dysregulated infant. In addition, we hope that the broader context of the neurorelational framework exposes the harm done by such default presuppositions. A blamed parent becomes a dysregulated parent; a parent who cannot implement the program properly has "failed" and becomes similarly dysregulated. In any such scenario, the parent is even less able to interactively regulate the infant.

If you have found a fair number of risk factors in the history worksheet, it is likely that you will find corresponding impingements in the following worksheets that identify each brain system's current capacities. The combined information from the History and Current Capacities Worksheets allows you to conceptualize an informed working hypothesis.

Step 2: Assess Each Brain System's Current Capacities

In the second step of the assessment and intervention process, we explore how these risk factors affect brain system capacities. In considering the capacities of all the brain systems, practitioners can use two different tools: Table 12.3 (also available on the CD-ROM, Section 12.3) lists all the brain capacities to prepare the practitioner for making use of the Current Capacities Worksheet in Figure 12.4. Keep in mind that current capacities are best understood within the context of development. If capacities were not expressed consistently at earlier developmental stages, then those factors must be considered when assessing current functioning.

Figure 12.4 is a filled-in version of the Current Capacities Worksheet (available on the CD-ROM, Section 12.4). The reader might notice that the figure lists the brain capacities noted in Table 12.3, here in shorthand form, which allows the practitioner to look at the patterns of strengths and concerns in a family system (in this case, Danny's) in a visually accessible way. Notice that the directions for use and the legend for the symbols (P1 and P2 = parent; C = child) are included under the instructions. The columns are labeled as to Triggers/Concerns and Preferences/Strengths as a way to organize the needs for intervention in concert with a strength-based approach.

Danny is in load. He is crying up to 2 hours at a time and sometimes up to 6 hours cumulatively per day. His stress recovery system is seriously overtaxed (i.e., taking too long to recover back to baseline, having too many stress responses per day). The only capacity that this family as a group is not meeting is the sleep cycle (see three checks under Triggers/Concerns in the regulation system). Although disruptive, the sleep

Table 12.3.   A Summary of Each Brain System's Capacities

Brain System	Brain System Capacities
Regulation	1. The capacity for deep sleep cycling 2. The capacity for alert processing 3. The capacity for the adaptive expression of all stress responses 4. The capacity for distinct states of arousal and smooth transitions between them 5. The capacity for connection to visceral cues 6. The capacity for efficient stress recovery
Sensory	1. The capacity to receive, translate, associate, and elaborate sensory signals within and across sensory modalities in a developmentally appropriate way (sensory processing) 2. The capacity to balance the flow of sensory signals in a way that is appropriate to context (sensory modulation)
Relevance	1. The capacity to flexibly experience, express, and modulate a full range of emotions in ways that are appropriate to context 2. The capacity to learn from experience by scanning and accessing a full range of memories that are appropriate to the context 3. The capacity to create meanings that accurately reflect self and others
Executive	1. The capacity to express spontaneous, automatic, and consciously controlled behaviors in a flexible and purposeful manner 2. The capacity to integrate the bottom-up influences of emotions with the top-down control of thoughts 3. The capacity to assess, integrate, and prioritize one's own internal (self) needs in relation to external (context/other) needs

disturbance is certainly understandable. In fact, the parents' systems were quite robust in other areas. Despite the early months of disrupted sleep from having twins, they still have energy reserves available to them, as a couple, to cope with the stressors Danny brings to the family system. However, periodic day or night respite care, provided by other family members or friends, is in order, so that the parents can catch their breath and obtain the replenishing benefits of uninterrupted deep sleep.

As a way to track each of the modalities of information, the sensory system is organized according to four components in this figure: (1) the sensory modalities most related to the internal world, (2) those most related to the external world, (3) sensory parameters related to processing, and (4) sensory parameters related to modulation. In the list of sensory modalities, the point is to note any that serve as a preference/strength or a trigger/concern. We see that for both the mother (P1) and Danny (C), movement and sounds are identified as sensory triggers. Specifically, Barbara is sensitive to loud sounds, and she grows dizzy quickly from circular vestibular input (making her a poor candidate for the merry-go-round

Assessment of Load Conditions and Current Brain Capacities
for Child and Parents

Instructions:

1. Place a √ mark in each box that applies to the parents (P1 and P2) and the child (C) for both categories: triggers and concerns and preferences and strengths.
2. Place an N/A in capacities that do not apply to the child for developmental reasons.
3. The three highlighted items are the most salient intervention goals.

Name: **Danny, Barbara & Bill**

Date: **November 11, 2003 (3 months old)**

Four Load Conditions	TRIGGERS & CONCERNS			PREFERENCES & STRENGTHS		
	P1	C	P2			
1. Too frequent stress responses to real or perceived stressors		✓				
2. Inability to adjust (habituate) to initial challenges that, over time, should no longer be stressful						
3. Prolonged stress response after the stressor is removed		✓				
4. Inadequate stress recovery back to baseline						

Regulation	P1	C	P2	P1	C	P2
■ Deep sleep cycling	✓	✓	✓			
■ Stable and expanding alert processing state		✓		✓		✓
■ Expression of all three stress responses		✓		✓		✓
■ Distinct states w/ smooth transitions		✓		✓		✓
■ Connection to visceral cues		✓		✓		✓
■ Efficient stress recovery		✓		✓		✓

Sensory	P1	C	P2	P1	C	P2
■ Internal (body)						
○ Pain (visceral, hunger, pain, pressure)		✓		✓		✓
○ Balance/vestibular/movement	✓	✓			✓	✓
○ Proprioception (use of joints, muscles)				✓	✓	✓
■ External (world)						
○ Tactile (light and deep touch)		✓		✓		✓
○ Taste		✓		✓		✓
○ Smell		✓		✓		✓
○ Auditory	✓	✓				✓
○ Vision				✓	✓	✓
■ Processing				✓	✓	✓
■ Modulation		✓		✓		✓

Relevance	P1	C	P2	P1	C	P2
■ Full range of emotions (positive and negative)		✓		✓		✓
■ Appropriate access to full range of memories		✓		✓		✓
■ Accurate meanings of self and other		✓		✓		✓

Executive	P1	C	P2	P1	C	P2
■ Purposeful adaptive behavior						
○ Spontaneous format		✓		✓		✓
○ Automatic format		✓		✓		✓
○ Conscious control format		N/A		✓		✓
■ Integrating thoughts and emotions		N/A		✓		✓
■ Shifting between self and other/context		N/A		✓		✓

Lillas & Turnbull, © 2008

Figure 12.4. Current Capacities Worksheet for Danny and his parents (3-month mark) assessing brain system capacities.

any time soon). Although Danny loves the bouncer—indeed, it is a sensory preference—he likes *only* the bouncer, so his vestibular modality is still a concern because it is so narrow and rigid. Thus, both vestibular preference and trigger boxes are checked. The father (P2) has no problem

with vestibular input, so his tolerance provides a complement and a resource for Danny. Another family resource is that parents and child alike are comfortable with proprioceptive input. With professional help, this may be an additional way to consider calming Danny. Another family strength is that they all appear to track and process sensory information accurately. As noted, Danny has triggers across several sensory modalities, including touch.

We see that Danny shows potential concerns for both relevance and executive capacities as well, whereas the parents are functioning with coordination. The last two capacities in the executive system are not age-appropriate for Danny, which is signified by N/A.

When filling out the Current Capacities Worksheet for one of your families, you can make use of the material in Section 12.5 on the CD-ROM, where we have assembled all the assessment tables provided throughout this book. This is a very long section (pp. 59 to 101). The duplication of tables and worksheets follow the sequence of the four brain systems. There are three additional tables in this section (within the executive system) that are not in the text of the book.

The History Worksheet and the Current Capacities Worksheet help us hold the big picture of how the four brain systems are operating in child and parent(s). Now we begin to consider the interpersonal context in which these systems are operating.

Step 3: Assess the Interpersonal Modes of Interaction Between Child and Parent

Relational dynamics have been emphasized throughout the neurorelational framework. The interpersonal dynamics of the family system (as well as the professional's approach with the family) contribute to either coordination or load conditions, based primarily on the meaning that family members attribute to each other's initiations or responses. The following questions can be used as guidelines for assessing whether the relational dynamics are aiding family members' ability to maintain flexible, stable patterns or contributing to rigid or chaotic patterns:

- Depending on the child's developmental age, functional capacities, and context, which parenting modes are most needed with the child: responsiveness, directiveness, and/or reflectiveness? To what degree does each parent match the needed style or provide a necessary blend?
- Does the child lean toward reliance on one particular interpersonal mode?

- How does each parent respond to his or her child's responsive, directive, and reflective modes?
- With either parent or child, are there sudden shifts into overly accommodating, demanding, or detached behaviors?
- Does the parents' use of interpersonal modes produce harmonizing, complementary, and flexible interactions with each other and with the child?
- Does the parents' use of interpersonal modes result in rigid, polarizing, or chaotic interactions with each other and with the child?
- What type of professional reaction would be helpful for this family system's dynamics (e.g., following the parent's lead, following the child's lead, following both of their leads, setting up more structure and boundaries, providing more problem-solving skills)?

In Chapters 8 and 9 on the relevance system, we briefly mentioned that at times, parental interaction modes, even when weighted toward a single modality, may be adaptive and useful to the specific child, providing a helpful complement. Next, we will see how Barbara and Bill were in a helpful *complementary pattern* that supported them during the early phases of Danny's life. Danny's situation called for parenting skills (and professional skills) that were responsive to him and reflective about what do to, how to do it, and when to do it. Barbara's and Bill's strengths naturally lent themselves toward these modes. Barbara was more oriented toward the responsive mode in her relationships with others. Thus, it was natural for her to try and notice Danny's sensory preferences and use them in ways that could be calming for him. Her responsive approach was crucial in these early months because, although she lacked an understanding of the big picture, she certainly fostered a loving connection, and her persistent efforts revealed important insights along the way. Danny loved to be bounced in the bouncer with a fast rhythm that matched his intense crying; as the fast rhythm and high intensity of the bounce began to soothe him, Barbara would decrease the rate and lower the intensity. Whenever he was in a calm, alert processing state, Barbara was sure to engage Danny, offering smiles and bright eyes, babbling back and forth with him, and catching him in spontaneous moments where they could laugh together. She found her way in learning how to regulate Danny using his sensory preference (at least there was one!) by experimenting with the dimensions of intensity, duration, and rhythm with the bouncer, and she used her natural responsive style to connect to Danny during the times he was not crying. Her responsiveness combined a hands-on style of parenting in conjunction with a willingness to seek professional advice. This type of action orientation combined a directive mode with her responsive orientation.

Bill was naturally more oriented toward the reflective interpersonal mode. He was able to focus his energies on keeping track of what was helpful to Danny, helping Barbara notice when Danny was most "organized" in his behavior. He was the first to figure out that the bouncer was the best way to soothe Danny. Bill provided a steady presence for Barbara and was good at organizing the information that came from all of the different professionals whom Barbara was consulting. Although Barbara felt that they were in the middle of chaos, Bill's strong executive skills supported his ability to reflect on exactly what and who was helping them. Bill was able to compare and contrast what one professional said against another, and he attempted to weave a cohesive and coherent plan out of the professionals' differences and similarities. This big-picture reflection and the structure that resulted from it brought organization to Barbara's efforts and allowed her to settle down and maintain her own self-regulation.

Both Barbara and Bill experienced Danny as a "demanding" infant. Whereas Kenny, Danny's twin brother, was naturally responsive and able to initiate warm, joyful exchanges, Danny's intense, prolonged, and frequent crying jags were perceived as intrusive. At this early, 3-month juncture, both parents related his demands to his discomfort in being in the world, associated with his intrauterine growth retardation and prematurity. At times, they felt deflated and that they were bad parents, but usually one would help pull the other away from that negative meaning and its associated bad feeling. Barbara's and Bill's parenting styles were *complementary*, creating matches that supported their efforts toward their own and their baby's baseline coordination.

Step 4: Consider the Ideal Possibilities for Parental and Professional Intervention Strategies

For parents, knowing to whom to turn and when is often complicated and confusing. At first, Barbara and Bill's pediatrician said that Danny's crying episodes were due to colic and that he would outgrow his symptoms between 3 and 4 months of age. During this time, they consulted with lactation specialists, who used feeding tubes attached to Barbara's breasts to help increase the amount of milk he was getting. Although this technique is often used to help a premature infant not have to work (suck) so hard to get his or her mother's milk, increasing the flow of milk actually made things worse for Danny because he also had trouble controlling the swallow of the fast-moving fluid. After 3 months, when Danny's distress had not subsided, Barbara and Bill became alarmed that they were not getting the right type of help.

Using the neurorelational framework's part-to-whole map of different disciplines, we see that we could begin to prioritize the use of team members from several disciplines. Figure 12.5 shows the different disciplines associated with the different brain systems. (Another worksheet that summarizes the potential disciplines as well as parenting and professional strategies can be found on the CD-ROM, Section 12.6.)

Danny's complex picture involved feeding problems, a reflux condition, and sensory modulation difficulties that, from an ideal perspective, needed to be addressed in tandem. The hope would be that his primary threats of choking, pain, and sensory triggers would be allayed sufficiently to allow him to experience longer periods of calm in the alert processing state, building on his sensory preferences into longer periods of positive engagement. There was an urgent need to find nontraumatic ways for Danny to feed because his memory system was now sensitized toward a flooded response. He arched, splayed his fingers, and screamed in a high-pitched cry with the approach of a bottle or breast—all signs of intense distress. Second, we needed to (a) reduce the pain he experienced from feedings, (b) reduce his sensory triggers, and (c) increase his sensory preferences.

Table 12.4 synthesizes the information gathered thus far on Danny: (1) the history risk factors, (2) the difficulties in the brain capacities, (3) preliminary working hypotheses, and (4) the types of professionals who would provide options for shifting Danny as quickly as possible out of load conditions. Ideally, all professionals on the team would make use of arousal regulation benchmarks (support sleep cycling, promote and expand the

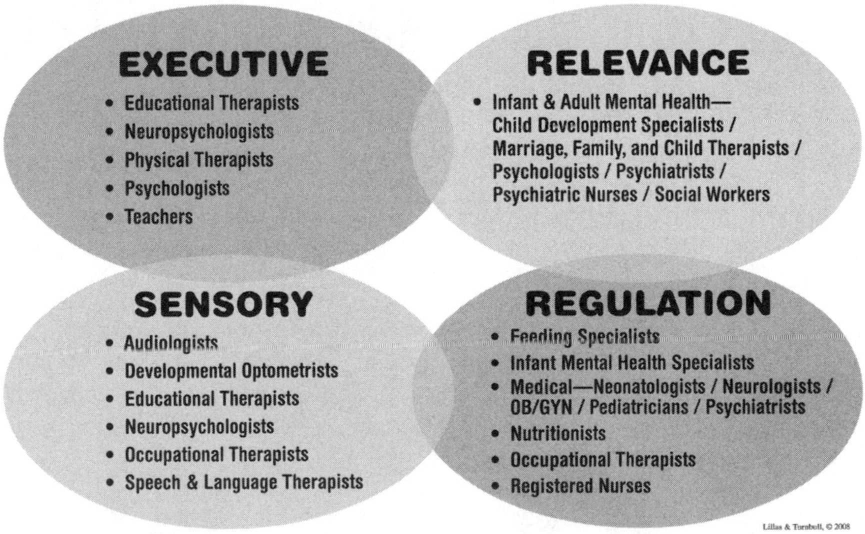

EXECUTIVE
- Educational Therapists
- Neuropsychologists
- Physical Therapists
- Psychologists
- Teachers

RELEVANCE
- Infant & Adult Mental Health—Child Development Specialists / Marriage, Family, and Child Therapists / Psychologists / Psychiatrists / Psychiatric Nurses / Social Workers

SENSORY
- Audiologists
- Developmental Optometrists
- Educational Therapists
- Neuropsychologists
- Occupational Therapists
- Speech & Language Therapists

REGULATION
- Feeding Specialists
- Infant Mental Health Specialists
- Medical—Neonatologists / Neurologists / OB/GYN / Pediatricians / Psychiatrists
- Nutritionists
- Occupational Therapists
- Registered Nurses

Lillas & Turnbull, © 2008

Figure 12.5. Professional disciplines associated with different brain systems.

Table 12.4 Danny's Risk Factors, Triggers, and Concerns in Current Brain Capacities, Working Hypotheses, and Professional Help Needed

History Risk Factors	Triggers and Concerns in Current Brain Capacities	NRF's Working Hypothesis	Professional Help Needed to Facilitate Interactive Regulation
Regulation			
• Prematurity • Multiple birth • Intrauterine growth retardation (IUGR) • Feeding problems • Medical concern (reflux)	✓ The capacity for deep sleep cycling ✓ The capacity for alert processing ✓ The capacity for the adaptive expression of all stress responses ✓ The capacity for distinct states of arousal and smooth transitions between them ✓ The capacity for connection to visceral cues ✓ The capacity for efficient stress recovery	• Prematurity (immaturity) and IUGR likely contributing to low vagal tone with subsequent difficulties related to poor vagal tone: • inadequate control in sucking, swallowing, and breathing, which leads to choking • inadequate inhibition with arousal regulation, resulting in flooded states and poor state transitions • reflux from gastrointestinal immaturity	• Feeding specialist (a variety of professionals may have this expertise) who could understand the implications of a poor inhibitory system across all brain systems • Medical specialist to treat the reflux • These professionals comprehend the emotional–memory implications of choking episodes and the effects of pain on feeding
Sensory			
• Overreactive to sensory information	✓ The capacity to balance the flow of sensory signals in a way that is appropriate to context (*sensory modulation*)	• Prematurity, IUGR, and poor vagal tone contribute to hypersensitivities • These need to be further delineated into triggers/preferences	• Sensory integration specialist who could (1) help delineate the sensory modalities that were acting as triggers; (2) provide treatment for sensory triggers; (3) identify sensory preferences; (4) help parents create a "sensory diet" at home; (5) teach parents how to use sensory preferences to prevent or interrupt escalations

Relevance			
• Rapid swing into high-intensity emotions • Traumatic memories (implicit)	✓ The capacity to flexibly experience, express, and modulate a full range of emotions in ways that are appropriate to context ✓ The capacity to learn from experience by scanning and accessing a full range of memories that are appropriate to the context ✓ The capacity to create meanings that accurately reflect self and others	• A cascade effect is occurring wherein poor coordination and inhibition, pain from reflux, and hypersensitivities create an overly negative experience of the world and relationships as being threatening • Procedural memories trigger fear and flooded arousal through crying and screaming related to daily routines and habits • The meanings with respect to self and others that Danny is creating may be negatively skewed	• This professional could comprehend the emotional–memory implications of how sensory triggers relate to experiences of threat from the world and relationships • If socioemotional milestones are not improving as underlying causes of threat are addressed, refer to a relationship specialist to facilitate interactions during the alert processing window.
Executive			
• Poor ability to shift • Poor ability to inhibit behaviors	✓ The capacity to express spontaneous, automatic, and consciously controlled behaviors in a flexible and purposeful manner	• Poor ability to modulate and smoothly shift from spontaneous excitement to a calmer condition, which is related to a weak "brake" and poor inhibitory capacities	• All professionals understand the effect of a weak inhibitory system, and all share the contributory triggers to arousal escalation with other team members so reducing threat, expanding the alert processing state, and enhancing stress recovery are coordinated efforts

alert processing state, and enhance efficient stress recovery) and the socioe-motional milestones as guideposts to the progress of the interventions in relation to the child, the parent, and the dyad.

Once initial assessments have been completed, the professional should consider the big picture and set priorities by holding the ideal set of team members and interventions in relation to the real-world practi-calities of the family's situation and available (geographically) professional resources.

Step 5: Determine Intervention Priorities in Relation to Real-World Practicalities

While the practitioner is holding in mind the multiple possibilities of whom should be consulted, who should be on the team, and what inter-vention strategies should be used, he or she should consider real-world practicalities—any limitations in financial, emotional, or professional arenas—in making intervention decisions. A few of the following ques-tions can help a professional begin to hone in on what is really possible and what sequence of events is most likely:

- Do the family members need sleep or respite care first?
- Does this situation require several interventions immediately?
- Are the ideal team members identified and available?
- Can the parents afford a "full-scope" team approach?
- Can the parents cope with information from, and interactions with, more than one provider at this time?
- Are the parents willing to explore a variety of approaches (i.e., is there an open learning system?), or do they have discernible biases for or against certain categories of intervention (e.g., medication, occupational therapy, mental health)?
- Are the parents weighted toward one maladaptive/inefficient style or pattern (e.g., permissive, demanding, detached, rigid, or chaotic) in parenting their children such that working with them individu-ally is as much as a priority as working with the parent–child dyad?

Barbara and Bill began the intervention process with emotional and financial resources—but what if this were not the case? What if they had financial resources but could not cope with so many practitioners weigh-ing in with opinions at the same time? Even though sleep is usually the first need to address, in this case, because these parents were functioning well despite having twins in the early months of sleep dysregulation, the

first priority would probably be to deal with Danny's sensitized feeding difficulties. When the engagement of multiple practitioners is not feasible, the professional with the strongest bond with the family is often the one who will problem solve treatment priorities with the parents. This role might include making calls to other professionals for consultation and suggestions about possible solutions (of course, following legal/ethical guidelines with respect to confidentiality). For families who cannot tolerate "too much, too fast," the pacing needs to be titrated accordingly—for example, the addition of new team members would occur much more slowly. Sometimes, once the top-priority needs begin to resolve, the family can tolerate cutting back to an every-other-week session with one practitioner and then incorporate the services of another needed professional. This transition can sometimes be made more smoothly if the current practitioner connected to the family works on a team with other practitioners that he or she knows and trusts. Having relationships across disciplines allows the practitioner who is most connected to the family to do his or her best job in achieving a good fit between the incoming practitioners and the family.

Unfortunately, Barbara and Bill's long-term experience was one of going from one professional to the next in an attempt to deal with each subsequent crisis. The reason for this "professional hopping" had very little to do with the parents' dissatisfaction; rather, it was motivated by the need to find a professional who could address each symptom. Although the professionals who provided help were experts in their discrete domains, they were not using a shared knowledge base and did not communicate with each other. As a result, there was no comprehensive and cohesive framework. Each professional provided new information and new ways of helping but also, quite inadvertently, created more fragmentation. The information and treatment guidance they provided were, at worst, blatantly contradictory and, at best, just different enough to be difficult for the parents to reconcile or gain an understanding of how one symptom was actually related to another.

For example, one professional along the way stated that Danny had "an attachment disorder," a conclusion that was shared with Barbara at the closing of an initial 1.5-hour consultation while gathering a history from both parents. Clearly upset and anxiety-stricken, Barbara asked for further clarification and was told that they could discuss it at their next meeting. As Barbara headed for the door, the professional gave her a handful of literature. As she pored over the literature at home that night, she found herself sinking into a hole of self-blame and despair—everything she read seemed to imply that she was to blame for this "new" disorder. It was unfortunate that this event coincided with a time when Barbara was especially vulnerable concerning her sense of inadequacy

with Danny. Her feelings of failure took hold and led to months of self-doubt, inhibited responses, and inefficient decision making.

By the time Barbara and Bill came to me (CL), when Danny was 3 years old, their strengths had turned into risk factors. Barbara overused her responsiveness and action tendencies, and Bill shifted into shutdown; they both became more rigid, and because of chronic load conditions, they were now in a polarized stress pattern with each other. What happened to them is not uncommon. We can begin to understand this process best by first taking a look at a second version of the Current Capacities Worksheet that was completed at the 3-year mark (see Figure 12.6).

At 3 years, the parents had shifted into load. They had lost their ability to self-regulate and, despite the fact that they had regained an adequate sleep cycle, in the face of constant daily stress with repeated hits the awake cycle was continually stressful. Recall that when we left the case in the regulation chapter, Danny's sensory system was much more flexible with regard to movement and vestibular activities, and the 2-hour crying episodes related to his diaper changes had abated. However, at this juncture, he still was tactilely sensitive. He hated to change his clothes, often sleeping in his day clothes because changing into pajamas would trigger a rage. He hated getting his hair washed and couldn't stand getting his hands wet or putting them in contact with glue or other sticky substances. He was still sensitive to smells and tastes, preferring only a narrow range of foods. Everyone in the family had become sensitized to his high-pitched screaming. Danny's crying and screaming now surrounded most transitions; he did not want to leave the house or change an activity in which he was engaged. Anything abrupt or surprising was met with resistance. He handled disappointments very poorly. If he lost a game, he fell apart; if things were not done in the sequence he wanted, he screamed for them to be redone. He could sustain attention for long periods of time, but shifting attention to something he did not want to do would induce a strong negative emotional reaction. Danny's escalations involved hitting his parents, occasionally hitting his brother, and pounding on the wall with his fist. He perceived his family members as intentionally trying to hurt him if something disappointed him or was not done exactly how he wanted it to be done. He would not accept that a disappointment was the result of a mistake or an accident. In parallel fashion, if he himself could not do something perfectly the first time, or very quickly, he would fall apart. In particular, he struggled with fine motor coordination and would erupt in frustration, tearing a piece of paper into many little pieces, for example, if he could not draw the way he wanted to.

Kenny continued to progress well but was getting lost in the family's constant vigilance of Danny. So much energy went into trying to avoid triggering Danny that little energy was left for Kenny. Although Barbara

Assessment of Load Conditions and Current Brain Capacities
for Child and Parents

Instructions:

1. Place a √ mark in each box that applies to the parents (P1 and P2) and the child (C) for both categories: triggers and concerns and preferences and strengths.
2. Place an N/A in capacities that do not apply to the child for developmental reasons.
3. The three highlighted items are the most salient intervention goals.

Name: **Danny, Barbara, & Bill**

Date: **May 21, 2006 (3 years old)**

Four Load Conditions	TRIGGERS & CONCERNS P1	C	P2			
1. Too frequent stress responses to real or perceived stressors	✓	✓	✓			
2. Inability to adjust (habituate) to initial challenges that, over time, should no longer be stressful	✓	✓	✓			
3. Prolonged stress response after the stressor is removed	✓	✓	✓			
4. Inadequate stress recovery back to baseline						

Regulation	TRIGGERS & CONCERNS P1	C	P2	PREFERENCES & STRENGTHS P1	C	P2
▪ Deep sleep cycling				✓	✓	✓
▪ Stable and expanding alert processing state	✓	✓	✓			
▪ Expression of all three stress responses	✓	✓	✓			
▪ Distinct states w/ smooth transitions	✓	✓	✓			
▪ Connection to visceral cues		✓		✓		✓
▪ Efficient stress recovery	✓	✓	✓			

Sensory	TRIGGERS & CONCERNS P1	C	P2	PREFERENCES & STRENGTHS P1	C	P2
▪ Internal (body)						
○ Pain (visceral, hunger, pain, pressure)		✓		✓		✓
○ Balance/vestibular/movement	✓				✓	✓
○ Proprioception (use of joints, muscles)				✓	✓	✓
▪ External (world)						
○ Tactile (light and deep touch)		✓		✓		✓
○ Taste		✓		✓		✓
○ Smell		✓		✓		✓
○ Auditory	✓	✓	✓			
○ Vision		✓		✓		✓
▪ Processing				✓	✓	✓
▪ Modulation	✓	✓	✓			

Relevance	TRIGGERS & CONCERNS P1	C	P2	PREFERENCES & STRENGTHS P1	C	P2
▪ Full range of emotions (positive and negative)	✓	✓	✓			
▪ Appropriate access to full range of memories	✓	✓	✓			
▪ Accurate meanings of self and other	✓	✓	✓			

Executive	TRIGGERS & CONCERNS P1	C	P2	PREFERENCES & STRENGTHS P1	C	P2
▪ Purposeful adaptive behavior						
○ Spontaneous format	✓	✓	✓			
○ Automatic format	✓	✓	✓			
○ Conscious control format	✓	✓	✓			
▪ Integrating thoughts and emotions	✓	✓	✓			
▪ Shifting between self and other/context	✓	✓	✓			

Lillas & Turnbull, © 2008

Figure 12.6. Current Capacities Worksheet for Danny and his parents (3-year mark) assessing brain system capacities.

and Bill celebrated Kenny's successes, in some situations, they had to be cautious about praising Kenny to avoid triggering Danny. In the sibling relationship, Kenny had to maintain his own form of vigilance with his brother, which likely detracted from his optimal functioning.

As Barbara and Bill each became more stressed and worn out from their journey for help, which seemed to be endless, the load side to each of their strengths began to emerge. Strengths can typically flip into concerns and even triggers under conditions of load. What were first strengths of responsiveness, nurturance, and action for Barbara changed into hypervigilance and anxiety (a load condition). As Danny's crying and screaming continued into year 2, at any sign of his escalation, Barbara slipped into a stress response pattern in which two responses co-occurred: She would shift into a mild dissociative state (hypoalert) in conjunction with being in her usual hyperalert stress response state. Barbara herself, already sensitive to loud sounds, was now sensitized to Danny's high-pitched scream. As soon as she sensed any sign that Danny might start to scream, she began to anticipate not being able to soothe him and having to withstand a potential 1- to 2-hour siege. That anticipation launched an internal activation (increased heart rate) that led to external inhibition (immobilization of her motor system). Emotionally, she was feeling more confused than ever regarding to whom to turn next, and she was utterly depleted in her efforts to soothe her child. Although gains had been definitely been made, new and distressing scenarios kept popping up. In fact, she felt like she was in a never-ending nightmare (loss of temporal integration) because as soon as one issue seemed to be resolved, another one would loom, leaving her exhausted and anxious. She felt totally lost even though she still searched for answers. As a way to attempt to stave off triggering Danny, she was becoming increasingly controlling of everyone on the family. Her anxious control in trying to circumvent Danny's screaming was experienced as both suffocating of others and too permissive toward Danny.

Barbara, who had relied on Bill's stronger executive capacities, now felt criticized by him as their parental dyad began to show the wear and tear of load. The chronic stress of an inconsolable child, who now seemed like a tyrannical child, was taking its toll on Bill. His stress response pattern was an oscillating one: He shifted into spurts of anger, with much longer periods of being tuned out and shut down. His anger was fueled by his observation that Barbara's vigilance led her to accommodate Danny too much. He felt that she responded too quickly to Danny's needs at the expense of ignoring her own needs and those of others in the family, while trying to control everyone else's actions. What he had appreciated as Barbara's initial spontaneity, he saw had now became laden with too much of her anxiety. He was also angry about the fact that she kept going from one professional to another, always getting excited about some new approach to try. Chiding her for losing sight of the bigger picture, his favorite cynical quip during his flooded rants was, "Who are you listening to this week?"

Bill's primary stress default mode, however, was to shut down into a hypoalert state. As he coped by tuning out more, he was not as available; he withdrew into his own world, choosing to focus on work and to zone out with the sports channel on the weekends.

In addition, Barbara and Bill became more sensitized to each other as partners, each triggering the other. In an angry tone of voice, Bill would accuse Barbara of catering to Danny too much, and she would respond, with a sarcastic retort, about how much help she was getting with the twins while he was watching TV. One could see the deterioration that took place. By now, the load conditions had eroded the regulatory, sensory, relevance, and executive strengths they had shown at Danny's 3-month mark. Table 12.5 juxtaposes Barbara's and Bill's early (3-month) parenting profile with their later (3-year) one.

Eventually, Bill suggested that perhaps they needed to get some family help and that what was missing were some agreed-on requirements and consequences that needed to be brought into the picture for Danny. Barbara was concerned that the requirements would be too harsh for Danny, whereas Bill was concerned that they would never have any expectations for Danny, viewing him as perpetually vulnerable. Having received widely varying advice from friends and family (from spanking to ignoring), Barbara was protective about any new approach for Danny. Yet for Bill to suggest that they get help from another professional was unusual—and a welcome change from the rut they were in. When they came to my (CL) office for consultation, I first commented that they were "both right." This awareness began to neutralize the escalating polarizations that had emerged between them. If they both were right, then perhaps they could find a way to meet in the middle. Barbara's concerns about being too demanding as parents could be honored, as could Bill's need to increase structure, expectations, limits, and consequences. They began to agree on ways they could begin to set boundaries and consequences for Danny

Table 12.5. Barbara's and Bill's Coordination and Load Relationship Patterns

Coordinated Relationship Pattern		Load Relationship Pattern	
Complementary		Polarizing	
Barbara	*Bill*	*Barbara*	*Bill*
Responsive	Reflective	Overaccommodating	Detached
Directive		and anxiously	
		controlling	

when he threw tantrums, which now seemed to be his automatic way of expressing himself, regardless of the situation. Instead of vigilantly trying to avoid his rages by walking on eggshells, Barbara had to learn how to deal with the tantrums in new ways. Because Danny was now 3 (i.e., old enough), I suggested strategies for enhancing arousal regulation that I knew would draw on the executive system (i.e., a top-down approach). Barbara began to use a white board on which she pictured the events of the day by using Velcro pictures. She began to use a timer that helped Danny antici- pate (executive) a transition; this system helped him learn to trust that a transition would not occur too abruptly for him. Barbara began to trust that she could provide Danny with nurturance and sensory comfort while allowing him to learn to tolerate disappointments (relevance). The speech and language therapist and I both began to help Danny develop more of an emotional language for his needs and disappointments (relevance). Both Barbara and Bill worked with me to develop clear guidelines for when to say *no* and for reliably following through with consequences for Danny (relevance). As Bill helped Danny anticipate what was expected of him and what the consequences would be (executive), he reengaged in the parenting effort, returning his executive resources to both Barbara and Danny. Bill led the way in setting healthy requirements for Danny while following through with the consequences; Barbara began to appreciate his taking the lead in this area—which helped her begin to let go of her hypervigilance.

During this same time, Barbara and Bill decided to try a modified ver- sion of an unconventional protocol for Danny's tactile sensitivities. Often referred to as "brushing," the technique actually involves deep-pressure touch and proprioceptive manipulation. This protocol, which was developed by Wilbarger and requires training (Parents' Place, n.d.; Wilbarger, n.d.), proved to be very helpful.[1] At this juncture, Barbara and Bill were using sensory, relevance, and executive interventions in a more comprehensive manner, all at the same time. In addition, their parenting modes began to blend in a beneficial way, such that their response, direct, and reflect approaches cre- ated an effective, integrated parental system. As the whole family system became more coordinated, Barbara and Bill regained their executive ca- pacities and were able to begin to integrate and flexibly apply all the things they had learned through a very long, arduous process. In hindsight, we realized that even when they were functioning in their earlier coordinated states, they were still headed toward polarization in their parenting modes, which then became extreme when they entered into load conditions. The blending of their parenting modes strengthened the robustness of all their brain systems and thus their abilities to return to coordination—and to continue to nurture and structure their family life.

We have seen how Barbara and Bill found their way out of their polarizing pattern. Table 12.6 provides examples of interpersonal load patterns and corresponding intervention approaches for dyadic relationships that may be useful. It is important to remember that any of these stress responses can be adaptive, and a load condition is defined by too lengthy or too frequent stress responses. These descriptions in the table are not meant to be exhaustive by any means. Although the examples in this table are weighted toward adult partners, these patterns can be applied to any type of dyad: parent–parent, parent–child, teacher–child, therapist–child, therapist–parent, and so on.

APPLYING THE NEURORELATIONAL FRAMEWORK IN THE PROFESSIONAL COMMUNITY

We hope this book will provide a framework that can be applied across diverse disciplines, thereby promoting the building of truly interdisciplinary team–based relationships. Our dream is that professionals who have the vision and drive for interdisciplinary collaboration would find this framework to be a useful tool and resource for coming together and building bridges within their own research, academic, and clinical communities. In our experience, expanding learning through relationships with colleagues who know something different from what we already know is invaluable—and exciting. This type of interchange stimulates connections within one's own thinking, as well as across relationships, and even across previously isolated service systems.

Groups that function in an open learning system are characterized by several key features that would be important to implement when using the neurorelational framework as a guide. Group formations are often contingent upon a "catalyst" (Brafman & Beckstrom, 2006)—the type of person or persons who may want to organize an open learning community. In our context, this catalyst would initiate the connections but not "lead" in the traditional sense. This type of inspirational leader has a vision to get things started, yet knows when to let go and allow group members to run on their own. Groups interested in implementing the neurorelational framework can use the following guidelines, which outline the assumptions on which this framework operates:

1. Group members share three values:

    a. Development is viewed as inherently the product of underlying complexities that are connected by multiple, rather than singular, causal agents.

    b. Sound neurodevelopmental principles should serve as guides for comprehending developmental processes and evaluating clinical strategies.

    c. Early relationships and the quality of all relationships, regardless of age, are recognized as a necessary consideration in any successful intervention.

2. Group members acknowledge that other disciplines have specialized knowledge that they themselves lack or know less about.

3. Group members believe that everyone has something to contribute and see value in adding diversity to their group.

4. Group members honor a nonhierarchical approach to relationships across disciplines; no one discipline has more power or prestige than another within the group.

5. Group members believe that it is imperative to share knowledge and expertise, not withhold knowledge as the exclusive property of the self or one's discipline.

6. Group members implement the open learning model, which allows for both positive and negative emotions to emerge while learning. This type of learning anticipates disagreements and emotional reactions and views the *respectful* bumping into others as part of the nature of healthy learning, rather than a competitive or unhealthy endeavor.

One such learning community in Los Angeles is using the neurorelational framework to shape the clinical model for their service delivery system and guide continuing education training curriculum for their network of three community agencies. The Westside Infant Family Network (WIN) is a pilot project that was selected under the 2007 Robert Wood Johnson Foundation Local Funding Partners granting cycle as an innovative health-related program and potential national model. By servicing both the concrete needs (e.g., for food, housing, transportation) of families through case managers, medical care through available physicians, and professional home visitation, the families receive the support they need to shift from load conditions into conditions of coordination.

    By using a Personal Knowledge Inventory (available on the CD-ROM, Section 12.8), each clinician can gain an overview of the areas of knowledge in which he or she is strong and those they still need to acquire. Then, using the form Mapping the Content of Workshop Presentations (on the CD-ROM, Section 12.9), each practitioner can map the presentations, workshops, and conferences he or she attends in terms of the brain systems and clinical modes wherein they are weighted. Figure 12.7 presents a sample filled-in version of this form.

Table 12.6. Examples of Interpersonal Load Patterns for Dyadic Relationships and Corresponding Intervention Approaches

Co-Occurring (too much of the same thing)	Polarizing (modes that become rigid)	Oscillating (modes that are chaotic)
Both partners use the same load version of an interpersonal mode with each other: • Too much dependence on each other (overaccommodating) • Too frequent opposing of each other (demanding) • Too much avoidance of each other (detaching)	Two different modes become rigidly entrenched between partners, creating triggered reactions; partners become more extreme in reactions to "counterbalance" the other: • Extremely compliant (overaccommodating) partner with an extremely demanding partner • Highly detached partner with a highly demanding partner (the more one chases, the more the other dodges; passive–aggressive expressions of anger may ensue). Often, the avoidant partner appears more "powerful" because his or her neglect invalidates the other's impassioned expression of emotions and demands • Overaccommodating partner with a highly avoidant partner (one always accommodates to the other's lack of initiative)	One or both partners oscillate between one extreme interpersonal mode and another: • For example, a parent oscillates between being strict with structure and limit setting to being accommodating and lax with boundaries (e.g., sets harsh limits and then intermittently ignores imposing any consequences) • Both partners oscillate between accommodating and demanding extremes at different times (e.g., child screams and fights when he cannot get what he wants when he wants it immediately and later collapses into tears, repeatedly saying "I'm sorry" while parent oscillates between setting up hostile, demanding consequences and then not following through) • Couple oscillates between being detached and demanding. Partners alternate between making hostile demands and when things don't go their way, shutting down and stonewalling

(Continued)

Table 12.6.   Continued

Co-Occurring (too much of the same thing)	Polarizing (modes that become rigid)	Oscillating (modes that are chaotic)

Intervention Approaches

Highly accommodating partners are likely to need interventions that are based in all the brain systems. The following are examples from a bottom-up perspective. Consider teaching partners to do the following:

1. Develop a private self, which includes paying attention to internal, visceral cues related to self-needs (e.g., hunger, satiety) and visceral cues giving negative emotional feedback (regulation system with relevance and executive systems).

2. Notice what sensory triggers from others, in particular, induce the tendency to accommodate and give "too much" (sensory system).

3. Learn to hold onto his or her own needs, desires, and wants in relation to others (relevance and executive systems).

4. Tolerate the conflict between asserting and giving modes (relevance and executive systems).

The most extreme profile of a demand–accommodate couple occurs in cycles of domestic violence, a topic too broad for this book. See CD-ROM, Section 12.7 for a brief overview (Babcock, Green, & Robie, 2004; Egeland, Jacobvitz, & Sroufe, 1988; Frank & Rodiwski, 1999; Lederman & Osofsky, 2004; Osofsky, 2003; Osofsky & Lederman, 2004; Stith, Rosen, McCollum, & Thomsen, 2004; Thobaben, 1998; Walker, 1977, 2000).

Often, this type of coupling polarization becomes more extreme when one partner who values boundaries becomes alarmed that the other partner is too lenient, thus moving more into a rigid pattern to compensate for the other. On the other hand, the partner who is more lenient becomes alarmed that the other partner is too rigid, becoming too permissive in parenting. In actuality, the structure that a demanding person can offer needs to be integrated with the flexibility an accommodating partner can offer. Both partners need to learn from each other. The demanding partner's challenge is to down-regulate into more assertiveness while becoming more flexible and giving with his or her need for structure. The

For the couple with oscillations into high demand and high accommodation, the following suggestions may apply:

1. Increase the emotional muscle to tolerate and modulate disappointments (regulation and relevance systems).

2. Encourage, and teach partners how, to blend expressing empathy while enforcing pertinent self-boundaries (relevance system).

3. Set reasonable expectations (not so excessive that they cannot be achieved) (relevance system).

4. Develop a problem-solving process that includes ways to anticipate possible triggers and disappointments and a plan for how to deal with them (executive system).

5. Learn to express each of his or her "true" needs and desires, acquiring assertiveness skills (relevance and executive systems).
6. Acquire problem-solving skills (executive system).

A demand–demand couple is at risk for abuse; they may need to be separated as a couple for a time. This dynamic requires an intervention that addresses processes in all four brain systems. Consider teaching partners to do the following:

1. Exercise more restraint ("putting on the brakes") in behavior (both regulation- and executive-based interventions).
2. Recognize sensory triggers (e.g., tone of voice, look, gesture) that contribute to escalations (relevance system) and begin to minimize them (executive system).
3. Increase any domains of positive regard and enjoyment (relevance system).
4. Provide one another with mirroring, empathy, and perspective taking on how each partner disappoints the other (relevance system).

overaccommodating partner's challenge is to up-regulate into assertiveness while becoming more structured and restrained with his or her need for flexibility.

See information in column 1 on demanding and accommodating styles.

The demanding partner in a polarized couple is at risk for abuse, and the avoidant partner needs to become more engaged in the process, both essentially learning to give more of what his or her partner needs, moving toward an assertive, middle position in terms of arousal and behavior. If the avoidant partner is content with "less" in the relationship, the demanding partner is often left wanting. A passive-aggressive style (Benjamin, 2003) may be prevalent with the detached partner in which, for example, his or her smile may be perceived by the demanding partner as being an angry one, but he or she denies it. Hostility comes in different shapes and sizes. The demanding partner may have to realize that his or her aggressiveness is shutting down the partner's assertiveness; the detached partner may have to realize that his or her avoidance and delays communicate hostility.

The demanding partner not only needs to down-regulate to assertiveness, he or she also may need to learn how to meet needs on his or her own, establish better boundaries, have a wider

Extreme oscillating patterns of demandingness and detachment can occur with a partner who alternates between being abusive and neglectful. The double bind hypothesis may apply to this type of oscillating situation wherein a child (or adult) who tries to comply with parental demands may experience that he (or she) is "damned if he does and damned if he doesn't" (Bateson, Jackson, Haley, & Weakland, 1956; Ringstrom, 1998). When a partner's compliance to a parental demand is met with detachment (or further contradictory demands), the partner may feel that he or she cannot please the parent no matter what (Gibney, 2006).

See information in column 1 on demanding and detaching styles.

(Continued)

Table 12.6. Continued

Co-Occurring (too much of the same thing)	Polarizing (modes that become rigid)	Oscillating (modes that are chaotic)
5. Build an emotional muscle to tolerate the disappointment each partner stimulates (relevance system). 6. Transform aggression into assertion, using top-down inhibition skills (executive system). 7. Increase reflection (hindsight) on the triggers each partner engages from past relationships (relevance and executive systems). 8. Develop problem-solving skills to resolve or negotiate conflicts with more flexibility (executive system).	span of relationships, and have a broader repertoire of hobbies and activities. Learning how to give to others may be a crucial part of the process in changing this pattern. Because both partners are usually disappointing each other, learning to be empathetic and respectful about differences is important. The detached partner often has to become more connected to his or her emotional self. Often, ambivalent feelings are present so his or her indecisiveness is fueled by conflicted emotions (Slavik, Carlson, & Sperry, 1998). As these ambivalent feelings are sorted through for clarity, feelings of loss may need to be tolerated with the help of a loving connection so, paradoxically, he or she can care about wanting more (Guntrip, 1969, 1973). See information in column 1 on demanding and detaching styles.	
Highly detached partners are likely to need interventions based in all the brain systems. Consider teaching partners to do the following:	Within a polarized couple with accommodating and detached styles, both partners are being evasive and unclear as to his or her own needs. Each partner may need to move toward more healthy	An oscillating accommodate–detach pattern may reflect a "push–pull" dynamic in relationships. This dynamic has been clinically identified in people with borderline personality disorders (Salzman,

1. Connect to visceral self (regulation system).
2. Recognize subtle state and emotional shifts between each other by learning to read nonverbal cues (sensory system).
3. Engage genuine interests and motivations (relevance system).
4. Learn how to trust that sharing feelings, ideas, wants, and needs can be fulfilling rather than frightening (relevance system; with entrenched detached patterns, this trust often doesn't develop unless there is a new/therapeutic relationship that offers and facilitates that new experience; Guntrip, 1969, 1973).
5. Mature in their capacity to act in a nurturing and giving way toward others, accurately reading others' cues and inferences (relevance and executive systems).

assertiveness and ownership of feelings and needs as well as reasonable expectations from each other.
See information in column 1 on accommodating and detaching styles.

Salzman, & Wolfson, 1997) and ambivalent attachments (Salzman, 1997). Dialectical behavioral therapy provides a complex synthesis of multiple strategies (Linehan, 1993) that has been shown to be a promising treatment for borderline personality disorder (Bohus et al., 2000; Verheul et al., 2003).
See information in column 1 on accommodating and detaching styles.

On another level, catalyst clinicians within networks, such as WIN, can use the form to systematically determine which trainings are needed, which disciplines to seek for consultation, and which local courses to recommend within the network. Different networks can begin to form consortiums, within which training needs can be coordinated on a large scale. At this phase in the use of the neurorelational framework, for example, the WIN participants note that their next step is to build collaborations with professionals working within the agencies and schools that provide services under the Individuals with Disabilities Education Act for developmental

Instructions: 1. Place a √ in the boxes that pertain to the predominant orientation of the presentation

Schedule	Regulation Brain System	Sensory Brain System	Relevance Brain System	Executive Brain System (includes motor)	Heart (respond)	Hand (direct)	Head (reflect)
September, 2007 Orientation to the Big Picture	√	√	√	√	√	√	√
October, 2007 Building Healthy Minds & Relationships			√				√
October, 2007 Post-partum Depression	√		√		√		
November, 2007 Typical and Atypical Developmental Milestones	√	√		√		√	√
December 3, 2007 Breast Feeding: Joys and Complications	√		√		√	√	
January, 2008 Strength-Based Approaches to Home Visiting			√		√		
February, 2008 Working with	√	√	√	√		√	

(Continued)

Autistic Spectrum Disorders							
March, 2008 Culturally-Sensitive Treatment Approaches to Working with Immigrant and Traumatized Families		√	√	√			√
April, 2008 Early Speech Delays		√	√		√	√	
May, 2008 Learning Disabilities		√		√		√	√
June, 2008 Case Presentations with a Full-Scope Interdisciplinary Panel	√	√	√	√	√	√	√

Figure 12.7. A sample of how to map workshop content using the neurorelational framework.

delays. They are also interested in delving deeper into understanding developmental milestones/delays and educational delays. Filling in the gaps becomes much more organized when individuals and groups can see for themselves where their knowledge is deficient.

For those who are new to the concept of creating a team and building relationships across disciplines, the following national organizations and Web sites can form a basic foundation of information from diverse fields.

Educational Practitioners

Association of Educational Therapists: www.aetonline.org

Early Head Start: www.ehsnrc.org

Head Start: www.headstartinfo.org/infocenter/ehs_tkit1.htm

National Association for the Education of Young Children: www.naeyc.org

National Association of Special Education Teachers: www.naset.org

Infant Mental Health Practitioners

Interdisciplinary Council for Developmental and Learning Disorders: www.icdl.com

World Association for Infant Mental Health: www.waimh.org

ZERO TO THREE: www.zerotothree.org

Medical Practitioners

American Academy of Child and Adolescent Psychiatry: www.aacap.org

American College of Obstetricians and Gynecologists: www.acog.org

National Association of Pediatric Nurse Practitioners: www.napnap.org

Society for Developmental and Behavioral Pediatrics: www.sdbp.org

Neuropsychology

International Neuropsychological Society (INS): www.the-ins.org

National Academy of Neuropsychology (NAN): www.nanonline.org

Occupational Therapists

American Occupational Therapy Association (AOTA): www.aota.org

Physical Therapists

American Physical Therapy Association (APTA): www.apta.org

Speech and Language Therapists

American Speech Language Hearing Association (ASHA): www.asha.org

Gaining facility in applying the neurorelational framework can be expedited by specialized training in learning how to observe behaviors across

the brain systems in infants and young children. The following site provides links for training in the neurorelational framework: www.the-nrf.com

ENVISIONING THE FUTURE

In an ideal world, the current renewed interest in and influence of interdisciplinary approaches to complex questions would evolve to a critical mass within research, academic, and clinical settings, wherein the absence of an interdisciplinary approach would be seen as substandard. By breaking down barriers that circumscribe knowledge within specific disciplinary boundaries, we can create an open learning system where the language we use supports the sharing of knowledge across research, academic, and clinical communities. In this context, professionals would expect to collaborate with others and learn within a multidimensional model from the start of their research, academic, and clinical training, rather than after the fact. It would seem likely that such a development would greatly improve the quality of service delivery.

In an ideal world, the neurorelational framework would continue to support and spawn other clinical frameworks that consider multiple developmental factors and integrate them into a cohesive network of assessment and intervention strategies that hold complexity. Ours is an example of one type of synthesis that we anticipate (and hope) will undergo continued iterations. We look forward to the emergence of many more developmental syntheses from diverse collaborations.

In an ideal world, developmental research efforts would continue to reflect increasing degrees of complexity in design and execution, building on efforts already in place (Lewis & Granic, 2000; Sameroff & Fiese, 2000a; Wachs, 2000). In our view, the dynamic nature of development itself begs for such multidimensional and complex analyses. Dynamic systems theory offers an exciting new horizon of scientific investigation that uses complex statistical and experimental models across multiple levels of analysis (Cicchetti & Blender, 2006; Wachs, 2000) that can also capture real-time, real-world interactions (e.g., for the use of state–space grids to plot dyadic interactions in real time, see Granic & Hollenstein, 2003; Hollenstein, 2007; Hollenstein & Lewis, 2006).

The need for research that better encompasses the complexities inherent in what is being researched is well articulated by Weisz and Gray (2008, pp. 59–60), who note the problems that exist with the current gold standard of randomized control trials for evidence-based treatments (EBTs):

> Various writers have suggested that EBTs (a) have been developed and tested with relatively simple, often subclinical cases, and thus may not work well

with the complex and severe cases often seen in usual clinical care; (b) have been designed for single problems or diagnoses and thus may not fare so well when they confront co-occurring problems and comorbid diagnoses, which are common in usual clinical care; (c) are so strictly and uniformly structured that they make it hard to individualize treatment to meet to meet distinctive client needs, (d) are so formulaic that they constrain therapist creativity in addressing unusual or unexpected events in client's lives; and (e) are so lacking in spontaneity and flexibility that they interfere with rapport-building and development of a good therapeutic relationship. Several of the concerns reflect the view that evidence-based treatments may not be well-suited to the challenge of treating clinically-referred individuals in the context of usual clinical care (Addis & Krasnow, 2000; Addis & Waltz, 2002; Garfield, 1996; Havik & VandenBos, 1996; Strupp & Anderson, 1997; Westen, Novotny, & Thompson-Brenner, 2004a, 2004b). Further, experts on culture and ethnicity have voiced concerns that EBTs may not have been adequately adapted for, and may not work so well with, members of ethnic minority groups (Bernal & Scharron-Del-Rio, 2001; Gray-Little & Kaplan, 2000; Hall, 2001; Sue, 2003).

At this point in our research history, Weisz and Gray note that "we cannot assume that all evidence-based treatments are superior to what clinicians are doing routinely in usual care" (2008, p. 61) and summarize this juncture with the reflection that "a critical question for the field is what *approach* to empirical testing will give us the strongest treatments that are most robust in actual clinical practice" (2008, p. 62). Weisz and colleagues (Weisz & Gray, 2008; Weisz, Hawley, & Doss, 2004) propose a "development-focused model" that values use of published case studies developed by clinicians in real-world settings as the place to start, creating a process wherein these can be tested early in their development and in a sequential manner. Regardless of the specific approach used, its ability to accommodate complexity is essential. In Wachs's words, "whether one is involved in research, intervention, or public policy, we need models and intervention strategies that honor existing complexities that underlie individual human developmental variability. Through understanding of these complexities, we will better be able to promote both competence and resilience for a greater number of individuals" (2000, p. 334).

At the same time, it is important to note that pointing out the flaws of EBTs does not rationalize ignorance or wholesale rejection of them. The foregoing criticisms point out the need for greater flexibility and adaptability that leave room for clinical wisdom and sensitivity to the needs of the individual child, dyad, and family. An example of an error in this direction is seen in the professional who outright rejects all behaviorally oriented treatments (e.g., discrete trial training) on the grounds that

they are too restrictive or rigid. What is missing in this perspective is a recognition of the importance of automatic routines. Many children and families can benefit from both structured and unstructured treatments, and there are times in the course of treatment where the structured treatment may well be the appropriate priority. In other words, value and relevance can be found in all our clinical approaches.

In an ideal world, catalysts would inspire interdisciplinary efforts in research, academic, and clinical fronts that would flourish around the world. Networking and dialoguing on national and international professional levels would become common. Most professional organizations have some type of system for sharing disciplinary knowledge with the public; however, interdisciplinary collaboration takes knowledge sharing to a level that requires reciprocity. That is, knowledge must be received, as well, and efforts made to understand the similarities and differences in language and underlying theory. There will be points of convergence and divergence, and both are equally fruitful in yielding insights and ideas. This practice of reciprocal knowledge sharing would lead to the development of interdisciplinary competencies, which in turn, would positively affect training, service delivery, and public policy.

In an ideal world, not only would practitioners be in discourse, creating an interdiscipline for the early childhood field, but relationships would build among researchers, academics, practitioners, and family members who share an understanding of the complexity inherent in development (the Interdisciplinary Council for Developmental and Learning Disorders community is an excellent example of such an effort). Discussion and reflection across these venues would begin to shape the types of research questions that are asked. Answering these questions will help support efforts to create an integrated knowledge base across disciplines. Such a knowledge base can then exponentially facilitate the refinement of additional research and clinical frameworks that truly reflect the children and families we serve.

NOTE

1. As noted in Chapter 1, it is important to hold a balance among evidence-based treatments, clinical expertise, and family values. While research literature regarding treatment efficacy is important, it must be held in tension with the other two variables. When research-validated approaches do not exist or have been exhausted, the professional should rely on approaches that fit within the context of sound neurodevelopmental theory and guiding principles.

References

Abel, E. (1980). Smoking during pregnancy: A review on growth and development of offspring. *Human Biology, 52,* 593–625.

Acolet, D., Modi, N., Giannakoulopoulos, X., Bond, C., Weg, W., Clow, A., et al. (1993). Changes in plasma cortisol and catecholamine concentrations in response to massage in preterm infants [special issue]. *Archives of Disease in Childhood, 68*(1), 29–31.

Addis, M. E., & Krasnow, A. D. (2000). A national survey of practicing psychologists' attitudes toward psychotherapy treatment manuals. *Journal of Consulting and Clinical Psychology, 68,* 331–339.

Addis, M. E., & Waltz, J. (2002). Implicit and untested assumptions about the role of psychotherapy treatment manuals in evidence based mental health practice. *Clinical Psychology: Science and Practice, 9,* 421–424.

Aksan, N., Van Voorhis, L. L., Weber, E. S., & Georgeson-Dunn, H. (1999, April). *Developmental progression of embarrassment and self-development in the second year.* Paper presented at the biennial meeting of the Society for Research in Child Development in Albuquerque, New Mexico.

Alexander, P. A., Jetton, T. L., & Kulikowich, J. M. (1995). Interrelationship of knowledge, interest, and recall: Assessing a model of domain learning. *Journal of Educational Psychology, 87,* 559–575.

Als, H. (1982). Toward a synactive theory of development: Promise for the assessment and support of infant individuality. *Infant Mental Health Journal, 3*(4), 229–243.

Als, H. (1984). *Manual for the naturalistic observation of newborn behavior (preterm and full term).* Boston: Children's Hospital.

Als, H. (2002). *Program guide—Newborn Individualized Developmental Care and Assessment Program (NIDCAP): An education and training program for health care professionals* (rev. ed.). Boston: Children's Medical Center.

Als, H., Duffy, F. H., McAnulty, G. B., Rivkin, M. J., Vajapeyam, S., Mulkern, R. V., et al. (2004). Early experience alters brain function and structure. *Pediatrics, 113*(4), 846–857.

Als, H., & Gibes, R. (1986). *Newborn Individualized Developmental Care and Assessment Program (NIDCAP).* Unpublished training guide. Boston: Children's Hospital.

Als, H., Gilkerson, L., Duffy, F. H., McAnulty, G. B., Buehler, D. M., Vandenberg, K., et al. (2003). A three-center, randomized, controlled trial of individualized developmental care for very low birth weight preterm infants: Medical, neurodevelopmental parenting and caregiving effects. *Journal of Developmental and Behavioural Pediatrics, 24*(6), 399–408.

Als, H., Lawhon, G., Duffy F., McAnulty, G. B., Gibes-Grossman, R., & Blickman, J. G. (1994). Individualized developmental care for the very low-birth-weight preterm infant: Medical and neurofunctional effects. *Journal of the American Medical Association, 272*(11), 853–858.

Amaral, D. (2000). The functional organization of perception and movement. In E. R. Kandel, J. H. Schwartz, & T. M. Jessell (Eds.), *Principles of neural science* (4th ed., pp. 337–348). New York: McGraw-Hill.

American Association on Intellectual and Developmental Disabilities (2008, March 7). Low maternal education linked to intellectual disabilities in offspring. *ScienceDaily.* Retrieved May 15, 2008, from www.sciencedaily.com/releases/2008/03/080305121015.htm

American Psychiatric Association. (1994). *Diagnostic and statistical manual of mental disorders* (4th ed.) (*DSM-IV-TR*). Washington, DC: APA.

Ammen, S. A., & Limberg, B. (2005). Play therapy with preschoolers using the ecosystem model. In K. M. Finello (Ed.), *The handbook of training and practice in infant and preschool mental health* (pp. 207–232). San Francisco, CA: Wiley.

Anderson, S. J., Cohen, G., & Taylor, S. (2000). Rewriting the past: Some factors affecting the variability of personal memories. *Applied Cognitive Psychology, 14*(5), 435–454.

Anderson, V., & Catroppa, C. (2007). Memory outcome at 5 years post-childhood traumatic brain injury. *Brain Injury, 21,* 1399–1409.

Aslin, R. N. (1981). Development of smooth pursuit in human infants. In D. F. Fisher, R. A. Monty, & J. W. Senders (Eds.), *Eye movements: Cognition and visual perception* (pp. 31–51). Hillsdale, NJ: Lawrence Erlbaum.

Associated Press. (2008, April 3). In Egypt, children bear weight of poverty. Retrieved April 16, 2008, from www.cbsnews.com/stories/2008/04/03/world/main3992011.shtml

Astington, J. W. (2000). *Language and metalanguage in children's understanding of mind.* Malden, MA: Blackwell.

Astington, J. W. (2003). *Sometimes necessary, never sufficient: False-belief understanding and social competence.* New York: Psychology Press.

Astington, J. W., & Jenkins, J. M. (1999). A longitudinal study of the relation between language and theory-of-mind development. *Developmental Psychology, 35*(5), 1311–1320.

Atkinson, J., & Braddick, O. (2007). Visual and visuocognitive development in children born very prematurely. In C. von Hofsten & K. Rosander (Eds.), *From action to cognition* (Progress in Brain Research no. 164, pp. 123–149). Amsterdam: Elsevier.

Ayres, A. J. (1989). *Sensory integration and praxis test.* Los Angeles: Western Psychological Services.

Babcock, J. C., Green, C. E., & Robie, C. (2004). Does batterers' treatment work? A meta-analytic review of domestic violence treatment outcome research. *Clinical Psychology Review, 23,* 1023–1053.

Backhaus, J., Hoeckesfeld, R., Born, J., Hohagen, F., & Junghanns, K. (2008). Immediate as well as delayed post learning sleep but not wakefulness enhances declarative memory consolidation in children. *Neurobiology of Learning and Memory, 89*(1), 76–80.

Backs, R.W. (1998). A comparison of factor analytic methods of obtaining cardiovascular autonomic components for the assessment of mental workload. *Ergonomics, 41*(5), 733–745.

Bagnato, S. J., Neisworth, J. T., & Munson, S. M. (1997). *Linking assessment and early intervention: An authentic curriculum-based approach.* Baltimore: Paul H. Brookes.

Baharav, A., Kotagal, S., Gibbons, V., Rubin, B. K., Pratt, G., Karin, J., et al. (1995). Fluctuations in autonomic nervous activity during sleep displayed by power spectrum analysis of heart rate variability. *Neurology, 45*(6), 1183–1187.

Ballabriga, A. (1990). Malnutrition and the central nervous system. In R. Suskind & L. Lewinter-Suskind (Eds.), *The malnourished child* (pp. 177–192). New York: Raven Press.

Baranek, G. T., David, F. J., Poe, M. D., Stone, W. L., & Watson, L. R. (2006). Sensory experiences questionnaire: Discriminating sensory features in young children with autism, developmental delays, and typical development. *Journal of Child Psychology and Psychiatry, 47*(6), 591–601.

Barker, D. J. (1995). Intrauterine programming of adult disease. *Molecular Medicine Today, 1,* 418–423.

Barkley, R. A. (1997). *ADHD and the nature of self-control.* New York: Guilford Press.

Barnard, K. E. (1979). *Nursing Child Assessment Satellite Training (NCAST) teaching and feeding scales.* Seattle: Nursing Child Assessment Satellite Training, University of Washington.

Barnard, K. E. (1999). *Beginning rhythms. The emerging process of sleep-wake behavior and self-regulation.* Seattle: Nursing Child Assessment Satellite Training, University of Washington.

Barnett, S., Jung, K., Yaroz, D., Thomas, J., & Hornbeck, A. (2008). Educational effects of the Tools of the Mind curriculum: A randomized trial. *Early Childhood Research Quarterly, 1*(3), 293–301.

Bart, O., Katz, N., Weiss, P. T., & Josman, N. (2006). Street crossing by typically developed children in real and virtual environments. *Proceedings of the 5th International Workshop on Virtual Rehabilitation,* pp. 42–46.

Bartsch, K., & Wellman, H. M. (1995). *Children talk about the mind.* New York: Oxford University Press.

Bateson, G., Jackson, D. D., Haley, J., & Weakland, J. (1956). Towards a theory of schizophrenia. *Behavioral Science, 1*, 251–264.

Baumeister, R. F. (2005). *The cultural animal: Human nature, meaning, and social life.* New York: Oxford University Press.

Baumeister, R. F., Bratslavsky, E., Finkenauer, C., & Vohs, K. D. (2001). Bad is stronger than good. *Review of General Psychology, 5*, 323–370.

Baumeister, R. F., DeWall, C. N., Ciarocco, N. J., & Twenge, J. M. (2005). Social exclusion impairs self-regulation. *Journal of Personality and Social Psychology, 88*(4), 589–604.

Baumeister, R. F., Twenge, J. M., & Nuss, C. K. (2002). Effects of social exclusion on cognitive processes: Anticipated aloneness reduces intelligent thought. *Journal of Personality and Social Psychology, 83*(4), 817–827.

Baumeister, R. F., Vohs, K. D., DeWall, C. N., & Zhang, L. (2007). How emotion shapes behavior: Feedback, anticipation, and reflection, rather than direct causation *Personality and Social Psychology Review, 11*, 167.

Baumeister, R. F., Vohs, K. D., & Tice, D. M. (2006). *Emotional influences on decision making.* New York: Psychology Press.

Baumrind, D. (1971). Current patterns of parental authority. *Developmental Psychology Monographs, 4*, 1–103.

Baumrind, D. (1991). The influence of parenting style on adolescent competence and substance use. *Journal of Early Adolescence, 11*(1), 56–95.

Bayley, N. (2005). *Bayley scales of infant and toddler development—Third edition (BSID-III).* San Antonio: Psychological Corporation.

Baylor, P., Mouton, A., Shamoon, H. H., & Goebel, P. (1995). Increased norepinephrine variability in patients with sleep apnea syndrome. *American Journal of Medicine, 99*, 611–615.

Bechara, A., & Damasio, A. (2005). The somatic marker hypothesis: A neural theory of economic decision. *Games and Economic Behavior, 52*(2), 336–372.

Bechara, A., Damasio, H., Tranel, D., & Damasio, A. R. (2005). The Iowa gambling task (IGT) and the somatic marker hypothesis (SMH): Some questions and answers. *Trends in Cognitive Sciences, 9*(4), 159–162.

Beebe, B., & Lachmann, F. M. (2002). *Infant research and adult treatment: Co-constructing interactions.* Hillsdale, NJ: Analytic Press.

Beebe, B., Stern, D., & Jaffe, J. (1979). The kinesic rhythm of mother-infant interactions. In A. Siegman & S. Feldstein (Eds.), *Of speech and time* (pp. 23–34). Hillsdale, NJ: Erlbaum.

Beeghly, M., & Cicchetti, D. (1996). Child maltreatment, attachment, and the self system: Emergence of an internal state lexicon in toddlers at high social risk. In M. E. Hertzig & E. A. Farber (Eds.), *Annual progress in child psychiatry and child development 1995* (pp. 127–166). New York: Brunner/Mazel.

Bellinger, D., Titlebaum, L., Hu, H., & Needleman, H. (1994). Attentional correlates of dentin and bone lead levels in adolescents. *Archives of Environmental Health, 49*, 98–105.

Bellugi, U., Litchenberger, L., Jones, W., Lai, Z., & St. George, M. (2000). The neurocognitive profile of Williams syndrome: A complex pattern of strengths and weaknesses. *Journal of Cognitive Neuroscience, 12*(Suppl. 1), 7–29.

Benes, F. M. (2001). The development of prefrontal cortex: The maturation of neurotransmitter systems and their interactions. In C. A. Nelson & M. Luciana (Eds.), *Handbook of developmental cognitive neuroscience* (pp. 79–92). Cambridge, MA: MIT Press.

Benjamin, L. S. (2003). *Interpersonal diagnosis and treatment of personality disorders*. New York: Guilford Press.

Bennett, D. S., Benderksy, M., & Lewis, M. (2005). Does the organization of emotional expression change over time? Facial expressivity from 4 to 12 months. *Infancy, 8*(2), 167–187.

Ben-Sasson, A., Cermak, S. A., Orsmond, G. I., Carter, A. S., & Fogg, L. (2007). Can we differentiate sensory over-responsivity from anxiety symptoms in toddlers? Perspectives of occupational therapists and psychologists. *Infant Mental Health Journal, 28*(5), 536–558.

Berg, B. (2004a). *The anger control game (8 years and up)*. Los Angeles: Western Psychological Services.

Berg, B. (2004b). *The social conflict game (8 years and up)*. Los Angeles: Western Psychological Services.

Bernal, G., & Scharron-Del-Rio, M. R. (2001). Are empirically supported treatments valid for ethnic minorities? Toward an alternative approach for treatment research. *Cultural Diversity and Ethnic Minority Psychology, 7,* 328–342.

Bernstein, V. J., Hans, S. L., & Percansky, C. (1991). Advocating for the young child in need through strengthening the parent-child relationship. *Journal of Clinical Child Psychology, 20,* 28–41.

Berntson, G. G., Bechara, A., Damasio, H., Tranel, D., & Cacioppo, J. T. (2007). Amygdala contribution to selective dimensions of emotion. *Social Cognitive and Affective Neuroscience, 2,* 123–129.

Berntson, G. G., Boysen, S. T., & Cacioppo, J. T. (1991). Cardiac orienting and defensive responses: Potential origins in autonomic space. In B. A. Campbell (Ed.), *Attention and information processing in infants and adults* (pp. 163–200). Hillsdale, NJ: Erlbaum.

Berntson, G. G., & Cacioppo, J. T. (2000). From homeostasis to allodynamic regulation. In J. T. Cacioppo, L. G. Tassinary, & G. G. Berntson (Eds.), *Handbook of psychophysiology* (2nd ed., pp. 459–481). New York: Cambridge University Press.

Berntson, G. G., & Cacioppo, J. T. (2004). Heart rate variability: Stress and psychiatric conditions. In M. Malik & A. J. Camm (Eds.), *Dynamic electrocardiography* (pp. 57–64). New York: Futura.

Berntson, G. G., & Cacioppo, J. T. (2007). Integrative physiology: Homeostasis, allostasis and the orchestration of systemic physiology. In J. T. Cacioppo, L. G. Tassinary, & G. G. Berntson (Eds.), *Handbook of psychophysiology* (3rd ed., pp. 433–452). New York: Cambridge University Press.

Berntson, G. G., Cacioppo, J. T., & Grossman, P. (2007). Whither vagal tone. *Biological Psychology, 74*(2), 295–300.

Berntson, G. G., Cacioppo, J. T., & Quigley, K. S. (1991). Autonomic determinism: The modes of autonomic control, the doctrine of autonomic space, and the laws of autonomic constraint. *Psychological Review, 98,* 459–487.

Berntson, G. G., Cacioppo, J. T., Quigley, K. S., & Fabro, V. T. (1994). Autonomic space and psychophysiological response. *Psychophysiology, 31,* 44–61.

Berntson, G. G., Cacioppo, J. T., & Sarter, M. (2003). Bottom-up: Implications for neurobehavioral models of anxiety and autonomic regulation. In R. J. Davidson, K. R. Sherer, & H. H. Goldsmith (Eds.), *Handbook of affective sciences* (pp. 1105–1116). New York: Oxford University Press.

Berntson, G. G., Sarter, M., & Cacioppo, J. T. (2003a). Ascending visceral regulation of cortical affective information processing. *European Journal of Neuroscience, 18,* 2103–2109.

Berntson, G. G., Sarter, M., & Cacioppo, J. T. (2003b). Autonomic nervous system. In L. Nadel (Ed.), *Encyclopedia of cognitive science* (Vol. 1, pp. 301–308). London: Nature Publishing Group.

Bertalanffy, L., von. (1968). *General system theory: Foundations, development, applications* (Rev. ed.). New York: George Braziller.

Bertenthal, B. I., Campos, J. J., & Haith, M. M. (1980). Development of visual organization: The perception of subjective contours. *Child Development, 51*(4), 1072–1080.

Bierdman, J., Rosenbaum, J. F., Hirshfeld, D. R., Faraone, S. V., Bolduc, E. A., Gersten, M., et al. (1991). Psychiatric correlates of behavioral inhibition in young children of parents with and without psychiatric disorders. In S. Chess & M. E. Hertzig (Eds.), *Annual progress in vhild psychiatry and child development* (pp. 269–284). New York: Brunner/Mazel.

Bierman, K. L. & Erath, S. A. (2006). *Promoting social competence in early childhood: Classroom curricula and social skills coaching programs.* Malden, MA: Blackwell.

Bierman, K. L., & Welsh, J. A. (2000). Assessing social dysfunction: The contributions of laboratory and performance-based measures. *Journal of Clinical Child Psychology, 29*(4), 526–539.

Bischof-Köhler, D. (2000). Empathie, prosoziales verhalten und bindungsqualität bei zweijährigen [Empathy, prosocial behavior and security of attachment in two-year-olds]. *Psychologie in Erziehung und Unterricht, 47*(2), 142–158.

Bjorklund, D. (1985). The role of conceptual knowledge in the development of organization in children's memory. In C. Brainerd & M. Pressley (Eds.), *Basic processes in memory development* (pp. 103–142). New York: Springer.

Bjorklund, D. (1987). How changes in knowledge base contribute to the development of organization in children's memory: An interpretive review. *Developmental Review, 7,* 93–130.

Blackburn, S. (1986a). Sleep and awake states of the newborn. In K. E. Barnard (Ed.), *NCAST Instructor's Learning Manual* (pp. 25–27). Seattle, WA: NCAST Publications.

Blackburn, S. (1986b). State related behaviors and individual differences. In K. E. Barnard (Ed.), *NCAST Instructor's Learning Manual* (pp. 28–39). Seattle, WA: NCAST Publications.

Blairs, S., & Slater, S. (2007). The clinical application of deep touch pressure with a man with autism presenting with severe anxiety and challenging behavior. *British Journal of Learning Disabilities, 35,* 214–220.

Blanche, E., & Schaaf, R. (2001). Proprioception: A cornerstone of sensory integrative intervention. In S. Roley, E. Blanche, & R. Schaaf (Eds.), *Understanding the nature of sensory integration with diverse populations* (pp. 109–124). Austin, TX: PRO-ED.

Block, J., & Kremen, A. M. (1996). IQ and ego-resiliency: Conceptual and empirical connections and separateness. *Journal of Personality and Social Psychology, 70,* 349–360.

Bodrova, E., & Leong, D. J. (2001). Tools of the mind: A case study of implementing the Vygotskian approach in American early childhood and primary classrooms (UNESCO Innodata Monographs: Educational Innovations in Action no. 7). Geneva: International Bureau of Education, UNESCO.

Bodrova, E., & Leong, D. (2007). *Tools of the mind: The Vygotskian approach to early childhood education* (2nd ed.). Upper Saddle River, NJ: Prentice Hall.

Bohus, M., Haaf, B., Stiglmayr, C., Pohl, U., Bohme, R., & Linehan, M. (2000). Evaluation of inpatient dialectical-behavioral therapy for borderline personality disorder: A prospective study. *Behaviour Research and Therapy, 38*(9), 875–887.

Bollas, C. (1983). Expressive uses of the countertransference—notes to the patient from oneself. *Contemporary Psychoanalysis, 19,* 1–33.

Bollas, C. (1987). *The shadow of the object: Psychoanalysis of the unthought known.* New York: Columbia University Press.

Botvinick, M. M., Braver, T. S., Barch, D. M., Carter, C. S., & Cohen, J. D. (2001). Conflict monitoring and cognitive control. *Psychological Review, 108*(3), 624–652.

Bower, G. H. (1981). Mood and memory. *American Psychologist, 36*(2), 129–148.

Bowlby, J. (1969). *Attachment and loss: Vol. 1. Attachment.* New York: Basic Books.

Bowlby, J. (1973). *Attachment and loss: Vol. 2. Separation, anxiety, and anger.* New York: Basic Books.

Bowlby, J. (1978). Attachment theory and its therapeutic implications. In S. C. Feinstein & P. L. Giovacchini (Eds.), *Adolescent psychiatry* (Vol. 6, pp. 5–33). Chicago: University of Chicago Press.

Bozarth, M. A. (1994). Pleasure systems in the brain. In D. M. Warburton (Ed.), *Pleasure: The politics and the reality* (pp. 5–14). New York: Wiley.

Brafman, O., & Beckstrom, R. A. (2006). *The starfish and the spider: The unstoppable power of leaderless organizations.* New York: Penguin.

Brainerd, C. J., & Reyna, V. F. (1990). Gist is the grist: Fuzzy-trace theory and the new intuitionism [Special Issue: Limited resource models of cognitive development]. *Developmental Review, 10*(1), 3–47.

Brandchaft, B. (1994, March). *Structures of pathologic accommodation and change in psychoanalysis.* Paper presented at the Association for Psychoanalytic Self Psychology, New York.

Brandt, T., & Dieterich, M. (1999). The vestibular cortex: Its locations, functions, and disorders. *Annals of the New York Academy of Sciences, 871,* 293–312.

Brazelton, T. B. (1973). *Neonatal behavioral assessment scale: Clinics in developmental medicine no. 50.* Philadelphia: Lippincott.

Brazelton, T. B. (1984). *Neonatal behavioral assessment scale* (2nd ed.). Philadelphia: Lippincott.

Brazelton, T. B. (1992). *Touchpoints: Your child's emotional and behavioral development.* New York: Addison-Wesley.

Bricker, D., & Squires, J. (1999). *Ages & Stages Questionnaires: A parent-completed, child monitoring system* (2nd ed.). Baltimore: Paul H. Brookes.

Briggs, D. C. (1975). *Your child's self-esteem.* Garden City, NY: Doubleday.

Brooks, R., & Meltzoff, A. N. (2002). The importance of eyes: How infants interpret adult looking behavior. *Developmental Psychology, 38*(6), 958–966.

Brooks, R., & Meltzoff, A. N. (2005). The development of gaze following and its relation to language. *Developmental Science, 8*(6), 535–543.

Brooks-Gunn, J., & Lewis, M. (1984). The development of early visual self-recognition. *Developmental Review, 4*(3), 215–239.

Brown, A. L., Palincsar, A. S., & Purcell, L. (1986). Poor readers: Teach, don't label. In U. Neisser (Ed.), *The school achievement of minority children: New perspectives* (pp. 105–143). Hillsdale, NJ: Erlbaum.

Brown, C., & Dunn, W. (2002). *Adolescent/adult sensory profile self questionnaire.* San Antonio, TX: Harcourt Assessment.

Browne, J. V., MacLeod, A. M., & Smith-Sharp, S. (1999). *Family infant relationship support training (FIRST): Developmentally supportive care: Hospital to home for community professionals and care providers.* Denver, CO: Children's Hospital Association Center for Family and Infant Interaction.

Brubakken, D. M., & Lui, B. J. (2005). *Talk blocks.* Seattle, WA: Innovative Interactions.

Buchanan, T. W., Tranel, D., & Adolphs, R. (2006). Impaired memory retrieval correlates with individual differences in cortisol response but not autonomic response. *Learning & Memory, 13*(3), 382–387.

Buckley, K. E., Winkel, R. E., & Leary, M. R. (2004). Reactions to acceptance and rejection: Effects of level and sequence of relational evaluation. *Journal of Experimental Social Psychology, 40*(1), 14–28.

Buron, K. D. (2008). *A "5" could make me lose control: An activity-based method for evaluating and supporting highly anxious students.* Shawnee Mission, KS: Autism Asperger Publishing.

Buros Institute. (2007). *The seventeenth mental measurements yearbook.* In K. F. Geisinger, R. A. Spies, A. S. Carlson, & B. S. Plake (Eds.), Lincoln: University of Nebraska Press.

Butterfield, B., & Metcalfe, J. (2001). Errors made with high confidence are hypercorrected. *Journal of Experimental Psychology: Learning, Memory, and Cognition, 27,* 1491–1494.

Buysee, V., & Wesley, P. W. (2006). *Evidence-based practice in the early childhood field.* Washington, DC: ZERO TO THREE.

Bryanton, C., Bossé, J., Brien, M., McLean, J., McCormick, A. & Sveistrup, H. (2006). Feasibility, motivation and selective motor control: Virtual reality compared to conventional home exercise in children with cerebral palsy. *CyberPsychology & Behavior, 9*(2), 123–128.

Cacioppo, J. T. (1998). Somatic responses to psychological stress: The reactivity hypothesis. In M. Sabourin, F. Craik, & M. Robert (Eds.), *Advances in psychological*

science: Vol. 2. Biological and cognitive aspects (pp. 87–114). East Sussex, UK: Psychology Press.

Cacioppo, J. T. (2000). Autonomic, neuroendocrine, and immune responses to psychological stress. *Psychologische Beitrage, 42,* 4–23.

Cacioppo, J. T., & Berntson, G. G. (1999). The affect system: Architecture and operating characteristics. *Current Directions in Psychological Science, 8,* 133–137.

Cacioppo, J. T., & Berntson, G. G. (2002). Social neuroscience. In J. T. Cacioppo, G. G. Berntson, R. Alophs, C. S. Carter, R. J. Davidson, M. K. McClintock, et al. (Eds.), *Foundations in social neuroscience* (pp. 3–10). Cambridge, MA: MIT Press.

Cacioppo, J. T., & Berntson, G. G. (2007). The brain, homeostasis, and health: Balancing demands of the internal and external milieu. In H. S. Friedman & R. Cohen Silver (Eds.), *Foundations of health psychology* (pp. 73–91). New York: Oxford University Press.

Cacioppo, J. T., Berntson, G. G., Adolphs, R., Carter, C. S., Davidson, R. J., McClintock, M. K., et al., Eds. (2002). *Foundations in social neuroscience.* Cambridge, MA: MIT Press.

Cacioppo, J. T., Berntson, G. G., Larsen, J. T., Poehlmann, K. M., & Ito, T. A. (2000). The psychophysiology of emotion. In R. Lewis & J. M. Haviland-Jones (Eds.), *The handbook of emotion* (2nd ed., pp. 173–191). New York: Guilford Press.

Cacioppo, J. T., Berntson, G. G., Malarkey, W. B., Kiecolt-Glaser, J. K., Sheridan, J. F., Poehlmann, K. M., et al. (1998). Autonomic, neuroendocrine, and immune responses to psychological stress: The reactivity hypothesis. *Annals of the New York Academy of Sciences, 840,* 664–673.

Cacioppo, J. T., Ernst, J. M., Burleson, M. H., McClintock, M. K., Malarkey, W. B., Hakley, L., et al. (2002). Lonely traits and concomitant physiological processes: The MacArthur social neuroscience studies. In J. T. Cacioppo, G. G. Berntson, R. Alophs, C. S. Carter, R. J. Davidson, M. K. McClintock, et al. (Eds.), *Foundations in social neuroscience* (pp. 839–852). Cambridge, MA: MIT Press.

Cacioppo, J. T., & Gardner, W. L. (1999). Emotion. *Annual Review of Psychology, 50,* 191–214.

Cacioppo, J. T., Gardner, W. L., & Berntson, G. G. (1997). Beyond bipolar conceptualizations and measures: The case of attitudes and evaluative space. *Personality and Social Psychology Review, 1,* 3–25.

Cacioppo, J. T., Gardner, W. L., & Berntson, G. G. (1999). The affect system has parallel and integrative processing components: Form follows function. *Journal of Personality and Social Psychology, 76*(5), 839–855.

Cacioppo, J. T., Hawkley, L. C., & Berntson, G. G. (2003). The anatomy of loneliness. *Current Directions in Psychological Science, 12,* 71–74.

Cacioppo, J. T., Larsen, J. T., Smith, N. K., & Berntson, G. G. (2004). The affect system: What lurks below the surface of feelings? In A. S. R. Manstead, N. H. Frijda, & A. H. Fischer (Eds.), *Feelings and emotions: The Amsterdam conference* (pp. 223–242). New York: Cambridge University Press.

Caldwell, B. M. (1973). The importance of beginning early. In M. B. Karnes (Ed.), *Not all little wagons are red: The exceptional child's early years* (pp. 2–10). Arlington, VA: Council for Exceptional Children.

Camp, B. W., Blom, G. E., Hebert, F., & van Doornick, W. J. (1977). "Think aloud": A program for developing self-control in young aggressive boys. *Journal of Abnormal Child Psychology, 5*(2), 157–169.

Campbell, S. B. (1995). Behavior problems in preschool children: A review of recent research. *Journal of Child Psychology and Psychiatry, 36*(1), 113–149.

Campbell, S. B. (2002). *Behavior problems in preschool children: Clinical and developmental issues.* New York: Guilford Press.

Campbell, S. B., & Ewing, L. J. (1990). Follow-up of hard-to-manage preschoolers: Adjustment at age 9 and predictors of continuing symptoms. *Journal of Child Psychology and Psychiatry, 31*(6), 871–889.

Camras, L. A. (2000). Surprise! Facial expressions can be coordinative motor structures. In M. Lewis & I. Granic (Eds.), *Emotion, development, and self-organization: Dynamic systems approaches to emotional development* (pp. 100–124). New York: Cambridge University Press.

Canfield, R. L., & Haith, M. M. (1991). Young infants' visual expectations for symmetric and asymmetric stimulus sequences. *Developmental Psychology, 27,* 198–208.

Canli, T., Zhao, Z., Brewer, J., Gabrieli, J. D., & Cahill, L. (2000). Event-related activation in the human amygdala associates with later memory for individual emotional experience. *Journal of Neuroscience, 20*(RC99), 1–5.

Cannon, W. B. (1927). The James-Lange theory of emotions: A critical examination and an alternative. *American Journal of Psychology, 39,* 106–124.

Cannon, W. B. (1929). Organization for physiological homeostasis. *Physiological Reviews, 9,* 399–431.

Carlson, N. R. (2001). *Physiology of behavior* (7th ed.). Boston: Allyn and Bacon.

Carlson, S. M. (2005). Developmentally sensitive measures of executive function in preschool children. *Developmental Neuropsychology, 28*(2), 595–616.

Carpenter, M., Nagell, K., & Tomasello, M. (1998). Social cognition, joint attention, and communicative competence from 9 to 15 months of age. *Monographs of the Society for Research in Child Development, 63*(4), 1–166.

Carter, C. S., Braver, T. S., Barch, D. M., Botvinick, M. M., Noll, D., & Cohen, J. D. (1998). Anterior cingulate cortex, error detection, and the online monitoring of performance. *Science, 280,* 747–749.

Carter, C. S., & Van Veen, V. (2007). Anterior cingulate cortex and conflict detection: An update of theory and data. *Cognitive, Affective & Behavioral Neuroscience, 7*(4), 367–379.

Caspi, A., Moffitt, T. E., Newman, D. L., & Silva, P. A. (1996). Behavioral observations at age 3 predict adult psychiatric disorders: Longitudinal evidence from a birth cohort. *Archives of General Psychiatry, 53,* 1033–1039.

Cepeda, N. J., Pashler, H., Vul, E., Wixted, J. T., & Rohrer, D. (2006). Distributed practice in verbal recall tasks: A review and quantitative synthesis. *Psychological Bulletin, 132*(3), 354–380.

Changjun, S., & Michael, D. (1999). Pain pathways involved in fear conditioning measured with fear-potentiated startle: Lesion studies. *Journal of Neuroscience, 19*(1), 420–430.

Charness, N., Milberg, W., & Alexander, M. P. (1988). Teaching an amnesic a complex cognitive skill. *Brain Cognition, 8,* 253–272.

Chase, J. E., & Gidal, B. E. (1997). Melatonin: Therapeutic use in sleep disorders. *Annals of Pharmacotherapy, 31,* 1218–1225.

Chess, S., & Thomas, A. (1999). *Goodness of fit: Clinical applications from infancy through adult life.* Philadelphia: Brunner/Mazel.

Chi, M. T. H. (1978). Knowledge structures and memory development. In R. Siegler (Ed.), *Children's thinking: What develops?* (pp. 73–96). Hillsdale, NJ: Erlbaum.

Churchill, J. D., Galvez, R., Colcombe, S., Swain, R. A., Kramer, A. F., & Greenough, W. T. (2002). Exercise, experience and the aging brain. *Neurobiology of Aging, 23,* 941–955.

Churchland, P. S., Ramachandran, V. S., & Sejnowski, T. J. (1994). A critique of pure vision. In C. Koch & J. Davis (Eds.), *Large scale neuronal theories of the brain* (pp. 23–60). Cambridge, MA: MIT Press.

Cicchetti, D. (1991). Fractures in the crystal: Developmental psychopathology and the emergence of self. *Developmental Review, 11*(3), 271–287.

Cicchetti, D., & Blender, J. A. (2006) A multiple-levels-of-analysis perspective on resilience: Implications for the developing brain, neural plasticity, and preventive interventions. *Annals of the New York Academy of Sciences, 1094*(1), 248–258.

Cicchetti, D., & Cohen, D. J. (1995) Perspectives in developmental psychopathology. In D. Cicchetti & D. J. Cohen (Eds.), *Developmental psychopathology. Vol. 1: Theory and methods* (pp. 3–20). New York: Wiley.

Claparède, E. (1903). *L'association des idées.* Paris: Doin.

Clark, A. (1997). *Being there: Putting brain, body, and world together again.* Cambridge, MA: Bradford Books.

Clark, A. (2003). *Natural-born cyborgs: Minds, technologies, and the future of human intelligence.* New York: Oxford University Press.

Coe, C. L., & Lubach, G. R. (2008). Fetal programming: Prenatal origins of health and illness. *Associations for Psychological Science, 17*(1), 36–41.

Cohen, N. J., & Squire, L. R. (1980). Preserved learning and retention of pattern-analyzing skill in amnesia: Dissociation of "knowing how" and "knowing that." *Science, 210,* 207–209.

Compas, B. E. (2006). Psychobiological processes of stress and coping: Implications for resilience in children and adolescents—Comments on the papers of Romeo & McEwen and Fisher et al. *Annals of the New York Academy of Sciences, 1094*(1), 226–234.

Conduct Problems Prevention Research Group. (1999). Initial impact of the fast track prevention trial for conduct problems: II. Classroom effects. *Journal of Consulting and Clinical Psychology, 67*(5), 648–657.

Connors, M. E. (2000). Chapter 11 dimensions of experience in relationship seeking. *Progress in Self Psychology, 16,* 199–216.

Consumer Reports Health. (2006). How to help your child get a good night's sleep. Retrieved March 22, 2008, from www.consumerreports.org/health/free-highlights/manage-your-health/child_sleep_problems.htm

Cotman, C. W., & Berchtold, N. C. (2002). Exercise: A behavioral intervention to enhance brain health and plasticity. *Trends in Neuroscience, 25*(6), 295–301.

Courage, M. L., & Howe, M. L. (2002). From infant to child: The dynamics of cognitive change in the second year of life. *Psychological Bulletin, 128*(2), 250–277.

Courage, M. L., & Howe, M. L. (2004). Advances in early memory development research: Insights about the dark side of the moon. *Developmental Review, 24,* 6–32.

Covert, M. V., Tangney, J. P., Maddux, J. E., & Heleno, N. M. (2003). Shame-proneness, guilt-proneness, and interpersonal problem solving: A social cognitive analysis. *Journal of Social and Clinical Psychology, 22*(1), 1–12.

Cowan, N. (2001). The magical number 4 in short-term memory: A reconsideration of mental storage capacity. *Behavioral and Brain Sciences, 24*(1), 87–185.

Cowardt, M. (2006). Embodied cognition vs. classicism/cognitivism. In J. Fieser & B. Dowden (Eds.), *The Internet encyclopedia of philosophy*. Retrieved March 19, 2008, from www.iep.utm.edu/e/embodcog.htm

Craik, F. I., & Lockhart, R. S. (1972). Levels of processing: A framework for memory research. *Journal of Verbal Learning and Verbal Behavior, 17,* 671–684.

Crawford, L. E., & Cacioppo, J. T. (2002). Learning where to look for danger: Integrating affective and spatial information. *Psychological Science, 13,* 449–453.

Crick, N. R., & Dodge, K. A. (1994). A review and reformulation of social information-processing mechanisms in children's social adjustment. *Psychological Bulletin, 115*(1), 74–101.

Crick, N. R., & Dodge, K. A. (1996). Social-information processing mechanisms in reactive and proactive aggression. *Child Development, 67*(3), 993–1002.

Cullen-Powell, L. A., Barlow, J. H., & Cushway, D. (2005). Exploring a massage intervention for parents and their children with autism: The implications for bonding and attachment. *Journal of Child Health Care, 9*(4), 245–255.

Custers, R., & Aarts, H. (2005a). Beyond priming effects: The role of positive affect and discrepancies in implicit processes of motivation and goal pursuit. *European Review of Social Psychology, 16,* 257–300.

Custers, R., & Aarts, H. (2005b). Positive affect as implicit motivator: On the nonconscious operation of behavioral goals. *Journal of Personality and Social Psychology, 89*(2), 129–142.

Dahl, R. (1998). Common sleep problems in children. In J. S. Poceta & M. M. Mitler (Eds.), *Sleep disorders: Diagnosis and treatment* (pp. 161–186). Totowa, NJ: Humana Press.

Dalgleish, T., Taghavi, R., Neshat Doost, H., Moradi, A., Canterbury, R., & Yule, W. (2003). Patterns of processing bias for emotional information across clinical disorders: A comparison of attention, memory, and prospective cognition in children and adolescents with depression, generalized anxiety, and posttraumatic stress disorder. *Journal of Clinical Child and Adolescent Psychology, 32,* 10–21.

Dalgleish, T., & Watts, F. N. (1990). Biases of attention and memory in disorders of anxiety and depression. *Clinical Psychology Review, 10,* 589–604.

Dalterio, S., & Fried, P. (1992). The effects of marijuana use on offspring. In T. Sonderegger (Ed.), *Perinatal substance abuse* (pp. 161–183). Baltimore: Johns Hopkins University Press.

Damasio, A. R. (1994). *Descartes' error: Emotion, reason, and the human brain.* New York: Grossett/Putnam.

Damasio, A. R. (1996). The somatic marker hypothesis and the possible functions of the prefrontal cortex. *Philosophical Transactions of the Royal Society B, 351,* 1413–1420.

Damasio, A. R. (1999). *The feeling of what happens: Body and emotion in the making of consciousness.* New York: Harcourt Brace.

Damasio, A. (2003). *Looking for Spinoza: Joy, sorrow, and the feeling brain.* Orlando, FL: Harcourt.

D'Apolito, K. (1991). What is an organized infant? *Neonatal Network, 10,* 23–29.

Dapretto, M. (2006). Understanding emotions in others: Mirror neuron dysfunction in children with autism spectrum disorders. *Nature Neuroscience, 9*(1), 28–30.

Darwin, C. (1877). A biographical sketch of an infant. *Mind: Quarterly Review of Psychology and Philosophy, 2,* 285–294.

Dawson, M. E., Schell, A. M., & Filion, D. L. (2007). The electrodermal system. In J. T. Cacioppo, L. G. Tassinary, & G. G. Berntson (Eds.), *Handbook of psychophysiology* (pp. 159–181). New York: Cambridge University Press.

Davidson, M. C., Amso, D., Anderson, L. C., & Diamond, A. (2006). Development of cognitive control and executive functions from 4 to 13 years: Evidence from manipulations of memory, inhibition, and task switching. *Neuropsychologia, 44,* 2037–2078.

Davidson, R., & Fox, N. (1982). Asymmetrical brain activity discriminates between positive versus negative affective stimuli in human infants. *Science, 218,* 1235–1237.

Davis, H. L., & Pratt, C. (1996). The development of children's theory of mind: The working memory explanation. *Australian Journal of Psychology, 47,* 25–31.

DeGangi, G. (2000). *Pediatric disorders of regulation in affect and behavior: A therapist's guide to assessment and treatment.* San Diego, CA: Academic Press.

DeGangi, G., & Balzer-Martin, L. A. (2000). Appendix C: The sensorimotor history questionnaire for preschoolers. In G. DeGangi (Ed.), *Pediatric disorders of regulation in affect and behavior: A therapist's guide to assessment and treatment* (pp. 361–365). San Diego, CA: Academic Press.

DeGangi, G. A., DiPietro, J. A., Greenspan, S. I., & Porges, S. W. (1991). Psychophysiological characteristics of the regulatory disordered infant. *Infant Behavior and Development, 14,* 37–50.

DeGangi, G. A., & Greenspan, S. I. (1989). *Test of sensory functions in infants (4–18 months).* Los Angeles: Western Psychological Services.

DeGangi, G. A., Poisson, S., Sickel, R. Z., & Wiener, A. S. (1995). *Infant-toddler symptom checklist.* Tucson, AZ: Therapy Skill Builders.

de Haan, M., & Johnson, M. H. (2003). Mechanisms and theories of brain development. In M. de Hann & M. H. Johnson (Eds.), *The cognitive neuroscience of development* (pp. 1–18). New York: Psychology Press.

Delis, D. C., Kaplan, E., & Kramer, J. H. (2001). *Delis-Kaplan executive function system.* San Antonio, TX: Harcourt Assessment.

Delis, D., Lansing, A., Houston, W. S., Wetter, S., Duke Han, S., Jacobson, M., et al. (2007). Creativity lost: The importance of testing higher-level executive functions in school-age children and adolescents. *Journal of Psychoeducational Assessment, 25,* 29–40.

Denham, S. A., Blair, K. A., DeMulder, E., Levitas, J., Sawyer, K., Auerbach-Major, S., et al. (2003). Preschool emotional competence: Pathway to social competence. *Child Development, 74*(1), 238–256. DOI:10.1111/1467-8624.00533

de Oliveira, L. F., Camboim, C., Diehl, F., Consiglio, A. R., & Quillfeldt, J. A. (2007). Glucocorticoid-mediated effects of systemic oxytocin upon memory retrieval. *Neurobiology of Learning and Memory, 87*(1), 67–71.

Derryberry, D., & Rothbart, M. K. (1997). Reactive and effortful processes in the organization of temperament. *Development and Psychopathology, 9*(4), 633–652.

DeWall, C. N., & Baumeister, R. F. (2006). Alone but feeling no pain: Effects of social exclusion on physical pain tolerance and pain threshold, affective forecasting, and interpersonal empathy. *Journal of Personality and Social Psychology, 91*(1), 1–15.

de Weerth, C., & van Geert, P. (2000). The dynamics of emotion-related behaviors in infancy. In M. Lewis & I. Granic (Eds.), *Emotion, development, and self-organization: Dynamic systems approaches to emotional development* (pp. 324–348). New York: Cambridge University Press.

Diamond, A. (1985). Development of the ability to use recall to guide action, as indicated by infants' performance on A-not-B. *Child Development, 56,* 868–883.

Diamond, A., Barnett, W. S., Thomas, J., & Munro, S. (2007). Preschool program improves cognitive control. *Science, 318*(5855), 1387–1388.

Diamond, A., & Taylor, C. (1996). Development of an aspect of executive control: Development of the abilities to remember what I said and to "do as I say, not as I do." *Developmental Psychobiology, 29*(4), 315–334.

Diamond, A., Werker, J. F., & Lalonde, C. (1994). Toward understanding commonalities in the development of object search, detour navigation, categorization, and speech perception. In G. Dawson & K. W. Fischer (Eds.), *Human behavior and the developing brain* (pp. 380–426). New York: Guilford Press.

Diamond, D. M., Park, C. R., Campbell, A. M., & Woodson, J. C. (2005). Competitive interactions between endogenous LTD and LTP in the hippocampus underlie the storage of emotional memories and stress-induced amnesia. *Hippocampus, 15,* 1006–1025.

Dicker, S., & Gordon, E. (2000). Connecting healthy development and permanency: A pivotal role for child welfare professionals. *Permanency Planning Today, 1*(1), 12–15.

Dicker, S., & Gordon, E. (2002). Building a pathway to well-being: The story of the "healthy development checklist for children in foster care." *ZERO TO THREE*, April/May, 26–32.

Dicker, S., Gordon, E., & Knitzer, J. (2001). *Improving the odds: Promoting health, developmental, and emotional well-being of young children in foster care*. National Center for Children in Poverty.

Diego, M., Field, T., & Hernandez-Reif, M. (2006). Vagal activity, gastric motility and weight gain in massaged preterm infants. *Journal of Pediatrics, 147,* 50–55.

Dijkstra, K., Kaschak, M., & Swaan, R. (2007). Body posture facilitates retrieval of autobiographical memories. *Cognition, 102,* 139–149.

DiPietro, J. A., & Porges, S. W. (1991). Vagal responsiveness in gavage feeding as an index of preterm status. *Pediatric Research, 29,* 231–236.

Dobbs, T. M. (2000). *The three personalities of the three schools of psychology*. Unpublished manuscript, Pacific Oaks College, Pasadena, CA.

Dodge, K. A., Pettit, G. S., & Bates, J. E. (1997). How the experience of early physical abuse leads children to become chronically aggressive. In D. Cicchetti (Ed.), *Developmental perspectives on trauma: Theory, research, and intervention, Rochester Symposium on Developmental Psychology, 8* (pp. 263–288). Rochester, NY: University of Rochester Press.

Dodge, K. A., & Somberg, D. R. (1987). Hostile attributional biases among aggressive boys are exacerbated under conditions of threats to the self. *Child Development, 58,* 213–224.

Dolan, R. J. (2007). *Keynote address: Revaluing the orbital prefrontal cortex*. Malden, MA: Blackwell.

Downer, C. L. J. (1962). Interhemispheric integration in the visual system. In V. B. Mountcastle (Ed.), *Interhemispheric relations and cerebral dominance* (pp. 87–100). Baltimore: Johns Hopkins University Press.

Downing, G. (2008, July). *Video intervention therapy (VIT)* [Lecture series]. Infant-Parent Mental Health Post-Graduate Certificate Program, Napa Valley, CA.

Dowsett, S., & Livesey, D. J. (2000). The development of inhibitory control in pre-school children: Effects of "executive skills" training. *Developmental Psychobiology, 36*(2), 161–174.

Dozier, M., Dozier, D., & Manni, M. (2002). Attachment and biobehavioral catch-up: The ABC's of helping infants in foster care cope with early adversity. *ZERO TO THREE*, April/May, 7–13.

Drinka, T. J. K., Miller, T. F., & Goodman, B. M. (1996). Characterizing motivational styles of professionals who work on interdisciplinary healthcare teams. *Journal of Interprofessional Care, 10*(1), 51–61.

Drummey, A. B., & Newcombe, N. S. (2002). Developmental changes in source memory. *Developmental Science, 5,* 502–513.

Dumas, J. E., LaFreniere, P. J., & Serketich, W. J. (1995). "Balance of power": A transactional analysis of control in mother-child dyads involving socially competent, aggressive, and anxious children. *Abnormal Psychology, 104*(1), 104–113.

Dunn, W. (1997). The impact of sensory processing abilities on the daily lives of young children and their families: A conceptual model. *Infants and Young Children, 9*(4), 23–35.

Dunn, W. (1999). *Sensory profile manual.* San Antonio, TX: Psychological Corporation.

Dunn, W. (2002). *The infant/toddler sensory profile manual.* San Antonio, TX: Psychological Corporation.

Dunn, W. (2004). A sensory processing approach to supporting infant-caregiver relationships. In A. J. Sameroff, S. C. McDonough, & K. L. Rosenblum (Eds.), *Treating parent-infant relationship problems: Strategies for intervention* (pp. 152–187). New York: Guilford Press.

Dunn, W., & Daniels, D. (2002). Infant/toddler sensory profile caregiver questionnaire. San Antonio, TX: Psychological Corporation.

Dworkin, B. R. (2000). Interoception. In J. T. Cacioppo, L. G. Tassinary, & G. G. Bernston (Eds.), *Handbook of psychophysiology* (2nd ed., pp. 482–506). New York: Cambridge University Press.

Dworkin, B. R. (2007). Interoception. In J. T. Cacioppo, L. G. Tassinary, & G. G. Bernston (Eds.), *Handbook of psychophysiology* (3rd ed., pp. 482–506). New York: Cambridge University Press.

Edelson, S. M., Edelson, M.G., Kerr, D. C., & Grandin, T. (1999). Behavioral and physiological effects of deep pressure on children with autism: A pilot study evaluating the efficacy of Grandin's hug machine. *American Journal of Occupational Therapy, 53,* 145–151.

Egeland, B., Jacobvitz, D., & Sroufe, A. (1988). Breaking the cycle of abuse. *Child Development, 59,* 1080–1088.

Ehri, L. C. (1998). Grapheme-phoneme knowledge is essential for learning to read words in English. In J. Metsala & L. Ehri (Eds.), *Word recognition in beginning reading* (pp. 3–40). Hillsdale, NJ: Erlbaum.

Eisenberg, N., Guthrie, I. K., Fabes, R. A., Reiser, M., Murphy, B. C., Holgren, R., et al. (1997). The relations of regulation and emotionality to resiliency and competent social functioning in elementary school children. *Child Development, 68*(2), 295–311.

Eisenberg, N., Spinrad, T. L., Fabes, R. A., Reiser, M., Cumberland, A., Shepard, S. A., et al. (2004). The relations of effortful control and impulsivity to children's resiliency and adjustment. *Child Development, 75*(1), 25–46.

Eisenberg, N., Valiente, C., Fabes, R. A., Smith, C. L., Reiser, M., Shepard, S. A., et al. (2003). The relations of effortful control and ego control to children's resiliency and social functioning. *Developmental Psychology, 39*(4), 761–776.

Eisenberg, N., Zhou, Q., Spinrad, T. L., Valiente, C., Fabes, R. A., & Liew, J. (2005). Relations among positive parenting, children's effortful control, and externalizing problems: A three-wave longitudinal study. *Child Development, 76*(5), 1055–1071.

Ekman, P. (2003). *Emotions revealed: Recognizing faces and feelings to improve communication and emotional life.* New York: Times Books.

Elliott, R. (1998). The neuropsychological profile in unipolar depression. *Trends in Cognitive Science, 2,* 447–454.

Emde, R., & Harmon, R. (Eds.). (1984). *Continuities and discontinuities in development.* New York: Plenum Press.

Faber, A., & Mazlish, E. (2002). *How to talk so kids will listen and listen so kids will talk.* New York: HarperCollins.

Fabes, R. A., Gaertner, B. M., & Popp, T. K. (2006). *Getting along with others: Social competence in early childhood.* Malden, MA: Blackwell.

Fadiga, L., Craighero, L., & Olivier, E. (2005). Human motor cortex excitability during the perception of others' action. *Current Opinion in Neurobiology, 15*(2), 213–218.

Fadiga, L., Fogassi, L., Pavesi, G., & Rizzolatti, G. (1995). Motor facilitation during action observation: A magnetic stimulation study. *Journal of Neurophysiology, 73*(6), 2608–2611.

Farroni, T., Csibra, G., Simion, F., & Johnson, M. H. (2002). Eye contact detection in humans from birth. *Proceedings of the National Academy of Sciences of the United States of America, 99,* 9602–9605.

Farroni, T., Johnson, M. H., Brockbank, M., & Simion, F. (2000). Infants' use of gaze direction to cue attention: The importance of perceived motion. *Visual Cognition, 7,* 705–718.

Feldman, R. (2006). From biological rhythms to social rhythms: Physiological precursors of mother-infant synchrony. *Developmental Psychology, 42,* 175–188.

Feldman, R. (2007). Parent-infant synchrony: Biological foundations and developmental outcomes. *Association for Psychological Science, 16*(6), 340–345.

Feldman, R., & Eidelman, A. I. (1998). Intervention methods for premature infants: How and do they affect development. *Clinical Perinatology, 25,* 613–626.

Feldman, R., & Eidelman, A. I. (2003). Skin-to-skin contact (kangaroo care) accelerates autonomic and neurobehavioral maturation in preterm infants. *Developmental Medicine & Child Neurology, 45,* 274–281.

Feldman, R., Weller, A., Sirota, L., & Eidelman, A. I. (2003). Testing a family intervention hypothesis: The contribution of mother-infant skin-to-skin contact (kangaroo care) to family interaction, proximity, and touch. *Journal of Family Psychology, 17*(1), 94–107.

Ferber, R. (1985). *Solve your child's sleep problems.* New York: Simon & Schuster.

Field, T., Diego, M., & Hernandez-Reif, M. (2007). Massage therapy research. *Developmental Review, 27,* 75–89.

Field, T., Grizzle, N., Scafidi, F., Abrams, S., Richardson, S., Kuhn, C., et al. (1996). Massage therapy for infants of depressed mothers. *Infant Behavior and Development, 19,* 107–112.

Field, T., Pickens, J., Fox, N. A., Nawrocki, T., & Gonzalez, J. (1995). Vagal tone in infants of depressed mothers. *Development and Psychopathology, 7,* 227–231.

Finello, K. M. (Ed.). *The handbook of training and practice in infant and preschool mental health.* San Francisco: Jossey-Bass.

Finkelstein, N., & Ramey, C. (1977). Learning to control the environment. *Child Development, 48,* 806–819.

Fisher, A. G., & Murray, E. A. (1991). Introduction to sensory integration theory. In A. G. Fisher, E. A. Murray, & A. C. Bundy (Eds.), *Sensory integration: Theory and practice* (pp. 3–26). Philadelphia: F. A. Davis.

Fisher, P. A., Gunnar, M. R., Dozier, M., Bruce, J., & Pears, K. C. (2006). Effects of therapeutic interventions for foster children on behavioral problems, caregiver attachment, and stress regulatory neural systems. *Annals of the New York Academy of Sciences, 1094,* 215–225.

Flavell, J., Miller, P., & Miller, S. (1993). *Cognitive development.* Englewood Cliffs, NJ: Prentice Hall.

Flom, R., & Bahrick, L. E. (2007). The development of infant discrimination of affect in multimodal and unimodal stimulation: The role of intersensory redundancy. *Developmental Psychology, 43*(1), 238–252.

Fogassi, L., Ferrari, P. F., Gesierich, B., Rozzi, S., Chersi, F., & Rizzolatti, G. (2005). Parietal lobe: From action organization to intention understanding. *Science, 308,* 662–667.

Fogassi, L., Gallese, V., Fadiga, L., Luppino, G., Matelli, M., & Rizzolatti, G. (1996). Coding of peripersonal space in inferior premotor cortex (area F4). *Journal of Neurophysiology, 76,* 141–157.

Fogel, A. (1993). *Developing through relationships: Origins of communication, self, and culture.* Chicago: University of Chicago Press.

Fogel, A., & Melson, G. F. (1988). *Child development.* New York: West.

Fraiberg, S. (Ed.). (1980). *Clinical studies in infant mental health.* New York: Basic Books.

Francis, D. J., Shaywitz, S. E., Stuebing, K. K., Shaywitz, B. A., & Fletcher, J. M. (1996). Developmental lag versus deficit models of reading disability: A longitudinal, individual growth curves analysis. *Journal of Educational Psychology, 88*(1), 3–17.

Frank, J., & Rodiwski, M. (1999). Review of psychological issues in victims of domestic violence seen in emergency settings. *Emergency Medicine Clinics of North America, 17,* 657–677.

Freeman, W. J. (2000). *How brains make up their minds.* New York: Columbia University Press.

Friedman, R. J., & Chase-Lansdale, P. L. (2002). Chronic adversities. In M. Rutter & E. Taylor (Eds.), *Child and adolescent psychiatry: Modern approaches* (4th ed., pp. 261–276). London: Blackwell.

Friedman, W. J. (2007). The development of temporal metamemory. *Child Development, 78,* 1472–1491.

Frost, J. L., Wortham, S. C., & Reifel, S. (2001). *Play and child development.* Upper Saddle River, NJ: Prentice Hall.

Frye, D., Zelazo, P. D., & Burack, J. A. (1998). Cognitive complexity and control: I. Theory of mind in typical and atypical development. *Current Directions in Psychological Science, 7*(4), 116–121.

Funder, D. C. (in press). Personality, situations, and person-situation interactions. In O. P. John, R. W. Robins, & L. A. Pervin (Eds.), *Handbook of personality* (3rd ed.). New York: Guilford Press.

Fuster, J. (2002). Physiology of executive functions: The perception-action cycle. In D. T. Stuss & R. T. Knight (Eds.), *Principles of frontal lobe function* (pp. 96–108). New York: Oxford University Press.

Gais, S., Lucas, B., & Born, J. (2006). Sleep after learning aids memory recall. *Learning and Memory, 13,* 259–262.

Gal, E., Goren-Bar, D., Bauminger, N., Stock, O., Zancanaro, M., & Weiss, P. L. (2006, June). *A pilot study of enforced collaboration during computerized story-telling to enhance social communication of children with high-functioning autism.* Paper presented at the 11th Annual CyberTherapy Conference, Gatineau, Canada.

Gallese, V., & Goldman, A. (1998). Mirror neurons and the simulation theory of mindreading. *Trends in Cognitive Sciences, 2,* 493–501.

Galton, F. (1892). *Hereditary genius: An inquiry into its laws and consequences.* London: Macmillan.

Gardner, E. P., & Kandel, E. R. (2000). Touch. In E. R. Kandel, J. H. Schwartz, & T. M. Jessell (Eds.), *Principles of neural science* (4th ed., pp. 451–471). New York: McGraw-Hill.

Gardner, E. P., & Martin, J. H. (2000). Coding of sensory information. In E. R. Kandel, J. H. Schwartz, & T. M. Jessell (Eds.), *Principles of neural science* (4th ed., pp. 411–429). New York: McGraw-Hill.

Gardner, E. P., Martin, J. H., & Jessell, T. M. (2000). The bodily senses. In E. R. Kandel, J. H. Schwartz, & T. M. Jessell (Eds.), *Principles of neural science* (4th ed., pp. 430–450). New York: McGraw-Hill.

Garfield, S. L. (1996). Some problems associated with "validated" forms of psychotherapy. *Clinical Psychology: Science and Practice, 3,* 218–229.

Garon, N., Bryson, S. E., & Smith, I. M. (2008). Executive function in preschoolers: A review using an integrative framework. *Psychological Bulletin, 134*(1), 31–60.

Gathercole, S. E. (1998). The development of memory. *Journal of Child Psychology and Psychiatry, 39*(1), 3–27.

Gazzola, V., Rizzolatti, G., Wicker, B., & Keysers, C. (2007). The anthropomorphic brain: The mirror neuron system responds to human and robotic actions. *NeuroImage, 35*(4), 1674–1684.

Gentilucci, M., Scandolara, C., Pigarev, I. N., & Rizzolatti, G. (1983). Visual responses in the postarcuate cortex (area 6) of the monkey that are independent of eye position. *Experimental Brain Research, 50,* 464–468.

Gesell, A. (1929). *Infancy and human growth.* New York: Macmillan.

Gibney, P. (2006). The double bind theory: Still crazy-making after all these years. *Psychotherapy in Australia, 12*(3), 48–55.

Ginsburg, G. S., Grover, R. L., & Ialongo, N. (2005). Parenting behaviors among anxious and non-anxious mothers: Relation with concurrent and long-term child outcomes. *Child and Family Behavior Therapy, 26*(4), 23–41.

Glascoe, F. P. (1997). *Parents' evaluation of developmental status* (PEDS). Nashville, TN: Ellsworth & Vandermeer Press.

Glascoe, F. P., & Robertshaw, N. S. (2006). *Parents' evaluation of developmental status: Developmental milestones (PEDS: DM).* Nashville, TN: Ellsworth & Vandermeer Press.

Gleick, J. (1987). *Chaos: Making a new science.* New York: Viking.

Glenberg, A. M., Gutierrez, T., Levin, J. R., Japuntich, S., & Kaschak, M. P. (2004).

Activity and imagined activity can enhance young children's reading comprehension. *Journal of Educational Psychology, 96*(3), 424–436.

Gold, J. I., Kim, S. H., Kant, A. J., & Rizzo, A. A. (2005). Virtual anesthesia: The use of virtual reality for pain distraction during acute medical interventions. *Seminars in Anesthesia, Perioperative Medicine and Pain, 24,* 203–210.

Goleman, D. (2006a, October 10). Friends for life: An emerging biology of emotional healing. *New York Times.* Retrieved May 14, 2007, from www.nytimes.com/2006/10/10/health/psychology/10essa.html?_r=1&oref=slogin

Goleman, D. (2006b). *Social intelligence: The new science of human relationships.* New York: Bantam Dell.

Gopnik, A., Glymour, C., Sobel, D. M., Schulz, L. E., Kushnir, T., & Danks, D. (2004). A theory of causal learning in children: Causal maps and Bayes nets. *Psychological Review, 111*(1), 3–32.

Gopnik, A., & Graf, P. (1988). Knowing how you know: Young children's ability to identify and remember the sources of their beliefs. *Child Development, 59,* 1366–1371.

Gopnik, A., Sobel, D. M., Schulz, L. E., & Glymour, C. (2001). Causal learning mechanisms in very young children: Two-, three-, and four-year-olds infer causal relations from patterns of variation and covariation. *Developmental Psychology, 37,* 620–629.

Gordon, J., Chilardi, M. F., & Ghez, C. (1995). Impairments of reaching movements in patients without proprioception, I. Spatial errors. *Journal of Neurophysiology, 73,* 347–360.

Gozal, D., & Molfese, D. (2005). *Attention deficit hyperactivity disorder: From genes to patients.* Totowa, NJ: Humana Press.

Graf, P., & Schacter, D. L. (1985). Implicit and explicit memory for new associations in normal and amnesic patients. *Journal of Experimental Psychology: Learning, Memory, & Cognition, 11,* 501–518.

Gralinski, J. H., & Kopp, C. B. (1993). Everyday rules for behavior: Mothers' requests to young children. *Developmental Psychology, 29,* 573–584.

Grandin, T. (1992). Calming effects of deep touch pressure in patients with autistic disorder, college students and animals. *Journal of Child and Adolescent Psychopharmacology, 2,* 63–72.

Granic, I. (2000). Self-organization of parent-child relations. In M. Lewis & I. Granic (Eds.), *Emotion, development, and self-organization: Dynamic systems approaches to emotional development* (pp. 267–297). Cambridge: Cambridge University Press.

Granic, I., & Hollenstein, T. (2003). A survey of dynamic systems methods for developmental psychopathology. *Development and Psychopathology, 15*(3), 641–669.

Gray-Little, B., & Kaplan, D. (2000). Race and ethnicity in psychotherapy research. In C. R. Snyder & R. E. Ingram (Eds.), *Handbook of psychological change: Psychotherapy processes and practices for the 21st century* (pp. 591–613). New York: Wiley.

Graziano, M. S. A., Reiss, L. A. J., & Gross, C. G. (1999). A neuronal representation of the location of nearby sounds. *Nature, 397,* 428–430.

Grealy, M., Johnson, D., & Rushton, S. (1999). Improving cognitive function after

brain injury: The use of exercise and virtual reality. *Archives of Physical Medicine and Rehabilitation, 80,* 661–667.

Greenberg, M. T. (2006). Promoting resilience in children and youth: Preventive interventions and their interface with neuroscience. *Annals of the New York Academy of Sciences, 1094,* 139–150.

Greenberg, M. T., & Kusché, C. A. (1993). *Promoting social and emotional development in deaf children: The PATHS project.* Seattle: University of Washington Press.

Greenberg, M. T., & Kusché, C. A. (1998). Preventive interventions for school-age deaf children: The PATHS curriculum. *Journal of Deaf Studies and Deaf Education, 3*(1), 49–63.

Greenberg, M. T., Kusché, C. A., Cook, E. T., & Quamma, J. P. (1995). Promoting emotional competence in school-aged children: The effects of the PATHS curriculum [Special Issue: Emotions in developmental psychopathology]. *Development and Psychopathology, 7*(1), 117–136.

Greene, G. (1999). Mnemonic multiplication fact instruction for students with learning disabilities. *Learning Disabilities Research and Practice, 14*(3), 141–148.

Greene, R. L. (1989). Spacing effects in memory: Evidence for a two-process account. *Journal of Experimental Psychology: Learning, Memory, and Cognition, 15*(3), 371–377.

Greene, R. W. (2001). *The explosive child: A new approach for understanding and parenting easily frustrated, chronically inflexible children.* New York: Harper Paperback.

Greene, R. W., Ablon, J. S., & Goring, J. C. (2003). A transactional model of oppositional behavior: Underpinnings of the Collaborative Problem Solving approach. *Journal of Psychosomatic Research, 55*(1), 67–75.

Greenough, W., & Alcantara, A. (1993). The roles of experience in different developmental information stage processes. In B. de Boysson-Bardies, S. de Schonen, P. Jusczyk, P. MacNeilage, & J. Morton (Eds.), *Developmental neurocognition: Speech and face processing in the first year of life* (pp. 3–16). Dordrecht: Kluwer.

Greenspan, S. I. (1985). *First feelings: Milestones in the emotional development of your baby and child.* New York: Viking Penguin.

Greenspan, S. I. (1992). *Infancy and early childhood: The practice of clinical assessment and intervention with emotional and developmental challenges.* Madison, CT: International Universities Press.

Greenspan, S. I. (1996). Assessing the emotional and social functioning of infants and young children. In S. J. Meisels & E. Fenichel (Eds.), *New visions for the developmental assessment of infants and young children* (pp. 231–266). Washington, DC: ZERO TO THREE.

Greenspan, S. I. (1999). *Building healthy minds.* New York: Da Capo Press.

Greenspan, S. I. (2005). Social-emotional scale. *Bayley Scales of Infant and Toddler Development* (3rd ed., Bayley-III). San Antonio, TX: Harcourt Assessment.

Greenspan, S. I., DeGangi, G. A., & Wieder, S. (2001). *The functional emotional assessment scale (FEAS) for infancy and early childhood: Clinical and research applications.* Bethesda, MD: Interdisciplinary Council on Developmental and Learning Disorders.

Greenspan, S. I., & Lourie, R. S. (1981). Developmental structuralist approach to the classification of adaptive and pathologic personality organizations: Application to infancy and early childhood. *American Journal of Psychiatry, 138*, 6–14.

Greenspan, S. I., & Meisels, S. J. (with the Zero To Three Work Group on Developmental Assessment). (1996). Toward a new vision for the developmental assessment of infants and young children. In S. J. Meisels & E. Fenichel (Eds.), *New visions for the developmental assessment of infants and young children* (pp. 11–26). Washington, DC: ZERO TO THREE: National Center for Infants, Toddlers, and Families.

Greenspan, S. I., & Wieder, S. (1998). *The child with special needs: Encouraging intellectual and emotional growth.* Reading, MA: Addison-Wesley.

Gross, J. J. (1998). Antecedent- and response-focused emotion regulation: Divergent consequences for experience, expression, and physiology. *Journal of Personality and Social Psychology, 74*(1), 224–237.

Gruber, J., Johnson, S. L., Oveis, C., & Keltner, D. (2008). Risk for mania and positive emotional responding: Too much of a good thing? *Emotion, 8*(1), 23–33.

Gunnar, M. R. (2000). Early adversity and the development of stress reactivity and regulation. In C. A. Nelson (Ed.), *Minnesota Symposia on Child Psychology: Vol. 31. The effects of adversity on neurobehavioral development* (pp. 163–200). Mahwah, NJ: Erlbaum.

Gunnar, M. R., Bruce, J., & Donzella, B. (2001). Stress physiology, health and behavioral development. In A. Thornton (Ed.), *The well-being of children and families: Research and data needs* (pp. 188–212). Ann Arbor: University of Michigan Press.

Gunnar, M. R., & Fisher, P. A. and the Early Experience, Stress, and Prevention Science Network. (2006). Bringing basic research on early experience and stress neurobiology to bear on preventive interventions for neglected and maltreated children. *Development and Psychopathology, 18*, 651–677.

Gunnar, M. R., & Quevedo, K. (2007). The neurobiology of stress and development. *Annual Review of Psychology, 38*, 145–173.

Gunnar, M. R., & Quevado, K. M. (2008). Early care experiences and HPA axis regulation in children: A mechanism for later trauma vulnerability. In E. R. de Kloet, M. S. Oitzl, & E. Vermetten (Eds.), *Progress in brain research, 167* (pp. 137–149). Amsterdam: Elsevier.

Gunnar, M. R., Van Dulmen, M. H. M., & The International Adoption Project Team. (2007). Behavior problems in postinstitutionalized internationally adopted children. *Development and Psychopathology, 19*, 129–148.

Guntrip, H. (1969). *Schizoid phenomenon, object-relations, and the self.* New York: International Universities Press.

Guntrip, H. (1973). *Psychoanalytic theory, therapy, and the self.* New York: Basic Books.

Guralnick, M. J. (1996). Second-generation research in the field of early intervention. In M. M. Guralnick (Ed.), *The effectiveness of early intervention* (pp. 3–20). Baltimore: Paul H. Brookes.

Guralnick, M. J. (2000). *Interdisciplinary clinical assessment of young children with developmental disabilities.* Baltimore: Paul H. Brookes.

Hagerman, R. (1996). Biomedical advances in developmental psychology: The case of fragile X syndrome. *Developmental Psychology, 32*, 416–424.

Haith, M. M., Benson, J. B., Roberts, R. J., & Pennington, B. F. (1994). *The development of future oriented processes.* Chicago: University of Chicago Press.

Haith, M. M., Hazen, C., & Goodman, G. S. (1988). Expectation and anticipation of dynamic visual events by 3.5-month-old babies. *Child Development, 59*, 467–479.

Halfon, N., & Hochstein, M. (2002). Life course health development: An integrated framework for developing health, policy, and research. *Milbank Quarterly, 60*(3), 433–479.

Hall, G. C. N. (2001). Psychotherapy research with ethnic minorities: Empirical, ethical, and conceptual issues. *Journal of Consulting and Clinical Psychology, 69*, 502–510.

Hall, M., Vasko, R., Buysse, D., Ombao, H., Chen, Q., Cashmere, J. D., et al. (2004). Acute stress affects heart rate variability during sleep. *Psychosomatic Medicine, 66*, 56–62.

Happaney, K., Zelazo, P. D., & Stuss, D. T. (2004). Development of orbitofrontal function: Current themes and future directions. *Brain and Cognition, 55*, 1–10.

Hasher, L., & Zacks, R. T. (1979). Automatic and effortful processes in memory. *Journal of Experimental Psychology: General, 108*, 356–389.

Hasselhorn, M., Mähler, C., & Grube, D. (2005). *Theory of mind, working memory, and verbal ability in preschool children: The proposal of a relay race model of the developmental dependencies.* Mahwah, NJ: Erlbaum.

Harkness, K. L., & Tucker, D. M. (2000). Motivation of neural plasticity: Neural mechanisms in the self-organization of depression. In M. Lewis & I. Granic (Eds.), *Emotion, development, and self-organization: Dynamic systems approaches to emotional development* (pp. 186–208). New York: Cambridge University Press.

Hart, C. H., Gunnar, M. R., & Cicchetti, D. (1996). Altered neuroendocrine activity in maltreated children related to symptoms of depression. *Development and Psychopathology, 8*(1), 201–214.

Havik, O. E., & VandenBos, G. R. (1996). Limitations of manualized psychotherapy for everyday clinical practice. *Clinical Psychology: Science and Practice, 3*, 264–267.

Hawkley, L., & Cacioppo, J. T. (2004). Stress and the aging immune system. *Brain, Behavior, and Immunity, 18*(2), 114–119.

Hebb, D. (1949). *The organization of behavior.* New York: Wiley.

Heller, S. (2002). *Too loud, too bright, too fast, too tight: What to do if you are sensory defensive in an overstimulating world.* New York: HarperCollins.

Hendler, T., Rotshtein, P., Yeshurun, Y., Weizmann, T., Kahn, I., Ben-Bashat, D., et al. (2003). Sensing the invisible: Differential sensitivity of visual cortex and amygdala to traumatic context. *NeuroImage, 19*, 587–600.

Henson, M. A., Roberts, A. C., Salimi, K., Vadlamudi, S., Hamer, R. M., Gilmore, J. H., et al. (2008). Developmental regulation of the NMDA receptor subunits, NR3A and NR1, in human prefrontal cortex. *Cerebral Cortex.* Retrieved March 20, 2008, from www.cercor.oxfordjournals.org/cgi/content/abstract/bhn017

Hepper, P. G. (1997a). Fetal habituation: Another Pandora's box? *Developmental Medicine and Child Neurology, 39*, 274–278.

Hepper, P. G. (1997b). Memory in utero. *Developmental Medicine and Child Neurology, 39*, 343–346.

Hernandez-Reif, M., Diego, M., & Field, T. (2007). Preterm infants show reduced stress behaviors and activity after 5 days of massage therapy. *Infant Behavior & Development, 30*, 557–561.

Hernandez-Reif, M., Field, T., Diego, M., & Ruddock, M. (2006). Greater arousal and less attentiveness to face/voice stimuli by neonates of *depressed* mothers on the Brazelton Neonatal Behavioral Assessment Scale. *Infant Behavior and Development, 29*(4), 594–598.

Hillier, S. (2007). Intervention for children with developmental coordination disorder: A systematic review. *Internet Journal of Allied Health Sciences and Practice, 5*(3). Available at ijahsp.nova.edu/articles/vol5num3/hillier.htm

Hinkley, J. J., Patterson, J. P., & Carr, T. H. (2001). Differential effects of context- and skill-based treatment approaches: Preliminary findings. *Aphasiology, (15)*5, 463–476.

Hirshfeld-Becker, D. R., Biederman, J., Henin, A., Faraone, S. V., Dowd, S. T., De Petrillo, L. A., et al. (2006). Psychopathology in the young offspring of parents with bipolar disorder: A controlled pilot study. *Psychiatry Research, 145*, 155–167.

Hirt, E. R., Devers, E. E., & McCrea, S. M. (2008). I want to be creative: Exploring the role of hedonic contingency theory in the positive mood-cognitive flexibility link. *Journal of Personality and Social Psychology, 94*(2), 214–230.

Hobel, C. J., Arora, C. P., & Korst, L. M. (1999). Corticotrophin-releasing hormone and CRH-binding protein: Differences between patients at risk for preterm birth and hypertension. *Annals of the New York Academy of Sciences, 897*, 54–65.

Hoffman, M. L. (1978). Toward a theory of empathic arousal and development. In M. Lewis & L. A. Rosenblum (Eds.), *The development of affect* (pp. 227–256). New York: Plenum.

Holden, G. W., & West, M. J. (1989). Proximate regulation by mothers: A demonstration of how differing styles affect young children's behavior. *Child Development, 60*(1), 64–69.

Hollenstein, T. (2007). State-space grids: Analyzing dynamics across development. *International Journal of Behavioral Development, 31*(4), 384–396.

Hollenstein, T., Granic, I., Stoolmiller, M., & Snyder, J. (2004). Rigidity in parent-child interactions and the development of externalizing and internalizing behavior in early childhood. *Journal of Abnormal Child Psychology, 32*, 595–607.

Hollenstein, T., & Lewis, M. (2006). A state space analysis of emotion and flexibility in parent-child interactions. *Emotion, 6*, 656–662.

Hongcai, W. (2007). Education: A discipline or a field? *Frontiers of Education in China, 2*(1), 63–73.

Hongwanishkul, D., Happaney, K. R., Lee, W. S. C., & Zelazo, P. D. (2005). Assessment of hot and cool executive function in young children: Age-related changes and individual differences. *Developmental Neuropsychology, 28*, 617–644.

Horney, K. (1945). *Our inner conflicts.* New York: Norton.

Horney, K. (1950). *Neurosis and human growth.* New York: Norton.

House, J. S., Landis, K. R., & Umberson, D. (1988). Social relationships and health. *Science, 241,* 540–545.

Howe, M. L., Cicchetti, D., & Toth, S. L. (2006). Children's basic memory processes, stress, and maltreatment. *Development and Psychopathology, 18,* 759–769.

Howe, M. L., & Courage, M. L. (1993). On resolving the enigma of infantile amnesia. *Psychological Bulletin, 113,* 305–326.

Howe, M. L., & Courage, M. L. (1997a). The emergence and early development of autobiographical memory. *Psychological Review, 104,* 499–523.

Howe, M. L., & Courage, M. L. (1997b). Independent paths in the development of infant learning and forgetting. *Journal of Experimental Child Psychology, 67,* 131–163.

Howe, M. L., Courage, M. L., & Edison, S. C. (2003). When autobiographical memory begins. *Developmental Review, 23,* 471–494.

Howe, M. L., & Lewis, M. D. (2005). The importance of dynamic systems approaches for understanding development. *Developmental Review, 25,* 247–251.

Howe, M. L., & O'Sullivan, J. T. (1990). The development of strategic memory: Coordinating knowledge, metamemory, and resources. In D. F. Bjorklund (Ed.), *Children's strategies: Contemporary views of cognitive development* (pp. 129–155). Hillsdale, NJ: Erlbaum.

Howe, M. L., & O'Sullivan, J. T. (1997). What children's memories tell us about recalling our childhoods: A review of storage and retrieval processes in the development of long-term retention. *Developmental Review, 17*(2), 148–204.

Howe, M. L., Toth, S. L., & Cicchetti, D. (2006). Memory and developmental psychopathology. In D. Cicchetti & D. J. Cohen (Eds.), *Developmental psychopathology: Vol. 2. Developmental neuroscience* (2nd ed., pp. 629–655). Series on Personality Process. New York: Wiley.

Hulme, C., Thomson, N., Muir, C., & Lawrence, A. (1984). Speech rate and the development of short-term memory span. *Journal of Experimental Child Psychology, 38*(2), 241–253.

Hurlemann, R., Hawellek, B., Maier, W., & Dolan, R. J. (2007). Enhanced emotion-induced amnesia in borderline personality disorder. *Psychological Medicine, 37,* 971–981.

Huttenlocher, J. (1998). Language input and language growth. *Preventive Medicine, 27*(2), 195–199.

Huttenlocher, P. R. (1990). Morphometric study of human cerebral cortex development. *Neuropsychologia, 28*(6), 517–527.

Huttenlocher, P. R. (2002). *Neural plasticity: The effects of the environment on the development of the cerebral cortex.* Cambridge, MA: Harvard University Press.

Huttenlocher, P. R., & Dabholkar, A. S. (1997). Developmental anatomy of prefrontal cortex. In N. A. Krasnegor, G. R. Lyon, & P. S. Goldman-Rakic (Eds.), *Development of the prefrontal cortex* (pp. 69–83). Baltimore: Paul H. Brookes.

Interdisciplinary Council on Developmental and Learning Disorders–Diagnostic Manual for Infancy and Early Childhood (ICDL-DMIC) Work Groups. (2005).

Diagnostic manual for infancy and early childhood: Mental health, developmental, regulatory-sensory processing, language and learning disorders. Bethesda, MD: Interdisciplinary Council on Developmental and Learning Disorders.

Inman, D., Loge, K., & Leavens, J. (1997). VR education and rehabilitation. *Communications of the ACM, 40*(8), 53–58.

Ireton, H. (1992). *The Child Development Inventory.* Minneapolis, MN: Behavior Science Systems.

Isaacs, E. B., & Vargha-Khadem, F. (1989). Differential course of development of spatial and verbal memory span: A normative study. *British Journal of Developmental Psychology, 7*(4), 377–380.

Ito, T. A., & Cacioppo, J. T. (2005). Variations on a human universal: Individual differences in positivity offset and negativity bias. *Cognition and Emotion, 19,* 1–26.

Ito, T. A., Larsen, J. T., Smith, N. K., & Cacioppo, J. T. (1998). Negative information weighs more heavily on the brain: The negativity bias in evaluative categorizations. *Journal of Personality and Social Psychology, 75,* 887–900.

Ivanenko, A., McLaughlin Crabtree, V., & Tauman, R. (2003). Melatonin in children and adolescents with insomnia: A retrospective study. *Clinical Pediatrics, 42*(1), 51–58.

Iversen, S., Iversen, L., & Saper, C. B. (2000). The autonomic nervous system and the hypothalamus. In E. R. Kandel, J. H. Schwartz, & T. M. Jessell (Eds.), *Principles of neural science* (pp. 960–981). New York: McGraw-Hill.

Iversen, S., Kupfermann, I., & Kandel, E. R. (2000). Emotional states and feelings. In E. R. Kandel, J. H. Schwartz, & T. M. Jessell (Eds.), *Principles of neural science* (pp. 982–995). New York: McGraw-Hill.

Izard, C. E., Ackerman, B. P., Schoff, K. M., & Fine, S. E. (2000). Self-organization of discrete emotions, emotion patterns, and emotion-cognition relations. In M. Lewis & I. Granic (Eds.), *Emotion, development, and self-organization: Dynamic systems approaches to emotional development* (pp. 15–36). New York: Cambridge University Press.

Izard, C. E., King, K. A., Trentacosta, C. J., Morgan, J. K., Laurenceau, J-P., Krauthamer-Ewing, E. S., et al. (2008). Accelerating the development of emotion competence in Head Start children: Effects on adaptive and maladaptive behavior. *Development and Psychopathology, 20,* 369–397.

Izard, C. E., Trentacosta, C. J., King, K. A., & Mostow, A. J. (2004). An emotion-based prevention program for Head Start children. *Early Education & Development, 15*(4), 407–422.

Jacobson, L., & Pianta, R. (2007, April). *Children's executive functioning and adjustment to middle school: Do elementary classroom experiences make a difference?* Poster presented at the Society for Research in Child Development Biennial Meeting, Boston, MA.

Jaffe, A. V., & Gardner, L. (2008). *My book of feelings: How to control and react to the SIZE of your emotions.* Shawnee Mission, KS: Autism Asperger Publishing.

Jenkins, J. M., & Astington, J. W. (1996). Cognitive factors and family structure associated with theory of mind development in young children. *Developmental Psychology, 32,* 70–78.

Jernberg, A. M., & Booth, P. B. (1999). *Theraplay: Helping parents and children build better relationships through attachment-based play* (2nd ed.). San Francisco: Jossey-Bass.

Johnson, C. N., & Wellman, H. M. (1980). Children's developing understanding of mental verbs: Remember, know, and guess. *Child Development, 51,* 1095–1102.

Johnson, G. M. (2004). Constructivist remediation: Correction in context. *International Journal of Special Education, (19)*1, 72–88.

Johnson, M. H. (1995). The inhibition of automatic saccades in early infancy. *Developmental Psychobiology, 28*(5), 281–291.

Johnson, M. H. (2005). *Developmental cognitive neuroscience* (2nd ed.). Malden, MA: Blackwell.

Johnson, M. H., & Morton, J. (1991). *Biology and cognitive development: The case of face recognition.* Oxford: Blackwell.

Jolibert, B. (1993). Sigmund Freud (1856–1939). *Prospects: Quarterly Review of Comparative Education, 23*(3/4), 459–472.

Jones, E. G. (1990). The role of afferent activity in the maintenance of primate neocortical function. *Journal of Experimenal Biology, 153,* 155–176.

Juel, C. (1988). Learning to read and write: A longitudinal study of 54 children from first through fourth grades. *Journal of Educational Psychology, 80,* 437–447.

Kagan, J. (1981). *The second year: The emergence of self-awareness.* Cambridge, MA: Harvard University Press.

Kagan, J., Reznick, J. S., & Snidman, N. (1987). The physiology and psychology of behavioral inhibition in children. *Child Development, 58,* 1459–1473.

Kagan, J., Reznick, J. S., & Snidman, N. (1999). Biological basis of childhood shyness. In A. Slater & D. Muir (Eds.), *The Blackwell reader in developmental psychology* (pp. 65–78). Malden, MA: Blackwell.

Kaler, S. R., & Kopp, C. B. (1990). Compliance and comprehension in very young toddlers. *Child Development, 61,* 1997–2003.

Kaltsas, G. A., & Chrousos, G. P. (2007). The neuroendocrinology of stress. In J. T. Cacioppo, L. G. Tassinary, & G. G. Berntson (Eds.), *Handbook of psychophysiology* (2nd ed., pp. 303–318). New York: Cambridge University Press.

Kam, C., Greenberg, M. T., & Kusché, C. A. (2004). Sustained effects of the PATHS curriculum on the social and psychological adjustment of children in special education. *Journal of Emotional and Behavioral Disorders, 12,* 66–78.

Kandel, E. R. (2000). Nerve cells and behavior. In E. R. Kandel, J. H. Schwartz, & T. M. Jessell (Eds.), *Principles of neural science* (pp. 19–35). New York: McGraw-Hill.

Kandel, E. R. (2007). *In search of memory: The emergence of a new science of mind.* New York: Norton.

Kapp, B., & Cain, M. (2001). The neural basis of arousal. In N. Smelser & P. Baltes (Eds.), *The international encyclopedia of social and behavioral sciences* (pp. 1463–1466). Oxford: Elsevier Science.

Karen, R. (1994). *Unfolding the mystery of the infant-mother bond and its impact on later life: Becoming attached.* New York: Warner Books.

Kaufer, D. I. (2007). The dorsolateral and cingulate cortex. In B. L. Miller & J. L. Cummings (Eds.), *The human frontal lobes: Functions and disorders* (pp. 44–58). New York: Guilford Press.

Kaufman, J., Birmaher, B., Perel, J., Dahl, R., Moreci, P., Nelson, B., et al. (1997). The cortcotropin-releasing hormone challenge in depressed abused, depressed nonabused, and normal control children. *Biological Psychiatry, 42,* 669–679.

Kawai, N., Morokuma, S., Tomonaga, M., Horimoto, N., & Taanaka, M. (2004). Associative learning and memory in a chimpanzee fetus. *Developmental Psychobiology, 44,* 116–122.

Keating, D. P. (1999). Developmental health as the wealth of nations. In D. P. Keating & C. Hertzman (Eds.), *Developmental health and the wealth of nations: Social, biological, and educational dynamics* (pp. 337–347). New York: Guilford Press.

Keating, D. P., & Miller, F. K. (2000). Commentary. The dynamics of emotional development: Models, metaphors, and methods. In M. Lewis & I. Granic (Eds.), *Emotion, development, and self-organization: Dynamic systems approaches to emotional development* (pp. 373–392). Cambridge: Cambridge University Press.

Kelly, J. F., & Barnard, K. E. (2000). Assessment of parent-child interaction: Implications for early intervention. In J. P. Shonkoff & S. J. Meisels (Eds.), *Handbook of early childhood intervention* (pp. 258–289). New York: Cambridge University Press.

Keltner, D., & Harker, L. A. (1998). The forms and functions of the nonverbal signals of shame. In P. Gilbert & B. Andrews (Eds.), *Shame, interpersonal behavior, psychopathology, and culture* (pp. 78–98). New York: Oxford University Press.

Kemper, H. C. G. (2001). Is physical exercise good for the brain of a child? *Developmental Neurorehabilitation, 4*(3), 145–147.

Kendall, P. C., & Hedtke, K. (2006). *Cognitive-behavioral therapy for anxious children: Therapist manual* (3rd ed.). Ardmore, PA: Workbook Publishing.

Kensinger, E. A., & Corkin, S. (2004). Two routes to emotional memory: Distinct processes for valence and arousal. *Proceedings of the National Academy of Sciences, 101,* 3310–3315.

Kerns, J. G., Cohen, J. D., MacDonald, A. W. III, Cho, R. Y., Stenger, V. A., & Carter, C. S. (2004). Anterior cingulate conflict monitoring and adjustments in control. *Science, 303,* 1023–1026.

Kiecolt-Glaser, J. K., Glaser, R., Cacioppo, J. T., & Malarkey, W. B. (1998). Marital stress: Immunologic, neuroendocrine, and autonomic correlates. *Annals of the New York Academy of Sciences, 840,* 656–663.

Kilpatrick, L., & Cahill, L. (2003). Amygdala modulation of parahippocampal and frontal regions during emotionally influenced memory storage. *NeuroImage, 20,* 2091–2099.

Kirkham, Z. K., Cruess, L., & Diamond, A. (2003). Helping children apply their knowledge to their behavior on a dimension switching task. *Developmental Science, 6,* 449–476.

Kiyokawa, S., Izawa, T., & Ueda, K. (2007). Role exchange between task-doing and observing others as a means of facilitating insight problem-solving. *Japanese Journal of Educational Psychology, 55*(2), 255–265.

Klein, J. T. (2005). Interdisciplinary teamwork: The dynamics of collaboration and integration. In S. J. Derry, C. D. Schunn, & M. A. Gernsbacher (Eds.), *Interdisciplinary collaboration: An emerging cognitive science* (pp. 23–50). Hillsdale, NJ: Erlbaum.

Klein, M. (2001). *Envy and gratitude: A study of unconscious sources.* London: Routledge. (Original work published 1957)

Kleitman, N. (1963). *Sleep and wakefulness.* Chicago: University of Chicago Press.

Klingberg, T., Fernell, E., Olesen, P., Johnson, M., Gustafsson, P., Dahlström, K., et al. (2005). Computerized training of working memory in children with ADHD—a randomized, controlled trial. *Journal of the American Academy of Child and Adolescent Psychiatry, 44,* 177–186.

Kloo, D., & Perner, J. (2003). Training transfer between card sorting and false belief understanding: Helping children apply conflicting descriptions. *Child Development, 74,* 1823–1839.

Kochanska, G., Murray, K. T., & Harlan, E. T. (2000). Effortful control in early childhood: Continuity and change, antecedents, and implications for social development. *Developmental Psychology, 36*(2), 220–232.

Koenig, K. P. (2007, February). *Personal perspectives of sensory integration and praxis issues in individuals with autism.* Paper presented at the R2K: Research 2007 Conference in Long Beach, CA.

Koivisto, M., & Revonsuo, A. (2007). How meaning shapes seeing. *Psychological Science, 18*(10), 845–849.

Koizumi, K., & Kollai, M. (1992). Multiple modes of operation of cardiac autonomic control: development of the ideas from Cannon and Brooks to the present. *Journal of the Autonomic Nervous System, 41,* 19–30.

Kopp, C. B. (1982). The antecedents of self-regulation: A developmental perspective. *Developmental Psychology, 18,* 199–214.

Korkman, M., Kirk, U., & Kemp, S. (2007). *NEPSY-II.* San Antonio, TX: Harcourt Assessment.

Kort, B., Reilly, R., & Picard, R. W. (2001). *An affective model of interplay between emotions and learning: Reengineering educational pedagogy—Building a learning companion.* Paper presented at the International Conference on Advanced Learning Technologies, University of Madison, Wisconsin. Retrieved September 10, 2007, from affect.media.mit.edu/projectpages/lc/icalt.pdf

Kranowitz, C. S. (1998). *The out-of-sync child: Recognizing and coping with sensory integration dysfunction.* New York: Berkley Publishing.

Kray, J., Eber, J., & Karbach, J. (2008). Verbal self-instructions in task switching: A compensatory tool for action-control deficits in childhood and old age? *Developmental Science, 11*(2), 223–236.

Kuhl, P. K., Williams, K. A., Lacerda, F., & Stevens, K. N. (1992). Linguistic experience alters phonetic perception in infants by 6 months of age. *Science, 255*(5044), 606–608.

Kusché, C. A., & Greenberg, M. T. (1995). *The PATHS (promoting alternative thinking strategies) curriculum.* South Deerfield, MA: Channing-Bete.

LaBar, K. S., & Cabeza, R. (2006). Cognitive neuroscience of emotional memory. *Nature Reviews Neuroscience, 7,* 54–62.

Lagattuta, K. H. (2007). Thinking about the future because of the past: Young children's knowledge about the causes of worry and preventative decisions. *Child Development, 78*(5), 1492–1509.

Lalonde, C. E., & Chandler, M. J. (2002). Children's understanding of interpretation [Special Issue: Folk Epistemology]. *New Ideas in Psychology, 20*(2–3), 163–198.

Larsen, J. T., Hemenover, S. H., Norris, C. J., & Cacioppo, J. T. (2003). Turning adversity to advantage: On the virtues of the coactivation of positive and negative emotions. In L. G. Aspinwall & U. M. Staudinger (Eds.), *A psychology of human strengths: Perspectives on an emerging field* (pp. 211–226). Washington, DC: American Psychological Association.

Larsen, J. T., McGraw, P., & Cacioppo, J. T. (2001). Can people feel happy and sad at the same time? *Journal of Personality and Social Psychology, 81,* 684–696.

Larsen, J. T., McGraw, A. P., Mellers, B. A., & Cacioppo, J. T. (2004). The agony of victory and the thrill of defeat: Mixed emotional reactions to disappointing wins and relieving losses. *Psychological Science, 15,* 325–330.

Lederman, C. S., & Osofsky, J. D. (2004). Infant mental health interventions in juvenile court. *Psychology, Public Policy, and Law, 10*(1), 162–177.

LeDoux, J. E. (1996). *The emotional brain: The mysterious underpinnings of emotional life.* New York: Touchstone.

LeDoux, J. E. (2000). Emotion circuits in the brain. *Annual Review of Neuroscience, 23,* 155–184.

LeDoux, J. E. (2002). Emotion: Clues from the brain. In J. T. Cacioppo, G. G. Berntson, R. Alophs, C. S. Carter, R. J. Davidson, M. K. McClintock, et al. (Eds.), *Foundations in social neuroscience* (pp. 389–410). Cambridge, MA: MIT Press.

Leftwich, M., & Collins, F. (1994). Parental smoking, depression and child-development. *Journal of Pediatric Psychology, 19,* 557–569.

Léger, D., Annesi-Maesano, I., Carat, F., Rugina, M., Chanal, I., Pribil, C., et al. (2006). Allergic rhinitis and its consequences on quality of sleep. *Archives of Internal Medicine, 166,* 1744–1748.

Leonard, C. M. (2003). Neural substrate of speech and language development. In M. H. Johnson & M. de Haan (Eds.), *The cognitive neuroscience of development* (pp. 127–156). Milton Park, UK: Routledge.

Lester, B. M., Zachariah Boukydis, C. F., Garcia-Coll, C. T., Peucker, M., McGrath, M. M., Vohr, B. R., et al. (1995). Developmental outcome as a function of the goodness of fit between the infant's cry characteristics and the mother's perception of her infant's cry. *Pediatrics, 95,* 516–521.

Levanen, S., & Hamdorf, D. (2001). Feeling vibrations: Enhanced tactile sensitivity incongenitally deaf humans. *Neuroscience Letters, 301,* 75–77.

Levine, L. J., & Pizarro, D. A. (2004). Emotion and memory research: A grumpy overview. *Social Cognition, 22,* 530–554.

Levine, P. A. (1997). *Waking the tiger: Healing trauma.* Berkeley, CA: North Atlantic Books.

Levine, P. A., & Kline, M. (2008). *Trauma-proofing your kids: A parent's guide for instilling confidence, joy, and resilience.* Berkeley, CA: North Atlantic Books.

Levitsky, D., & Strupp, B. (1995). Malnutrition and the brain. *Journal of Nutrition, 125*(Suppl. 85), 2212S–2220S.

Lewis, M. (2000). Emotional self-organization at three time scales. In M. Lewis & I. Granic (Eds.), *Emotion, development, and self-organization: Dynamic systems approaches to emotional development* (pp. 37–69). New York: Cambridge University Press.

Lewis, M. (2005). Bridging emotion theory and neurobiology through dynamic systems modeling. *Behavioral and Brain Science, 28,* 169–245.

Lewis, M., & Granic, I. (2000). Introduction: A new approach to the study of emotional development. In M. Lewis & I. Granic (Eds.), *Emotion, development, and self-organization: Dynamic systems approaches to emotional development* (pp. 1–12). New York: Cambridge University Press.

Lezak, M. (1995). *Neuropsychological assessment* (3rd ed.). New York: Oxford University Press.

Liberman, I. Y., Shankweiler, D., & Liberman, A. M. (1989). The alphabetic principle and learning to read. In D. Shankweiler & I. Y. Liberman (Eds.), *Phonology and reading disability: Solving the reading puzzle* (pp. 1–33). Ann Arbor: University of Michigan Press.

Lieberman, A. F. (1991). Attachment theory and infant-parent psychotherapy: Some conceptual, clinical and research considerations. In D. Cicchetti (Ed.), *Rochester symposium on developmental psychopathology* (Vol. 3, pp. 261–287). Rochester, NY: University of Rochester Press.

Lieberman, A. F., Silverman, R., & Pawl, J. H. (2000). Infant-parent psychotherapy: Core concepts and current approaches. In C. H. Zeanah, (Ed.), *Handbook of infant mental health* (2nd ed., pp. 472–484). New York: Guilford Press.

Lieberman, A. F., Weston, D., & Pawl, J. H. (1991). Preventive intervention and outcome with anxiously attached dyads. *Child Development, 62,* 199–209.

Lieberman, M. D., & Eisenberg, N. (2005). A pain by any other name (rejection, exclusion, ostracism) still hurts the same: The role of dorsal anterior cingulate cortex in social and physical pain. In J. T. Cacioppo, P. S. Visser, & C. L. Pickett (Eds.), *Social neuroscience: People thinking about people* (pp. 167–188). Cambridge, MA: MIT Press.

Lindamood, C. H., & Lindamood, P. C. (1984). *Auditory discrimination in depth.* Austin, TX: PRO-ED.

Lindhiem, O., & Dozier, M. (2007). Caregiver commitment to foster children: The role of child behavior. *Child Abuse and Neglect, 31*(4), 361–374.

Linehan, M. (1993). *Cognitive-behavioral treatment of borderline personality disorder.* New York: Guilford Press.

Loftus, E. F. (1994). The repressed memory controversy. *American Psychologist, 49,* 443–445.

Loftus, E. F. (1997). Creating false memories. *Scientific American, 277*(3), 70–75.

Loftus, E. F., Loftus, G. R., & Messo, J. (1987). Some facts about weapon focus. *Law and Human Behavior, 11,* 55–62.

Lozoff, B., Jimenez, E., Hagen, J., Mollen, E., & Wolf, A. W. (2000). Poorer behavioral and developmental outcome more than 10 years after treatment for iron deficiency in infancy. *Pediatrics, 105*(4), e51. Available at www.pediatrics .org/egi/content/full/105/4/e51

Lozoff, B., Klein, N. K., Nelson, E. C., McClish, D. K., Manuel, M., & Chacon, M. E. (1998). Behavior in infants with iron-deficient anemia. *Child Development, 69,* 24–36.

Ludington-Hoe, S. M., & Swinth, J. Y. (1996). Developmental aspects of kangaroo care. *Journal of Obstetric, Gynecologic, and Neonatal Nursing, 25,* 691–703.

MacArthur, J. (1998). *Successful Christian parenting.* Nashville, TN: Thomas Nelson.

Maccoby, E. E., & Martin, J. A. (1983). Socialization in the context of the family: Parent-child interaction. In P. H. Mussen (Series Ed.) & E. M. Hetherington (Vol. Ed.), *Handbook of child psychology: Vol. 4. Socialization, personality, and social development* (4th ed., pp. 1–101). New York: Wiley.

MacLean, P. D. (1955). The limbic system ("visceral brain") in relation to central gray and reticulum of the brain stem: Evidence of interdependence in emotional processes. *Psychosomatic Medicine, 27*(5), 355–366.

Mahler, M., Pine, F., & Bergman, A. (1975). *The psychological birth of the human infant.* New York: Basic Books.

Mahler, M. S. (1967). On human symbiosis and the vicissitudes of individuation. *Journal of the American Psychoanalytic Association, 15,* 740–763.

Mahoney, M. J. (1991). *Human change processes: The scientific foundations of psychotherapy.* New York: Basic Books.

Majnemer, A. (1998). Benefits of early intervention for children with developmental disabilities. *Seminars in Pediatric Neurology, 5,* 62–69.

Maltese, J. (2005). Dyadic therapy with very young children and their primary caregivers. In K. M. Finello (Ed.), *The handbook of training and practice in infant and preschool mental health* (pp. 93–113). San Francisco: Jossey-Bass.

Mancuso, R. A., Schetter, C. D., Rini, C. M., Roesch, S. C., & Hobel, C. J. (2004). Maternal prenatal anxiety and corticotrophin-releasing hormone associated with timing of delivery. *Psychosomatic Medicine, 66,* 762–769.

Mangeot, S. D., Miller, L. J., McIntosh, D. N., McGrath-Clarke, J., Simon, J., Hagerman, R., et al. (2001). Sensory modulation dysfunction in children with attention-deficit-hyperactivity disorder. *Developmental Medicine & Child Neurology, 43,* 399–406.

Manian, N., Strauman, T. J., & Denney, N. (1998). Temperament, recalled parenting style, and self-regulation: Testing the developmental postulates of self-discrepancy theory. *Journal of Personality and Social Psychology, 75,* 1321–1332.

Mant, C. M., & Perner, J. (1988). The child's understanding of commitment. *Developmental Psychology, 24,* 343–351.

Markowitsch, H. J. (2000). Memory and amnesia. In M. M. Mesulam (Ed.), *Principles of behavioral and cognitive neurology* (pp. 257–293). New York: Oxford University Press.

Martel, M., Nikolas, M., & Nigg, J. T. (2007). Executive function in adolescents with ADHD. *Journal of the American Academy of Child & Adolescent Psychiatry, 46*(11), 1437–1444.

Martel, M. M., Nigg, J. T., Wong, M. M., Fitzgerald, H. E., Jester, J. M., Puttler, L. I., et al. (2007). Childhood and adolescent resiliency, regulation, and executive functioning in relation to adolescent problems and competence in a high-risk sample. *Development and Psychopathology, 19*(2), 541–563.

Mauss, I. B., Levenson, R. W., McCarter, L., Wilhelm, F. H., & Gross, J. J. (2005). The tie that binds? Coherence among emotion experience, behavior, and autonomic physiology. *Emotion, 5*(2), 175–190.

McClure, E. B., Brennan, P., Hammen, C., & LeBrocque, R. (2001). Perceived parenting behavior as a mediator of the relationship between parent and child anxiety disorders in a high-risk sample. *Journal of Abnormal Child Psychology, 29*, 1–10.

McCormick, D. A., & Thompson, R. F. (1984) Cerebellum: Essential involvement in the classically conditioned eyelid response. *Science, 223*, 296–299.

McDonough, S. C. (1995). Promoting positive early parent-infant relationships through interaction guidance. *Child and Adolescent Psychiatric Clinics of North America, 4*, 661–672.

McDonough, S. C. (2000). Interaction guidance: An approach for difficult to engage families. In C. H. Zeanah (Ed.), *Handbook of infant mental health* (2nd ed., pp. 185–493). New York: Guilford Press.

McDonough, S. C. (2004). Interaction guidance: Promoting and nurturing the caregiving relationship. In A. J. Sameroff, S. C. McDonough, & K. L. Rosenblum (Eds.), *Treating parent-infant relationship problems: Strategies for intervention* (pp. 79–96). New York: Guilford Press.

McEwen, B. (2002). *The end of stress as we know it.* Washington, DC: Joseph Henry Press.

McIntosh, D. N., Miller, L. J., Shyu, V., & Hagerman, R. J. (1999). Sensory-modulation disruption, electrodermal responses, and functional behaviors. *Developmental Medicine & Child Neurology, 41*, 608–615.

McKenna, J. J. (1986). An anthropological perspective on the sudden infant death syndrome (SIDS). The role of parental breathing cues and speech breathing adaptations. *Medical Anthropology, 10*, 9–53.

McKenna, J. J. (1993). Infant-parent co-sleeping in an evolutionary perspective: Implications for understanding infant sleep development and the sudden infant death syndrome. *Sleep 16*(3), 263–282.

McKenna, J. J., & McDade, T. (2005). Why babies should never sleep alone: A review of the co-sleeping controversy in relation to SIDS, bedsharing and breast feeding. *Paediatric Respiratory Review, 6*, 134–152.

McNamara, F., Lijowska, A. S., & Thach, B. T. (2002). Spontaneous arousal activity in infants during NREM and REM sleep. *Journal of Physiology, 538*, 263–269.

Meisels, S. J., & Shonkoff, J. P. (2000). Early childhood intervention: A continuing evolution. In J. P. Shonkoff & S. J. Meisels (Eds.), *Handbook of early childhood intervention* (pp. 3–34). Cambridge: Cambridge University Press.

Mellin, L. (2004). *The pathway.* New York: Regan Books.

Mellin, L. (2009). *Wired for joy: How to be happy regardless of circumstances.* Carlsbad, CA: Hay House.

Meltzoff, A. N. (1988a). Imitation of televised models by infants. *Child Development, 59,* 1221–1229.

Meltzoff, A. N. (1988b). Infant imitation after a 1-week delay: Long-term memory for novel acts and multiple stimuli. *Developmental Psychology, 24,* 470–476.

Meltzoff, A. N. (1988c). Infant imitation and memory: Nine-month-olds in immediate and deferred tests. *Child Development, 59,* 217–225.

Meltzoff, A. N. (1995). What infant memory tells us about infantile amnesia: Long-term recall and deferred imitation. *Journal of Experimental Child Psychology, 59,* 497–515.

Meltzoff, A. N. (2002). Elements of a developmental theory of imitation. In A. N. Meltzoff & W. Prinz (Eds.), *The imitative mind: Development, evolution, and brain bases* (pp. 19–41). Cambridge: Cambridge University Press.

Meltzoff, A. N. (2007). "Like me": A foundation for social cognition. *Developmental Science, 10,* 126–134.

Meltzoff, A. N., & Brooks, R. (2007). Eyes wide shut: The importance of eyes in infant gaze following and understanding others minds. In R. Flom, K. Lee, & D. Muir (Eds.), *Gaze following: Its development and significance* (pp. 217–241). Mahwah, NJ: Erlbaum.

Mercer, J. (2001). Attachment therapy using deliberate restraint: An object lesson on the identification of unvalidated treatments. *Journal of Child and Adolescent Psychiatric Nursing, 14*(3), 105–114.

Mercer, J. (2002). Child psychotherapy involving physical restraint: Techniques used in four approaches. *Child and Adolescent Social Work Journal, 19*(4), 303–314.

Mercer, J., Sarner, L., & Rosa, L. (2003). *Attachment therapy on trial: The torture and death of Candace Newmaker.* Westport, CT: Greenwood.

Mesibov, G. B. (1984). Social skills training with verbal autistic adolescents and adults: A program model. *Journal of Autism and Developmental Disorders, 14*(4), 395–404.

Mesulam, M. M. (1998). From sensation to cognition. *Brain, 121,* 1013–1052.

Mesulam, M. M. (2000a). Aging, Alzheimer's disease, and dementia: Clinical and neurobiological perspectives. In M. M. Mesulam (Ed.), *Principles of behavioral and cognitive neurology* (pp. 439–522). New York: Oxford University Press.

Mesulam, M. M. (2000b). Behavioral neuroanatomy: Large-scale networks, association cortex, frontal syndromes, the limbic system, and hemispheric specializations. In M. M. Mesulam (Ed.), *Principles of behavioral and cognitive neurology* (pp. 1–120). New York: Oxford University Press.

Mesulam, M. M. (2002). The human frontal lobes: Transcending the default mode through contingent encoding. In D. T. Stuss & R. T. Knight (Eds.) *Principles of frontal lobe function* (pp. 8–30). New York: Oxford University Press.

Miller, B. L., & Cummings, J. L. (2007). Conceptual and clinical aspects of the frontal lobes. In B. L. Miller & J. L. Cummings (Eds.), *The human frontal lobes: Functions and disorders* (pp. 12–24). New York: Guilford Press.

Miller, L. J. (2007). *Sensational kids: Hope and help for children with sensory processing disorder.* New York: Penguin Books.

Miller, L. J., & Lane, S. J. (2000). Toward a consensus in terminology in sensory integration theory and practice: Part 1. Taxonomy of neurophysiological processes. *Sensory Integration Special Interest Section Quarterly, 23*(1), 1–4.

Miller, L. J., McIntosh, D. N., McGrath, J., Shyu, V., Lampe, M., Taylor, A. K., et al. (1999). Electrodermal responses to sensory stimuli in individuals with fragile X syndrome: A preliminary report. *American Journal of Medical Genetics, 83*(4), 268–279.

Miller, L. J., Reisman, J. E., McIntosh, D. N., & Simon, J. (2001). An ecological model of sensory modulation: Performance of children with fragile X syndrome, autistic disorder, attention-deficit/hyperactivity disorder, and sensory modulation dysfunction. In S. S. Roley, E. I. Blanche, & R. C. Schaaf (Eds.), *Understanding the nature of sensory integration with diverse populations* (pp. 57–88). Austin, TX: PRO-ED.

Miller, L. J., Robinson, J., & Moulton, D. (2004). Sensory modulation dysfunction: Identification in early childhood. In R. DelCarmen-Wiggins & A. Carter (Eds.), *Handbook of infant, toddler, and preschool mental health assessment* (pp. 247–270). New York: Oxford University Press.

Miller, L. J., Schoen, S. A., James, K., & Schaaf, R. C. (2007). Lessons learned. A pilot study of occupational therapy effectiveness for children with sensory modulation disorder. *American Journal of Occupational Therapy, 61,* 161–169.

Miller, L. J., & Summers, C. (2001). Clinical applications in sensory modulation dysfunction. In S. S. Roley, E. I. Blanche, & R. C. Schaaf (Eds.), *Understanding the nature of sensory integration with diverse populations* (pp. 247–274). Austin, TX: PRO-ED.

Mills, R. S. L. (2005). Taking stock of the developmental literature on shame. *Developmental Review, 25*(1), 26–63.

Mischel, W., Shoda, Y., & Peake, P. K. (1988). The nature of adolescent competencies predicted by preschool delay of gratification. *Journal of Personality and Social Psychology, 54*(4), 687–696.

Mishkin, M., Ungerleider, L. G., & Macko, K. A. (1983). Object vision and spatial vision: Two cortical pathways. *Trends in Neurosciences, 6*(10), 414–417.

Modell, A. (1993). *The private self.* Cambridge, MA: Harvard University Press.

Molfese, D. (2000). Predicting dyslexia at 8 years of age using neonatal brain responses. *Brain and Language, 72,* 238–245.

Molfese, D. L., & Molfese, V. J. (1985). Electrophysiological indices of auditory discrimination in newborn infants: The bases for predicting later language development? *Infant Behavior & Development, 8*(2), 197–211.

Mollett, G. A., & Harrison, D. W. (2007). Affective verbal learning in hostility: An increased primacy effect and bias for negative emotional material. *Archives of Clinical Neuropsychology, 22,* 53–61.

Mollo, K., Schaaf, R. C., & Benevides, T. (2007, April). *The use of Kripalu yoga to decrease sensory reactivity and increase participation in individuals with sensory defensiveness.* Poster presented at American Occupational Therapy Annual Conference, Thomas Jefferson University, Charlotte, NC.

Monastra, V. J. (2005). Electroencephalographic biofeedback (neuropathy) as a treatment for attention deficit hyperactivity disorder: Rationale and empirical foundation. *Child and Adolescent Psychiatric Clinics of North America, 14,* 55–82.

Montague, D. P. F., & Walker-Andrews, A. S. (2001). Peekaboo: A new look on infants' perception of emotion expressions. *Developmental Psychology, 37,* 826–838.

Montague, D. P. F., & Walker-Andrews, A. S. (2002). Biobehavioral development, perception, and action. Mothers, fathers, and infants: The role of person familiarity and parental involvement in infants' perception of emotion expressions. *Child Development, 73,* 1339–1352.

Montague, P. R., & Quartz, S. R. (1999). Computational approaches to neural reward and development. *Mental Retardation & Developmental Disabilities Research Reviews, 5,* 86–99.

Moore, C. (1996). Theories of mind in infancy. *British Journal of Developmental Psychology, 14,* 19–40.

Moore, P. J., Adler, N. E., Williams, D. R., & Jackson, J. S. (2002). Socioeconomic status and health: The role of sleep. *Psychosomatic Medicine, 64,* 337–344.

Moore, R. Y., & Eichler, V. B. (1972). Loss of circadian adrenal corticosterone rhythm following suprachiasmatic lesions in the rat. *Brain Research, 42,* 201–206.

Morgan, G. A., Harmon, R. J., & Maslin-Cole, P. M. (1990). Mastery motivation: Its definition and measurement. *Early Education and Development, 1,* 318–339.

Morgan, M. A., & Pfaff, D. W. (2001). Effects of estrogen on activity and fear-related behaviors in mice. *Hormones and Behavior 40,* 472–482.

Moriguchi, Y., Decety, J., Ohnishi, T., Maeda, M., Mori, T., Nemoto, K., et al. (2007). Empathy and judging other's pain: An fMRI study of alexithymia. *Cerebral Cortex, 17,* 2223–2234.

Moscolo, M. F., Harkins, D., & Harakal, T. (2000). The dynamic construction of emotion: Varieties in anger. In M. Lewis & I. Granic (Eds.), *Emotion, development, and self-organization: Dynamic systems approaches to emotional development* (pp. 125–154). New York: Cambridge University Press.

Mukamel, R., Ekstrom, A. D., Kaplan, J. T., Iacoboni, M., & Fried, I. (2007). *Mirror properties of single cells in human medial frontal cortex.* Paper presented at the Society for Neuroscience, San Diego, CA.

Multimodal Treatment Study of Children with ADHD Cooperative Group, US. (1999a). A 14-month randomized clinical trial of treatment strategies for attention-deficit/hyperactivity disorder. *Archives of General Psychiatry, 56*(12), 1073–1086.

Multimodal Treatment Study of Children with ADHD Cooperative Group, US. (1999b). Moderators and mediators of treatment response for children with attention-deficit/hyperactivity disorder: The multimodal treatment study of

children with attention-deficit/hyperactivity disorder. *Archives of General Psychiatry, 56*(12), 1088–1096.

Muraven, M., & Baumeister, R. F. (2000). Self-regulation and depletion of limited resources: Does self-control resemble a muscle? *Psychological Bulletin, 126,* 247–259.

Nahum, J. P. (2000). An overview of Louis Sander's contribution to the field of mental health. *Infant Mental Health Journal, 21,* 29–41.

National Institutes of Health, Office of Portfolio Analysis and Strategic Initiative. (2008). *Overview of the NIH roadmap.* Retrieved January 30, 2008, from nihroadmap.nih.gov/overview.asp

National Research Council & Institute of Medicine. (2000). *From neurons to neighborhoods: The science of early childhood development* (J. P. Shonkoff & D. A. Phillips, Eds.). Committee on Integrating the Science of Early Childhood Development; Board on Children, Youth, and Families; Commission on Behavioral and Social Sciences and Education. Washington, DC: National Academies Press.

NCAST-AVENUW. (2003). *BabyCues: A child's first language.* Seattle: University of Washington Press.

Nelson, C. A. (1995). The ontogeny of human memory: A cognitive neuroscience perspective. *Developmental Psychology, 31,* 723–735.

Nelson, C. A. (1997). The neurobiological basis of early memory development. In N. Cowan (Ed.), *The development of memory in childhood* (pp. 41–82). Hove, UK: Psychology Press.

Nelson, C. A., & Collins, P. F. (1992). Neural and behavioral correlates of visual recognition memory in 4-and 8-month-old infants. *Brain and Cognition, 19,* 105–121.

Neylan, T. C., Lenoci, M., Maglione, M. L., Rosenlicht, N. Z., Metzler, T. J., Otte, C., et al. (2003). Delta sleep response to metyrapone in post-traumatic stress disorder. *Neuropsychopharmacology, 28,* 1666–1676.

Nolan, M. A., Redoblado, M. A., Lah, S., Sabaz, M., Lawson, J. A., Cunningham, A. M., et al. (2004). Memory function in childhood epilepsy syndromes. *Journal of Paediatrics and Child Health, 40,* 20–27.

Ochs, M., & Frasson, C. (2004). Optimal emotional conditions for learning with an intelligent tutoring system. In SpringerLink (Ed.), *Intelligent tutoring systems* (pp. 845–847). Berlin: Springer.

Ogden, P., Minton, K., & Pain, C. (2006). *Trauma and the body: A sensorimotor approach to psychotherapy.* New York: Norton.

Olds, J., & Milner, P. (1954). Positive reinforcement produced by electrical stimulation of septal area and other regions of rat brain. *Journal of Comparative and Physiological Psychology, 47,* 419–427.

O'Leary, D. D. M. (1989). Do cortical areas emerge from a protocortex? *Trends in Neuroscience, 12,* 400–406.

Olesen, P. J., Westerberg, H., & Klingberg, T. (2004). Increased prefrontal and parietal activity after training of working memory. *Nature Neuroscience, 7,* 75–79.

Olson, H., Streissguth, A., Bookstein, F., Barr, H., & Sampson, P. (1994). Developmental research in behavioral teratology. In S. Friedman & H. C. Haywood

(Eds.), *Developmental follow-up* (pp. 67–112). San Diego, CA: Academic Press.

Olson, J. M., & Janes, L. M. (2002). Asymmetrical impact: Vigilance for differences and self-relevant stimuli. *European Journal of Social Psychology, 32,* 383–393.

Olson, S. L., & Hoza, B. (1993). Preschool developmental antecedents of conduct problems in children beginning school. *Journal of Clinical Child Psychology, 22*(1), 60–67.

O'Neill, D. K., Astington, J. W., & Flavell, J. H. (1992). Young children's understanding of the role that sensory experiences play in knowledge acquisition. *Child Development, 63*(2), 474–490.

Ornstein, P. A., & Hayden, C. A. (2001). Memory development or the development of memory? *Current Directions in Psychological Science, 10*(6), 202–205.

Oser, C., & Cohen, J. (2003). *America's babies: The ZERO TO THREE policy center data book.* Washington, DC: ZERO TO THREE.

Osofsky, J. D. (2003). Prevalence of children's exposure to domestic violence and child maltreatment: Implications for prevention and intervention. *Clinical Child and Family Psychology Review, 6*(3), 161–170.

Osofsky, J. D., & Lederman, C. (2004). Healing the child in juvenile court. In J. D. Osofsky (Ed.), *Young children and trauma: Intervention and treatment* (pp. 221–241). New York: Guilford Press.

Ostfeld, B. M., Perl, H., Esposito, L., Hempstead, K., Hinnen, R., Sandler, A., et al. (2006). Sleep environment, positional lifestyle, and demographic characteristics associated with bed sharing in sudden infant death syndrome cases: A population-based study. *Pediatrics, 118,* 2051–2059.

Overton, W. F., & Horowitz, H. A. (1991). Developmental psychopathology: Integrations and differentiations. In D. Cicchetti & S. L. Toth (Eds.), *Rochester symposium on developmental psychopathology. Vol. 3: Models and integrations* (pp. 1–42). Rochester, NY: University of Rochester Press.

Panksepp, J. (2000). The neurodynamics of emotions: An evolutionary-neurodevelopmental view. In M. Lewis & I. Granic (Eds.), *Emotion, development, and self-organization: Dynamic systems approaches to emotional development* (pp. 236–266). New York: Cambridge University Press.

Papoušek, M. (2008). Disorders of behavioral and emotional regulation: Clinical evidence for a new diagnostic concept. In M. Papoušek, M. Schieche, & H. Wurmser, (Eds.), *Disorders of behavioral and emotional regulation in the first years of life: Early risks and intervention in the developing parent-infant relationship* (pp, 53–84). Washington, DC: ZERO TO THREE.

Papoušek, M., & Hofacker, N. von. (2008). Clinging, romping, throwing tantrums: Disorders of behavioral and emotional regulation in older infants and toddlers. In M. Papoušek, M. Schieche, & H. Wurmser, (Eds.), *Disorders of behavioral and emotional regulation in the first years of life: Early risks and intervention in the developing parent-infant relationship* (pp, 169–200). Washington, DC: ZERO TO THREE.

Parents' Place. (n.d.). *Newsletter 3.* Retrieved April 30, 2008, from www.thetherapyplace.net/newsletter/newsletter3.pdf

Parker, A., Gellatly, A., & Waterman, M. (1999). The effect of environmental context manipulation on memory: Dissociation between perceptual and conceptual implicit tests. *European Journal of Cognitive Psychology 11*, 555–570.

Parker, S. W., & Nelson, C. A. and The Bucharest Early Intervention Project Core Group. (2005). The impact of early institutional rearing on the ability to discriminate facial expressions of emotion: An event-related potential study. *Child Development, 76*(1), 54–72.

Parsons, S., Beardon, L., Neale, H. R., Reynard, G., Eastgate, R., Wilson, J. R., et al. (2000) Development of social skills amongst adults with Asperger's Syndrome using virtual environments: The "AS Interactive" project. In P. Sharkey, A. Cesarani, L. Pugnetti, & A. Rizzo (Eds.), *Proceedings of the 3rd International Conference on Disability, Virtual Reality, and Associated Technology.* Alghero, Sardinia, Italy, September, 23–25.

Parsons, T., Bowerly, T., Buckwalter, J. G., & Rizzo, A. A. (2007). A controlled clinical comparison of attention performance in children with ADHD in a virtual reality classroom compared to standard neuropsychological methods. *Child Neuropsychology. 13*, 363–381.

Pascual-Leone, A., Grafman, J., & Hallet, M. (1995). Procedural learning and the prefrontal cortex. *Annals of the New York Academy of Sciences, 769*, 61–70.

Pathways. (2008). *Newborn individualized developmental care and assessment program.* Retrieved January 25, 2008, from www.pathwaystooutcomes.org/index .cfm?fuseaction=Page.viewPage&pageId=529

Pearson, D., & Dietrich, K. (1985). The behavioral toxicology and teratology of childhood. *Neurotoxicology, 6*, 165–182.

Pelphrey, K., & Reznick, J. (2002). Working memory in infancy. *Advances in Child Development and Behavior, 31*, 173–227.

Perry, B. D. (1998, September). *Physiological measurements in the assessment of maltreated children: The physical impact on the developing brain.* Keynote presentation at the 12th International ISPCAN Congress on Child Abuse and Neglect, Protecting children: Innovation and Inspiration, Auckland, New Zealand.

Perry, B. D. (2006). Applying principles of neurodevelopment to clinical work with maltreated and traumatized children: The neurosequential model of therapeutics. In N. Boyd Webb (Ed.), *Working with traumatized youth in child welfare* (pp. 27–52). New York: Guilford Press.

Perry, B. D., Pollard, R., Blakely, T., Baker, W., & Vigilante, D. (1995). Childhood trauma, the neurobiology of adaptation and "use-dependent" development of the brain: How "states" become "traits." *Infant Mental Health Journal, 16*(4), 271–291.

Perry, B., & Szalavitz, M. (2006). *The boy who was raised as a dog and other stories from a child psychiatrist's notebook: What traumatized children can teach us about loss, love, and healing.* New York: Basic Books.

Peskin, J. (1992). Ruse and representations: On children's ability to conceal information. *Developmental Psychology, 28*(1), 84–89.

Petri, H. L., & Mishkin, M. (1994). Behaviorism, cognitivism and the neuropsychology of memory. *American Scientist, 82*, 30–37.

Pfaff, D. (2006). *Brain arousal and information theory: Neural and genetic mechanisms.* Cambridge, MA: Harvard University Press.

Piaget, J. (1960). *The psychology of intelligence.* New York: Littlefield Adams. (Original work published in 1947 in French)

Picton, T. W., Alain, C., & McIntosh, A. R. (2002). The theatre of the mind: Physiological studies of the human frontal lobes. In D. T. Stuss & R. T. Knight (Eds.), *Principles of frontal lobe function* (pp. 109–126). New York: Oxford University Press.

Pigliucci, M. (2001). *Phenotypic plasticity: Beyond nature and nurture.* Baltimore: Johns Hopkins University Press.

Pivik, R. T. (2007). Sleep and dreaming. In J. T. Cacioppo, L. G. Tassinary, & G. G. Berntson (Eds.), *Handbook of psychophysiology* (2nd ed., pp. 633–662). New York: Cambridge University Press.

Polak-Toste, C. P., & Gunnar, M. R. (2006). Temperamental exuberance: Correlates and consequences. In P. J. Marshall & N. A. Fox. (Eds.), *The development of social engagement: Neurobiological perspectives* (pp. 19–41). New York: Oxford University Press.

Polikarov, A. (1995). Concerning the integration of science: Kinds and stages. *Journal for General Philosophy of Science, 26*(2), 297–312.

Poppenk, J., Walia, G., Joanisse, M., Danckert, S., & Köhler, S. (2006, April). *Why is form information poorly remembered? An fMRI study on the role of novelty-encoding processes.* Paper presented at the annual meeting of the Cognitive Neuroscience Society, San Francisco, CA.

Porges, S. W. (1995): Orienting in a defensive world: Mammalian modifications of our evolutionary heritage. A polyvagal theory. *Psychophysiology, 32,* 301–318.

Porges, S. W. (2001). The polyvagal theory: Phylogenetic substrates of a social nervous system. *International Journal of Psychophysiology, 42,* 123–146.

Porges, S. W. (2003). Social engagement and attachment: A phylogenetic perspective. Roots of mental illness in children. *Annals of the New York Academy of Sciences, 1008,* 31–47.

Porges, S. W. (2004). Neuroception: A subconscious system for detecting threats and safety. *ZERO TO THREE,* May, 19–24.

Posner, M. I., Rafal, R. D., Choate, L. S., & Vaughan, J. (1985). Inhibition of return: Neural basis and function. *Cognitive Neuropsychology, 2*(3), 211–228.

Posner, M. I., & Rothbart, M. K. (2002). Attention, self-regulation, and consciousness. In J. T. Cacioppo, G. G. Berntson, R. Alophs, C. S. Carter, R. J. Davidson, M. K. McClintock, et al. (Eds.), *Foundations in social neuroscience* (pp. 215–234). Cambridge, MA: MIT Press.

Poulsen, M. K. (2005). Diagnosis in mental health in young children. In K. M. Finello (Ed.), *The handbook of training and practice in infant and preschool mental health* (pp. 71–92). San Francisco: Jossey-Bass.

Prechtl, H. (1977). *The neurological examination of the full-term newborn infant: A manual.* Philadelphia: Lippincott.

Premack, D. G., & Woodruff, G. (1978). Does the chimpanzee have a theory of mind? *Behavioral and Brain Sciences, 1,* 515–526.

Prencipe, A., & Zelazo, P. D. (2005). Development of affective decision making for self and other: Evidence for the integration of first- and third-person perspectives. *Psychological Science, 16,* 501–505.

Protopopescu, X., Pan, H., Tuescher, O., Cloitre, M., Goldstein, M., Engelien, W., et al. (2005). Differential time-courses and specificity of amygdala activation in PTSD subjects and normal controls. *Biological Psychology, 57,* 464–473.

Quartz, S. R., & Sejnowski, T. J. (1997). The neural basis of cognitive development: A constructivist manifesto. *Brain and Behavioral Sciences, 20,* 537–596.

Raloff, J. (2006). Virtual reality for earthquake fears. *Science News.* Retrieved May 4, 2008, from www.thefreelibrary.com/Virtual+reality+for+earthquake+fears-a0151188408

Rauschecker, J. P., & Tian, B. (2000). Mechanisms and streams for processing of "what" and "where" in auditory cortex. *Proceedings of the National Academy of Sciences of the United States of America, 97,* 11800–11806.

Rechtschaffen, A., & Siegel, J. (2000). Sleep and dreaming. In E. R. Kandel, J. H. Schwartz, & T. M. Jessell (Eds.), *Principles of neural science* (pp. 936–947). New York: McGraw-Hill.

Reed, C. L., Klatzky, R. L., & Halgren, E. (2005). What vs. where in touch: An fMRI study. *NeuroImage, 25,* 718–726.

Reed, M. A., Pien, D. L., & Rothbart, M. K. (1984). Inhibitory self-control in preschool children. *Merrill-Palmer Quarterly, 30*(2), 131–147.

Reisberg, D., & Heuer, F. (2004). Remembering emotional events. In D. Reisberg & P. Hertel (Eds.), *Memory and emotion* (pp. 3–41). New York: Oxford University Press.

Repacholi, B. M., & Gopnik, A. (1997). Early reasoning about desires: Evidence from 14- and 18-month-olds. *Developmental Psychology, 33*(1), 12–21.

Resch, F. (2008). Developmental psychopathology in early childhood: Interdisciplinary challenges. In M. Papoušek, M. Schieche, & H. Wurmser (Eds.), *Disorders of behavioral and emotional regulation in the first years of life: Early risks and intervention in the developing parent-infant relationship* (pp. 13–26). Washington, DC: ZERO TO THREE.

Resnick, M. B., Eyler, F. D., Nelon, R. M., Eitzman, D. V., & Bucciarelli, R. L. (1987). Developmental intervention for low birth weight infants: Improved early developmental outcome. *Pediatrics, 80,* 68–74.

Riggs, N. R., Greenberg, M. T., Kusché, C. A., & Pentz, M. A. (2006). The mediational role of neurocognition in the behavioral outcomes of a social-emotional prevention program in elementary school students: Effects of the PATHS curriculum. *Prevention Science, 7*(1), 91–102.

Ringstrom, P. A. (1998). Therapeutic impasses in contemporary psychoanalytic treatment: Revisiting the double bind hypothesis. *Psychoanalytic Dialogues, 8,* 297–316.

Rizzo, A. A., Klimchuk, D., Mitura, R., Bowerly, T., Buckwalter, J. G., & Parsons, T. (2006). A virtual reality scenario for all seasons: The virtual classroom. *CNS Spectrums, 11*(1), 35–44.

Rizzo, A. A., Strickland, D., & Bouchard, S. (2004). Issues and challenges for using virtual environments in telerehabilitation. *Telemedicine Journal and e-Health, 10*(2), 184–195.

Rizzo, T. (2001). Habituation technique in study of development of fetal behaviour. *Lancet, 357,* 328–329.

Rizzolatti, G., & Craighero, L. (2004). The mirror-neuron system. *Annual Review of Neuroscience, 27,* 169–192.

Rizzolatti, G., Fogassi, L., & Gallese, V. (2000). Cortical mechanisms subserving object grasping and action recognition: A new view on the cortical motor functions. In M. S. Gazzaniga (Ed.), *The cognitive neurosciences* (2nd ed., pp. 539–552). Cambridge, MA: MIT Press.

Rizzolatti, G., Fogassi, L., & Gallese, V. (2002). Motor and cognitive functions of the ventral premotor cortex. *Current Opinion in Neurobiology, 12,* 149–154.

Rizzolatti, G., Scandolara, C., Matelli, M., & Gentilucci, M. (1981). Afferent properties of periarcuate neurons in macaque monkeys. II. Visual responses. *Behavioral Brain Research, 2,* 147–163.

Roesch, E. B., Fontaine, J. R., Scherer, K. R., Ellsworth, P., & Shen, Y.-L. (2007, June). *Componential approach to the old question of the kind and number of emotional dimensions across cultures.* Paper presented at the Pierre Dasen Conference in Cross-Cultural Psychology, Geneva.

Roesch, S. C., Schetter, C. D., Woo, G., & Hobel, C. J. (2004). Modeling the types of timing of stress in pregnancy. *Anxiety, Stress, & Coping, 17*(1), 87–102.

Rogeness, G., & McClure, E. (1996). Development and neurotransmitter-environmental interactions. *Development and Psychopathology, 8,* 183–199.

Rogers, S. J. (2000). Interventions that facilitate socialization in children with autism. *Journal of Autism and Developmental Disorders, 30,* 399–409.

Rohrer, D., & Pashler, H. (2007). Increasing retention without increasing study time. *Current Directions in Psychological Science, 16*(4), 183–186.

Role, L. W., & Talmage, D. A. (2007). Neurobiology: New order for thought disorders. *Nature, 448,* 263–265.

Roley, S. S. (2006). Sensory integration theory revisited. In R. C. Schaaf & S. S. Roley (Eds.), *Sensory integration: Applying clinical reasoning to practice with diverse populations* (pp. 1–14). Austin, TX: PRO-ED.

Rolls, E. T. (2002) The functions of the orbitofrontal cortex. In D. T. Stuss & R. T. Knight (Eds.), *Principles of frontal lobe function* (pp. 354–375). New York: Oxford University Press.

Rose, S. A., Feldman, J. F., & Jankowski, J. J. (2002). Processing speed in the 1st year of life: A longitudinal study of preterm and full term infants. *Developmental Psychology, 38,* 895–902.

Rosenbaum, J. F., Biederman, J., Gertsen, M., Hirschfield, O. R., Menninger, S. R., Herman, J., et al. (1988). Behavioral inhibition in children of parents with panic disorder and agoraphobia: A controlled study. *Archives of General Psychiatry, 45,* 463–470.

Rosenblum, K. L. (2004). Defining infant mental health: A developmental relational perspective on assessment and diagnosis. In A. J. Sameroff, S. C. McDonough,

& K. L. Rosenblum (Eds.), *Treating parent-infant relationship problems: Strategies for intervention* (pp. 43–75). New York: Guilford Press.

Ross, S. M. (1983). Increasing the meaningfulness of quantitative material by adapting context to student background. *Journal of Educational Psychology, 75*, 519–529.

Rothbart, M. (2007). Temperament, development, and personality. *Current Directions in Psychological Science, 16*(4), 207–212.

Rothbart, M., Ziale, H., & O'Boyle, G. (1992). Self-regulation and emotion in infancy. *New Directions for Child Development, 55*(Spring), 7–23.

Rothschild, B. (2000). *The body remembers: The psychophysiology of trauma and trauma treatment.* New York: Norton.

Rotman, G., Troje, N. F., Johansson, R. S., & Flanagan, J. R. (2006). Eye movements when observing predictable and unpredictable actions. *Journal of Neurophysiology, 96*, 1358–1369.

Rovee-Collier, C. (1993). The capacity for long-term memory in infancy. *Current Directions in Psychological Science, 2*(4), 130–135.

Rovee-Collier, C., Hayne, H., & Colombo, M. (2001). *The development of implicit and explicit memory.* Philadelphia: John Benjamins.

Rubenstein, J., Lotspeich, L., & Ciaranello, R. (1990). The neurobiology of developmental disorders. In B. Lahey & A. Kazdin (Eds.), *Advances in clinical child psychology* (Vol. 13, pp. 1–52). New York: Plenum Press.

Ruddick, S. (1994). Thinking mothers/conceiving birth. In D. Bassin, M. Honey, & M. M. Kaplan (Eds.), *Representations of motherhood* (pp. 29–46). New Haven, CT: Yale University Press.

Rueda, M. R., Rothbart, M. K., McCandliss, B. D., Saccomanno, L., & Posner, M. I. (2005). Training, maturation, and genetic influences on the development of executive attention. *Proceedings of the National Academy of Sciences USA, 102*, 14931–14936.

Rutter, M. (1985). Resilience is the face of adversity: Protective factors and resistance to psychiatric disorder. *British Journal of Psychiatry, 147*, 598–631.

Rutter, M., Bailey, A., Bolton, P., & LeCouteur, A. (1993). Autism. In R. Plomin & G. McClearn (Eds.), *Nature, nurture, and psychology* (pp. 285–306). Washington, DC: American Psychological Association.

Sahar, T., Shalev, A. Y., & Porges, S. W. (2001). Vagal modulation of responses to mental challenge in posttraumatic stress disorder. *Society of Biological Psychiatry, 49*, 637–643.

Salzman, J. P. (1997). Ambivalent attachment in female adolescents: Association with affective instability and eating disorders. *International Journal of Eating Disorders, 21*(3), 251–259.

Salzman, J. P., Salzman, C., & Wolfson, A. N. (1997). Relationship of childhood abuse and maternal attachment to the development of borderline personality disorder. In M. C. Zanarini (Ed.), *Role of sexual abuse in etiology of borderline personality disorder* (pp. 71–92). Washington, DC: American Psychiatric Press.

Sameroff, A. J. (1989). Models of developmental regulations: The environtype. In D. Cicchetti (Ed.), *Development and psychopathology* (pp. 41–68). Hillsdale, NJ: Erlbaum.

Sameroff, A. J. (2004). Ports of entry and the dynamics of mother-infant interventions. In A. J. Sameroff, S. C. McDonough, & K. L. Rosenblum (Eds.), *Treating parent-infant relationship problems* (pp. 3–28). New York: Guilford Press.

Sameroff, A. J., & Emde, R. N. (1989). *Relationship disturbances in early childhood. A developmental approach.* New York: Basic Books.

Sameroff, A. J., & Fiese, B. H. (2000a). Models of development and developmental risk. In C. H. Zeanah (Ed.), *Handbook of infant mental health* (pp. 3–19). New York: Guilford Press.

Sameroff, A. J., & Fiese, B. H. (2000b). Transactional regulation: The developmental ecology of early intervention. In S. J. Meisels & J. P. Shonkoff (Eds.), *Handbook of early childhood intervention* (pp. 135–159). Cambridge: Cambridge University Press.

Sameroff, A. J., Seifer, R., Baldwin, A., & Baldwin, C. (1993). Stability of intelligence from preschool to adolescence: The influence of social and family risk factors. *Child Development, 64,* 80–97.

Sameroff, A. J., Seifer, R., Barocas, R., Zax, M., & Greenspan, S. (1987). Intelligence quotient scores of 4-year-old children: Social environmental risks. *Pediatrics, 79,* 343–350.

Sander, D., & Scherer, K. R. (2005). Amalgams and the power of analytical chemistry: Affective science needs to decompose the appraisal-emotion interaction. Commentary on M. D. Lewis, Bridging emotion theory and neurobiology through dynamic systems modeling. *Behavioral and Brain Sciences, 28,* 169–245.

Sander, L. W. (1988). The event-structure of regulation in the neonate-caregiver system. *Progress in Self Psychology, 3,* 64–77.

Sansone, C., & Smith, J. L. (2000). Interest and self-regulation: The relation between having to and wanting to. In C. Sansone & J. M. Harackiewicz (Eds.), *Intrinsic and extrinsic motivation: The search for optimal motivation and performance* (pp. 341–372). San Diego, CA: Academic Press.

Saper, C. B., Iversen, S., & Frakowiak, R. (2000). Integration of sensory and motor function. In E. R. Kandel, J. H. Schwartz, & T. M. Jessell (Eds.), *Principles of neural science* (pp. 349–380). New York: McGraw-Hill.

Sapolsky, R. M. (1994). *Why zebras don't get ulcers: A guide to stress, stress-related diseases, and coping.* New York: W. H. Freeman.

Schaaf, R. C., Miller, L. J., Seawell, D., & O'Keefe, S. (2003). Children with disturbance in sensory processing: A pilot study examining the role of the parasympathetic nervous system. *American Journal of Occupational Therapy, 57*(4), 442–449.

Schacter, D. L. (1996). *Searching for memory: The brain, the mind, and the past.* New York: Basic Books.

Schachter, S., & Dodson, C. S. (2002). Misattribution, false recognition and the sins of memory. In A. Baddeley, M. Conway, & J. Aggleton (Eds.), *Episodic memory: New directions in research* (pp. 77–85). London: Oxford University Press.

Schieche, M., Rupprecht, C., & Papoušek, M. (2008). Sleep disorders: Current results and clinical experience. In M. Papoušek, M. Schieche, & H. Wurmser, (Eds.), *Disorders of behavioral and emotional regulation in the first years of*

life: Early risks and intervention in the developing parent-infant relationship (pp. 117–140). Washington, DC: ZERO TO THREE.

Schneider, W., Lockl, K., & Fernandez, O. (2005). *Interrelationships among theory of mind, executive control, language development, and working memory in young children: A longitudinal analysis.* Mahwah, NJ: Erlbaum.

Schneider, W., & Pressley, M. P. (1997). *Memory development between two and twenty* (2nd ed.). Mahwah, NJ: Erlbaum.

Schore, A. N. (1994). *Affect regulation and the origin of the self: The neurobiology of emotional development.* Hillsdale, NJ: Erlbaum.

Schore, A. N. (1998). Early shame experiences and infant brain development. In P. Gilbert & B. Andrews (Eds.), *Shame, interpersonal behavior, psychopathology, and culture* (pp. 57–77). New York: Oxford University Press.

Schore, A. N. (2001). The effects of early relational trauma on right brain development, affect regulation, and infant mental health. *Infant Mental Health Journal, 22,* 201–269.

Schore, A. N. (2003a). *Affect dysregulation and disorders of the self.* New York: Norton.

Schore, A. N. (2003b). *Affect regulation and the repair of the self.* New York: Norton.

Schraw, G. (1998). Promoting general metacognitive awareness. *Instructional Services, 26*(1–2), 113–125.

Schubotz, R. I. (2007). Prediction of external events with our motor system: Towards a new framework. *Trends in Cognitive Sciences, 11*(5), 211–218.

Schulz, L. E., & Gopnik, A. (2004). Causal learning across domains. *Developmental Psychology, 40*(2), 162–176.

Schultz, W. (2000). Multiple reward signals in the brain. *Nature Review Neuroscience, 1,* 199–207.

Schumann-Hengsteler, R., & Pohl, S. (1996, July). *Children's temporary memory for spatial sequences in the Corsi blocks.* Paper presented at the International Conference on Memory, Padua, Italy.

Schwanenflugel, P. J., Hamilton, A. M., Kuhn, M. R., Wisenbaker, J. M., & Stahl, S. A. (2004). Becoming a fluent reader: Reading skill and prosodic features in the oral reading of young readers. *Journal of Educational Psychology, 96,* 119–129.

Scientific Learning Corporation. (n.d.). *Fast ForWord.* Retrieved March 3, 2008, from www.scilearn.com/index.php

Seligman, M. E. P. (1975). *Helplessness: On depression, development, and death.* San Francisco: W. H. Freeman.

Seligman, M. E. P., & Maier, S. F. (1967). Failure to escape traumatic shock. *Journal of Experimental Psychology, 74,* 1–9.

Sestieri, C., Di Matteo, R., Ferretti, A., Del Gratta, C., Caulo, M., Tartaro, A., et al. (2006). "What" versus "where" in the audiovisual domain: An fMRI study. *NeuroImage, 33,* 672–680.

Shahmoon-Shanok, R. (2000). The action is in the interaction: Clinical practice guidelines for work with parents of children with developmental disorders. In Interdisciplinary Council on Developmental and Learning Disorders Clinical Practice Guidelines Workgroup, *Clinical practice guidelines: Redefining the standards of care for infants, children, and families with special needs* (pp. 333–374). Bethesda, MD: ICDL Press.

Sharply, C. F. (1992). Children's, adolescents,' and young adults' heart rate reactivity to, and recovery from, a brief psychological stressor. *International Journal of Behavioral Development, 15*(3), 399–410.

Shaywitz, B. A., Shaywitz, S. E., Blachman, B., Pugh, K. R., Fulbright, R., Skudlarski, P., et al. (2004). Development of left occipito-temporal systems for skilled reading following a phonologically-based intervention in children. *Biological Psychiatry, 55*, 926–933.

Shaywitz, S. E., Fletcher, J. M., Holahan, J. M., Schneider, A. E., Marchione, K. E., Stuebing, K. K., et al. (1999). Persistence of dyslexia: The Connecticut longitudinal study at adolescence. *Pediatrics, 104*, 1351–1359.

Shechtman, Z. (2002). Cognitive and affective empathy in aggressive boys: Implications for counseling. *International Journal for the Advancement of Counselling, 24*, 211–222.

Shevell, M. I., Majnemer, A., Webster, R. I., Platt, R. W., & Birnbaum, R. (2005). Outcomes at school age of preschool children with developmental language impairment. *Pediatric Neurology, 32*(4), 264–269.

Shonkoff, J. (2000). Science, policy and practice: Three cultures in search of a shared mission. *Child Development, 71*, 181–187.

Siegel, D. J. (1999). *The developing mind: Toward a neurobiology of interpersonal experience.* New York: Guilford Press.

Siegel, D. J. (2007a). Mindfulness training and neural integration: Differentiation of distinct streams of awareness and the cultivation of well-being. *Social Cognitive and Affective Neuroscience, 2*(4), 259–263.

Siegel, D. J. (2007b). *The mindful brain: Reflection and attunement in the cultivation of well-being.* New York: Norton.

Siegel, D. J., & Hartzell, M. (2003). *Parenting from the inside out: How a deeper self-understanding can help you raise children who thrive.* New York: Penguin Putnam.

Sibley, C. P., Turner, M. A., Cetin, I., Ayuk, P., Boyd, C. A. R., D'Souza, S. W., et al. (2005). Placental phenotypes of intrauterine growth. *Pediatric Research, 58*(5), 827–832.

Sigel, I. E., McGillicuddy-De Lisi, A. V., & Goodnow, J. J. (1992). *Parental belief systems: The psychological consequences for children.* Hillsdale, NJ: Erlbaum.

Silverthorn, D. U. (2006). *Human physiology: An integrated approach* (4th ed.). San Francisco: Benjamin Cummings.

Silvia, P. J. (2006). *Exploring the psychology of interest.* New York: Oxford University Press.

Singer, L., Arendt, R., Farkas, K., Minnes, S., Huang, J., & Yamashita, T. (1997). Relationship of prenatal cocaine exposure and maternal postpartum psychological distress to child developmental outcome. *Development and Psychopathology, 9*, 473–489.

Singer, L., Yamashita, T., Hawkins, S., Cairns, D., Baley, J., & Kleigman, R. (1994). Increased incidence of intraventricular hemorrhage and developmental delay in cocaine-exposed very low birth weight infants. *Journal of Pediatrics, 124*, 765–771.

Skeels, H. M., & Dye, H. B. (1939). A study of the effects of differential stimulation on mentally retarded children. *Proceedings of the American Association of Mental Deficiency, 44,* 114–136.

Slamecka, N. J., & Graf, P. (1978). The generation effect: Delineation of a phenomenon. *Journal of Experimental Psychology: Human Learning and Memory, 4,* 592–604.

Slavik, S., Carlson, J., & Sperry, L. (1998). The passive-aggressive couple. In J. Carlson & L. Sperry (Eds.), *The disordered couple* (pp. 299–314). Bristol, PA: Brunner/Mazel.

Sleight, P. (1995). Physiology and pathophysiology of heart rate and blood pressure variability in humans: Is power spectral analysis largely an index of baroreflex gain? *Clinical Science, 88,* 103–109.

Snell, R. S. (2006). *Clinical neuroanatomy* (6th ed.). Baltimore: Lippincott Williams & Wilkins.

Sobel, D. M., Tenenbaum, J. B., & Gopnik, A. (2004). Children's causal inferences from indirect evidence: Backwards blocking and bayesian reasoning in preschoolers. *Cognitive Science: A Multidisciplinary Journal, 28*(3), 303–333.

Sodian, B. (2005). *Theory of mind: The case for conceptual development.* Mahwah, NJ: Erlbaum.

Sodian, B., & Wimmer, H. (1987). Children's understanding of inference as a source of knowledge. *Child Development, 58,* 424–433.

Solchany, J. E. (2001). *Promoting maternal mental health during pregnancy.* Seattle: NCAST-AVENUW, University of Washington.

Sonksen, P. M., & Dale, N. (2002). Visual impairment in infancy: Impact on neurodevelopmental and neurobiological processes. *Developmental Medicine & Child Neurology, 44,* 782–791.

Sparrow, S., Balla, D., & Cicchetti, D. (1998). *Vineland Social-Emotional Early Childhood Scale (SEEC).* Bloomington, MN: Pearson Assessments.

Sperber, A. D., & Tarasiuk, A. (2007). Disrupted sleep in patients with IBS: A wake-up call for further research? *Nature Clinical Practice Gastroenterology & Hepatology, 4,* 412–413.

Spitz, R. A. (1945). Hospitalism: An inquiry into the genesis of psychiatric conditions in early childhood. In R. S. Eissler (Ed.), *Psychoanalytic study of the child* (Vol. 1, pp. 53–74). New Haven, CT: Yale University Press.

Squires, J., Bricker, D., & Twombly, E. (2002). *Ages & stages questionnaires: social-emotional.* Baltimore: Paul H. Brookes.

Sroufe, L. A. (1996). *Emotional development: The organization of emotional life in the early years.* New York: Cambridge University Press.

Stanford Report. (2004, August 18). Portions of brain are smaller in children born prematurely: Genetics, hormones may shield girls' brains from adverse effects of early birth. Retrieved May 9, 2008, from news-service.Stanford.edu/news/2004/august18/med-reiss-818.html

Stephan, F. K., & Zucker, I. (1972). Circadian rhythms in drinking behavior and locomotor activity of rats are eliminated in hypothalamic lesions. *Proceedings of the National Academy of Sciences USA, 69,* 1583–1586.

Sterling, P., & Eyer, J. (1988). Allostasis: A new paradigm to explain arousal pathology. In S. Fisher & J. Reason (Eds.), *Handbook of life stress, cognition, and health* (pp. 629–649). New York: Wiley.

Stern, D. N. (1971). A microanalysis of the mother-infant interaction. *Journal of the American Academy of Child Psychiatry, 10,* 501–507.

Stern, D. N. (1982). Some interactive functions of rhythm changes between mother and infant. In M. Davis (Ed.), *Interaction rhythms* (pp. 101–117). New York: Human Sciences Press.

Stern, D. N. (1985). *The interpersonal world of the infant: A view from psychoanalysis and developmental psychology.* New York: Basic Books.

Stern, D. N. (1995). *The motherhood constellation: A unified view of parent-infant psychotherapy.* New York: Basic Books.

Stern, D. N. (2004). *The present moment in psychotherapy and everyday life.* New York: Norton.

Stevenson, D. K., Verter, J., Fanaroff, A. A., Oh, W., Ehrenkranz, R. A., Shankaran, S., et al. (for the National Institute of Child Health and Human Development Neonatal Research Network). (2000). Sex differences in outcomes of very low birthweight infants: The newborn male disadvantage. *Archives of Disease in Childhood. Fetal Neonatal Edition, 83,* 182–185.

Stith, S. M., Rosen, K. H., McCollum, E. E., & Thomsen, C. J. (2004). Treating intimate partner violence within intact couple relationships: Outcomes of multi-couple versus individual couple therapy. *Journal of Marital and Family Therapy, 30*(3), 305–318.

Strehl, U., Leins, U., Goth, G., Klinger, C., Hinterberger, T., & Birbaumer, N. (2006). Self-regulation of slow cortical potentials: A new treatment for children with attention-deficit/hyperactivity disorder. *Pediatrics, 118*(5), 530–540.

Strickland, D., Marcus, L. M., Mesibov, G. B., & Hogan, K. (1996). Brief report: Two case studies using virtual reality as a learning tool for autistic children. *Journal of Autism and Developmental Disorders, 26,* 651–659.

Strobl, M., Strametz, D., & Schumann-Hengsteler, R. (2002). *Effekte der Aufgaben Komplexität und Matrixgrösse auf die Matrix-Muster-Aufgabe* [The effects of task complexity and size on the matrix task]. Eichstatt, Germany: Catholic University of Eichstatt-Ingolstadt.

Strupp, H. H., & Anderson, T. (1997). On the limitations of therapy manuals. *Clinical Psychology: Science and Practice, 4,* 76–82.

Sue, S. (2003). In defense of cultural competency in psychotherapy and treatment. *American Psychologist, 38,* 964–970.

Sunderland, M. (2006). *The science of parenting: How today's brain research can help you raise happy, emotionally balanced children.* New York: DK Publishing.

Suzuki, W. A., & Amaral, D. G. (1994). Perirhinal and parahippocampal cortices of the macaque monkey: Cortical afferents. *Journal of Comparative Neurology, 350,* 497–533.

Swanson, H. L. (1993). Executive processing in learning-disabled readers. *Intelligence, 17*(2), 117–149.

Swanson, J., Arnold, L. E., Kraemer, H., Hechtman, L., Molina, B., Hinshaw, S., et al. (2008a). Evidence, interpretation, and qualification from multiple reports of

long-term outcomes in the multimodal treatment study of children with ADHD (MTA): Part I: Executive summary. *Journal of Attention Disorders, 12*(1), 4–14.

Swanson, J., Arnold, L. E., Kraemer, H., Hechtman, L., Molina, B., Hinshaw, S., et al. (2008b). Evidence, interpretation, and qualification from multiple reports of long-term outcomes in the multimodal treatment study of children with ADHD (MTA): Part II: Supporting details. *Journal of Attention Disorders, 12*(1), 15–43.

Tager-Flusberg, H., & Sullivan, K. (1994). A second look at second-order belief attribution in autism. *Journal of Autism and Developmental Disorders, 24*(5), 577–586.

Tangney, J. P., Wagner, P. E., Hill-Barlow, D., Marschall, D. E., & Gramzow, R. (1996). Relation of shame and guilt to constructive versus destructive responses to anger across the lifespan. *Journal of Personality and Social Psychology, 70*(4), 797–809.

Tartaro, A., & Cassell, J. (in press). Using virtual peer technology as an intervention for children with autism. In J. Lazar (Ed.), *Towards universal usability: Designing computer interfaces for diverse user populations.* Chichester, UK: Wiley.

Tarter, R. E., Kirisci, L., Mezzich, A., Cornelius, J. R., Pajer, K., Vanyukov, M., et al. (2003). Neurobehavioral disinhibition in childhood predicts early age at onset of substance use disorder. *American Journal of Psychiatry, 160*(6), 1078–1085.

Task Force on Sudden Infant Death Syndrome. (2005). The changing concept of sudden infant death syndrome: Diagnostic coding shifts, controversies regarding the sleeping environment, and new variables to consider in reducing risk. American Academy of Pediatrics Policy Statement. *Pediatrics, 116,* 1245–1255.

Taylor, G. H., Klein, N., Minich, N. M., & Hack, M. (2000). Verbal memory deficits in children with less than 750g birth weight. *Child Neuropsychology, 6*(1), 49–63.

Thelen, E. (2000). Motor development as foundation and future of developmental psychology. *International Journal of Behavioral Development, 24*(4), 385–397.

Thelen, E., & Smith, L. B. (1994). *A dynamic systems approach to the development of cognition and action.* Bradford Books Series in Cognitive Psychology. Cambridge, MA: MIT Press.

Thobaben, M. (1998). Survivors of violence or abuse. In N. Frisch & L. Frisch (Eds.), *Psychiatric mental health nursing* (pp. 559–605). New York: Delmar.

Tian, B., Reser, D., Durham, A., Kustov, A., & Rauschecker, J. P. (2001). Functional specialization in rhesus monkey auditory cortex. *Science, 292,* 290–293.

Tice, D. M., Baumeister, R. F., Shmueli, D., & Muraven, M. (2007). Restoring the self: Positive affect helps improve self-regulation following ego depletion. *Journal of Experimental Social Psychology, 43*(3), 379–384.

Tipper, S. P., Bourque, T. A., Anderson, S. H., & Brehaut, J. (1989). Mechanisms of attention: A developmental study. *Journal of Experimental Child Psychology, 48,* 353–378.

Tomasello, M., Carpenter, M., & Liszkowksi, U. (2007). A new look at infant pointing. *Child Development, 78,* 705–722.

Torgesen, J. K. (1999). Phonologically based reading disabilities: Toward a coherent theory of one kind of learning disability. In R. J. Sternberg & L. Spear-Swerling (Eds.), *Perspectives on learning disabilities* (pp. 231–262). Boulder, CO: Westview Press.

Torgesen, J. K., & Burgess, S. R. (1998). Consistency of reading-related phonological processes throughout early childhood: Evidence from longitudinal, correlational, and instructional studies. In J. Metsala & L. Ehri (Eds.), *Word recognition in beginning reading* (pp. 161–188). Hillsdale, NJ: Erlbaum.

Torgesen, J. K., Rashotte, C. A., & Alexander, A. (2001). Principles of fluency instruction in reading: Relationships with established empirical outcomes. In M. Wolf (Ed.), *Dyslexia, fluency, and the brain* (pp. 333–355). Parkton, MD: York Press.

Torgesen, J. K., Wagner, R. K., Rashotte, C. A., Alexander, A. W., & Conway, T. (1997). Preventive and remedial interventions for children with severe reading disabilities. *Learning Disabilities: An Interdisciplinary Journal, 8,* 51–62.

Tortora, S. (2006). *The dancing dialogue: Using the communicative power of movement with young children.* Baltimore: Paul H. Brookes.

Towse, J., & Cowan, N. (2005). *Working memory and its relevance for cognitive development.* Mahwah, NJ: Erlbaum.

Tranel, D. (2002). Emotion, decision making, and the ventromedial prefrontal cortex. In D. T. Stuss & R. T. Knight (Eds.), *Principles of frontal lobe function* (pp. 338–353). New York: Oxford University Press.

Trepagnier, C. Y., Sebrechts, M. M., Finkelmeyer, A., Stewart, W., Woodford, J., & Coleman, M. (2006). Stimulating social interaction to address deficits of autistic spectrum disorder in children. *CyberPsychology & Behavior, 9*(2), 213–217.

Tronick, E. (2007). *The neurobehavioral and social-emotional development of infants and children.* New York: Norton.

Truex, R., & Carpenter, B. A. (1964). *Strong and Elwyn's human neuroanatomy* (5th ed.). Baltimore: Williams & Wilkins.

Tulving, E. (1985). How many memory systems are there? *American Psychologist, 40,* 385–398.

Tweed, D. (2003). *Microcosms of the brain: What sensorimotor systems reveal about the mind.* Oxford: Oxford University Press.

Twenge, J. M., Baumeister, R. F., Tice, D. M., & Stucke, T. S. (2001). If you can't join them, beat them: Effects of social exclusion on aggressive behavior. *Journal of Personality and Social Psychology, 81*(6), 1058–1069.

Twenge, J. M., Catanese, K. R., & Baumeister, R. F. (2003). Social exclusion and the deconstructed state: Time perception, meaninglessness, lethargy, lack of emotion, and self-awareness. *Journal of Personality and Social Psychology, 85*(3), 409–423.

U.S. Department of Health and Human Services. (2003). *Exploratory centers (P20) for interdisciplinary research.* (RFA-RM-04-004) [A roadmap initiative].

Retrieved January 30, 2008, from grants.nih.gov/grants/guide/rfa-files/RFA-RM-04-004.html

van Praag, H., Shubert, T., Zhao, C., & Gage, F. H. (2005). Exercise enhances learning and hippocampal neurogenesis in aged mice. *Journal of Neuroscience, 25,* 8680–8685.

van Veen, V., & Carter, C. S. (2002). The timing of action-monitoring processes in the anterior cingulate cortex. *Journal of Cognitive Neuroscience, 14*(4), 593–602.

Verheul, R., Van Den Bosch, L. M. C., Koeter, M. W. J., De Ridder, M. A. J., Stijnen, T., & Van Den Brink, W. (2003). Dialectical behaviour therapy for women with borderline personality disorder. *British Journal of Psychiatry, 182,* 135–140.

von Hippel, W., & Gonsalkorale, K. (2005) "That is bloody revolting!" Inhibitory control of thoughts better left unsaid. *Psychological Science, 16,* 497–500.

Vygotsky, L. S. (1978). *Mind in society: The development of higher psychological processes.* Cambridge, MA: Harvard University Press.

Wachs, T. D. (2000). *Necessary but not sufficient: The respective roles of single and multiple influences on individual development.* Washington, DC: American Psychological Association.

Waisman Center, Language Processes Lab, University of Wisconsin–Madison. Early language learning project. Retrieved March 19, 2008, from www .waisman.wisc.edu/lpl/completed.html

Walant, K. (1995). *Creating the capacity for attachment: Treating addictions and the alienated self.* Northvale, NJ: Jason Aronson.

Walker, L. E. (1977). Who are the battered women? *Frontiers: A Journal of Women's Studies, 2*(1), 52–57.

Walker, L. E. (2000). *The battered woman syndrome.* New York: Springer.

Wallace, M. T. (2004). The development of multisensory integration. In G. A. Calvert, C. Spence, & B. E. Stein (Eds.), *The handbook of multisensory processes* (pp. 625–642). Cambridge, MA: MIT Press.

Watson, J. B. (1928). *Psychological care of infant and child.* New York: Norton.

Watson, R. I., Sr. (1978). *The great psychologists* (4th ed.). New York: J. B. Lippincott.

Weatherston, D. J. (2005). Returning the treasure to babies: An introduction to infant mental health service and training. In K. M. Finello (Ed.), *The handbook of training and practice in infant and preschool mental health* (pp. 3–30). San Francisco: Jossey-Bass.

Webster-Stratton, C., & Reid, M. J. (2006). *Treatment and prevention of conduct problems: Parent training interventions for young children (2–7 years old).* Malden, MA: Blackwell.

Wei, J. L., Mayo, M. S., Smith, H. J., Reese, M., & Weatherly, R. A. (2007). Improved behavior and sleep after adenotonsillectomy in children with sleep-disordered breathing. *Archives of Otolaryngololy—Head and Neck Surgery, 133,* 974–979.

Weiss, C., Singer, S., & Feigenbaum, L. (2006). *Too much, too little, just right: A social communication game (ages 5 to 12 years).* Creative Therapy Store.

Weisz, J. R., & Gray, J. S. (2008). Evidence-based psychotherapy for children and adolescents: Data from the present and a model for the future. *Child and Adolescent Mental Health, 13*(2), 54–65.

Weisz, J. R., Hawley, K. M., & Doss, A. J. (2004). Empirically test psychotherapies youth internalizing and externalizing problems and disorders. *Child and Adolescent Psychiatric Clinics of North America, 13,* 720–815.

Wellman, H. M., Cross, D., & Watson, J. (2001). Meta-analysis of theory-of-mind development: The truth about false belief. *Child Development, 72,* 655–684.

Wells, K. C., Pelham, W. E., Jr., Kotkin, R. A., Hoza, B., Abikoff, H. B., Abramowitz, A., et al. (2000). Psychosocial treatment strategies in the MTA study: Rationale, methods, and critical issues in design and implementation [Special Issue: Child and Family Characteristics as Predictors and Outcomes in the Multimodal Treatment Study of ADHD (MTA Study)]. *Journal of Abnormal Child Psychology, 28*(6), 483–505.

Werker, J. F., & Polka, L. (1993). Developmental changes in speech perception: New challenges and new directions. *Journal of Phonetics. Special Issue: Phonetic Development, 21*(1–2), 83–101.

Werker, J. F., & Tees, R. C. (1984). Cross-language speech perception: Evidence for perceptual reorganization during the first year of life. *Infant Behavior & Development, 7*(1), 49–63.

Westen, D., Novotny, C. M., & Thompson-Brenner, H. (2004a). The empirical status of empirically supported therapies: Assumptions, findings, and reporting in controlled trials. *Psychological Bulletin, 130,* 631–663.

Westen, D., Novotny, C. M., & Thompson-Brenner, H. (2004b). The next generation of psychotherapy research: Reply to Ablon and Marci (2004), Goldfried and Eubanks-Carter (2004), and Haaga (2004). *Psychological Bulletin, 130,* 677–683.

Weston, D. R., Ivins, B., Heffron, M. C., & Sweet, N. (1997). Applied developmental theory: Formulating the centrality of relationships in early intervention: An organizational perspective. *Infants and Young Children, 9*(3), 1–12.

Wetherby, A. M., & Prizant, B. M. (2002). *Communication and Symbolic Behavior Scales Developmental Profile (CSBS DP).* Baltimore: Paul H. Brookes.

What Works Clearinghouse. (2007, July). *Beginning reading: Fast ForWord.* Washington, DC: U.S. Department of Education, Institute of Education Sciences.

Wicker, B., Keysers, C., Plailly, J., Royet, J. P., Gallese, V., & Rizzolatti, G. (2003). Both of us disgusted in my insula: The common neural basis of seeing and feeling disgust. *Neuron, 40*(3), 655–664.

Wieder, S., & Greenspan, S. I. (2005). Developmental pathways to mental health: The DIR™ model for comprehensive approaches to assessment and intervention. In K. M. Finello (Ed.), *The handbook of training and practice in infant and preschool mental health* (pp. 377–401). San Francisco: Jossey-Bass.

Wiesel, T. N., & Hubel, D. H. (1965). Comparison of the effects of unilateral and bilateral eye closure on cortical unit responses in kittens. *Journal of Neurophysiology, 28,* 1029–1040.

Wilbarger, P. (n.d.). *Pediatric Building Blocks.* Retrieved April 30, 2008, from www.thetherapyplace.net/newsletter/newsletter3.pdf

Williams, M. S., & Shellenberger, S. (1996). *How does your engine run? A leader's guide to the alert program for self-regulation.* Albuquerque, NM: Therapy Works.

Williamson, G. G., & Anzalone, M. (1997). Sensory integration: A key component of the evaluation and treatment of young children with severe difficulties in relating and communicating. *ZERO TO THREE Bulletin, 17,* 29–36.

Williamson, G. G., & Anzalone, M. E. (2001). *Sensory integration and self-regulation in infants and toddlers: Helping very young children interact with their environment.* Washington, DC: ZERO TO THREE.

Wills, T. A., Sandy, J. M., & Yaeger, A. M. (2001). Time perspective and early-onset substance use: A model based on stress-coping theory. *Psychology of Addictive Behaviors, 15*(2), 118–125.

Wills, T. A., Sandy, J. M., Yaeger, A., & Shinar, O. (2001). Family risk factors and adolescent substance use: Moderation effects for temperament dimensions. *Developmental Psychology, 37*(3), 283–297.

Wimmer, H., & Perner, J. (1983). Beliefs about beliefs: Representation and constraining function of wrong beliefs in young children's understanding of deception. *Cognition, 13*(1), 103–128.

Winnicott, D. W. (1967). Mirror-role of mother and family in child development. *Playing and reality.* Middlesex, UK: Penguin.

Wise, R. A., & Bozarth, M. A. (1981). Brain substrates for reinforcement and drug-self-administration. *Progress in Neuropsychopharmacology, 5,* 467–474.

W. M. Keck Foundation. (2003). *"National Academies Keck Futures Initiative" to transform interdisciplinary research* [press release]. Retrieved January 30, 2008, from www.wmkeck.org/contentManagement/PR_3f03bb3c-84d6-4516-b67a-d9b9af47d0e9.htm

Wolpert, D. M., & Flanagan, J. R. (2001). Motor prediction. *Current Biology, 11*(18), R729–R732.

Wurmser, H., & Papoušek, M. (2008). Facts and figures: Database of the Munich Interdisciplinary Research and Intervention Program for Fussy Babies. In M. Papoušek, M. Schieche, & H. Wurmser (Eds.), *Disorders of behavioral and emotional regulation in the first years of life: Early risks and intervention in the developing parent-infant relationship* (pp. 27–52). Washington, DC: ZERO TO THREE.

Wurmser, H., Papoušek, M., & Hofacker, N. von. (2008). Long-term risks of persistent excessive crying in infants. In M. Papoušek, M. Schieche, & H. Wurmser (Eds.), *Disorders of behavioral and emotional regulation in the first years of life: Early risks and intervention in the developing parent-infant relationship* (pp. 273–298). Washington, DC: ZERO TO THREE.

Wycoff, E. B., & Pryor, B. (2003). Cognitive processing, creativity, apprehension, and the humorous personality. *North American Journal of Psychology, 5*(1), 31–44.

Ybarra, O., Burnstein, E., Winkielman, P., Keller, M. C., Manis, M., Chan, E., et al. (2008). Mental exercising through simple socializing: Social interaction promotes general cognitive functioning. *Personality and Social Psychology Bulletin, 34*(2), 248–259.

Yehuda, R. (2000). Biology of posttraumatic stress disorder. *Journal of Clinical Psychiatry, 61*(Suppl. 7), 15–21.

Yehuda, R. (2001). Biology of posttraumatic stress disorder. *Journal of Clinical Psychiatry, 62,* 41–46.

Yerkes, R. M., & Dodson, J. D. (1908). The relation of strength of stimulus to rapidity of habit-formation. *Journal of Comparative Neurology and Psychology, 18,* 459–482.

Zeanah, C. H., Nelson, C. A., Fox, N. A., Smyke, A. T., Marshall, P. M., Parker, S. W., et al. (2003). Designing research to study the effects of institutionalization on brain and behavioral development: The Bucharest Early Intervention Project. *Development and Psychopathology, 15,* 885–907.

Zelazo, P. D. (1999). Language, levels of consciousness, and the development of intentional action. In P. Zelazo, J. Astington, & D. Olson (Eds.), *Developing theories of intention: Social understanding and self-control* (pp. 95–117). Mahwah, NJ: Erlbaum.

Zelazo, P. D., & Frye, D. (1998). Cognitive complexity and control: II. The development of executive function in childhood. *Current Directions in Psychological Science, 7*(4), 121–126.

Zelazo, P. D., & Müller, U. (2002). Executive function in typical and atypical development. In U. Goswami (Ed.), *Handbook of childhood cognitive development* (pp. 445–469). Oxford: Blackwell.

Zelazo, P. D., Qu, L., & Müller, U. (2005). *Hot and cool aspects of executive function: Relations in early development.* Mahwah, NJ: Erlbaum.

ZERO TO THREE. (1994). *Diagnostic classification of mental health and developmental disorders of infancy and early childhood (DC: 0–3).* Arlington, VA: National Center for Clinical Infant Programs.

ZERO TO THREE. (2005). *Diagnostic classification of mental health and developmental disorders of infancy and early childhood, revised (DC: 0–3R).* Washington, DC: ZERO TO THREE.

ZERO TO THREE. (2008). *Early childhood mental health.* Retrieved January 18, 2008, from www.zerotothree.org/site/PageServer?pagename=key_mental

Ziegler, M., Wollwerth de Chuquisengo, R., & Papoušek, M. (2008), Excessive crying in infancy. In M. Papoušek, M. Schieche, & H. Wurmser (Eds.), *Disorders of behavioral and emotional regulation in the first years of life: Early risks and intervention in the developing parent-infant relationship* (pp. 85–116). Washington, DC: ZERO TO THREE.

Zucconi, M., Caprioglio, A., Calori, G., Ferini-Strambi, L., Oldani, A., Castronovo, C., et al. (1999). Craniofacial modifications in children with habitual snoring and obstructive sleep apnoea: A case-control study. *European Respiratory Journal 13,* 411–417.

Index

The following abbreviations are used following page numbers: f, figure; n, note; t, table; w, worksheet.